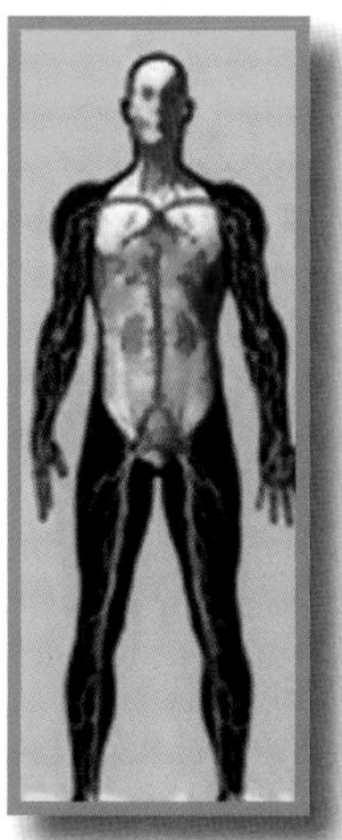

Illustrated Clinical Anatomy

2nd Edition

Peter H. Abrahams MB BS FRCS(Ed) FRCR DO (Hon)
Professor of Clinical Anatomy, Warwick Medical School, UK
Director of Anatomy, West Midlands Surgical Training Centre, UHCW NHS Trust
Extraordinary Professor, Department of Anatomy, University of Pretoria, South Africa
Fellow, Girton College, Cambridge
Professor of Clinical Anatomy, St George's University, Grenada, West Indies
Examiner to the Royal College of Surgeons, UK
Family Practitioner, Brent, London, UK

John L. Craven MD FRCS
Formerly Consultant Surgeon, York District Hospital and past Chairman of the Primary Examiners of the Royal College of Surgeons of England, UK

John S.P. Lumley MS FRCS FMAA (Hon) FGA
Emeritus Professor of Vascular Surgery, University of London
Past Council Member and Chairman of Primary Fellowship Examiners, Royal College of Surgeons of England, UK

Consultant Radiological Advisor: Jonathan D. Spratt BM BChir MA (Cantab) FRCS (Eng) FRCS(Glas) FRCR
Clinical Director of Radiology, University Hospital of North Durham; Honorary Lecturer in Anatomy, University of Durham; Examiner in Anatomy, Royal College of Surgeons of England, UK

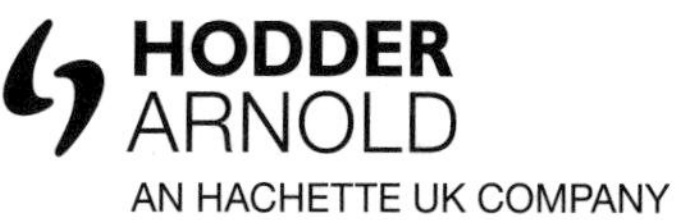

First published in Great Britain in 2005 by Hodder Arnold
This second edition published in 2011 by Hodder Arnold,
an imprint of Hodder Education, a division of Hachette UK,
338 Euston Road, London NW1 3BH

http://www.hodderarnold.com

British Library Cataloguing in Publication Data
A catalogue record for this book is available from the British Library

Library of Congress Cataloging-in-Publication Data
A catalog record for this book is available from the Library of Congress

ISBN: 9781 444109 252

1 2 3 4 5 6 7 8 9 10

Commissioning Editor: Joanna Koster
Project Editor: Stephen Clausard
Production Controller: Jonathan Williams
Cover Design: Amina Dudhia
Illustrations: Cactus Design and Illustration Ltd

Cover image: © Mehau Kulyk/Science Photo Library

Typeset in 9.5/12 pt Sabon by Phoenix Photosetting, Chatham, Kent
Printed in India

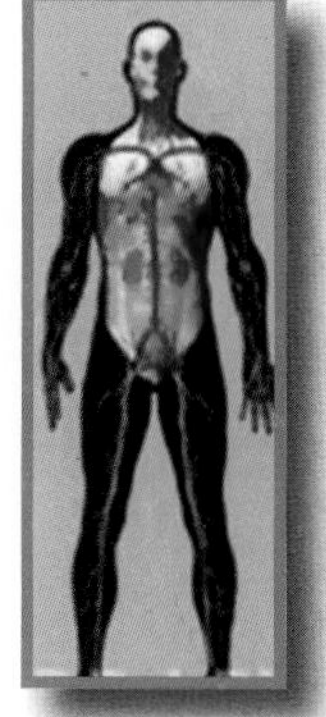

Illustrated Clinical Anatomy

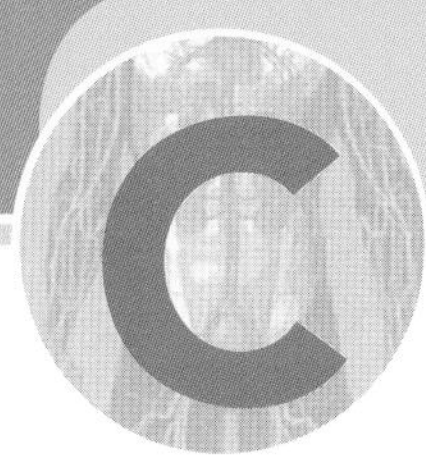

Contents

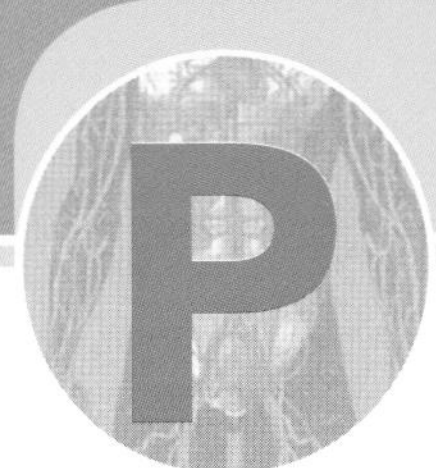

Preface to the second edition

Anatomy is an essential component of all clinical practice. In the first edition of this book our aim was to capitalize on our collective experience of over a century of teaching, publishing and practicing anatomy to produce a concise understandable and highly illustrated text, to pass on our personal enthusiasm for the subject to a future generation of doctors. So we were naturally delighted when it was awarded the Richard Asher Prize for the best new medical textbook at the Royal Society of Medicine/Society of Authors Book Awards, and was Highly Commended at the BMA Book Awards in 2005.

This second edition has taken notice of recommendations and reviews as well as the 2007 document of the education committee of the Anatomical Society of GB and Ireland (Eur J Anat 11 3–18 2007), which complements the earlier American Association of Clinical Anatomists document (Clin Anat 9 71–99 1996) – both of which define their view of the core knowledge of clinical anatomy required by medical students. With both of these documents to hand as well as our own personal clinical experience we have tried to cover the major anatomical factual content needed for a young physician or surgeon of the 21st century and we have included within the blue shaded columns illustration and explanation of hundreds of common clinical conditions, which each have an anatomical diagnostic basis. Suggestions from students and colleagues have contributed to these changes.

We have tried hard to keep the book short enough so as not to overwhelm students and have liberally illustrated it with clinical images and case presentations. The text is organized regionally but, since the basic clinical and diagnostic anatomy required for all doctors is essentially the same worldwide, it doesn't really matter which educational system your own medical school uses. So it is also easy to use for a systems approach or even in a problem-based curriculum as virtually every common anatomical problem has been illustrated – all these illustrations are available for your own personal use as part of the Vitalsource e-book.

It is irrelevant which exams you are preparing for; whether medical school, MRCS part A, or USMLE1. As examiners of decades of experience in each of these areas we know that the anatomy required is essentially the same. Details for postgraduates have been included in tables and with extra labeling on many illustrations as well as both clinical and radiological images. As in the first edition there are reasoned MCQs and applied problems at the end of every chapter, but we have now added extended multiple questions (EMQs) which are nowadays a common feature in all British postgraduate medical examinations.

We are most grateful to Jonathan Spratt for upgrading many of the radiological images that illustrate both normal and pathological anatomy using many different imaging modalities such as cross sectional MR and CT. All of these complement over four hundred original drawings and a similar number of surface anatomy and clinical conditions in this highly visual textbook. These can all be transferred into your own study files by using the simple password from the front of this book.

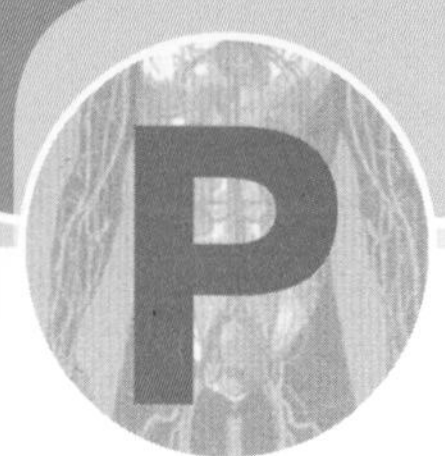

Preface to the first edition

This new textbook, focusing on clinically relevant anatomy, has been many years in the planning. Collectively we have over a century of experience teaching and examining in both medicine and anatomy, at undergraduate, postgraduate and specialist levels. This experience has allowed us to respond to the evolution of new integrated courses in medical schools worldwide and address the dichotomy between the needs of students and of trainee doctors.

We have followed the American Association of Clinical Anatomists' (AACA) core curriculum (*Clinical Anatomy* 1996 **9**: 71–99) as our guide to what is 'core', covering the clinical anatomy of most common diseases. So that medical students are not overwhelmed with detail we have kept the text simple and provided additional specialist anatomy in the illustrations and Tables. (For example, we have set out the details of muscular anatomy in a highly structured Table rather than describing them in the main text.) Clinical detail in the text has been clearly shaded blue so that our readers can easily identify it.

We have focused on normal and abnormal living anatomy of the whole body, excluding the nervous system as it is a book in itself and well covered in separate texts. Although we have not included a separate chapter on embryology, fetal development and paediatric anatomy have been integrated in the appropriate sections where clinically relevant.

Anatomy is a visually intense subject. Acknowledging the reduction in, or even disappearance of, dissection time in medical courses we have supplemented our text with a wealth of colour illustrations. Four hundred new anatomical drawings have been produced for the text; these include additional anatomical detail for specialist readers. With the help of Jonathan Spratt, we have taken advantage of new imaging techniques to show normal and abnormal living anatomy; each modality is well represented in its relevant area, particularly cross-sectional anatomy.

The book is organized topographically as this best relates to patient examination. Clinical examination requires a sound knowledge of surface anatomy. We have therefore included a comprehensive series of brand new surface anatomy photographs to complement the anatomical drawings and images, together with photographs of common clinical conditions on which anatomy has a bearing. We have endeavoured to provide a clinical photograph of each common condition listed in the AACA core curriculum.

Finally, we have included self-assessment material at the end of each section, providing MCQs and 'Applied Questions' that reflect examinations set at medical schools throughout the world. The answers and explanations can all be found within the text, but we have included specific responses alongside the questions as necessary.

We have enjoyed creating this book. We very much hope you enjoy reading and referring to it, and looking at the many illustrations. These are also available as electronic files on the website www.illustratedclinicalanatomy.com if you use your reader password at the front of the book.

P.A.
J.C.
J.S.P.L.
2005

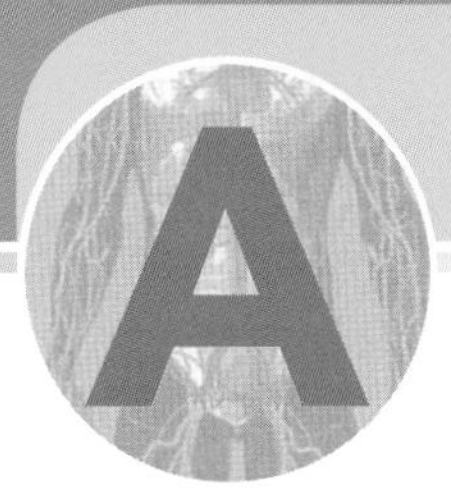

Acknowledgements

The authors and publisher thank the following individuals and institutions for kindly supplying figures for this book. Dr Tania Abrahams for tropical pathology. Dr Rosalind Ambrose for tropical radiology. Dr Ray Armstrong and ARC for musculoskeletal cases. Professor JM Boon for dissections from 'The Virtual Procedures Clinic' CD-ROM (www.primalpictures.com 2003). Section of Clinical Anatomy University of Pretoria, Dr L Van Heerden and the following students: Van Jaarsveld M; Joubert AT; Van Schoor AN; Phetla MV; Mbandlwa L; Mahlomoje ID; Deetlefs MEC; Schoonraad B; Van Blerk EM; Gichangi C; Smith AB; Van der Colff FJ; Connell A; Sitholimela SC for their beautiful dissections 2002/3. Mr S Dexter for laparoscopic shots. Professor R Ger for photos from 'Essentials of Clinical Anatomy', Parthenon, 1986. R Hutchings, freelance photographer. Professor Kubrick for lymphatic dissections. Dr Lahiri and the Wellington Hospital Cardiac Imaging and Research centre for EBCT scans of one of the authors. Miss Gilli Vafidis for ophthalmoscopy views. Dr Alan Hunter for a bronchoscopic view. Professor J Weir and team for images from *Imaging Atlas of Human Anatomy*, 4th edn, Elsevier 2010. Mr T Welch for tropical pathology. West Midlands Surgical Training Centre – plastinated prosection collection donated by the West Midlands SHA and produced in Gubin by Gunter von Hagens. Professor T Wright for auriscopic views.

Finally, we would like to thank Dr R Tunstall of Nottingham Postgraduate Medical School and Dr Jamie Roebuck of Warwick Medical School for their 'eagle-eyed' proof reading.

The following figures are reproduced with kind permission of Bart's Medical Illustration Collection, previously published in Lumley, JSP (ed), *Hamilton Bailey's Physical Signs: demonstrations of physical signs in clinical surgery* 18th edition (Arnold, 1997):

1.3, 1.6a, 1.12, 1.18, 1.20a, 2.20, 4.3a, 4.3b, 4.18, 5.8, 5.12, 5.14, 5.15, 6.8, 6.14, 7.8, 10.6, 12.5a, 12.5c, 12.5d, 12.6, 12.19a, 12.21, 14.4b, 14.8. 14.11, 15.6c, 15.7, 15.12c, 15.12d, 15.12e, 15.13, 15.18, 15.26a, 15.26b, 15.32b, 16.3a, 16.3b, 16.3c, 16.3d, 16.11a, 16.11b, 16.11c, 16.12, 17.6a, 17.6b, 17.6c, 17.6d, 17.10, 17.16, 19.6, 19.7b, 19.11, 19.26, 20.8, 20.9a, 20.18, 21.3, 22.12.

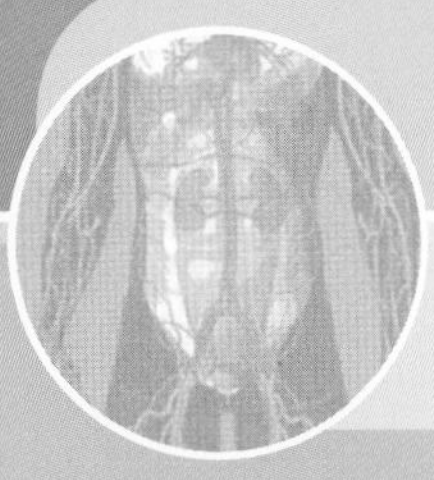

Introduction

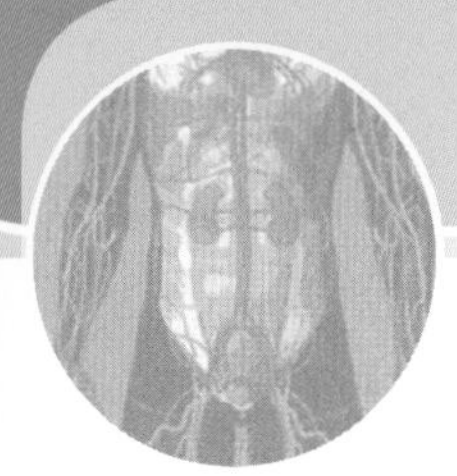

The structure of the body – the systems and organs

The systems and organs of the body are composed of epithelial, connective, muscular and nervous tissues.

EPITHELIAL TISSUE

Epithelium forms a protective covering over the internal and external surfaces of the body. It is derived from all three primitive embryonic layers. The ectoderm forms the skin; the mesoderm forms the pleura, pericardium and peritoneum; and the endoderm forms the endothelial lining of blood vessels and gut.

Most glands are epithelial in origin, as they are formed by invagination of an epithelial surface. Epithelium is resistant to physical and chemical damage and the effects of dehydration. It can serve as a selective barrier and can be resistant to harmful metabolites, chemicals and bacteria. It is characterized by a minimal amount of intercellular substance and a tendency to form sheets of cells of one or more layers, having a capability of continuous replacement. It may be simple, transitional or stratified.

Simple epithelium

This consists of a single layer of cells on a basement membrane (Fig. 0.1a–e). It is described as squamous (pavement), cuboidal or columnar, depending on the shape of its cells. Squamous cells are found lining the alveoli of the lungs, the blood vessels (endothelium) and the serous cavities (mesothelium). Cuboidal cells line the ducts of many glands. Columnar cells are often ciliated and may be modified as mucus-forming goblet cells; they line much of the alimentary, respiratory and reproductive tracts. Mucus, a glycoprotein, accumulates in the cell and is discharged from its free (luminal) surface.

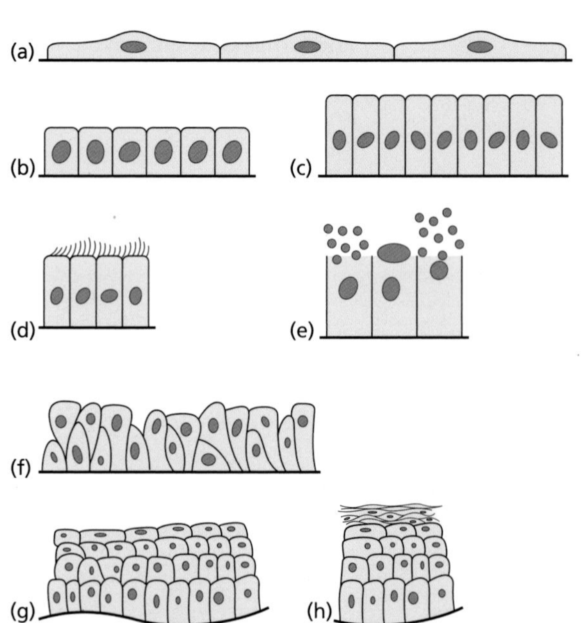

Figure 0.1 Epithelial tissue: (a) squamous; (b) cuboidal; (c) columnar; (d) columnar ciliated; (e) columnar with goblet cells; (f) transitional; (g) stratified epithelium; (h) stratified squamous epithelium

Transitional epithelium

This contains two or three layers of cells, most of which are attached to the basement membrane and are nucleated (Fig. 0.1f). It lines most of the urinary tract, is stretchable and does not desquamate. It contains few glands.

Stratified squamous epithelium

This also has two or more layers of cells (Fig. 0.1g,h). Those in contact with the basement membrane are columnar cells.

The more superficial cells are flattened and the surface cells have no nuclei (enucleate) and are continually being rubbed away (desquamated). This form of epithelium covers the exterior of the body, lines both ends of the alimentary tract, and is particularly suited to areas exposed to wear and tear. In the upper respiratory tract the differing lengths of the columnar cells gives the appearance of a double layer, and this is known as pseudostratified columnar epithelium; it contains numerous mucous cells.

Skin

This consists of two layers, an outer **epidermis** and an inner **dermis** (corium) (Fig. 0.2). The epidermis is composed of keratinized stratified squamous epithelium. **Hair follicles, sweat and sebaceous glands** and **nails** are modifications of the epidermis. The colour of the skin is determined by blood flow and the melanocytes, the pigment-producing cells that lie in the basal layer of the epidermis. The scales on the surface of the skin consist mainly of **keratin,** a sulphur-containing fibrous protein largely responsible for the protective and barrier properties of the skin.

The dermis is a layer of vascular connective tissue moulded tightly to the epidermis and merging in its deeper part with the subcutaneous tissues. Lying in the dermis are the coiled tubular sweat glands opening on to the skin surface and hair follicles, to each of which is attached an arrector pili muscle. The roots of the hairs and the sweat glands extend into the subcutaneous tissue.

Mucous and serous membranes

These line the wet internal surfaces of the body and consist of two layers, an epithelium and a corium. The epithelium of mucous membranes is usually of a simple variety with many mucous or serous cells, but the urinary tract is lined by transitional epithelium, and the respiratory tract by pseudostratified columnar ciliated epithelium with mucous cells. The serous membranes line most of the closed body cavities. The corium underlies the epithelium and is composed of connective tissue. In the alimentary tract it contains a thin sheet of smooth muscle – the **muscularis mucosa.**

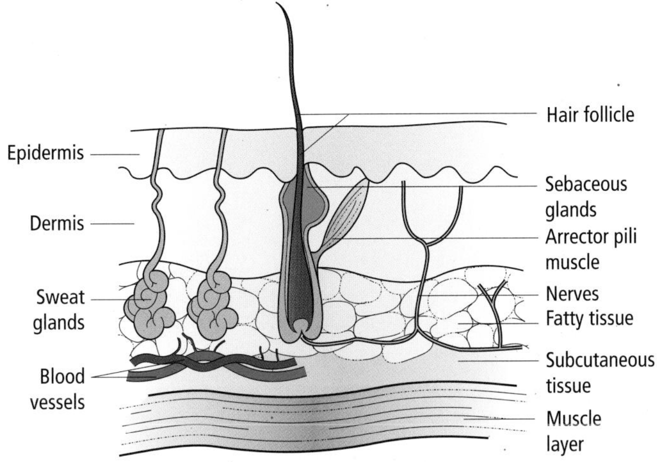

Figure 0.2 Diagram of cross-section through skin

Glands

These are epithelial ingrowths modified to produce secretions. These secretions may pass on to the epithelial surface (**exocrine** glands) or into the bloodstream (**endocrine** glands). Exocrine glands may be unicellular (goblet) or multicellular. The latter may be simple (containing one duct) or compound (branched) where numerous, small ducts open into a single main duct. The secretory part of the gland may be long and thin (tubular), globular (acinar), oval (alveolar) or intermediate, e.g. tubuloalveolar. The secretions of the exocrine glands may be formed by disintegration of the whole cell (holocrine, e.g. sebaceous glands), disintegration of the free end of the cell (**apocrine,** e.g. mammary glands), or without cellular damage (merocrine or **epicrine,** e.g. most other glands). Most endocrine glands are of the last type.

If the duct of an exocrine gland becomes blocked and the gland continues to secrete, the fluid accumulates and a cyst is formed. A generalized enlargement of glands is termed adenopathy.

CONNECTIVE TISSUE

This is characterized by having a large amount of intercellular substance. It forms areolar tissue, the packing material of the body, the supporting tissues (cartilage, bone) and blood (Fig. 0.3). Embryonic connective tissue is called mesenchyme.

Areolar tissue

The intercellular substance is semisolid and composed of proteins and mucopolysaccharides. Three types of fibres are found: coarse **collagen** fibres, which are white (in bulk), flexible, inelastic and arranged in bundles; **elastic** fibres, which are yellowish (in bulk), less frequent and branching;

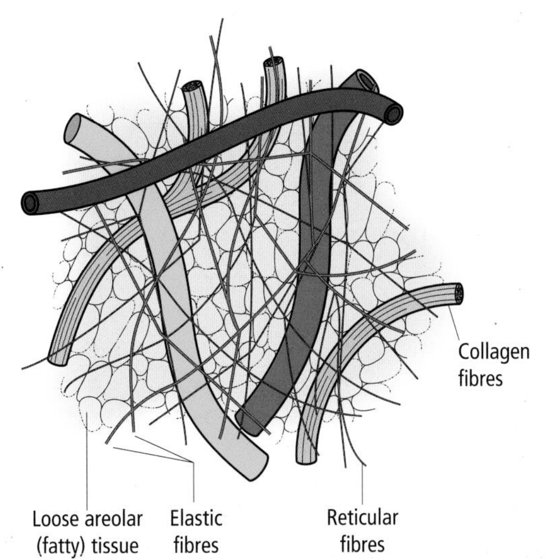

Figure 0.3 Connective tissue

and **reticular** fibres, which form a very fine silver-staining network throughout the tissues.

The cells are of five main varieties: large, slender poorly staining fibroblasts, closely concerned with the production of the three types of tissue fibre; tissue macrophages, which are phagocytic and can engulf particulate matter; oval plasma cells with their cartwheel-like staining nucleus, concerned with antibody production; granular basophilic mast cells, concerned with histamine and heparin production; and the cyst-like fat-containing cells.

The relative amounts of cellular and intercellular substance varies throughout the body. Subcutaneous tissue contains a variable amount of fat and loose fibrous tissue. Superficially, fat is usually predominant, but more deeply the fibrous tissue forms a well-defined superficial fascial sheet connecting it to the deep fascia which invests the limbs and trunk. In other places condensations of non-elastic fibrous tissue form **ligaments, tendons** and **aponeuroses,** and **retinacula.** Ligaments are usually attached to the bones on each side of a joint, maintaining its stability; tendons join the muscles to the bones by blending with the periosteum; aponeuroses are thin flattened tendinous sheets through which muscles gain wider attachments. Retinacula are usually thickenings of the deep fascia related to joints.

SUPPORTING TISSUE

Cartilage

This is an avascular firm tissue composed of cells (chondrocytes) in an abundant intercellular substance (matrix) (Fig. 0.4). It is formed from an overlying fibrous layer, the perichondrium, and classified, according to its predominant fibres, into hyaline cartilage, fibrocartilage and yellow elastic cartilage.

- **Hyaline cartilage** contains many cells, a few fine collagen-like fibres, and is found in the rib cartilages and over most articular surfaces. It also forms the precursor in cartilaginous ossification.
- **Fibrocartilage** contains many dense fibrous bundles, fewer cells, and is present in intervertebral discs, over the articular surface of bones that ossify in membranes, e.g. the mandible, and in intra-articular cartilages, e.g. the menisci of the knee.
- **Yellow elastic cartilage** contains elastic fibres and is found in the auricular, epiglottic and the apices of the arytenoid cartilages of the head.

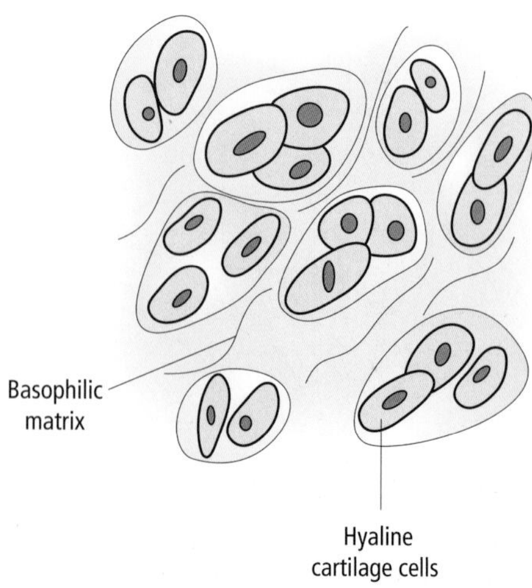

Figure 0.4 Hyaline cartilage

Bone

This is a hard supporting tissue composed mainly of inorganic calcium salts impregnating a network of collagen fibres (Fig. 0.5). The basic unit, composed of concentric layers around a central vessel, is known as a **Haversian system.** The bone cells (osteocytes) lie within spaces (lacunae) between the layers and their processes pass into canaliculi in the bone. **Compact bone** is dense and strong and forms the outer part of most bones. The **cancellous** (spongy) bone within consists of a network of thin partitions (trabeculae) around intercommunicating spaces; the osteocytes lie within lacunae in the trabeculae. The outer surface of a bone is covered by a thick fibrous layer, the **periosteum,** many of the cells of which are the granular, bone-forming **osteoblasts.** These cells, when enclosed in the hard intercellular substance, become osteocytes. The blood supply of bone is from the periosteum and muscular vessels and, in the case of long bones, from one or two nutrient arteries that enter the shaft.

The shape of the bones of the body, the proportion of compact to cancellous tissue and the architecture of the trabeculae are arranged to give maximum strength along with economy of material. Both genetic and local factors influence the shape and size of a bone. Adjacent muscles or organs (e.g. the brain) mould the bone to some extent.

Many of these factors can be investigated in the living person by means of X-rays.

Bones are classified as long, short, flat, sesamoid or irregular (Fig. 0.6a–d).

Long bones are present in the limbs. The body (shaft) is a cylinder of compact bone surrounding a medullary cavity which is filled with some cancellous bone and a large amount

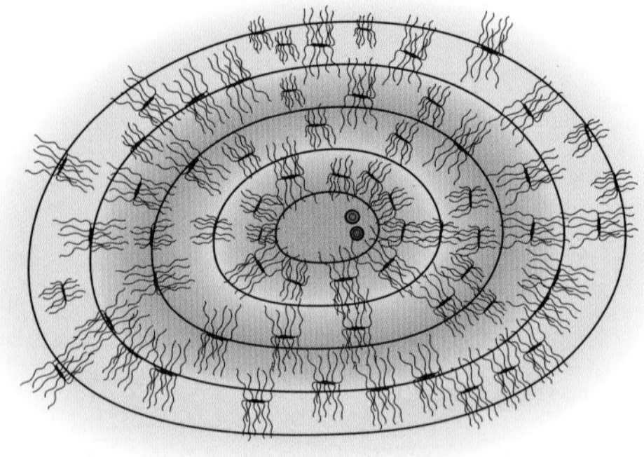

Figure 0.5 Haversian bony systems with osteoblasts in circular layers with central canals carrying nutrient vessels

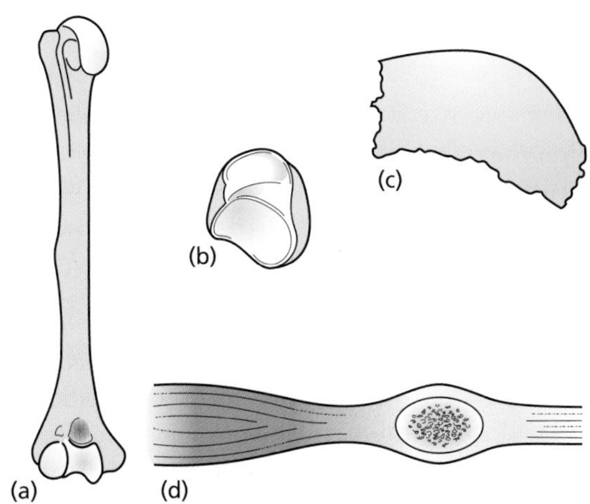

Figure 0.6 Bone types: (a) long bone (humerus); (b) irregular bone (lunate); (c) flat bone (from vault of skull); (d) sesamoid bone, a small pebble-like bone within a tendon, for example in the tendon of flexor hallucis longus beneath the head of the first metatarsal

of yellow fatty marrow. The two ends are formed of spongy bone with a thin outer shell of compact bone. The trabeculae in the cancellous bone are laid down along the lines of force. In the developing long bone of a child but not normally in the adult, blood-forming tissue is found in the marrow.

The **short bones** are found in the carpus and tarsus. They consist of spongy bone covered with a thin layer of compact bone.

The **flat bones,** e.g. the scapula, give attachment to muscles and form a protective covering (the bones of the skull vault). They consist of two layers of compact bone with a thin intervening spongy layer (the diplöe in the skull).

Sesamoid bones are formed within tendons and serve to relieve friction and to alter the line of pull of a muscle. The largest sesamoid bone is the patella.

The remaining **irregular bones** may contain red, blood-forming marrow (the vertebrae), or air spaces (sinuses) (Fig. 0.7a,b).

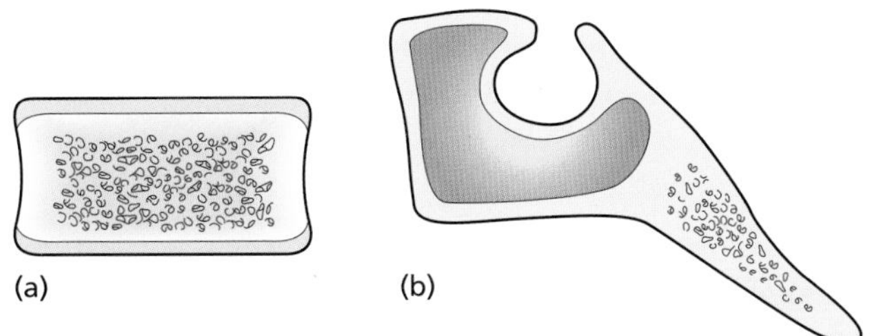

Figure 0.7 (a) Cancellous bone, for example within the centre of a vertebral body, surrounded with a layer of compact bone. (b) Pneumatized bone, for example the skull sinuses around the nasal cavity

Excessive force applied to a bone may cause it to break (fracture), and in such injuries the adjacent soft tissues may be damaged both by the force and by the broken ends of the bone. Knowledge of the anatomical relations of the bone enables the clinician to predict the likely association of nerve, artery and muscle injury with a fracture. A break in the overlying skin is a serious complication of fractures, as it permits the entry of infecting organisms. In these circumstances the fracture is said to be compound (Fig. 0.8a,b).

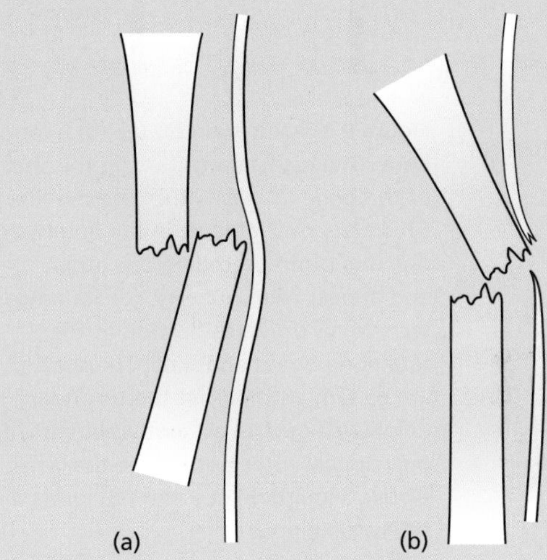

Figure 0.8 Fracture: (a) simple; (b) compound. In the latter the overlying skin has been lacerated. This is much more serious because bacterial infection can enter the bone with possible long-term sequelae

Ossification

Bone may develop either (i) in a condensed fibrous tissue model, when the process is called **membranous** (mesenchymal) ossification, or (ii) in a cartilage model which has replaced the mesenchyme, and the process is called **cartilaginous** (endochondral) ossification.

Mesenchymal ossification usually starts in the fifth to sixth weeks of intrauterine life and is found in the bones of the skull vault, the bones of the face and the clavicle (partly).

Cartilaginous ossification occurs in all long bones except the clavicle. A primary centre appears for the body of a long bone in about the eighth week of intrauterine life, and secondary centres for each end appear between birth and puberty. Fusion of the body and these centres occurs in about the 18th year in males. Secondary centres appear and fuse up to a year earlier in females. Further ossification centres may develop at puberty in areas of major muscle attachment, e.g. the processes of the vertebrae and the crests of the scapula and the hip. They fuse with the rest of the bone by about the 25th year.

Development of a long bone

A long bone develops from a cartilaginous model possessing an outer perichondrium and an irregular cartilaginous matrix; the deep layers of the perichondrium have bone-forming properties (Fig. 0.9a–e).

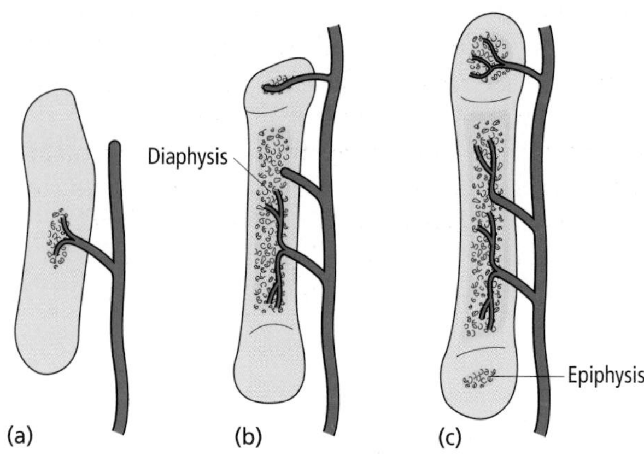

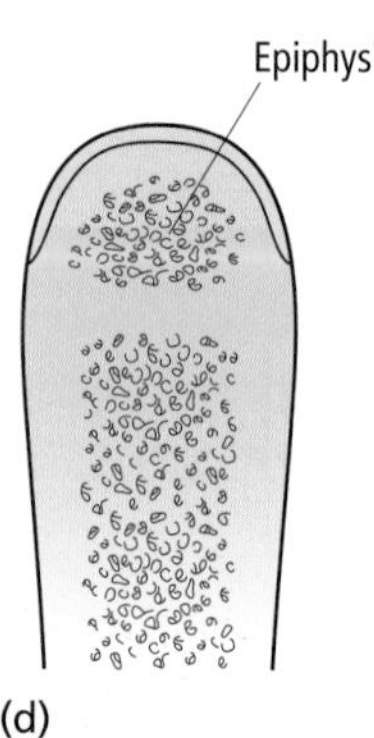

Figure 0.9 Ossification of: (a)–(d) a long bone. The ossification starts in the shaft of the bone usually within uterine life. Secondary centres start in the epiphysis, one end often preceding the other, and appear after puberty. (e) Staining techniques show ossification in the fetal long bones and skull. The shafts are already ossified but the secondary epiphyseal centres are not visible as they only appear after birth. Note the wrist, elbow, shoulder, knee and hip joints are still cartilaginous

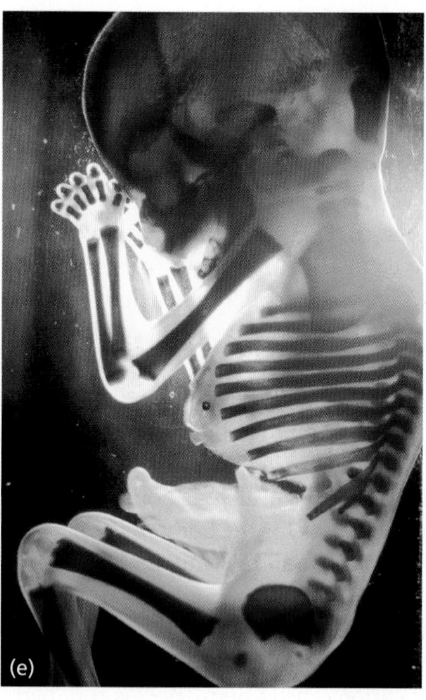

The first changes occur in the cartilage cells of the middle of the body (the **diaphysis**). They become greatly enlarged and the matrix is correspondingly reduced and calcified. The cells die and undergo shrinkage, leaving spaces known as primary alveoli. The deeper layer of **perichondrium** around the middle of the body starts to produce bone, and is then known as the **periosteum.** Blood vessels and bone cells (the bone-forming osteoblasts and the bone-removing osteoclasts) pass inwards from the periosteum to the calcified zone. The cartilage is not converted into bone but is replaced by it after its removal by the osteoclasts. The multinucleated osteoclasts initiate absorption of the calcified material, producing larger spaces, the secondary alveoli. Osteoblasts come to line the secondary alveoli and layers of bone are deposited. Some osteoblasts are incorporated into the bone, becoming the bone cells (**osteocytes**). Ossification extends up and down the body from this primary centre. The cells of the adjacent cartilage come to lie in parallel longitudinal rows and are subsequently replaced in the manner already described. This form of ossification is known as endochondral (cartilaginous).

Secondary centres of ossification (the **epiphyses**) appear later in life. Osteogenic cells invade the calcified cartilage after the cells have undergone hypertrophy, death and shrinkage. The layer of cartilage left between the epiphysis and the diaphysis is known as the **epiphyseal plate.** The part of the diaphysis bordering the plate is known as the **metaphysis;** the cartilage adjacent to the metaphysis is continually being ossified. New cartilage cells are formed in the epiphyseal plate. Growth in length of the bone continues until the cartilage cells stop multiplying, and fusion of the diaphysis and epiphysis then occurs. The internal architecture of the bone is remodelled by osteoclastic and osteoblastic activity. Simultaneous laying down of layers of bone around the body by the periosteum increases the girth of the bone and is known as **subperiosteal ossification;** it is a form of mesenchymal ossification. Growth and remodelling of the bone continues until adulthood by the continuous destruction by osteoclasts and replacement by osteoblasts.

Epiphyses may be classified into three types: **pressure** epiphyses, seen at the ends of weight-bearing bones, **traction** epiphyses occurring at the site of muscle attachments, and **'atavistic'** epiphyses, which are functionless skeletal remnants that may show on an X-ray and be mistaken for disease or injury.

Injury in a young person can dislodge the epiphysis from the metaphysis, e.g. a fall on the outstretched arm may produce a **slipped** epiphysis of the lower end of the radius. This injury may interfere with further growth at that end of the bone.

In summary, most primary ossification centres of long bones appear by the end of the second month of intrauterine life, and most epiphyseal centres before puberty. The epiphyses at the knee joint appear just before birth and are an indication of the age of the fetus. Most long bones cease to grow in length between the 18th and 20th years in men, and a year or so earlier in women.

The skeleton

The skeleton is divisible into an **axial** part (the bones of the head and trunk) and an **appendicular** part (the bones of the limbs). The upper limb is joined to the trunk by the mobile muscular pectoral girdle, and the lower limb by the stable bony pelvic girdle.

JOINTS

These are unions between two or more bones and may be of four types: bony, fibrous, cartilaginous or synovial.

Bony

The three elements of the hip bone are joined by bony union, as are the occipital and the sphenoid in the skull after completion of the second dentition (Fig. 0.10).

Fibrous

The bony surfaces are united by fibrous tissue. These comprise the skull sutures, the articulations of the roots of the teeth and the inferior tibiofibular joint (Fig. 0.11a,b).

Cartilaginous

These may be primary or secondary. In the primary cartilaginous joints the bony surfaces are united by hyaline cartilage, as seen in the union of the body and the ends in a developing long bone (Fig. 0.12a,b).

In the secondary cartilaginous joints, the symphyses (Fig. 0.13), the bony surfaces are covered with hyaline cartilage and united by a fibrocartilaginous disc. These joints all lie in the midline and comprise the intervertebral discs, the symphysis pubis and the manubriosternal and xiphisternal junctions.

Synovial

The bony articular surfaces (facets) are covered with **hyaline cartilage** (with the exception of the temporomandibular and sternoclavicular joints, where they are covered with fibrocartilage) (Fig. 0.14). A fibrous **capsule** is attached near to the articular margins of the bones. The surfaces of the interior of the joint, except those covered by cartilage, are lined by a delicate vascular **synovial membrane,** which secretes a lubricating **synovial fluid** into the joint cavity.

The capsule may possess **ligamentous thickenings,** and accessory extracapsular and intracapsular **ligaments** may pass across the joint. Fibrous intra-articular **discs** are present in some joints, occasionally completely dividing their cavity (e.g. temporomandibular joint). **Tendons** occasionally enter the

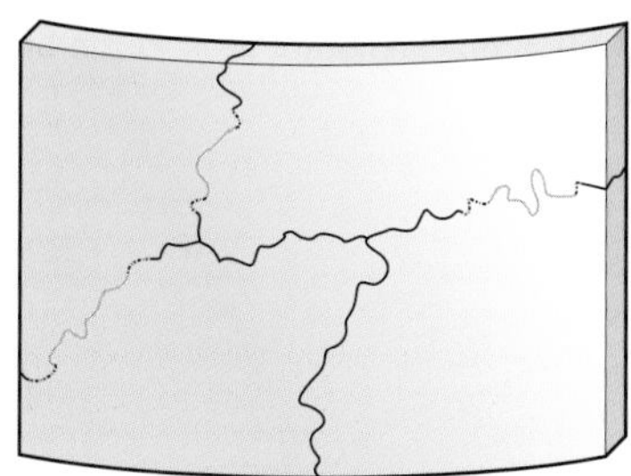

Figure 0.10 Bony joints between the skull bones. These ossify and disappear later in life

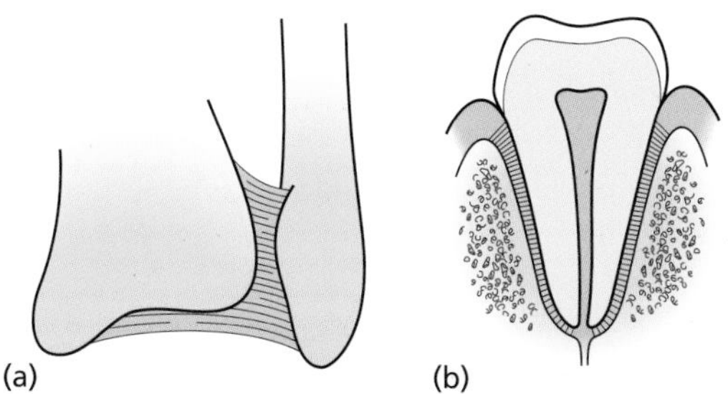

Figure 0.11 Fibrous joints where two bones are attached by fibrous tissue: (a) inferior tibiofibular joint; (b) tooth socket where the enamel is attached to the surrounding bone by fibres of the periodontal ligament

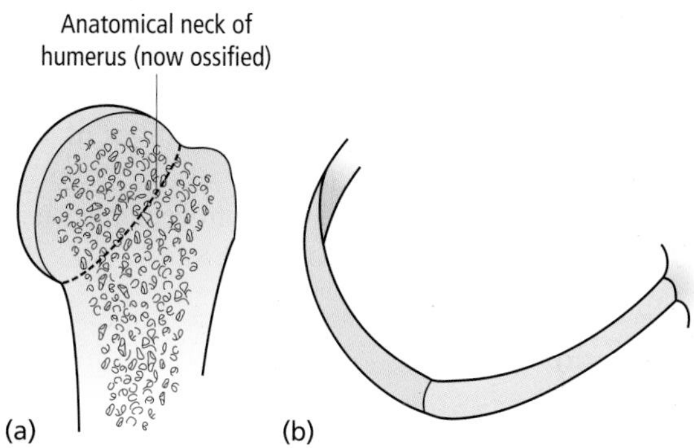

Figure 0.12 Primary cartilaginous joints: (a) union of epiphysis and metapysis (dotted line); originally hyaline cartilage, now ossified; (b) union between rib and costal cartilage

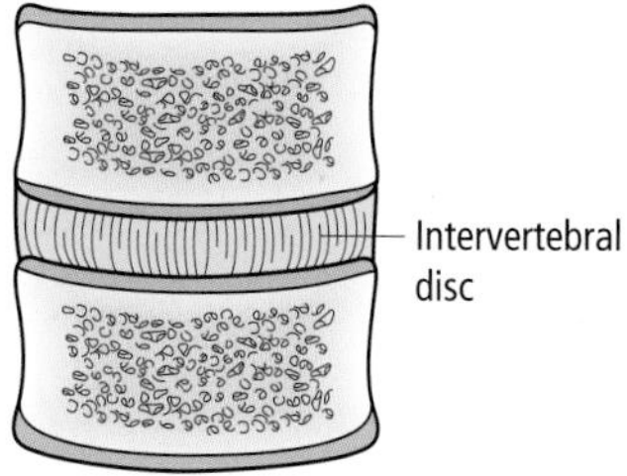

Figure 0.13 Secondary cartilaginous joint where the bone is covered by hyaline cartilage and two surfaces are joined by a fibrocartilaginous disc. These occur in the midline and include the intervertebral, the symphysis pubis and the manubriosternal joints

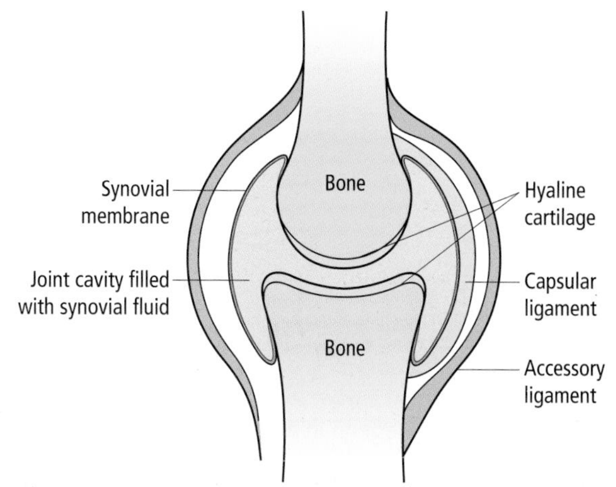

Figure 0.14 Synovial joints

joint cavity by piercing the capsule (biceps brachii), and **fat pads** may be present between the capsule and the synovial lining (knee joint).

Muscles or tendons crossing superficial to the joint may be protected by a synovial sheath or sac whose fluid prevents excessive friction. The sacs are known as **bursae,** and the cavity may communicate with that of the joint.

Functional aspects of joints

Movement

Bony, fibrous and primary cartilaginous joints are immobile, secondary cartilaginous joints are slightly mobile, and synovial joints are freely mobile.

Synovial joints are subdivided into a number of varieties according to the movements possible at the joint. These varieties are listed below and the movements are best understood by examining the examples given.

- **Hinge** – elbow, ankle and interphalangeal joints, the knee and temporomandibular joints are modified hinge joints (Fig. 0.15a–d)
- **Pivot** – the proximal radioulnar joint and the dens articulation of the atlantoaxial joint (Fig. 0.16)
- **Condyloid** – metacarpophalangeal joint (Fig. 0.17a)
- **Ellipsoid** – radiocarpal (wrist) joint (Fig. 0.17b)
- **Saddle** – carpometacarpal joint of the thumb (Fig. 0.18)
- **Ball and socket** – hip and shoulder joints (Fig. 0.19)
- **Plane** – intercarpal joints and joints between the articular processes of adjacent vertebrae (Fig. 0.20a,b).

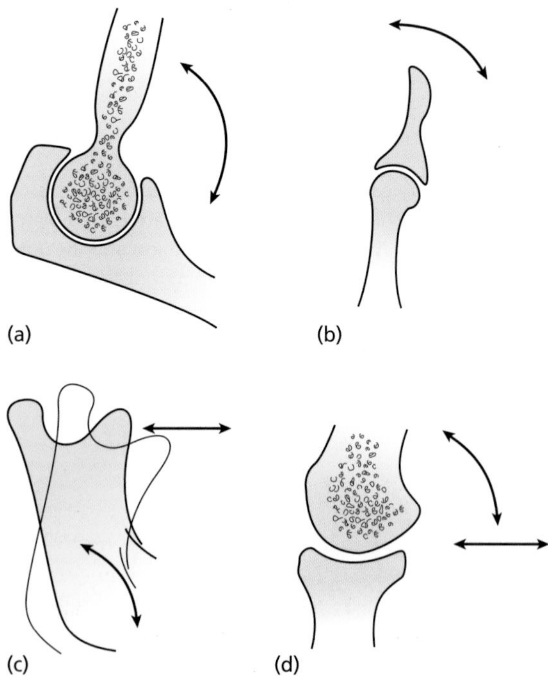

Figure 0.15 Hinge joints: (a) elbow; (b) interphalangeal joints allowing flexion, extension in a single plane; (c) temporomandibular joint; (d) knee joint, modified hinge joints with extension in a single plane but with a little rotation or gliding in the lax position of the capsules

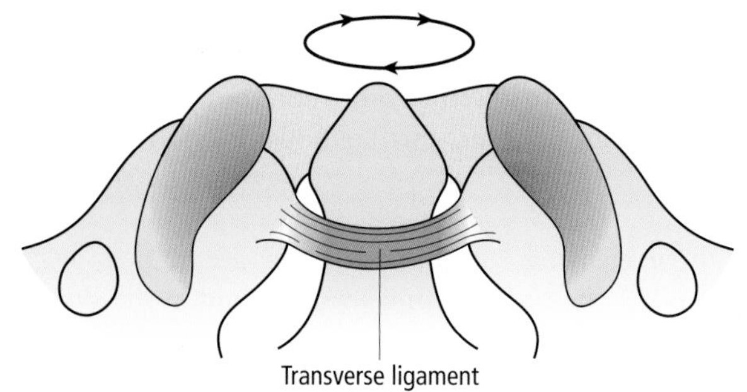

Figure 0.16 Pivot joint: horizontal view of the atlantoaxial joint. The odontoid process of the axis rotates with the anterior articular facet of the atlas anteriorly and transverse ligament posteriorly

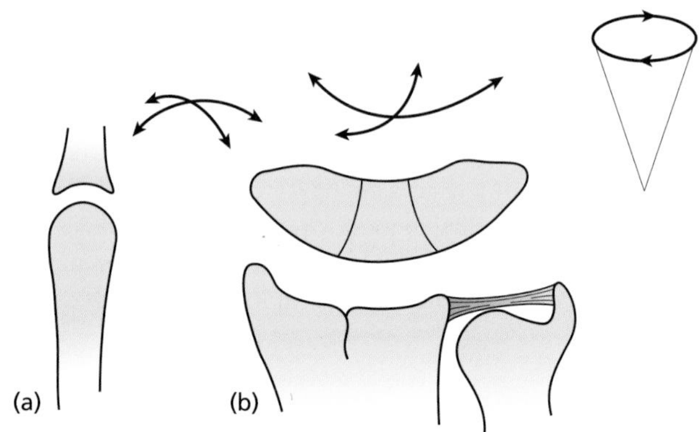

Figure 0.17 (a) Condyloid joint, for example, metacarpophalangeal joint. (b) Ellipsoid joint of the wrist (radiocarpal) joint. These joints move in two planes: flexion–extension and abduction–adduction. Circumduction is a combination of all of these movements where the distal part of the limb can rotate around the pivot point or the centre of the joint

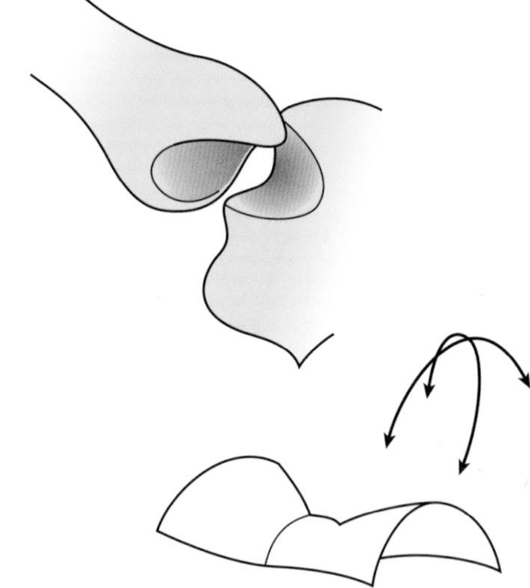

Figure 0.18 Saddle joint. The carpometacarpal joint of the thumb is shaped like the saddle of a horse where the rider can slide off from side to side as well as move backwards and forwards

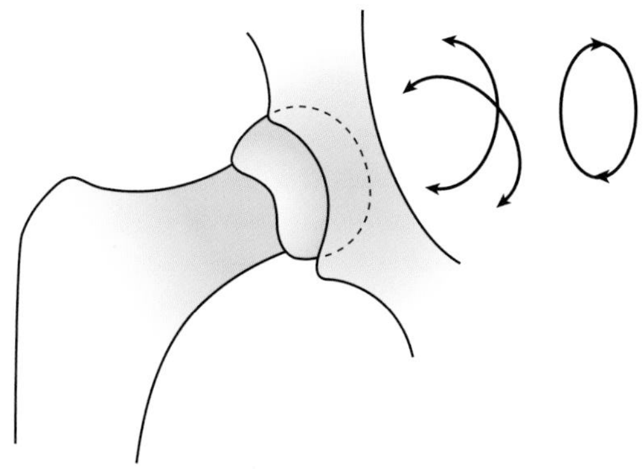

Figure 0.19 Ball and socket joint, for example, the hip. The hip joint has all the movements of the condyloid joint and in addition the head can rotate within the socket, i.e. additional medial and lateral rotation

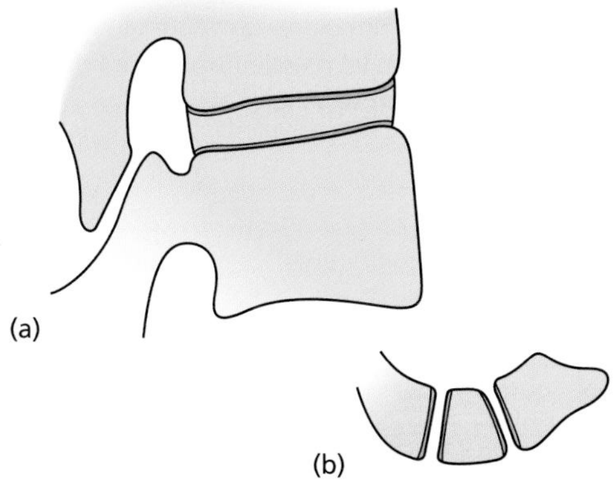

Figure 0.20 Joint movements. (a) In a secondary cartilaginous joint there is the possibility of slight stretching and movement, for example in the symphysis pubis and the intervertebral joints. The symphysis softens in pregnancy and allows slight adaptation of the pelvic form during parturition. (b) Plane joints allow a little gliding of the adjacent joints, for example in the carpus

Stability

Stability depends on bony, ligamentous or muscular factors. It is usually inversely related to the mobility of the joint.

Many of these functional aspects of joints may be assessed by radiology. Displacement of the articulating surfaces of a joint is known as dislocation. Partial displacement of the articulating surfaces is known as subluxation. Dislocation of a joint may follow severe injury and is always associated with damage to the capsular and accessory ligaments. There may also be fractures of the bony structures of the joint, and occasionally damage to closely related nerves and vessels. Chronic inflammatory processes are prone to affect the bone ends (osteoarthritis) and synovial membrane (rheumatoid arthritis), and joints thus affected may be deformed and painful, with marked limitation of movement.

Nerve supply

The capsule and ligaments of a joint contain pain, proprioceptive and stretch fibres: these provide information on the position of the joint and any abnormal forces. The nerve supply of a joint is from the nerves supplying the muscles acting on the joint.

MUSCULAR TISSUE

This is a contractile tissue. There are skeletal, smooth and cardiac varieties.

Skeletal (striated, voluntary) muscle

This acts mainly on the bony skeleton or as a diaphragm, but it is also found around the pharynx and larynx, and forms some sphincters (Fig. 0.21a–c). It is composed of unbranched fibres of sarcoplasm limited by a membrane, the sarcolemma, and contains many nuclei. Each fibre has a motor endplate and contains many contractile units, the myofibrils, which have alternating dark (A) and light (I) bands. A dark line (the Z disc) crosses the middle of the I band. The bands of adjacent myofibrils coincide, giving the muscle fibre its striated appearance. Each fibre is enveloped and attached to its neighbour by a fibrous endomysium, and bundles of fibres are enclosed by a fibrous perimysium. A muscle composed of many bundles is surrounded by an epimysium.

The motor nerve supply of the muscle comes from the anterior horn cells of the spinal cord and the motor nuclei of the brain stem. The sensory supply arises in the more specialized spindles and tendon organs as well as the simpler touch and pain endings. Impulses from the sensory endings pass into the posterior horn of the spinal cord.

Skeletal muscles are formed by voluntary fibres. The muscles are usually attached at each end to bone, by the periosteum, either directly or through **tendons** and **aponeuroses,** and cross one or more joints. Occasionally two muscles meet at a common stretchable union known as a **raphé,** e.g. mylohyoid muscles (Fig. 0.22g). Muscles have a very rich blood supply.

Muscle fibres are arranged either **parallel** (Fig 0.22a) to the direction of the action (sartorius), or **obliquely** to it and known as **pennate** muscles. **Unipennate** muscles (Fig. 0.22c) have oblique fibres inserted into one side of a side tendon (extensor digitorum longus). In **bipennate** muscles (Fig. 0.22d) oblique fibres are inserted into each side of the tendon (rectus femoris). A **multipennate** muscle has a number of parallel bipennate tendons (deltoid) or is a circular muscle with a central tendon (tibialis anterior). In muscles of equal volume, a parallel arrangement of fibres gives greater movement but less power than an oblique arrangement. The least mobile attachment of a muscle is often called its **origin,** and the more mobile attachment its **insertion.** But this is an arbitrary distinction, so reference in the text is made to muscle **attachments,** rather than to origin or insertion. An **aponeurosis** (Fig. 0.22f) is a flat, thin tendinous expansion providing a wide attachment, as seen in abdominal wall muscles.

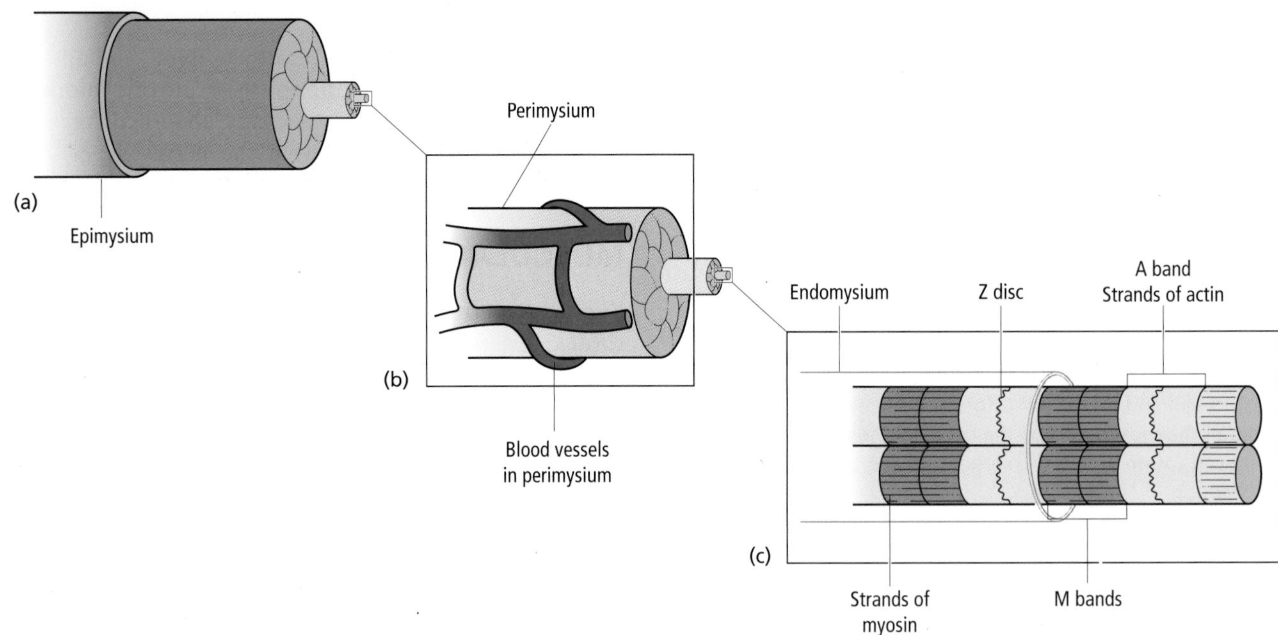

Figure 0.21 Muscle fibres of striated muscle ((a), (b) and (c) showing increasing magnification): (a) epimysium surrounding muscle bundles; (b) muscle bundles surrounded by perimysium containing nutrient blood vessels and nerves; (c) muscle fibres contained within endomysium. The strands of myosin and actin interlock during muscle contraction in a similar fashion to Velcro

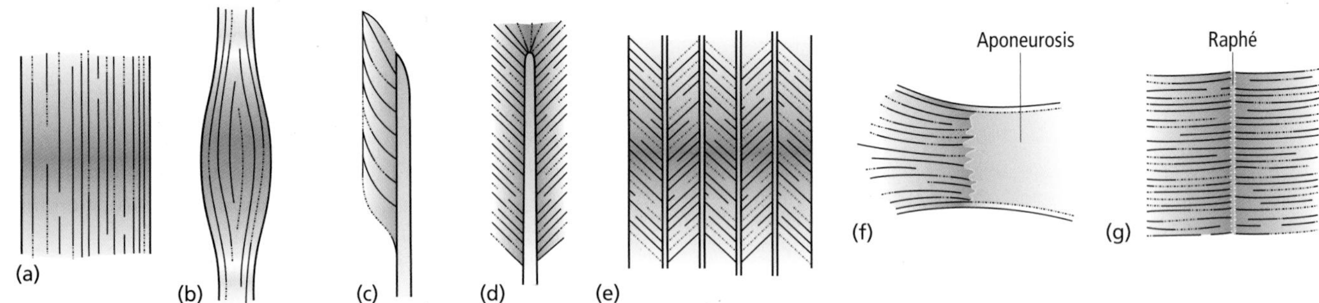

Figure 0.22 Types of striated muscle: (a) parallel (quadrate); (b) fusiform; (c) unipennate; (d) bipennate; (e) multipennate; (f) flat muscle inserted into a tendinous sheet (aponeurosis); (g) two muscles attached to each other along a raphé

When a movement occurs at a joint, the muscles concerned in producing it are known as the prime movers or agonists and those opposing it as antagonists. Muscles contracting to steady the joint across which movement is occurring are known as synergists. A further type of action is known as the action of paradox, in which a muscle gradually relaxes against the pull of gravity, e.g. bending forwards produced by relaxing the back muscles.

Smooth (unstriated, involuntary) muscle

This is present in the walls of most vessels and hollow organs of the body (Fig. 0.23). It is composed of unbranched spindle-shaped cells with a single central nucleus and containing many unstriated myofibrils. The fibres are arranged in interlacing bundles and are supplied by the autonomic nervous system.

Cardiac muscle

This is found in the heart. It consists of short, branched cylindrical fibres joined end to end (Fig. 0.24). The adherent ends of adjacent fibres form dark intercalated discs. Each fibre contains a single central nucleus and striated myofibrils resembling those of voluntary muscle. It is supplied by the autonomic nervous system, but heart muscle also has the properties of spontaneous and rhythmic activity. The conducting system of the heart is made up of modified cardiac muscle cells.

NERVOUS TISSUE

This is capable of excitability and conductivity. It consists of excitable cells (**neurons**) (Fig. 0.25) and supporting cells, which in the central nervous system are the **neuroglial cells,** and in the peripheral nervous system the **Schwann cells.**

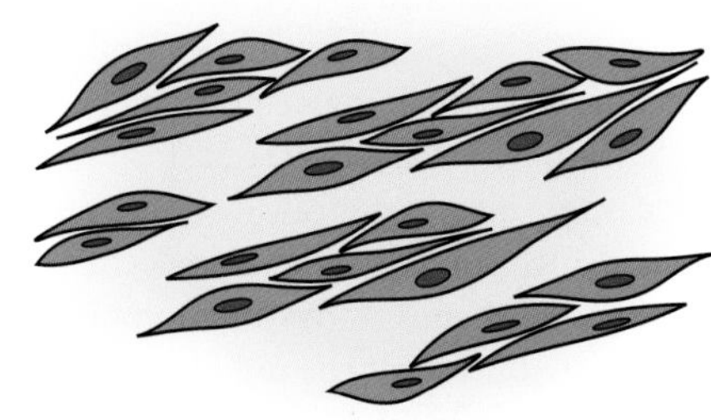

Figure 0.23 Smooth muscle fibres contained within a loose muscle bundle

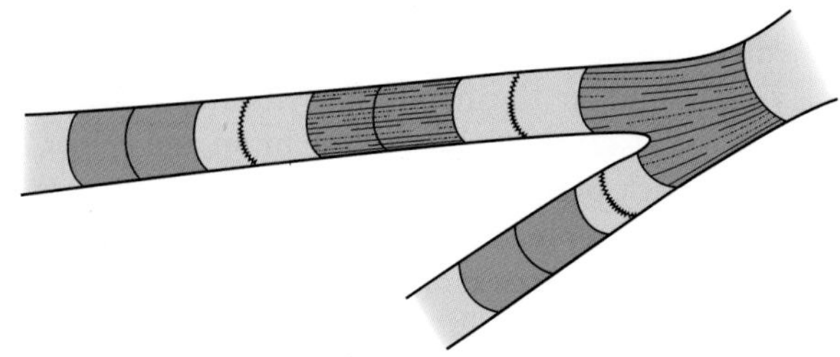

Figure 0.24 Cardiac muscle showing the striations of striated muscle and branching, producing a continuous network of muscle

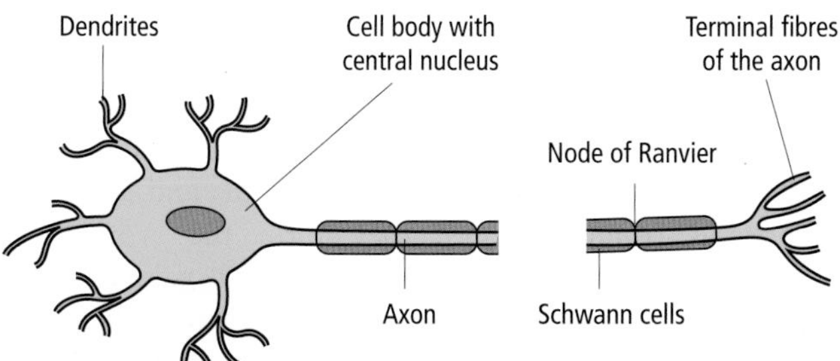

Figure 0.25 Neuron

The neuron is the functional unit of the nervous system and consists of a cell body and processes, usually an **axon** and one or more **dendrites.** The cell bodies are situated in the central nervous system or in peripheral ganglia. They possess a large nucleus and well-marked cellular inclusions. The axon (fibre) begins at a small axon hillock on the cell body and carries impulses away from the cell body. This often long, slender process ends by dividing into many branches which have small terminal knobs, the **boutons,** related to the cell bodies or branches of other neurons. The relationship is known as a **synapse** and may be either facilitatory or inhibitory, depending on the neuron of origin, and possibly on the receptor area of the second neuron. A rather specialized synapse is formed when a nerve ends on a muscle fibre at a **motor endplate.**

Axons may give off one or more short collateral branches. They are myelinated or unmyelinated. The myelin is interrupted about every millimetre or so, by a constriction called the **node of Ranvier.** In the peripheral nervous system each internodal segment of sheath is produced by a **Schwann cell,** the nucleus of which is seen on its surface. These cells play an important role in peripheral nerve regeneration. Fibres of the peripheral nervous system are also covered by a thin fibrous membrane, the **neurilemma.** In the central nervous system oligodendroglia take the place of the Schwann cells. Dendrites are usually short unmyelinated processes carrying membrane depolarizations to the cell body. The volume over which the dendrites of a single cell extend is known as the dendritic field.

Afferent neurons carry information towards the central nervous system and efferent neurons carry instructions away from it. Within the central nervous system afferent and efferent neurons are often connected by many intercalated (internuncial or intermediate) neurons.

The neurons are organized to form the central and peripheral nervous systems. The former comprises the brain and spinal cord (Fig. 0.26) and the latter the cranial nerves, spinal nerves and the autonomic nervous system (see below). A group of neurons in the central nervous system is called a **nucleus,** and outside the central nervous system (CNS) such a group is known as a **ganglion.** Within the CNS are neuroglial cells, variously known as **astrocytes, oligodendroglia** and **microglia,** and these make up almost half of the brain substance.

Astrocytes are stellate cells with large nuclei and numerous processes, which may be of the thick protoplasmic variety, as found mainly in the grey matter, or the thin fibrous variety found mainly in the white matter. Some of the processes end on blood vessels, and the astrocytes are thought to be concerned

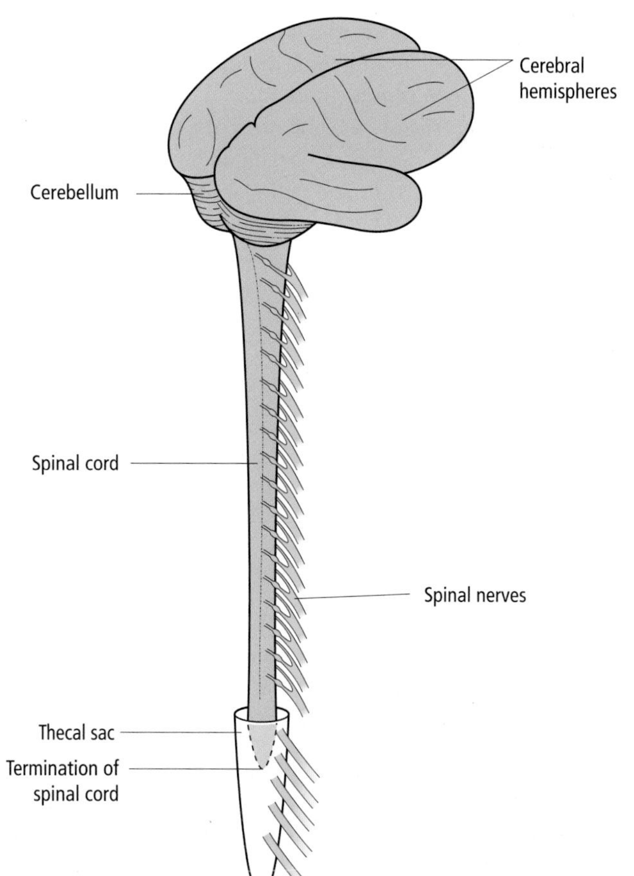

Figure 0.26 Brain and spinal cord

Introduction

with the fluid balance in the central nervous system and with the nutrition of the neurons. Oligodendroglia are oval dark-staining cells possessing few processes. They produce the myelin of the central nervous system. Microglia are small mobile phagocytic cells and form part of the macrophage system.

Ependymal cells are columnar in shape and line the cavities of the brain and spinal cord. In certain regions the ependyma is modified to form the choroid plexuses of the brain, which produce the cerebrospinal fluid.

Cranial nerves

Twelve pairs of nerves are attached to the brain (p. 333). Some are mainly sensory, some mainly motor, and others are mixed sensory and motor.

Spinal nerves

The 31 paired spinal nerves (8 cervical, 12 thoracic, 5 lumbar, 5 sacral and 1 coccygeal) (Fig. 0.26) are formed within the vertebral canal, each by the union of a ventral and a dorsal root. The roots are formed from a number of rootlets which emerge from the anterolateral and posterolateral sulci of the spinal cord. The **ventral root** carries efferent (motor) fibres from the cord, and the **dorsal root** carries afferent (sensory) fibres to the cord. The cell bodies of the sensory fibres are situated in a **ganglion** on the dorsal root (Fig. 0.27). The spinal nerves are therefore a mixture of motor and sensory fibres. Each nerve leaves the vertebral canal through an intervertebral foramen and soon divides into a large **ventral** and a smaller **dorsal ramus** (branch).

The adjacent ventral rami of most regions communicate to form **plexuses** (cervical, brachial and lumbosacral), whereas those of the thoracic region become the intercostal and subcostal nerves. The dorsal rami pass backwards into the postvertebral muscles and divide into medial and lateral branches. These rami supply the muscles and skin over the posterior aspect of the body, but give no branches to the limbs.

Tumours within the vertebral canal or a protrusion from a degenerate intervertebral disc may compress a spinal nerve and, occasionally, the spinal cord to produce segmental sensory and motor dysfunction. Knowledge of the anatomical distribution of the individual nerves enables the site of the disease to be identified.

Autonomic nervous system

The motor part of this system innervates glands, and smooth and cardiac muscle. Its fibres form a fine network on the blood vessels and in the nerves. All its fibres arise from neurons of the visceral columns of the brain and spinal cord and synapse with **peripheral ganglion** cells before reaching the organs they supply. This fine network is divisible into two complementary parts, **sympathetic** and **parasympathetic,** which leave the central nervous system at different sites. They usually have opposing effects on the structure they supply through endings, which are mainly adrenergic or cholinergic.

Sympathetic system

Each ventral ramus from the first thoracic to the second lumbar nerve gives a bundle of myelinated (preganglionic) fibres to the **sympathetic chain or trunk** (Fig. 0.27). The bundles arise near the formation of a ramus and are called **white rami communicantes;** they form the sympathetic outflow of the central nervous system. Each ventral ramus later receives a bundle of unmyelinated (postganglionic) fibres from the sympathetic trunk – a **grey ramus** communicans. (The myelinated and unmyelinated fibres are also termed the white and grey rami communicantes, respectively.)

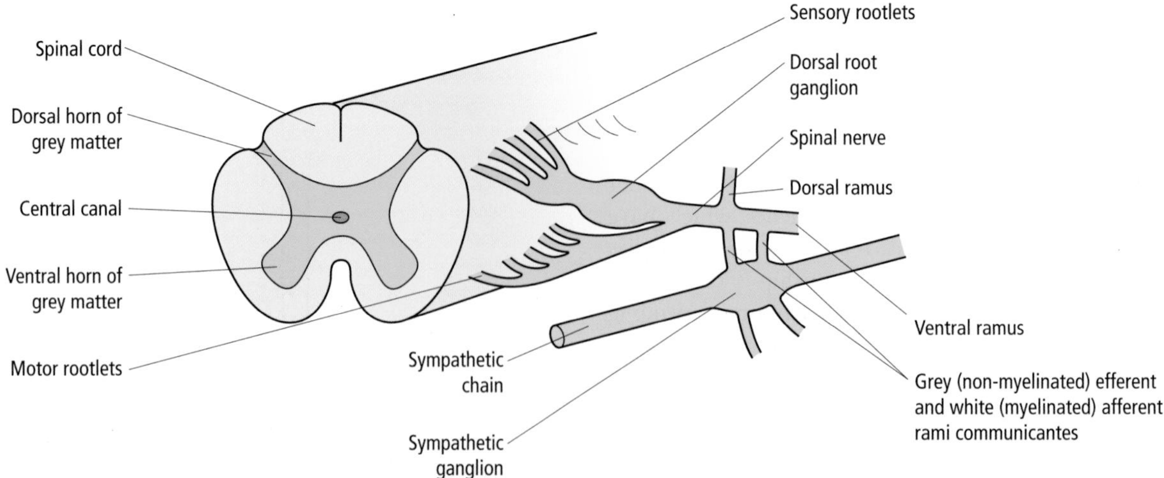

Figure 0.27 Typical spinal nerve formation and connections to the sympathetic ganglia and chain. The ventral motor rootlets unite to form a ventral motor root, joining with the dorsal sensory root which comes from the sensory rootlets and dorsal root ganglion of each spinal segment. The 'mixed' spinal nerve then divides into a dorsal and a ventral primary ramus. The dorsal rami supply the back whereas the larger ventral rami supply all the limbs and trunk. The sympathetic ganglia are connected to the ventral rami via white (presynaptic) rami communicantes and grey (postsynaptic) rami

The peripheral ganglia of the system lie within the two parallel sympathetic trunks alongside the vertebral column. The trunks extend from the base of the skull to the coccyx and have 3 cervical, 12 thoracic, 4 lumbar and 5 sacral ganglia. The preganglionic fibres from the thoracolumbar outflow may synapse (i) in the adjacent ganglion, (ii) in other ganglia higher or lower in the chain, or (iii) in the collateral ganglia situated in the plexuses around the aorta (e.g. coeliac). Each preganglionic fibre may synapse with 15 or more ganglionic cells, thus giving rise to widespread activity. A number of preganglionic fibres end in the medulla of the suprarenal gland.

Postganglionic (unmyelinated) fibres may (i) return to a spinal nerve in a grey ramus communicans to be distributed to peripheral smooth muscle, e.g. arterial walls, (ii) pass along the major arteries and their branches to be distributed to the organs these supply, or (iii) form named nerves, e.g. cardiac, running to the viscus concerned.

The cell bodies of the sympathetic fibres supplying the upper and lower limbs are situated in ganglia in the cervicothoracic and lumbosacral regions, respectively.

Chemical destruction or surgical removal of these ganglia may be undertaken to improve the cutaneous blood supply of the limb, or to reduce excessive sweating.

The visceral branches supply the smooth circular muscle, including the sphincters of the viscera.

Parasympathetic system

This system receives preganglionic fibres from four cranial nerves (oculomotor, facial, glossopharyngeal and vagus) and the second, third and fourth sacral spinal nerves (**craniosacral outflow**). The peripheral ganglia of this system are near the organs they supply, usually in its walls. There are, however, four well-defined, isolated, parasympathetic ganglia associated with the cranial nerves. The postganglionic fibres are usually short and unmyelinated. The visceral branches usually supply the smooth muscle responsible for emptying the organ, and also produce dilatation of the blood vessels. There is little evidence of parasympathetic supply to the limbs.

Afferent (e.g. pain) fibres from the viscera are present in both sympathetic and parasympathetic systems and pass to the central nervous system without synapsing. Their subsequent paths are similar to those of somatic pain. Afferent (reflex) fibres, e.g. from the lungs, heart, bladder, and visceral sensations of nausea, hunger, rectal distension, also reach the central nervous system, probably along parasympathetic pathways.

Most transmitter chemicals can be classified as adrenergic (for the sympathetic system) or cholinergic (for the parasympathetic system).

THE CARDIOVASCULAR SYSTEM

The cardiovascular system comprises the heart and blood vessels, **arteries, veins, capillaries** and **sinusoids.** The arteries and veins passing to organs and muscles are usually accompanied by the nerves, and together form a compact **neurovascular bundle.**

The walls of the arteries possess three coats (Fig. 0.28a): the intima, composed of an **endothelial** lining and a small amount of connective tissue; the **media** in the larger arteries which is composed mainly of elastic tissue, and almost entirely of smooth muscle in the small **arterioles** and medium-sized arteries; and the outer fibrous **adventitia.** The coats of the veins correspond to those of the arteries (Fig. 0.28b), but the media contains less smooth muscle and fewer elastic fibres. In the larger veins the adventitia is thicker than the media. In most veins, **valves** are present. These are formed of paired folds of endothelium and help to determine the direction of flow. Medium and smaller arteries are often accompanied by two veins rather than one, the **venae comitantes.** The smallest, postcapillary, veins are termed **venules.** The **capillaries,** which unite the arteries and veins, have their walls formed of a single endothelial layer of large angular flattened cells.

The direct union between two vessels is called an anastomosis. **Arteriovenous anastomoses** occur around the nail beds and are an important mechanism in controlling digital blood flow.

They may also exist as congenital abnormalities of the vascular system and can be created surgically when a large vein with an arterialized circulation is required for regular access to the circulation.

Sinusoids are thin-walled, dilated channels uniting arteries and veins and are found in the bone marrow, liver, spleen and suprarenal glands.

In some situations blood passes through two capillary beds before returning to the heart: this constitutes a **portal circulation.** The passage of blood from the stomach, intestine, pancreas and spleen through the liver exemplifies such a system. Short vessels passing through foramina in the skull and joining venous channels (**sinuses**) inside and veins outside are called **emissary** veins.

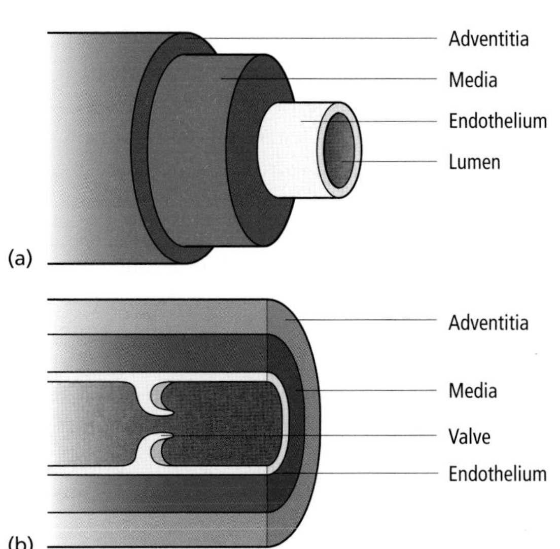

Figure 0.28 Structure of: (a) artery; (b) vein

Introduction

Reduction of the blood supply to a region is known as ischaemia, and this is of clinical importance in the heart and brain. One important degenerative arterial disease that can affect the vessels is arteriosclerosis, and this is very prevalent in developed countries. The arterial narrowing produced by the disease may cause local intravascular clotting (thrombosis) to occur. A **thrombus** may become detached and flushed into the bloodstream forming an **embolus** and block distal smaller vessels. Local death of an area of tissue or organ owing to reduction of its blood supply is known as an infarction. In situations where bacteria infect the infarcted area it undergoes putrefaction, a condition known as **gangrene.** In some instances it is possible surgically to bypass arterial blockages, thus re-establishing the distal blood supply and preventing infarction and gangrene.

The body responds to an injury, e.g. invading bacteria, by the process known as **inflammation.** The capillaries dilate and white blood cells pass out of the circulation to phagocytose the offending organisms. The area becomes red and hot because of the increased blood supply, and swollen with increased tissue fluid; it is also painful. A collection of dead tissue and dead white blood cells is called an **abscess.**

THE LYMPHATIC SYSTEM

Lymph consists of cells, mainly lymphocytes, and plasma.

The lymphatic system collects tissue fluid and conveys it to the bloodstream. It comprises the **lymph capillaries** and **vessels,** the lymph nodes, and aggregations of lymph tissue in the spleen, thymus and around the alimentary tract. The system forms an extensive network over the body, although its fine vessels are not easily identified (Fig. 0.29a,b).

The lymph capillaries are larger than those of the blood; they are composed of a single layer of **endothelial** cells. The lymph vessels resemble veins and possess many paired valves. The larger collecting vessels open into the venous system near the formation of the brachiocephalic veins.

A **lymph node** (Fig. 0.29c) is an aggregation of lymph tissue along the course of a lymph vessel. It is bean-shaped, with a number of afferent vessels (conveying lymph to the node) entering its convex surface and an efferent vessel (carrying lymph away from the node) leaving its hilus (opening). It is surrounded by a fibrous capsule from which fibrous trabeculae pass inwards. It is filled with a reticular network of fine collagen fibres, and the cells are either primitive (lymphocyte precursors) or fixed macrophages. Numerous lymphocytes and a few monocytes lie freely within the meshwork, but they are absent peripherally, leaving a subcapsular lymph space. The cells of the outer part of the node (cortex) are densely packed and known as germinal centres. The centre of the follicle and the hilar (medullary) regions of the node contain loosely packed lymphocytes.

Lymph aggregations elsewhere in the body consist of a mixture of follicles and loosely packed lymphocytes.

Bacterial infections produce inflammatory responses in the regional lymph nodes. In many malignant diseases neoplastic

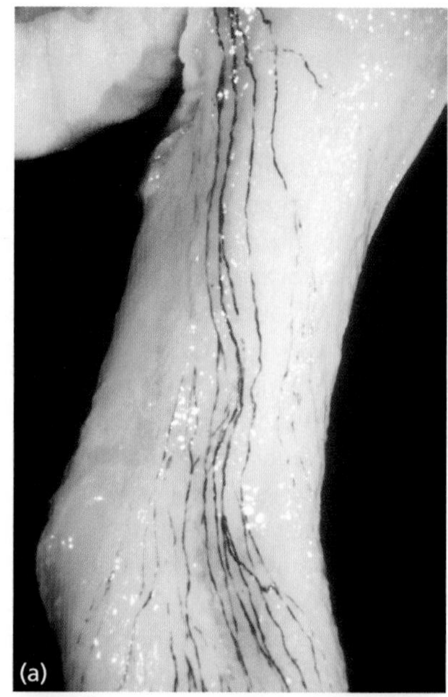

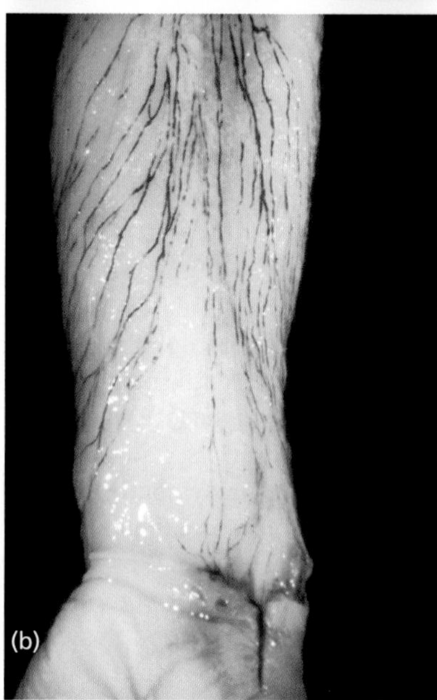

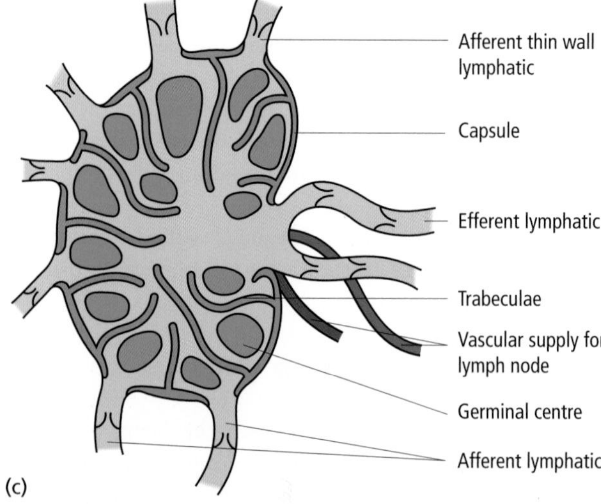

Figure 0.29 (a) and (b) Injection with Indian ink into palmar skin to show lymphatics of arm. (c) Lymph node structure

cells spread via the lymph vessels to the regional lymph nodes, and there develop to such an extent as to completely replace the normal tissue of the lymph node and occlude lymph flow. The stagnation of lymph within the tissues due to obstruction of flow produces a swelling of the tissues known as lymphoedema (Fig. 1.20b, p. 31). Lymphoedema may also occur in subjects who are born with a defective lymphatic system, this being termed primary lymphoedema; acquired obstruction is called secondary lymphoedema. The term lymphadenopathy is used to describe a generalized enlargement of the lymph nodes, although they are not glands in the strict definition of the term.

ORIENTATION

The **anatomical position** is that to which all anatomical descriptions refer. It is one in which the person stands upright with feet together, eyes looking forward and arms straight down the side of the body, with the palms facing forward (Fig. 0.30).

Structures in front are termed **anterior** (ventral) and those behind, **posterior** (dorsal). In the hands and feet the surfaces are referred to as **palmar** and dorsal, and **plantar** and dorsal, respectively. Structures above are **superior** (cranial, rostral) and those below, **inferior** (caudal). Structures may be nearer to (**medial**) or further from (**lateral**) the midline, and those in the midline are called **median. Paramedian** means alongside and parallel to the midline. **Superficial** and **deep** denote the position of structures in relation to the surface of the body. A **sagittal** plane passes vertically anteroposteriorly through the body and a **coronal** plane passes vertically at right-angles to a sagittal plane. **Transverse** (horizontal) planes pass horizontally through the body.

Proximal and **distal** are terms used to indicate the relation of a structure to the centre of the body. The ankle is distal to the knee joint; the shoulder is proximal to the elbow joint. Blood flows distally (peripherally) in the arteries and proximally (centrally) in the veins.

Movements

Forward movement in a sagittal plane is usually known as **flexion** (Fig. 0.31) and backward movement, **extension** (Fig. 0.32). Owing to rotation of the lower limb during development, backward movement of the leg extends the hip and flexes the knee; downward movement of the toes is flexion. Upward movement at the ankle joint is dorsiflexion (extension) and downward movement is plantar flexion (flexion) (Fig. 0.33a,b). Movement away from the midline in the coronal plane is **abduction** and movement towards the midline is **adduction** (Fig. 0.34). Abduction and adduction of the fingers and toes is taken in relation to the middle finger and second toe. During development of the thumb its axis is rotated in relation to the fingers, therefore movement is described in relation to the plane of the thumbnail. Side to side movement of the neck and trunk is termed **lateral flexion. Circumduction** (Fig. 0.34) is the movement when the distal

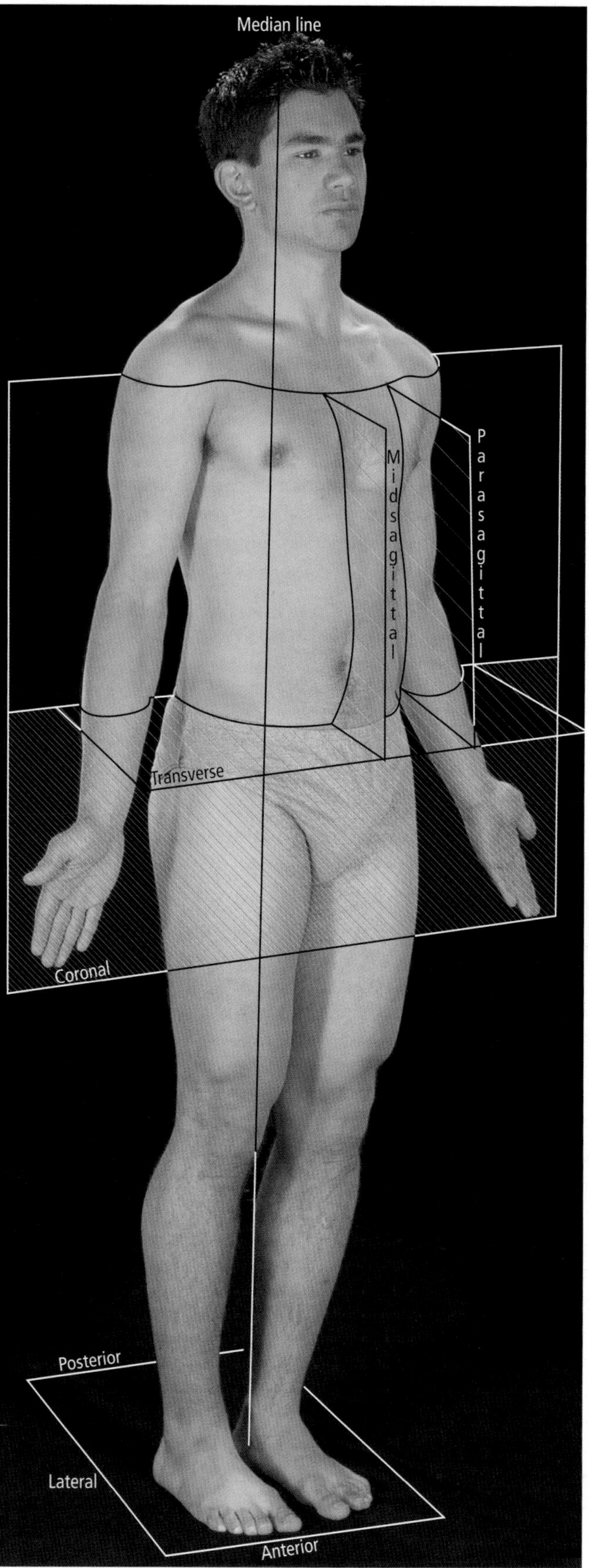

Figure 0.30 Anatomical position

end of a bone describes the base of a cone whose apex is at the proximal end. **Rotation** occurs in the long axis of a bone; in the limbs it may be **medial,** towards the midline, or **lateral,** away from it (Fig. 0.35a,b). Medial and lateral rotation of the forearm occurs through the axis drawn through the heads of the radius and ulna, and is termed **pronation** and **supination,** respectively (Fig. 0.36a,b). Rotation of the thumb and little finger so that their pulps meet is termed **opposition** of the two digits, the movement being particularly marked in the thumb. **Rotation** of the forefoot is termed **inversion** when the sole faces the midline and **eversion** when it is turned away from the midline (Fig. 0.37a,b).

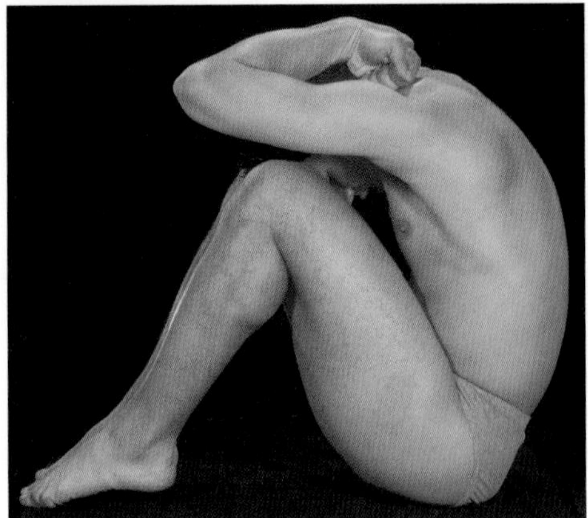

Figure 0.31 Flexion

IMAGING – THE ESSENTIALS

Since the discovery of X-rays over 100 years ago, the study of the normal and diseased human body has become one of the most rapidly expanding fields in medicine. In the 21st century, we now have ultrasound (US), computed tomography (CT), contrast studies, radionuclide scans and, during the last thirty years, huge advances in magnetic resonance imaging and angiography (MRI and MRA respectively) and, more recently, electron beam computed tomography (EBCT).

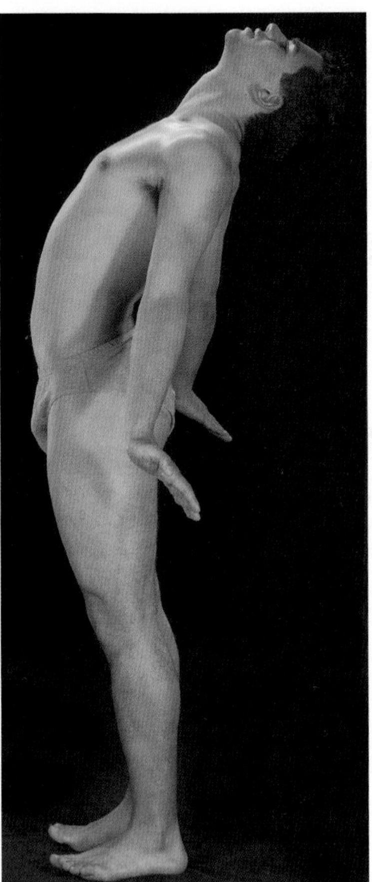

Figure 0.32 Extension

X-rays (Fig. 0.38)

X-rays pass easily through air or fatty tissues (radio-transparent) but substances such as bone, calcium stones or heavy metals absorb most of the X-rays (radio-opaque). X-rays that do not pass through to the X-ray plate release their energy inside the body, damaging the molecules they collide with. This is the mechanism by which X-rays are harmful – the effect is seen particularly on rapidly dividing cells especially those of the fetus and gonadal cells). Caution is therefore taken to shield the fetus when X-raying pregnant women and the gonads of those of reproductive age.

The direction that the beam passes through the subject determines the name of the view, i.e. a postero-anterior chest X-ray is taken with the subject's back towards the beam and the chest on the 'cold' X-ray plate. This view is ideal for judging heart size and lungs, whereas the antero-posterior chest X-ray is much better for viewing the vertebral bodies.

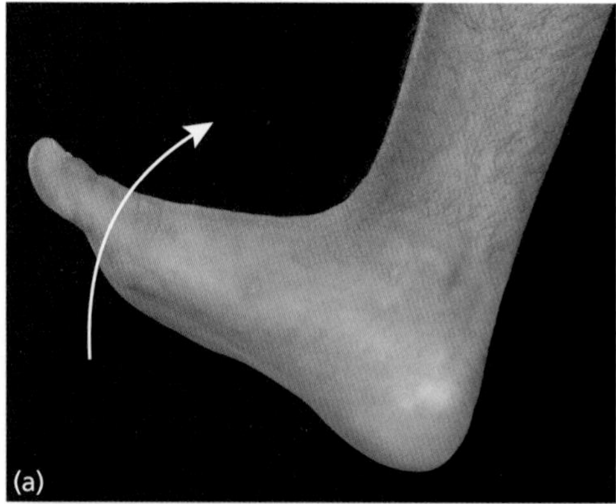

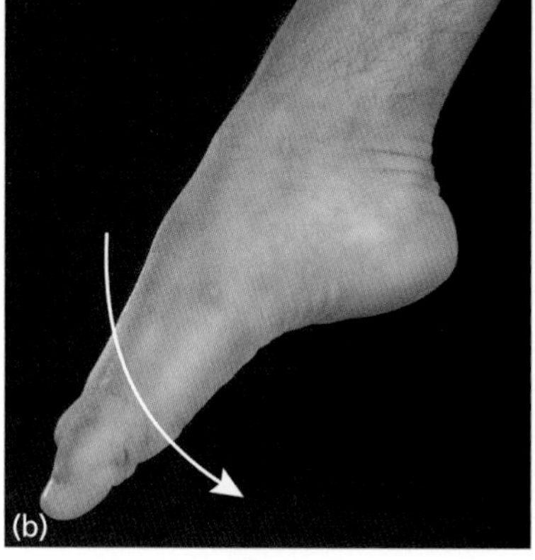

Figure 0.33 (a) Dorsiflexion (true extension). (b) Plantar flexion (true flexion)

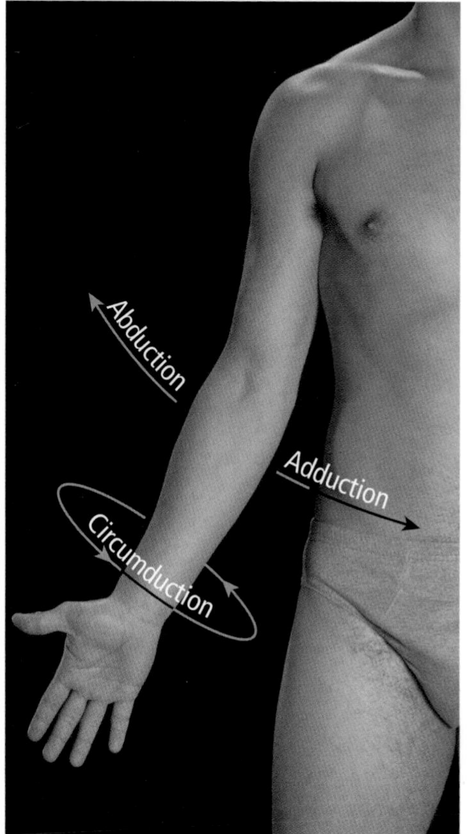

Figure 0.34 Abduction, adduction and circumduction

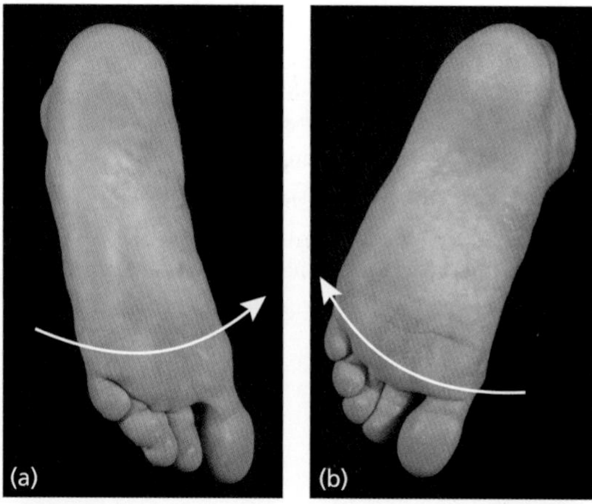

Figure 0.35 Rotation: (a) medial; (b) lateral

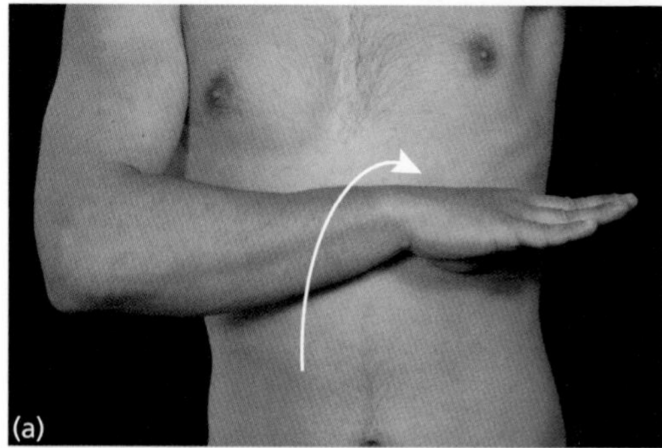

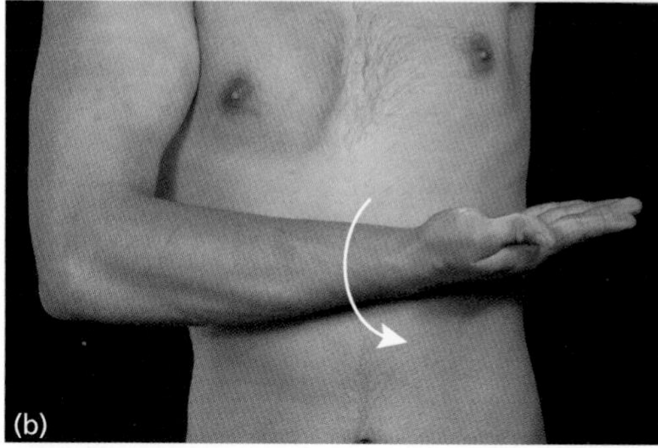

Figure 0.36 (a) Pronation. (b) Supination

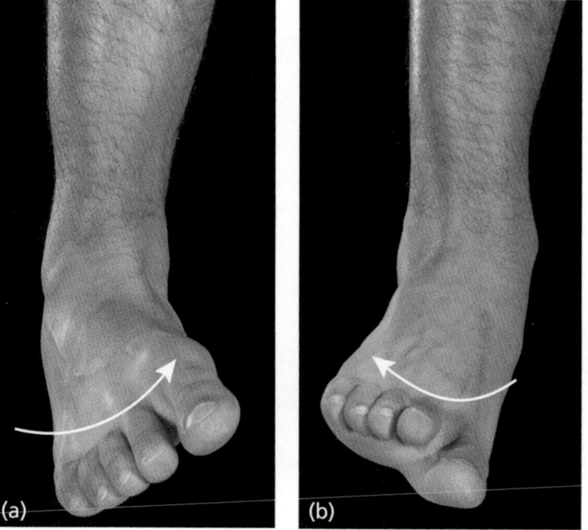

Figure 0.37 (a) Inversion. (b) Eversion

Contrast media

Body cavities, the lumen of vessels (e.g. arteries, veins), ureters or hollow viscera (e.g. bowel) can be outlined by the use of suspensions of heavy metals or halogens. These contrast media can be introduced in a variety of ways: by direct introduction (barium enema); by injection (arteriograms, venograms); or by injection into the bloodstream and then concentration by specific organs (e.g. intravenous urogram for outlining the kidneys and urinary tract, Fig. 039). Nowadays, the use of digital, computerized images allows the 'removal' of the images of soft tissues in the background and easier visualization of the system under investigation (digital subtraction angiography – DSA). More recently, the advent of non-invasive angiography, such as magnetic resonance angiography (MRA), will help to reduce the use of many invasive procedures.

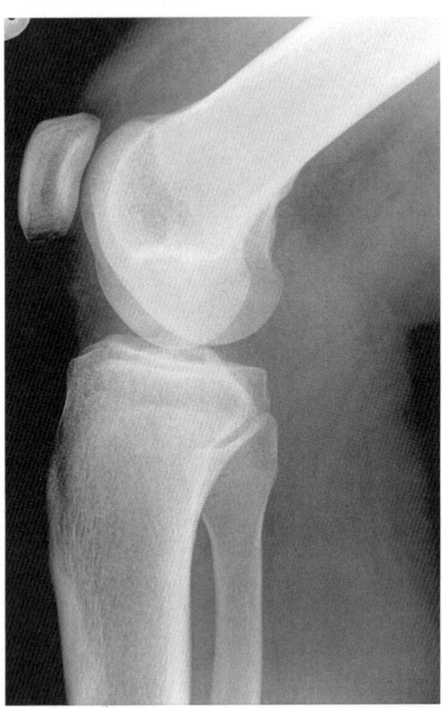

Figure 0.38 Lateral projection of plain X-ray of adult knee

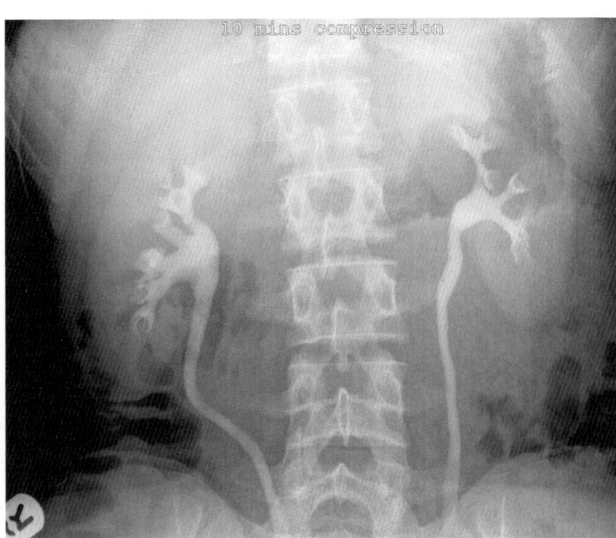

Figure 0.39 10-minute intravenous urogram (IVU) with abdominal compression

Nuclear medicine (Fig. 0.40)

Nuclear medicine uses radioactive isotopes, mainly for diagnosis but occasionally for therapeutic uses such as in hyperthyroid disease. In the diagnostic field, myocardial perfusion imaging, lung scans to detect pulmonary embolism and bone scans to find widespread metastases are now routine procedures.

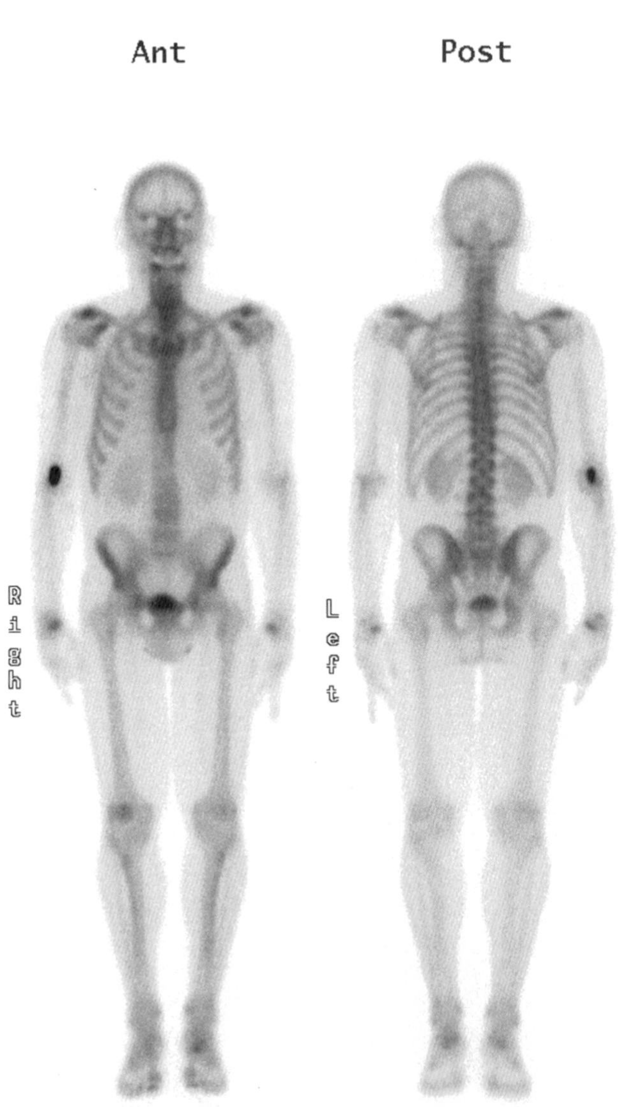

Figure 0.40 Whole body bone scan

Ultrasound (Fig. 0.41)

Much more easily performed, however, are ultrasound techniques that use high-frequency sound waves and their interaction with biological tissues to produce 'echograms'. Modern ultrasound hardware now allows real-time tomographic images, and the addition of the Doppler principle has led to duplex scanning which measures movement and blood flow in real-time and has the added attraction of providing easily interpreted colour images. Another really important advantage of ultrasound is that the technique is multi-planar and can be used at the bedside. These advantages now mean that many interventional procedures (e.g. biopsy and drainage of cysts or abscesses) can be done under ultrasound guidance. Usage of a variety of different transducers has improved the range of ultrasound imaging, but this technique is still totally operator-dependent and as it is a real-time interactive process, it is not best seen with hard-copy images. This explains why so few ultrasound images are included in this book.

Computed tomography (Fig. 0.42)

Computed tomography (CT) obtains a series of different angular X-ray projections that are processed by a computer to give X-ray views of a section or slice of specified thickness. The CT machine consists of a rigid metal frame with an X-ray tube sited opposite a set of detectors. All of the views per slice are collected simultaneously so that the tube and detectors rotate around the patient. One slice takes 15–30 seconds.

No specific preparation is required for examinations of the brain, spine, musculoskeletal system and chest. Studies of the abdomen and pelvis often require opacification of the gastrointestinal tract using a solution of dilute contrast medium (either a water-soluble or a barium compound). CT is especially useful in the analysis of bony structures and the most modern 64-slice units provide fantastically detailed 3D reconstructions that are prized by surgeons for their accurate pre-operative assessment.

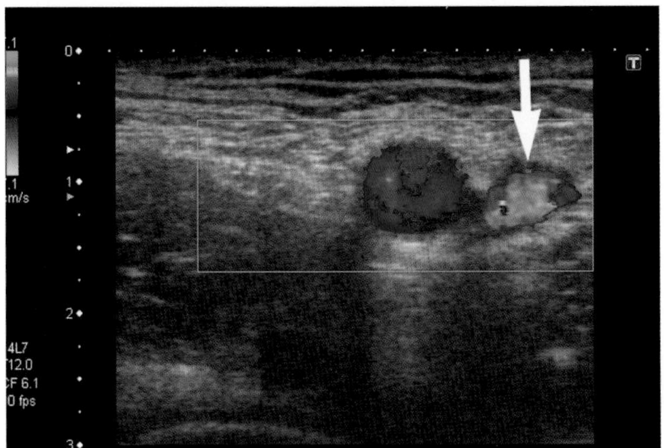

Figure 0.41 Colour Doppler ultrasound of the femoral vessels – the arrow points to the femoral artery which is red due to the direction of flow

Magnetic resonance imaging (Fig. 0.43)

Magnetic resonance imaging (MRI) combines a strong magnetic field and radio-frequency energy to study the distribution and behaviour of hydrogen protons in fat and water. MRI systems are graded according to the strength of the magnetic field they produce. High-field systems are those capable of producing a magnetic field strength of 1–2 Tesla. MRI does not cause any recognized biologic hazard, but patients who have any form of pacemaker or implanted electroinductive device must not be examined using MRI because of risks to its function. Other prohibited items include ferromagnetic intracranial aneurysm clips, certain types of cardiac valve replacement, and intraocular metallic foreign bodies. Generally, it is safe to examine patients who have extracranial vascular clips and orthopaedic prostheses, but these may cause local artefacts. Loose metal items must be excluded from the examination room and beware of your credit cards being wiped clean!

The real advantage of magnetic resonance imaging is that it provides vastly superior visualization of the soft tissues than CT. It also provides especially detailed imaging of soft tissues such as muscles, brain, fascial planes and intervertebral discs. An intravenous injection of contrast medium (a gadolinium complex) may be given to enhance tumours, inflammatory

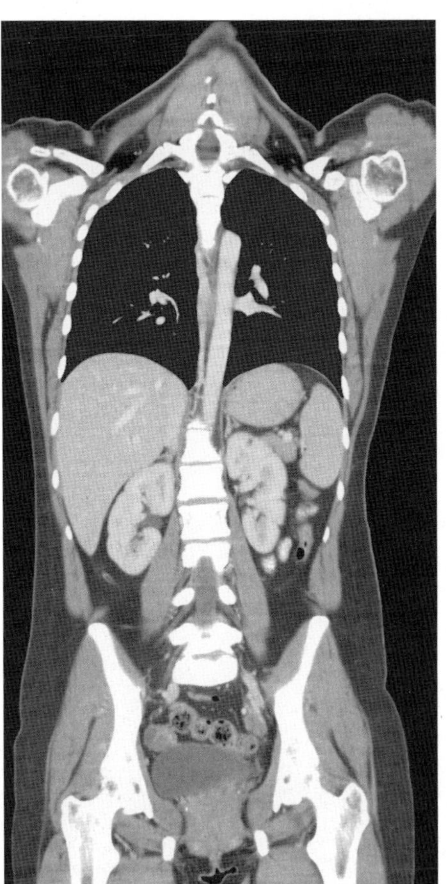

Figure 0.42 Coronal computed tomography scan of female thorax, abdomen and pelvis

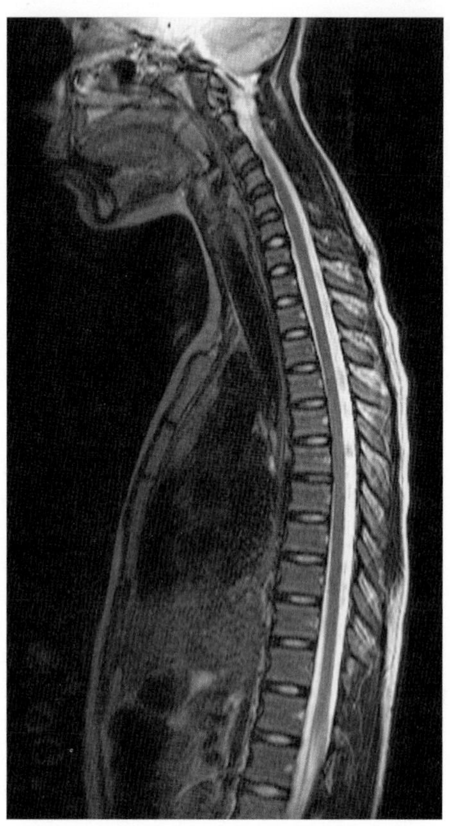

Figure 0.43 Sagittal magnetic resonance image of spine

and vascular abnormalities. The next decade will see the increased use of MR angiography (MRA), where the flow of blood in vessels is picked up without the use of contrast medium or any interventional procedure.

New techniques and future developments

Invasive techniques such as injections of contrast are unpopular with patients so it is only natural that non-invasive procedures quickly gain approval. However, it is not only this aspect that has pushed back the boundaries – it is also the ability to see images in three dimensions and perform reconstructions of the body in real-time that have brought us new imaging modalities. Modern machines are increasingly fast with their investigations: an electron-beam CT with high-speed sequencing of the cardiac cycle enables 3D chest reconstructions to be performed in a few minutes. A 64-slice CT has the ability to perform a whole torso scan in less than 15 seconds. This is particularly useful in trauma cases where there may be damage of more than one system. Resolution has now also improved as the computer-generated slices get thinner – down to 0.35 mm resolution; and with greater computer power, the ability to reconstruct images in three dimensions is ever advancing.

EMQs

Each question has an anatomical theme linked to the chapter, and a list of 10 related items (A–J) placed in alphabetical order: these are followed by five statements (1–5). Match **one or more** of the items A–J to each of the five statements.

Structure of the body

A. Ciliated columnar epithelium
B. Collagen fibre
C. Columnar epithelium
D. Elastic fibre
E. Endothelium
F. Osteoblast
G. Schwann cell
H. Squamous epithelium
I. Stratified squamous epithelium
J. Transitional epithelium

Match the following statements with the appropriate item(s) from the above list.

1. Lines the trachea
2. Lines the aortic arch
3. Surrounds peripheral nerves
4. Stretches without desquamation
5. A component of hyaline cartilage

Answers

1 A; 2 E; 3 G; 4 J; 5 B

Joints

A. Ball and socket
B. Bony
C. Condyloid
D. Ellipsoid
E. Fibrous
F. Hinge
G. Primary cartilaginous
H. Saddle
I. Secondary cartilaginous
J. Synovial

Match the following joints to the appropriate item(s) in the above list.

1. Inferior tibiofibular
2. Carpometacarpal of thumb
3. Sutures of the skull
4. Intervertebral disc
5. Manubriosternal

Answers

1 E; 2 HJ; 3 E; 4 I; 5 I

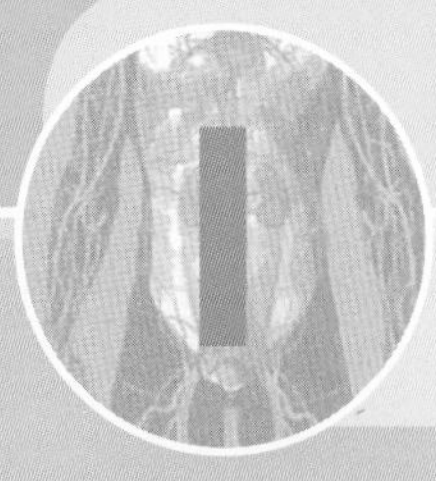

The thorax

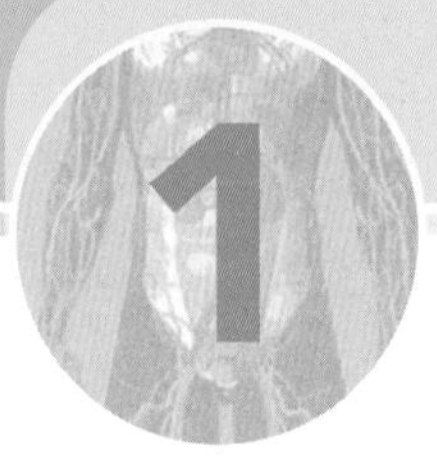

1 The thoracic wall and diaphragm

INTRODUCTION

The bony–cartilaginous skeleton of the thorax protects the heart, lungs and great vessels. It is conical, with a narrow inlet superiorly and a wide outlet inferiorly, and is formed of 12 thoracic vertebrae posteriorly, the sternum anteriorly, and 12 pairs of ribs with costal cartilages medially. The **thoracic inlet**, 10 cm wide and 5 cm anteroposteriorly, slopes downward and forwards and is bounded by the 1st thoracic vertebra posteriorly, the upper border of the manubrium anteriorly, and the first rib and costal cartilage anteriorly. It transmits the oesophagus, the trachea and the great vessels of the head and neck, and on each side lies the dome of the pleura. The **thoracic outlet** too is widest from side to side, and is bounded by the 12th thoracic vertebra posteriorly, the 11th and 12th ribs posteriorly, and the costal cartilages of the 7th, 8th, 9th and 10th ribs, which ascend to meet the sternum anteriorly (Fig. 1.1). The diaphragm separates the thorax from the abdomen.

The **sternum** is a flat bone, palpable throughout its length, with three parts, the manubrium, the body and the xiphoid process (Fig. 1.1). The **manubrium** is the thickest part, bearing

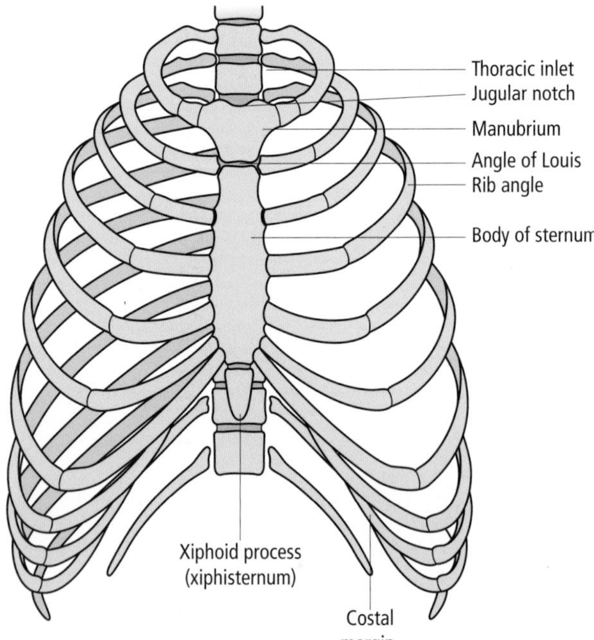

Figure 1.1 Thoracic cage

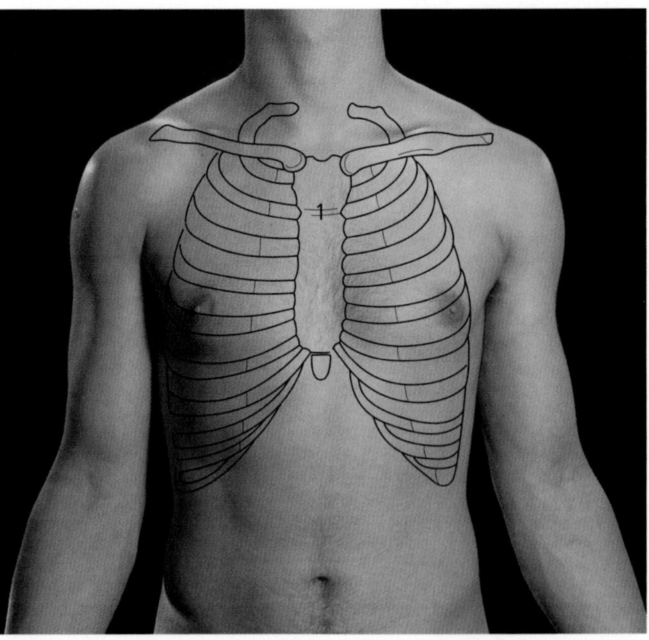

Figure 1.2 Anterior chest wall showing sternal angle (1)

on its upper border the **jugular notch** between the two lateral facets for articulation with the clavicles. Its inferior border articulates with the body at the palpable **sternal angle** (the **angle of Louis**; Fig. 1.2).

This readily palpable protuberance is an important landmark: here the 2nd costal cartilage articulates on the same plane as the 4th thoracic vertebra, the bifurcation of the trachea, and the beginning and end of the aortic arch.

The **body** of the sternum is some 10 cm long and articulates on its lateral borders with the 2nd to the 7th costal cartilages. Behind the body lie the heart valves, in the order from above downwards PAMT (pulmonary, aortic, mitral and tricuspid: see Fig. 2.1b, p. 35). The narrow lower end articulates with the **xiphoid cartilage**, which is cartilaginous in early life and gives attachment to the diaphragm and rectus abdominis.

In later life the xiphoid calcifies and can be mistaken for a gastric tumour by the inexperienced clinician. Sternal fractures have become more common because of the frequency of car accidents in which the driver's chest forcibly hits the steering column – less common with seatbelts. Pericardial, cardiac or aortic damage may then follow. A flail chest may also result from multiple rib fractures, when a whole section of the chest wall moves paradoxically during respiration (Fig. 1.3). Air bags and safety belts reduce the incidence of this injury. Although the procedure is less popular nowadays the sternum is still a useful site for bone marrow aspiration in adults if the iliac crest is unsuccessful.

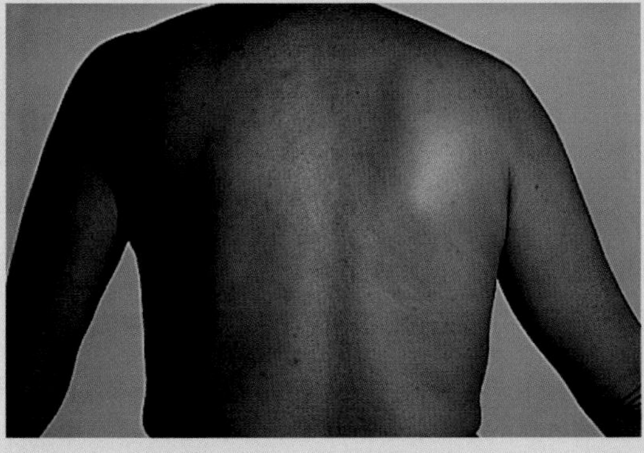

(a) Expiration

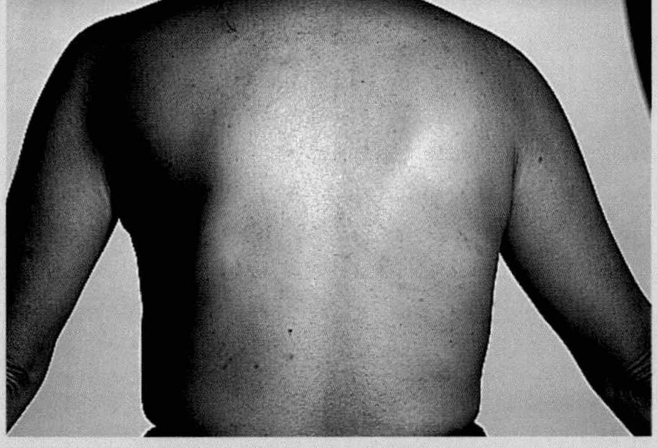

(b) Inspiration

Figure 1.3 (a) and (b) Multiple rib fractures, flail chest: note drawing in of left side of chest during inspiration

The **ribs**, usually 12 on each side, all articulate posteriorly with the thoracic vertebrae; the upper 7, known as true ribs, articulate through their costal cartilages with the sternum; the 8th to 10th ribs, 'false ribs', articulate through their cartilages with the cartilage above; and the 11th and 12th, the 'floating ribs', have free anterior ends (Fig. 1.1).

The costochondral and costosternal joints are tiny synovial joints reinforced with fibrous bands. Painful inflammation of these joints, sometimes known as Tietze's syndrome, can easily be misdiagnosed as cardiac disease. A special form of costochondritis known as the 'clicking-rib' syndrome is due to subluxation of a rib casing irritating the underlying intercostal nerve, and the pain it produces is easily confused with abdominal pathology.

A **typical rib** has a head, neck, tubercle and body (Fig. 1.4). The **head** articulates with adjacent vertebrae and is attached to the intervertebral disc. The **neck** gives attachment to the costotransverse ligaments, and the **tubercle** articulates with the transverse process. The flattened curved **body** has a rounded upper border and a sharper lower border, on the inside of which is the costal groove within which lie the intercostal nerve and vessels.

The 1st, 10th, 11th and 12th ribs are not typical. All articulate with only one vertebra. The **1st rib** is short, wide, and has superior and inferior surfaces (Fig. 1.5). The lower

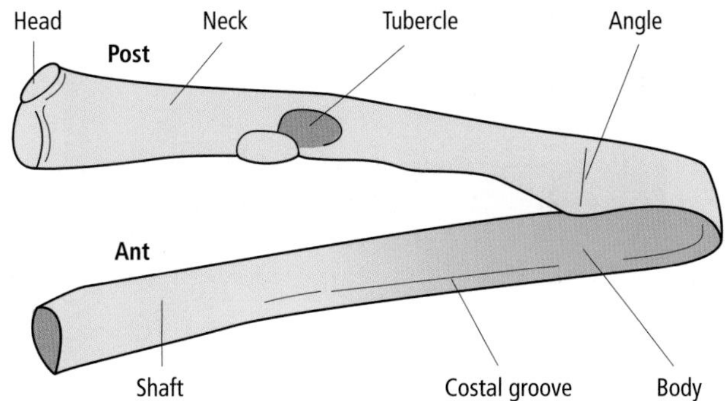

Figure 1.4 Typical right rib viewed from behind

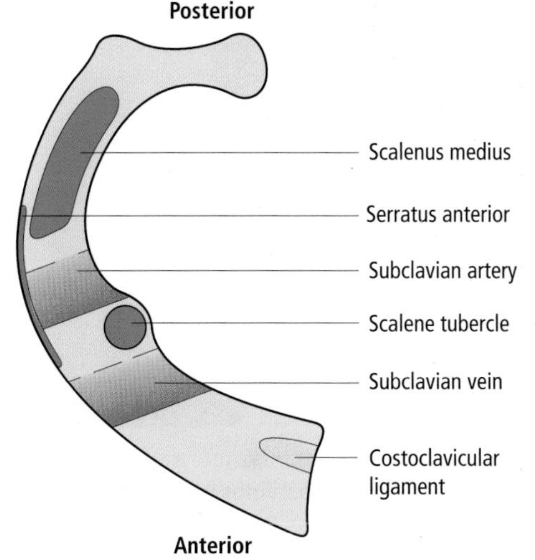

Figure 1.5 First rib – superior view

smooth surface lies on the pleura; the upper surface has two grooves separated by the **scalene tubercle,** to which scalenus anterior is attached; the anterior groove is for the subclavian vein and the posterior for the subclavian artery and the lower trunk of the brachial plexus. The **11th and 12th ribs** are short and have neither necks nor tubercles. Their costal cartilages lie free within the abdominal wall musculature.

The weakest part of the rib is the body anterior to the angle, and it is here that most fractures occur after blunt trauma. Direct trauma may produce fracture in any part of the rib. In both cases the fracture fragments may damage adjacent structures, such as intercostal vessels, pleura, lung or spleen. A pneumothorax, air in the pleural cavity, is a common complication of serious rib fractures rupturing the underlying lung (Fig. 1.6). In certain circumstances, the valvular nature of the tear in the lung tissue causes air to accumulate in the pleural cavity with each inspiration, and this accumulation will cause the mediastinum to shift across to the opposite side (tension pneumothorax; Fig. 1.6b).

(a)

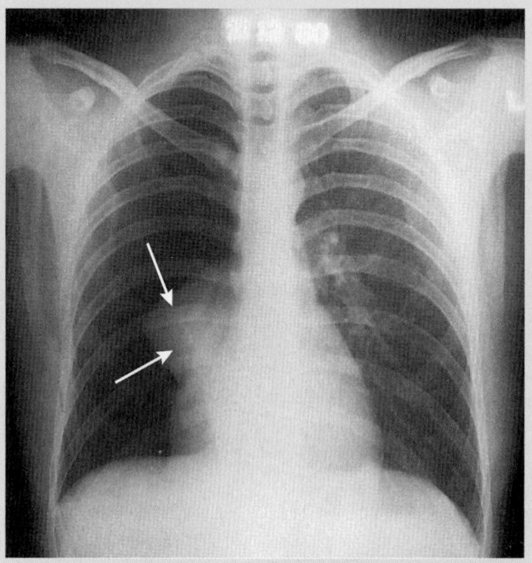

(b)

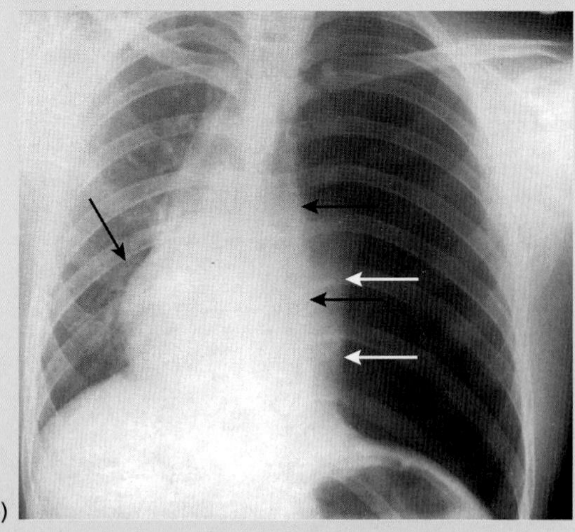

Figure 1.6 (a) Right pneumothorax: note dark shadow cast by air and the absence of lung markings in the right chest. The right lung is collapsed (arrows). (b) Left tension pneumothorax with mediastinal shift. Heart displaced to right (arrowed). White arrows show collapsed lung and black the left border of the heart

THE THORACIC CAGE

Note that:

- The cavity is kidney-shaped in cross-section because the vertebral column intrudes into the cage posteriorly.
- The ribs increase in length from the 1st to the 7th, and thereafter become shorter.
  - The ribs lie at an angle of about 45° to the vertebral column, the maximum obliquity being reached by the 9th rib.
  - The costal cartilages increase in length from above downwards – from ribs 1–10.
- The cage gives attachment to the muscles of the upper limb, the abdominal wall muscles, the extensor muscles of the back, the diaphragm and the intercostal muscles.

The **intercostal spaces**, bounded by ribs and costal cartilages, contain the intercostal vessels and nerves. The pleura is deep to them. The spaces contain three layers of muscles from without inwards: the external, the internal and the innermost intercostal muscles. They are supplied by their adjacent intercostal nerve and move the ribs (Fig. 1.7). When the 1st rib is anchored by contraction of the scalene muscles, approximation of the ribs by the intercostal muscles **raises** the sternum and air is drawn into the lungs. When the lower ribs are anchored by the abdominal muscles, approximation of the ribs **lowers** the sternum and air is forced out of the lungs.

Intercostal vessels and nerves

The **intercostal vessels and nerves** form a neurovascular bundle that passes forward in the subcostal groove deep to the internal intercostal muscle, separated from the pleura only by the innermost intercostal muscle.

Each intercostal space is supplied by posterior and anterior **intercostal arteries** which anastomose in the space. The first and second posterior arteries arise from branches of the subclavian artery, and all the remainder arise directly from the descending aorta; the anterior arteries are branches of the internal thoracic artery, a branch of the subclavian. The **intercostal veins**, lying above their arteries in the costal groove, drain to the internal thoracic and azygos veins.

The **intercostal nerves** are formed from the ventral rami of the upper 11 thoracic spinal nerves. Each is attached to the spinal cord by ventral and dorsal roots. The dorsal root bears a sensory ganglion in the intervertebral foramen. Once the roots have united the nerve divides into dorsal and ventral rami (Fig. 1.8). Each dorsal ramus supplies the extensor muscles of the back and, by cutaneous branches, the skin of the back. The ventral ramus forms the intercostal nerve, and this runs forward in the costal groove below the artery to supply the intercostal muscles and the skin of the lateral and anterior chest wall.

Insertion of a needle to obtain fluid or blood from the pleural cavity will be undertaken safely if the needle is introduced into the lower part of the intercostal space away from the intercostal neurovascular bundle lying in the subcostal groove (Figs 1.7a and 1.9).

The thorax

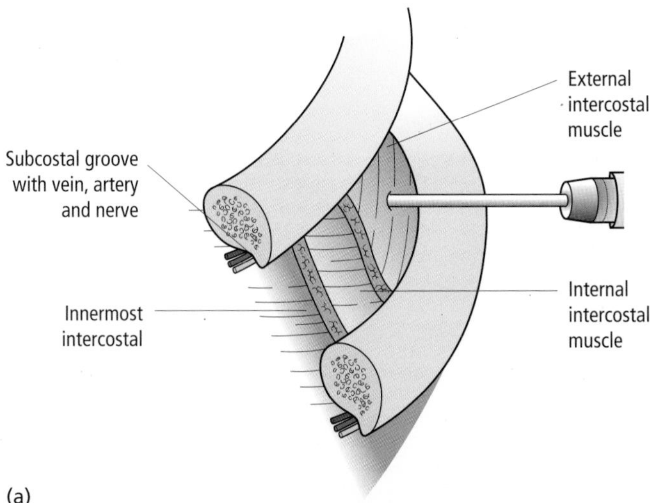

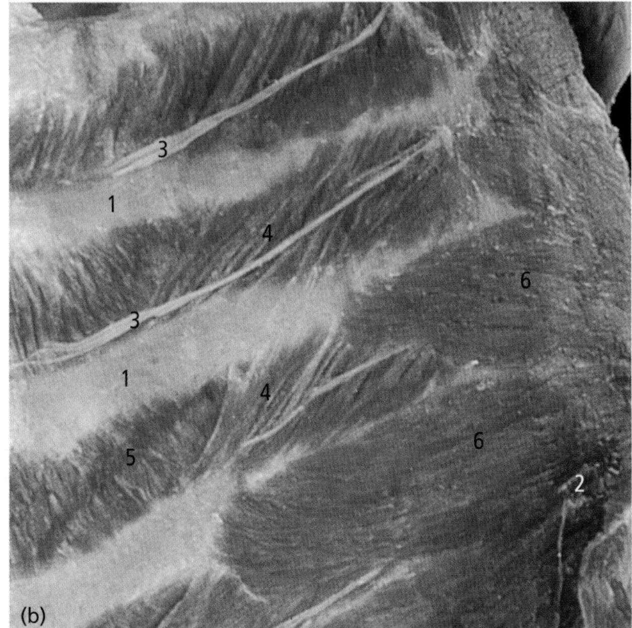

Figure 1.7 (a) Intercostal space showing the aspirating needle passed just above the rib, thus avoiding the vessels in the subcostal groove above. (b) Left thoracic wall showing details of intercostal muscles: 1, rib; 2, intercostal nerves; 3, lateral cutaneous branch of intercostal nerve; 4, external intercostals muscle; 5, internal intercostals muscle; 6, serratus anterior muscle

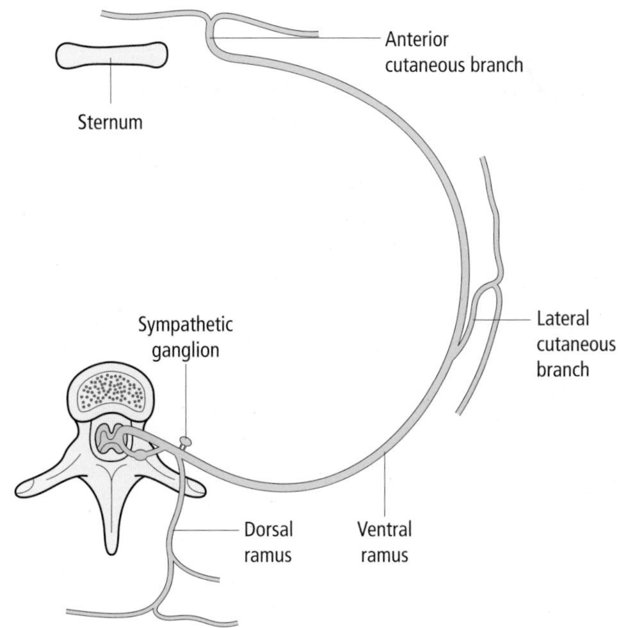

Figure 1.8 Typical spinal nerve

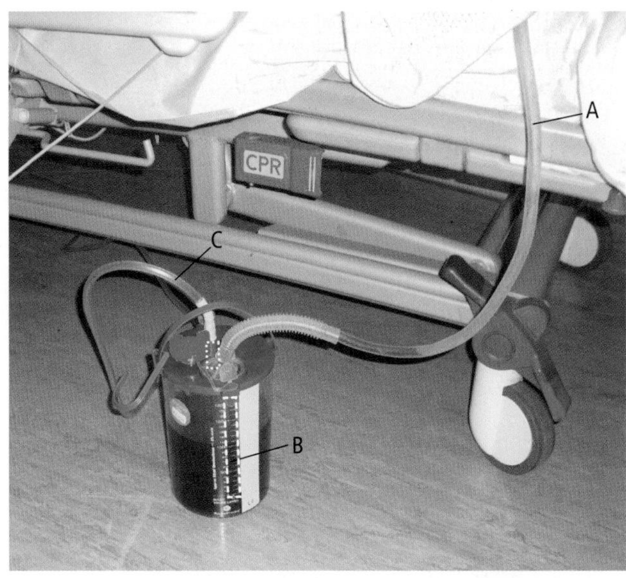

Figure 1.9 Underwater seal drain: A, tube passing to drain in the anterior mediastinum of patient; B, tube passing below the waterline of the container (white dashed line); C, exit tube above water line at atmospheric pressure (white dotted line). NB: the container must never be raised above the level of the patient, as fluid may otherwise siphon in the opposite direction

DERMATOMES

Through the cutaneous branches of the ventral and dorsal rami each spinal nerve supplies a **dermatome** – a strip of skin between the posterior and anterior midlines. These are arranged in segmental fashion because of their origin from segments of the spinal cord. There is overlapping of adjacent dermatomes.

Clinicians need a working knowledge of the dermatomal innervation of the skin in order to establish the normality or otherwise of the function of a particular segment of the spinal cord (Figs 1.10 and 1.11; see also Figs 12.17b, 17.12 and 17.13, pp. 176 and 270). Herpes zoster (shingles) is a viral infection of the dorsal root ganglia. Infection produces a sharp burning pain in the dermatome supplied by the infected segment. Several days later the affected dermatome becomes reddened and vesicular eruptions appear (Fig. 1.12).

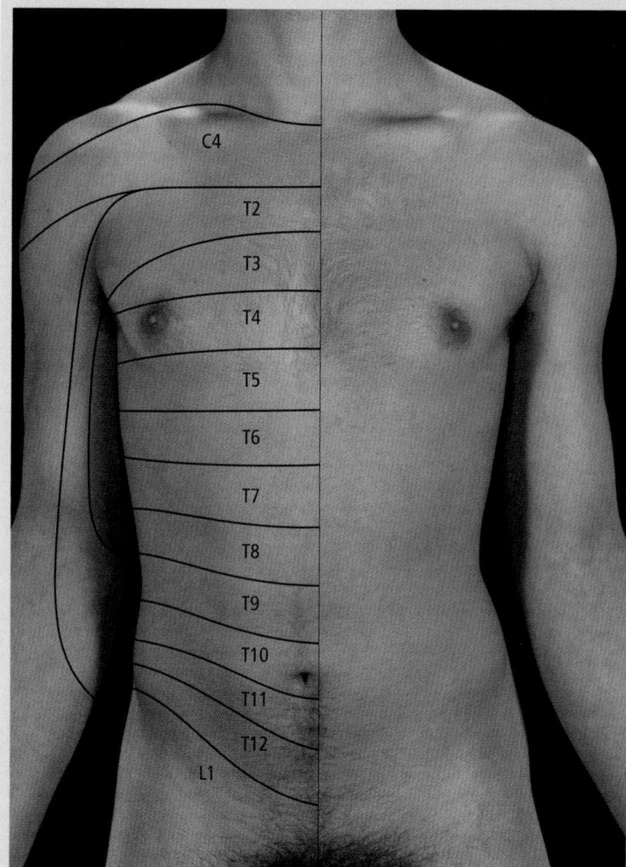

Figure 1.10 Cutaneous innervation of anterior trunk showing dermatomes: note the umbilicus is innervated by T10 and the groin by L1

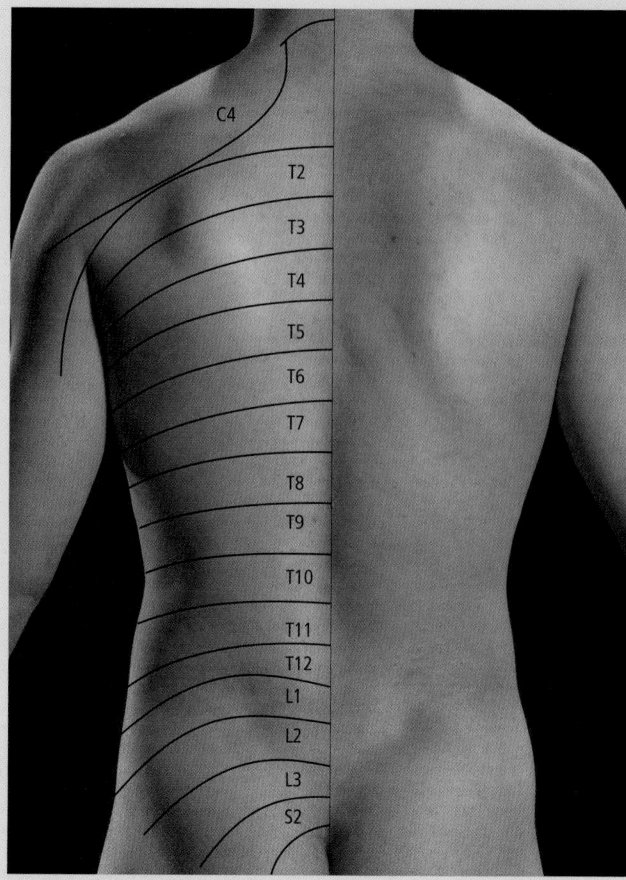

Figure 1.11 Cutaneous innervation of posterior trunk showing dermatomes

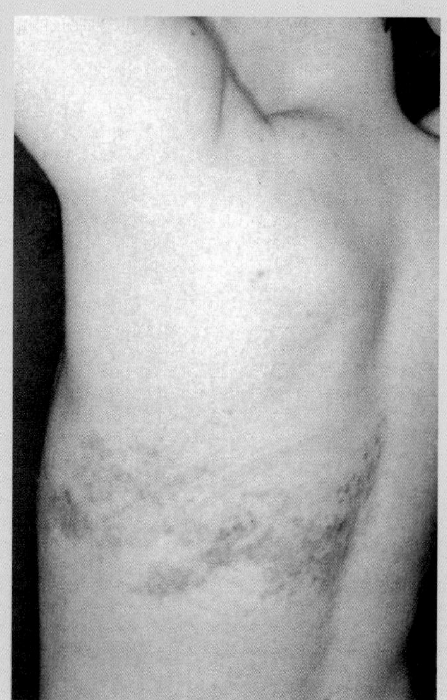

Figure 1.12 Lower thoracic Herpes zoster (shingles)

THE MEDIASTINUM

For the purposes of description, the mediastinum is divided into:

- The superior mediastinum extending from the thoracic inlet (Fig. 1.13) to the transverse plane, T4
- The posterior mediastinum below the plane and behind the heart
  - The anterior mediastinum below the plane and anterior to the heart
  - The middle mediastinum containing the pericardium, heart and main bronchi.

THE DIAPHRAGM

This musculotendinous septum separates the thoracic and abdominal cavities; it has a central tendinous part and a peripheral muscular part. It has peripheral attachments around the outlet of the thoracic cavity:

- **Sternal** – from the back of the xiphoid process
- **Costal** – from the inner surfaces of the lower six costal cartilages
- **Vertebral** – from the sides of the upper lumbar vertebrae by two crura and from medial and lateral arcuate ligaments.

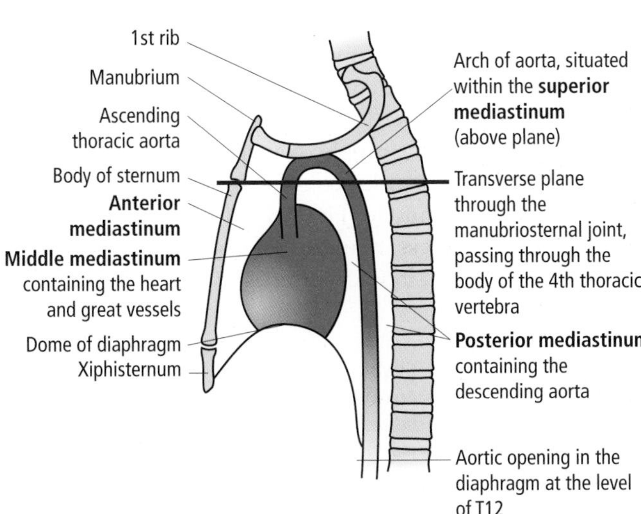

Figure 1.13 Thorax: sagittal section showing divisions of the mediastinum

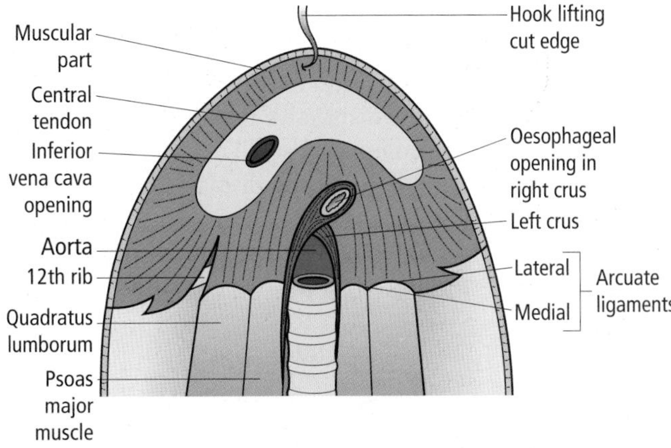

Figure 1.14 Inferior surface of the diaphragm. The anterior chest wall has been removed and the diaphragm lifted upwards to show its under surface whilst retaining its posterior attachments

The **right crus** arises from the bodies of the upper three vertebrae and the **left crus** from the first two. The **medial arcuate ligament**, the thickened upper edge of the psoas fascia, passes between the body of the 1st lumbar vertebra and its transverse process, the **lateral arcuate ligament**, is anterior to quadratus lumborum and extends between the 12th rib's transverse process and the tip of the 12th rib. Its central attachment is to the periphery of a trefoil central tendon. The diaphragm is the principal muscle of respiration. Contraction flattens the dome of the diaphragm and makes it descend, thereby increasing the vertical diameter of the chest; air is then drawn into the lungs. In expiration the diaphragm relaxes. The diaphragm curves upwards on each side, reaching the fifth intercostal space on the left side and slightly higher on the right (Figs 4.1, 4.2, pp 59 and 60).

Nerve supply

The two halves of the diaphragm are each supplied by a phrenic nerve and its periphery receives sensory branches from the lower intercostal nerves.

Openings

There are three large openings in the diaphragm (Fig. 1.14):

- The **caval opening** – at the level of the 8th thoracic vertebra. This transmits the inferior vena cava and the right phrenic nerve.
- The **oesophageal opening** – in the right crus, to the left of the **midline** at the level of the 10th thoracic vertebra. It transmits the oesophagus, the gastric branches of the vagus nerves and gastric vessels.
- The **aortic opening** – between the diaphragmatic crura in front of the 12th thoracic vertebra. It conveys the aorta, the thoracic duct and the azygos vein.

The left phrenic nerve pierces the dome of the left diaphragm. The heart and lungs, within the pericardial and pleural sacs, lie on its upper surface. The fibrous pericardium is firmly attached to its upper surface. Inferiorly on the right lie the liver, the right kidney and the suprarenal gland; on the left are the left lobe of the liver, gastric fundus, spleen, left kidney and suprarenal gland.

Respiration

Inspiration and expiration are produced by increasing and decreasing the volume of the thoracic cavity. In quiet respiration only the diaphragm is involved, and inspiration is aided by the weight of the liver attached to the underside of the diaphragm.

- **Inspiration** – the diaphragm contracts, descends, and the height of the thoracic cavity thus increases. The upper ribs are fixed by the scalenes and contraction of the intercostals thus raises the ribs, thereby increasing the anteroposterior and transverse diameters of the chest.
- **Expiration** – largely produced by relaxation of the diaphragm and elastic recoil of the lungs and the costal cartilages. Simultaneous contraction of the abdominal muscles forces the diaphragm upwards in forced expiration, such as in coughing and sneezing.

The diaphragm also helps in defecation. Straining involves deep inspiration and fixation of the contracted diaphragm and prevention of expiration by closure of the glottis. This action also assists in lifting heavy objects from the ground.

THE BREAST

The adult female breast is a soft, hemispherical structure. It is composed of glandular, and a variable amount of fat and fibrous tissue and lies in the superficial fascia of the upper anterior thoracic wall. The fascia invests it and forms radial septae, the suspensory ligaments (Cooper), which traverse the gland from the underlying fascia to be attached to the overlying skin. They divide the gland into 15–20 lobules. From the alveoli of each lobule the ducts unite to form a lactiferous duct. The breast lies on the fascia over pectoralis major but is separated from it by loose connective tissue. The male breast is a rudimentary organ comprising small ducts but no alveoli. It is, however, susceptible to all the diseases that afflict the female breast.

The female breast extends over the 2nd to the 6th ribs just lateral to the sternum as far as the midaxillary line, and lies mainly on the pectoralis major muscle (Fig. 1.15). For descriptive purposes it is divided into four quadrants; the upper outer quadrant extends laterally into the axilla as the **axillary tail**. Each of the 15 or so breast lobules drain by a lactiferous duct into the **nipple**, which is surrounded by thin pigmented skin, the **areola**, containing modified sebaceous glands and smooth muscle (Figs 1.15–1.17).

Blood supply is via branches of the internal thoracic, intercostal and lateral thoracic arteries.

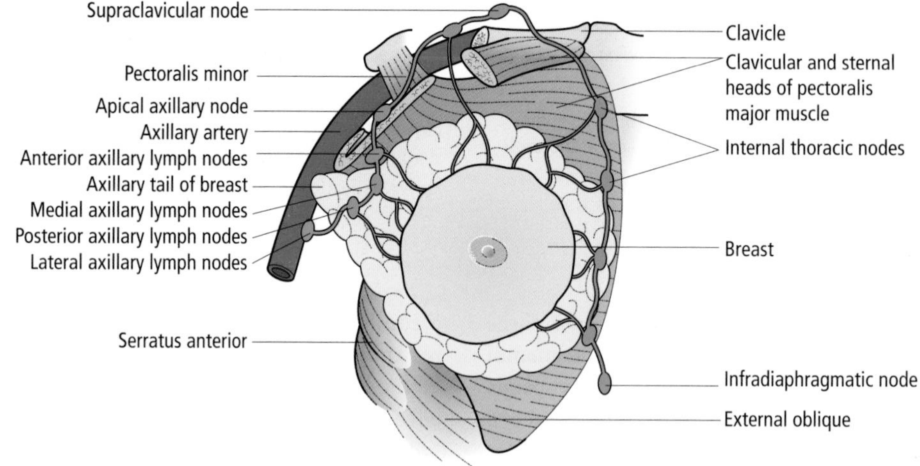

Figure 1.15 Relations and lymphatic drainage of female breast

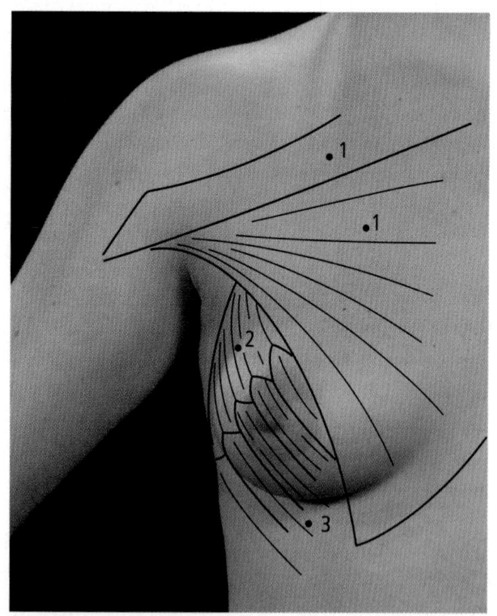

Figure 1.16 Surface anatomy of the breast: 1, clavicular and sternocostal parts of pectoralis major; 2, serratus anterior; 3, external oblique

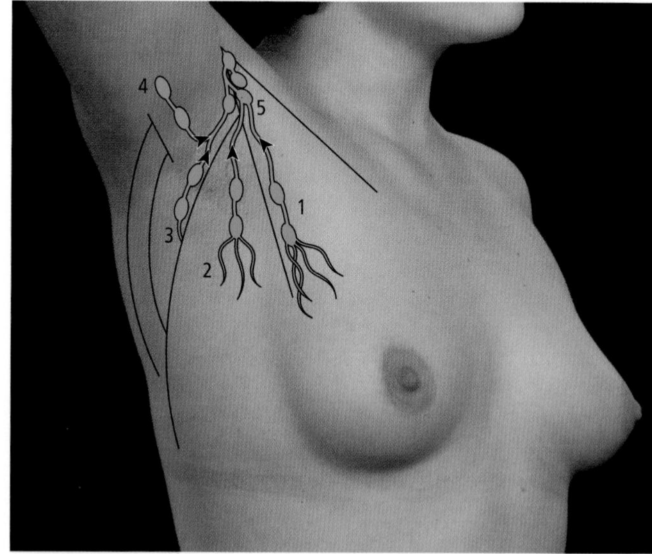

Figure 1.17 Lymphatic drainage of the breast. Axillary lymph nodes: 1, anterior; 2, medial; 3, posterior; 4, lateral; 5, apical

Lymph drains from the gland along vascular tributaries via two lymphatic plexuses: the subcutaneous subareolar plexus and the submammary plexus on pectoralis major. Although there is communication between lymphatics from these plexuses they mainly drain laterally to the axillary nodes, superiorly to infraclavicular and lower deep cervical nodes, inferiorly to lymphatics in the anterior abdominal wall, and medially to nodes around the internal thoracic artery. A small amount of lymph drains from the medial side of the breast into the opposite breast.

Supernumerary breasts or nipples may be formed anywhere along the 'milk line', which extends from axilla to groin (Fig. 1.18).

Pregnancy and lactation promote marked glandular proliferation, an increased pigmentation of the areola and nipple, and an increase in blood supply.

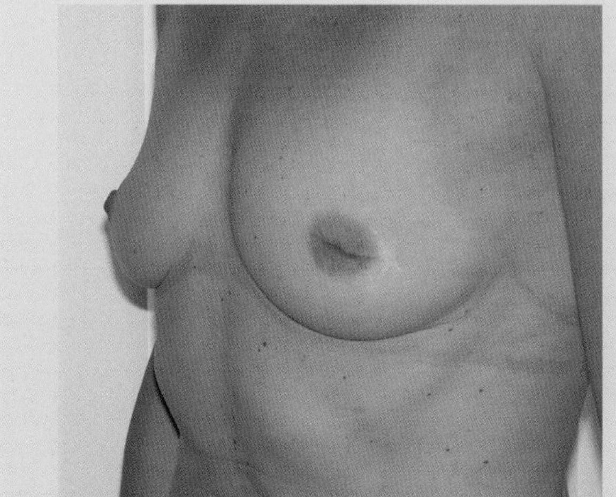

Figure 1.19 Retracted nipple

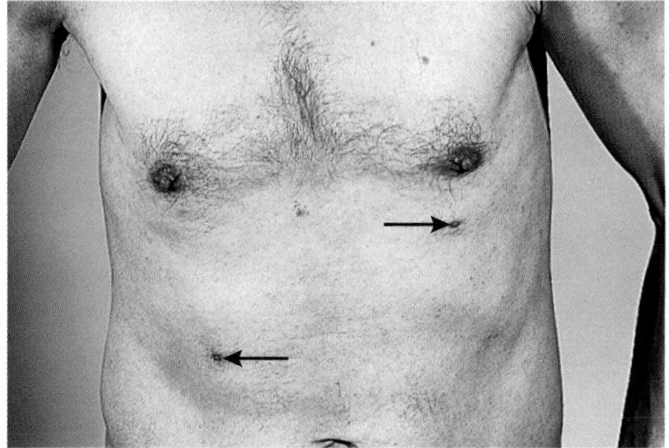

Figure 1.18 Accessory nipples (arrows)

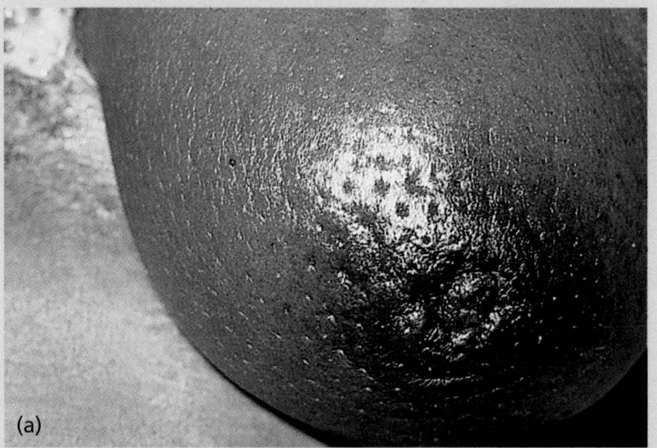

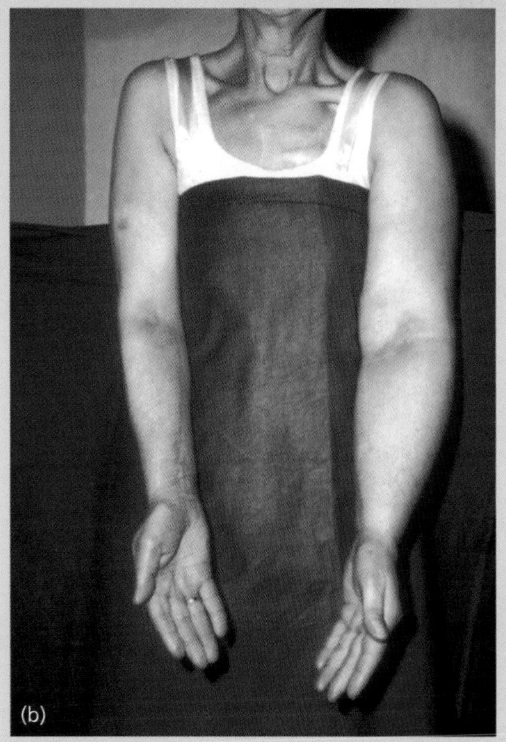

Figure 1.20 (a) Peau d'orange due to lymphatic obstruction. (b) Lymphoedema of the left arm due to breast malignancy

A lactating breast is susceptible to infection. Abscess drainage should be by a radial incision to avoid damage to the duct system. A breast cancer that has spread by infiltration may invade and become attached to the fascia and the pectoralis major muscle beneath it. If the suspensory ligaments are invaded then these contract and may produce retraction of the nipple (Fig. 1.19). If the spread has invaded and blocked the lymphatics of the breast then skin oedema will occur – *peau d'orange* (Fig. 1.20a). Cancerous infiltration of the axillary lymph nodes may produce arm swelling (lymphoedema) (Fig. 1.20b).

It is now realized that the former treatment of breast cancer – the attempted surgical removal of the whole breast with its contained cancer along with pectoralis major and all possibly involved lymph nodes – was based on the wrong assumption that it was possible to excise most breast cancers and the local lymphatic spread by surgical means. Nowadays it is accepted that in most cases the spread of the disease is wider than any possible surgical field could contain and so the surgical approach is limited to removal of the breast (or, in small cancers, the tumour and surrounding tissue) and the axillary nodes. Treatment of the wider spread of the cancer is undertaken with chemotherapy and/or radiotherapy.

MCQs

1. A typical rib: **T/F**

- **a** articulates with two vertebral bodies (___)
- **b** is attached to an intervertebral disc (___)
- **c** bears three facets for articulation with the vertebral column (___)
- **d** has a costal cartilage which articulates with the sternum by a synovial joint (___)
- **e** is grooved superiorly by the costal groove (___)

Answers

1.

a ***T*** – *Each typical rib bears two facets on its head for articulation with its own vertebra…*

b ***T*** – *… and the one above. The intervening crest is attached by an intra-articular ligament to the intervertebral disc.*

c ***T*** – *Two facets for articulation with two vertebral bodies and one for the transverse process.*

d ***T*** – *The joint between the 1st rib (which is not typical) and the sternum is a cartilaginous joint but the joints between the 2nd to the 7th costal cartilages and the sternum are synovial.*

e ***F*** – *The costal groove, conveying the intercostal vessels and nerve, lies inferiorly on the rib's inner surface.*

---

2. A typical intercostal nerve: **T/F**

- **a** is the ventral ramus of a thoracic spinal nerve (___)
- **b** lies, for most of its course, deep to the internal intercostal muscle (___)
- **c** lies, for the most part, in the subcostal groove (___)
- **d** supplies, amongst other structures, the skin of the back (___)
- **e** may supply the skin of the abdominal wall (___)

Answers

2.

a ***T*** – *It has cutaneous and muscular branches.*

b ***T*** – *Much of it is lying against the pleura.*

c ***T*** – *The artery and vein separate it from the rib.*

d ***F*** – *The skin of the back is supplied by branches of the dorsal rami.*

e ***T*** – *Anterior abdominal wall skin is supplied segmentally by the 7th to the 12th intercostal nerves.*

---

3. The diaphragm: **T/F**

- **a** is attached in part to the sternum (___)
- **b** is supplied by the phrenic and intercostal nerves (___)
- **c** increases the horizontal diameter of the chest when contracting (___)
- **d** has an opening in its central tendon for the inferior vena cava (___)
- **e** contracts during micturition (___)

Answers

3.

a ***T*** – *It gains attachment to the back of the xiphoid, the lowest six cartilages, the lateral and medial arcuate ligaments and by the right and left crura to the upper two or three lumbar vertebrae.*

b ***T*** – *Only the phrenic is motor; the intercostal nerves supply sensory branches to the periphery of the diaphragm.*

c ***F*** – *Contraction flattens the diaphragm thereby increasing the vertical diameter of the chest.*

d ***T*** – *The opening is slightly to the right of the midline and also conveys the right phrenic nerve.*

e ***T*** – *Expulsive acts, such as micturition and defecation, require a rise in intra-abdominal pressure which is usually produced by simultaneous contraction of the diaphragm and anterior abdominal wall.*

EMQs

Each question has an anatomical theme linked to the chapter, and a list of 10 related items (A–J) placed in alphabetical order: these are followed by five statements (1–5). Match **one or more** of the items A–J to each of the five statements.

Thoracic cage

A. 1st rib
B. 2nd rib
C. 5th rib
D. 7th rib
E. 9th rib
F. 10th rib
G. 12th rib
H. Body of sternum
I. Manubrium
J. Xiphisternum

Match the following statements with the appropriate item(s) from the above list.

1. Articulates at the sternal angle
2. Typical rib
3. Related to the subclavian artery
4. Atypical rib
5. Related to the right ventricle

Answers

1 BHI; 2 CDEF; 3 A; 4 ABG; 5 H

Diaphragm

A. Central tendon
B. Lateral arcuate ligament
C. Left crus
D. Left gastric nerve
E. Median arcuate ligament
F. Opening at the level of the 8th thoracic vertebra
G. Opening at the level of the 10th thoracic vertebra
H. Opening at the level of the 12th thoracic vertebra
I. Right crus
J. Right phrenic nerve

Match the following statements with the appropriate item(s) from the above list.

1. Gives passage to the inferior vena cava
2. Attached to the 12th rib
3. Overlies the aorta
4. Gives passage to the oesophagus
5. Attached to the 3rd lumbar vertebra

Answers

1 AF; 2 B; 3 CEHI; 4 GI; 5 I

APPLIED QUESTIONS

1. Where do ribs fracture? What may be the consequences?

1. The region of the angle of a rib is its weakest part and crushing injuries tend to fracture ribs just anterior to their angles. A direct blow may fracture the rib anywhere. Broken ends of fractured ribs may, when driven inwards, puncture the pleural sac and damage underlying viscera such as the lung, heart, spleen or kidney. The ribs of children, being mainly cartilaginous, are rarely fractured. A severe blow to the anterior chest may fracture the sternum and/or multiple ribs to produce a 'flail' anterior segment of the chest wall and respiratory embarrassment.

---

2. At which vertebral levels do the jugular notch, manubriosternal joint and inferior angle of the scapula usually lie?

2. These three palpable skeletal landmarks are reasonably constant and lie at T2, T4/5 and T7 respectively. The manubriosternal joint , also known as the sternal angle (of Louis), is also palpable and a useful point from which to count ribs – the 2nd rib articulates with the sternum at this point – and in this way provides a reliable method of identifying intercostal spaces.

---

3. Intradermal swelling and pitting of the skin may be seen in breast cancers. What is the anatomical explanation for this?

3. This is due to skin oedema and is known as peau d'orange. It is a classic sign of advanced breast cancer and is caused by blockage of the lymphatic drainage of the skin by cancer cells.

---

4. What special features may you see on examining the breasts of a pregnant woman?

4. The whole breast is enlarged and the axillary tail possibly noticed for the first time. Many dilated veins can be seen under the breast skin. The nipple and areola are more deeply pigmented and the areolar glands (Montgomery) larger and more numerous. Their function is to lubricate the nipple during lactation.

2 The thoracic cavity

The thoracic cavity is divided into right and left pleural cavities by the central mediastinum. The mediastinum is bounded behind by the vertebral column and in front by the sternum; it extends from the diaphragm below to become continuous above with the structures in the root of the neck. It contains the heart, great vessels, oesophagus, trachea and lymphatics.

THE HEART

The heart is the muscular pump of the systemic and pulmonary circulations. It has four chambers: two atria and two ventricles (Fig. 2.1a and Fig. 2.17a, p. 42). The direction of blood flow is controlled by unidirectional valves between the atria and ventricles, and between the ventricles and the emerging aorta and pulmonary trunk. The heart, the size of a clenched fist, weighs about 300 g and is the shape of a flattened cone with a base and an apex. It lies obliquely across the lower mediastinum behind the sternum within the pericardial sac, suspended by it from the great vessels.

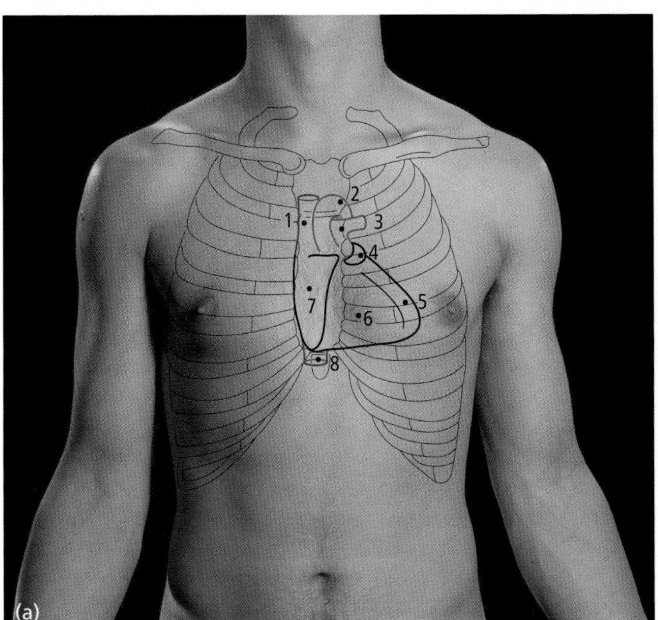

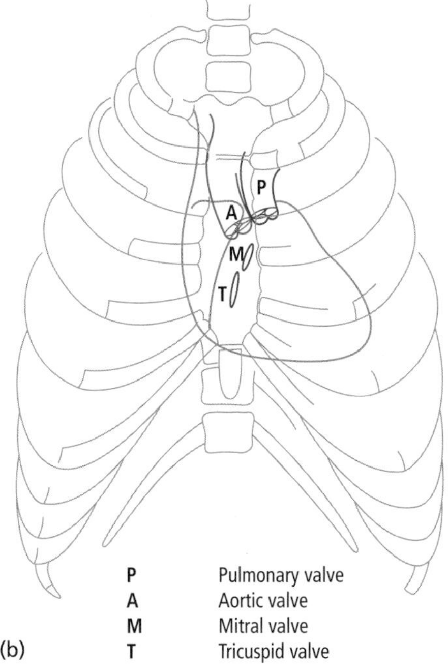

Figure 2.1 (a) Surface anatomy of chambers of the heart: 1, superior vena cava; 2, arch of aorta; 3, pulmonary trunk; 4, left auricle; 5, left ventricle; 6, right ventricle; 7, right atrium; 8, inferior vena cava. (b) Great vessels and position of valves

Its square base faces posteriorly and is formed from the left atrium and the four pulmonary veins (Fig. 2.2). The tip of the left ventricle forms the apex and is at the lower left extremity of the heart. The anterior surface is formed by the right atrium and the ventricles separated by the anterior interventricular grooves. The inferior surface rests on the central tendon of the diaphragm and is formed of both ventricles (mainly the left), separated by the posterior interventricular groove. The left surface, in contact with the left lung, is formed by the left ventricle and a small part of the left atrium. The right surface, in contact with the right lung, is formed by the right atrium, into which enter the superior and the inferior vena cavae.

Surface markings (Fig. 2.1b)

The right border of the heart extends between the 3rd and 6th right costal cartilages projecting just beyond the right sternal border. Its inferior border runs from the right 6th cartilage to the apex, situated in the 5th intercostal space in the midclavicular line. The left border extends from the apex to the left 2nd costal cartilage about 2 cm from the sternal edge.

THE CHAMBERS OF THE HEART

The right chamber pumps blood through the lungs and the left through the systemic circulation (Fig. 2.3).

The **right atrium**, a thin-walled chamber, receives blood from the superior and inferior venae cavae and the coronary sinus. Superomedially its small projection, the right auricle, overlaps the root of the aorta. On the right side a vertical ridge, the crista terminalis, passes between the cavae. The atrial wall behind the caval openings, the atrial septum, separates it from the left atrium, is smooth and bears a shallow central depression, the **fossa ovalis**. The wall is thicker anteriorly and formed of parallel muscular ridges which pass transversely to a vertical ridge, the crista terminalis. The superior caval orifice has no valves; that of the inferior vena cava has a rudimentary valve anteriorly, and between them, posteriorly, is the smaller opening of the coronary sinus.

The **right ventricle**, a thick-walled chamber, projects forward and to the left of the right atrium. An interventricular septum separates it from the left ventricle and bulges into the right cavity (Fig. 2.4). The ventricular walls are marked by interlacing muscular bands, except superiorly, where the smooth-walled infundibulum leads to the pulmonary orifice. The atrioventricular orifice lies posteroinferiorly and is guarded by the **tricuspid valve**, which has three cusps. Their ventricular surfaces are rough and anchored to the ventricular walls by fine tendinous cords arising from the ventricular septum or from two conical **papillary muscles**, which arise from the anterior and inferior ventricular walls. These cords and papillary muscles prevent eversion of the valve cusps into the atrial cavity during ventricular contraction and thus prevent regurgitation of blood into the atrium. The **pulmonary valve**, which lies at the upper end of the infundibulum, has three semilunar cusps; these are concave when viewed from above.

The **left atrium** is a rectangular chamber and lies behind the right atrium. Its appendix, the left auricular projection, overlies the left side of the pulmonary trunk. Four pulmonary veins enter its posterior surface, two on each side; their orifices possess no valves. The left atrioventricular orifice is on the anterior atrial wall. The posterior wall lies anterior to the oesophagus, left bronchus and descending thoracic aorta (Figs 2.2 and 2.5).

The **left ventricle** (Fig. 2.6), extending forwards and to the left of the left atrium, lies mainly behind the right ventricle. Its very thick walls (Fig. 2.4) are covered on the inside by muscular ridges, except for the smooth area below the aortic

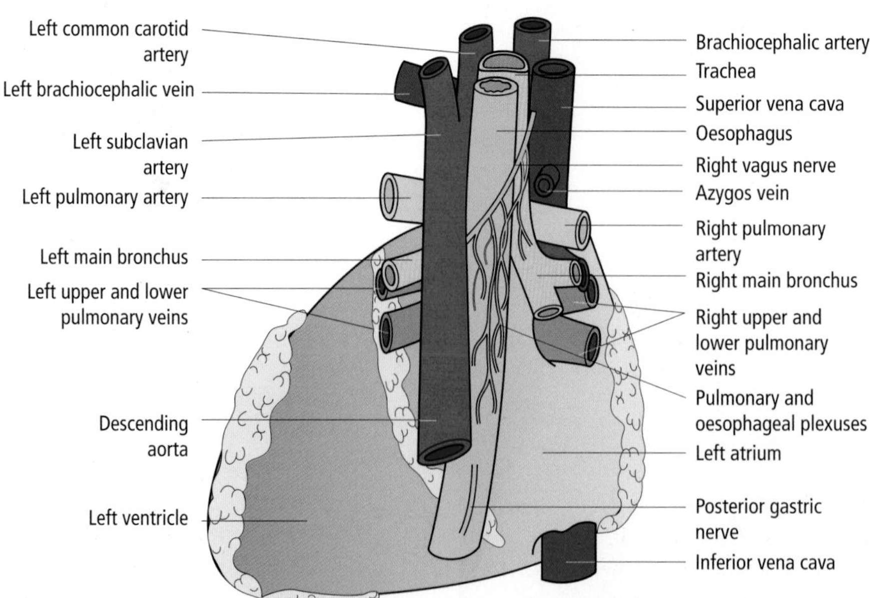

Figure 2.2 Posterior view of heart, great vessels and relationship to the oesophagus and trachea. Note that the posterior aspect of the heart contains the left atrium and pulmonary veins with the oesophagus in direct contact with the left atrium

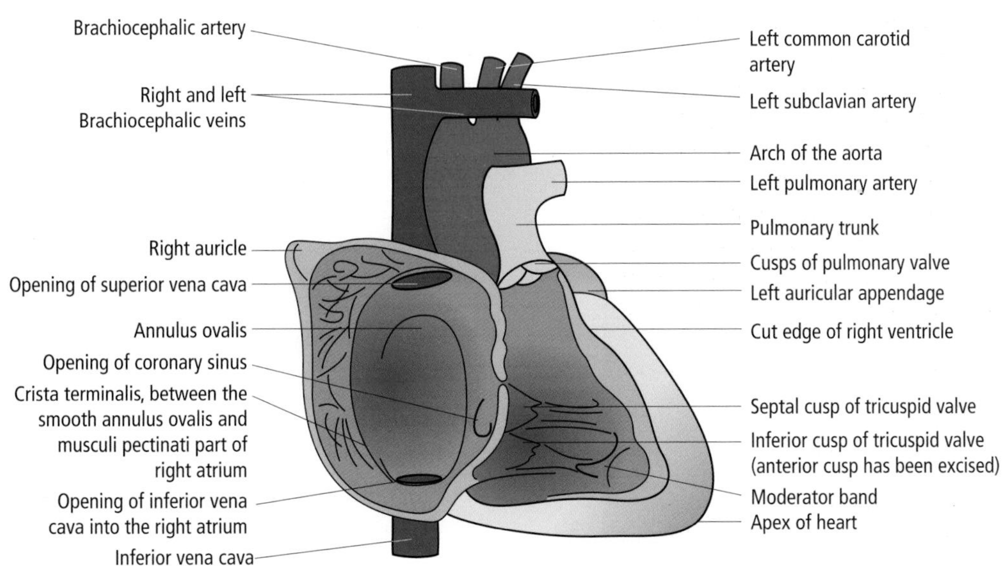

Figure 2.3 Anterior view of heart and great vessels to show the main chambers of the right side of the heart. The right atrial wall has been opened to reveal the internal structures and vessels draining into this chamber. The opened ventricle reveals the tricuspid valve and musculature

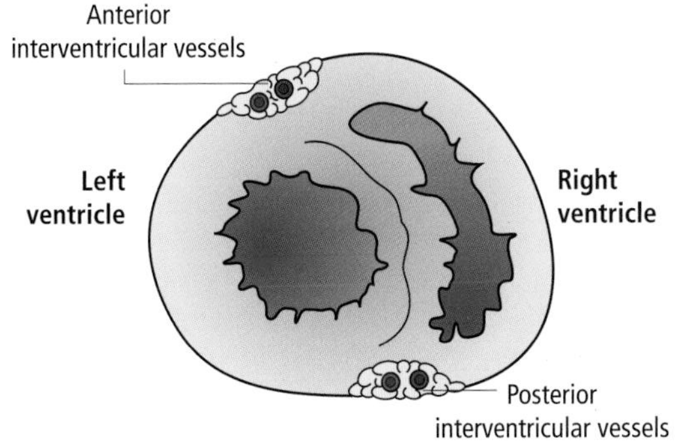

Figure 2.4 Transverse section through ventricles, showing relative thickness of walls

orifice, the vestibule. It has two orifices, the left atrioventricular posteriorly and the aortic superiorly. The left atrioventricular orifice is guarded by the **mitral valve**, which has two cusps, each anchored to papillary muscles by tendinous cords. The **aortic valve** has three cusps, above which are small dilatations, the aortic sinuses. The surface anatomy of the valves is shown in Fig. 2.7 and their relationships in Fig. 2.8.

The interventricular septum is thick, except for a thin membranous portion between the infundibulum and the vestibule. Both ventricular and atrial muscle fibres are anchored to a fibrous framework around the four valvular orifices, the fibrous skeleton of the heart (Fig. 2.8).

BLOOD SUPPLY

This is derived from the right and left coronary arteries. The **right coronary artery** (Figs 2.9 and 2.10) arises from the anterior aortic sinus and descends to the heart's anterior surface, in the atrioventricular groove supplying atrial and ventricular branches. It gains the posterior surface, where it gives off a marginal and a posterior interventricular artery, which may anastomose with the anterior interventricular branch of the left coronary artery. The **left coronary artery** (Figs 2.8, 2.9 and 2.11) is larger and arises from the left posterior aortic sinus. It passes forwards to supply atrial and ventricular branches. Its most important branch is the **anterior interventricular artery** (known clinically as the left anterior descending artery – LAD), which descends in the anterior

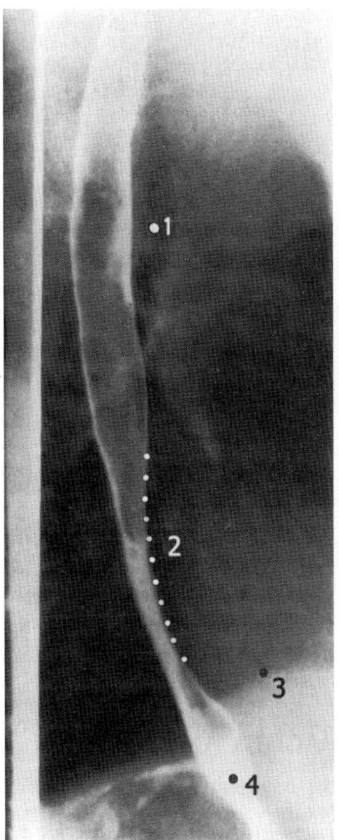

Figure 2.5 Barium swallow, right lateral view: 1, trachea; 2, cardiac impression (left atrium); 3, diaphragm; 4, gastro-oesophageal junction

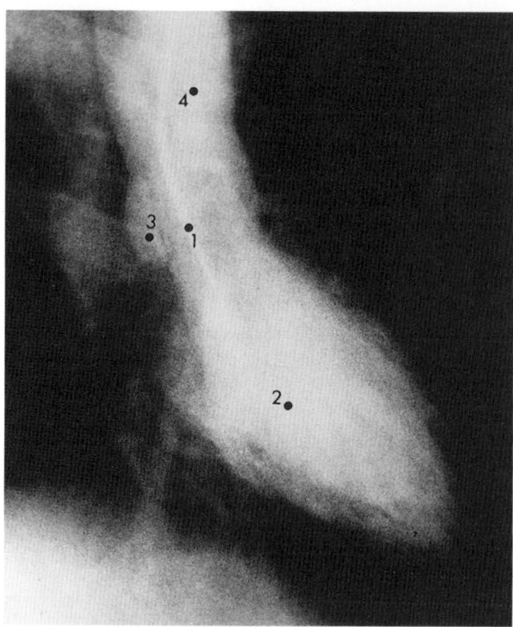

Figure 2.6 Left ventriculogram, right anterior oblique projection. The catheter (1) has been introduced into the right brachial artery and passed retrogradely into the left ventricle through the subclavian and brachiocephalic arteries, and the aorta and aortic valve. Contrast material has then been injected. 1, Catheter; 2, left ventricle; 3, right aortic sinus; 4, ascending aorta

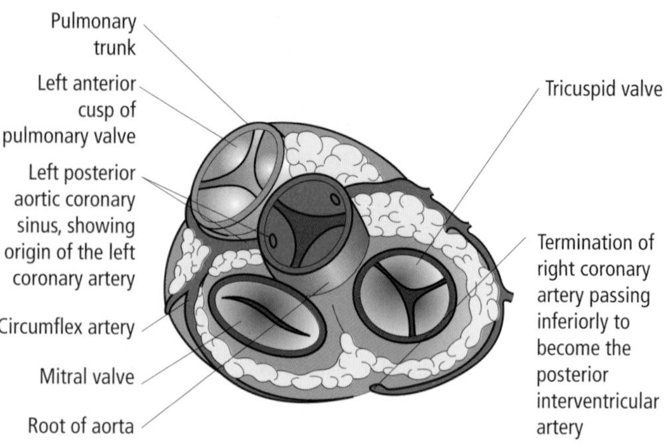

Figure 2.8 Upper aspect of heart with atria removed, showing aortic root, the pulmonary trunk, mitral and tricuspid valves, the fibrous skeleton and the right and left coronary arteries

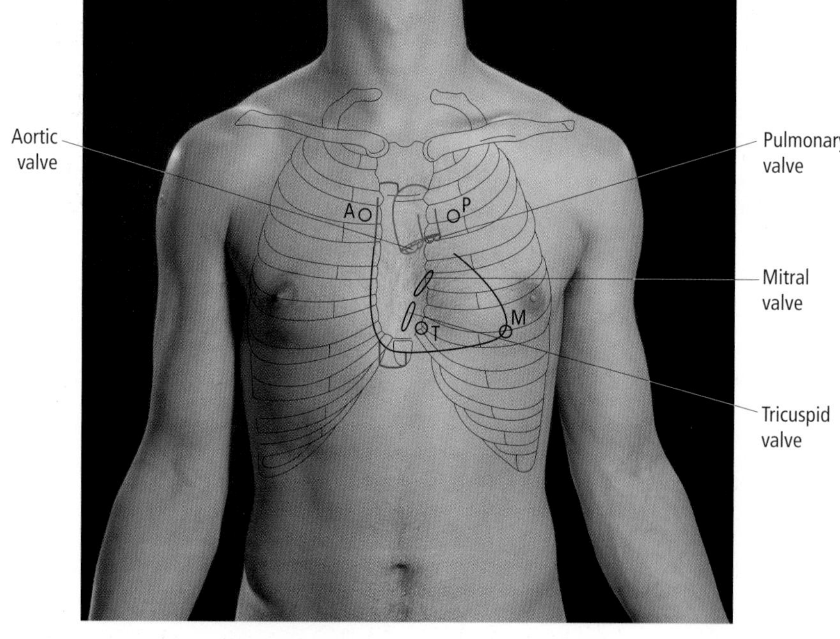

Figure 2.7 Surface markings of the four heart valves. The sites where the sounds coming from these valves are best heard with a stethoscope are indicated by a small circle with a corresponding letter

interventricular groove to the apex and the lower border to anastomose with the posterior interventricular branch of the right coronary artery. The circumflex branch passes posteriorly to supply much of the left ventricle. Usually the right ventricle is supplied by the right coronary artery, the left by the left, the interventricular septum by both, and the atria in a variable manner. The sinoatrial node and atrioventricular node are usually supplied by the right coronary artery (Figs 2.10 and 2.12).

The **mitral valve** is the most frequently diseased heart valve; fibrosis causes the cusps to shorten and causes incompetence and/or stenosis of the valve. Congenital stenosis of the pulmonary and the aortic valves may occur and result in hypertrophy of the right and left ventricles, respectively, and eventual cardiac decompensation. Although anastomoses exist between the two **coronary arteries**, sudden occlusion of a major branch may result in ischaemia and death of some heart muscle (**myocardial infarction**), and if

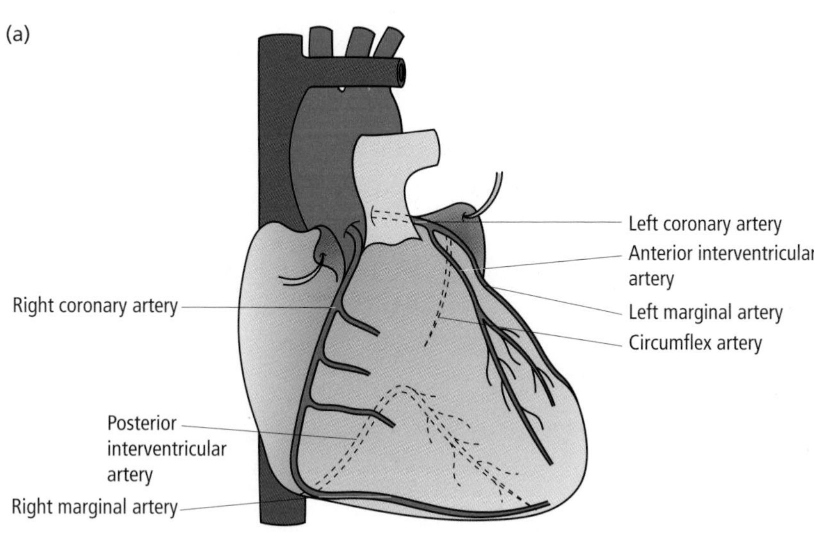

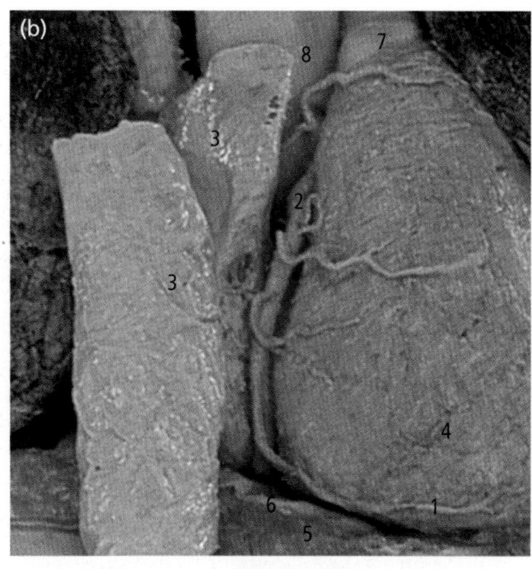

Figure 2.9 (a) Coronary arteries of the heart; those lying posteriorly are shown by dotted lines. (b) Anterior thorax, pericardium opened and retracted to the right: 1, right coronary artery, marginal branch; 2, right coronary artery; 3, retracted double layer of pericardium, shining parietal serous layer; 4, right ventricle, covered with visceral serous pericardium; 5, diaphragm; 6, fibrous pericardium attachment to central tendon of diaphragm; 7, pulmonary trunk; 8, aorta

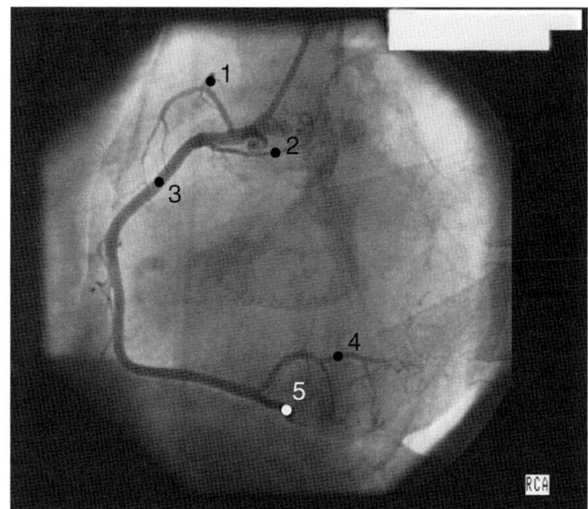

Figure 2.10 Right coronary arteriogram: 1, conus branch; 2, sinoatrial nodal artery; 3, right main coronary artery; 4. posterior interventricular artery; 5, origin of AV nodal branch

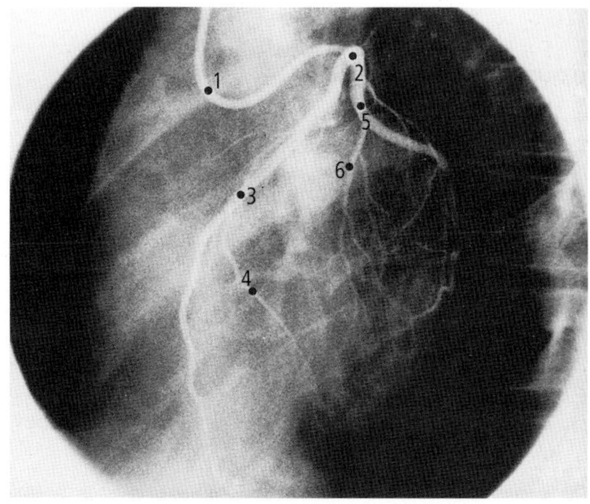

Figure 2.11 Left coronary arteriogram: 1, catheter; 2, common origin of L and R coronary arteries; 3, left anterior descending artery; 4, diagonal branch; 5, left main coronary artery; 6, anterior interventricular artery

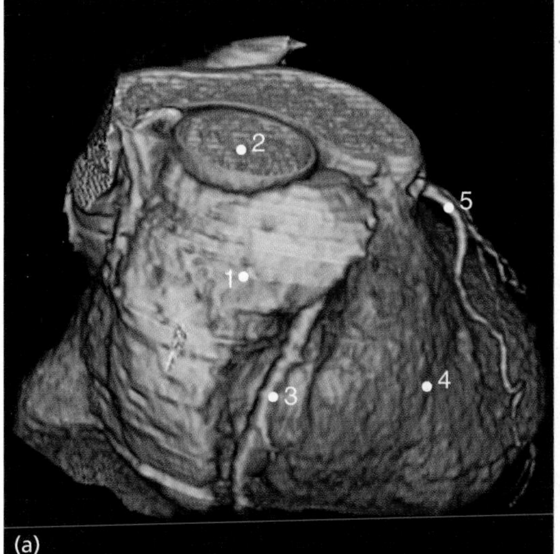

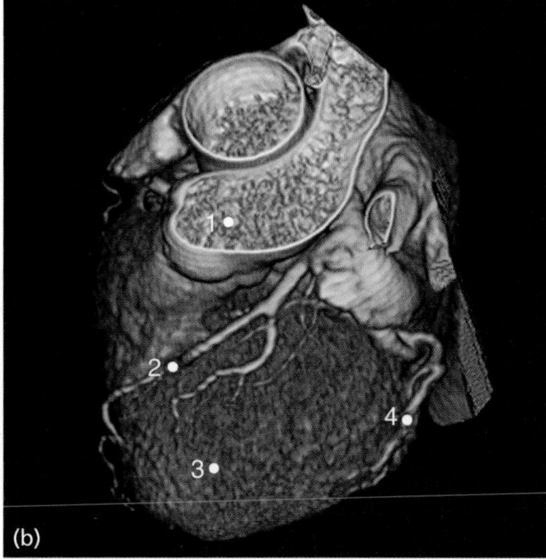

Figure 2.12 Electron beam CT. (a) Anterior view: 1, right atrium; 2, superior vena cava; 3, right coronary artery; 4, right ventricle; 5, anterior descending interventricular branch of left coronary artery (LAD). (b) Left lateral superior view: 1, aortic root; 2, anterior descending interventricular branch of the left coronary artery; 3, left ventricle; 4, circumflex branch of left coronary artery

the area affected includes the conducting system or is large, then the patient may die. Lesser degrees of ischaemic damage diminish the heart's work capacity, and pain (angina) may be felt on exertion. Narrowing of the coronary arteries may, by diminishing blood supply to the cardiac muscle, also cause angina, a pain usually felt in the substernal region. Ischaemia of the myocardium stimulates nerve endings within it. Sensory impulses are carried, largely on the left side, in the sympathetic branches to the thoracic segments T1–4. Pain arising in the heart is felt substernally but is often referred to the left arm and neck. This coronary narrowing is sometimes amenable to treatment by balloon dilatation, stenting or surgical bypass of the occlusion (Fig. 2.13) (CABG – coronary artery bypass graft). Rupture of a papillary muscle, for instance after ischaemic damage, may result in incompetence of the mitral or tricuspid valve. Valvular stenosis or incompetence may require surgical replacement of the valve.

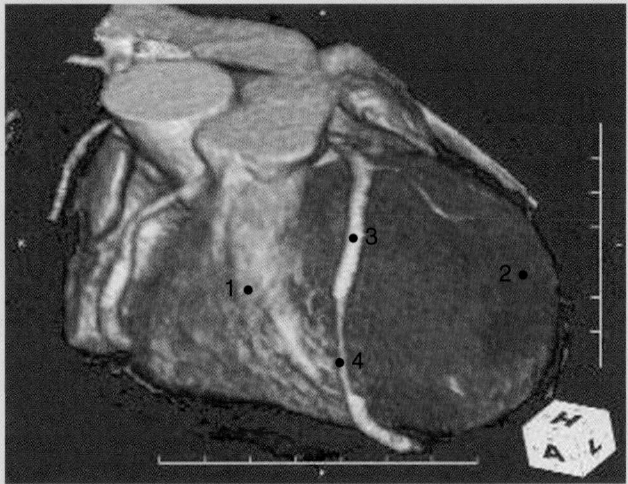

Figure 2.13 Electron beam CT of patient following insertion of a stent (small tube to open up blocked artery): 1, right ventricle; 2, left ventricle; 3, stent in descending interventricular branch of left coronary artery; 4, stenosis (narrowed segment) of coronary artery even after stenting

Venous drainage

This is largely via the **coronary sinus**, which drains into the right atrium near to the opening of the inferior vena cava (Fig. 2.14). It is about 3 cm long and receives the **great cardiac vein**, which ascends the anterior interventricular groove, the **middle cardiac vein** running in the posterior interventricular groove, a **small cardiac vein** which reaches it in the coronary sulcus, and branches from the posterior of the left ventricle and atrium. **Anterior cardiac veins**, several in number, draining the anterior right ventricle, drain directly into the right atrium. **Venae cordii minimae** drain much of the heart wall. They are small and open directly into the heart's chambers.

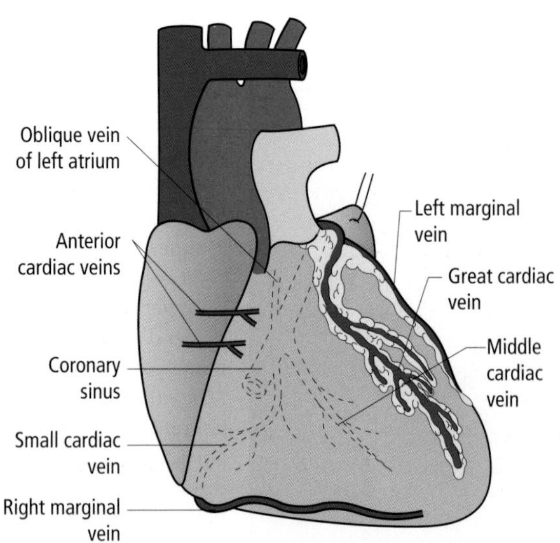

Figure 2.14 Coronary veins of the heart – those lying posteriorly are shown by dotted lines

LYMPHATIC DRAINAGE

This is to the tracheobronchial nodes.

NERVE SUPPLY

This is from the vagus (cardioinhibitory) and sympathetic (cardioexcitatory) nerves through the cardiac plexus (p. 67). The fibres pass with the branches of the coronary arteries. Parasympathetic ganglia lie in the heart wall. The vagus conveys sensory fibres; pain fibres run with the sympathetic nerves and traverse the cervical and upper thoracic sympathetic ganglia before entering the spinal nerves T1–T4.

Cardiac pain – this is produced by ischaemic heart tissue. Since the afferent sensory fibres pass through the cervical and upper thoracic ganglia before entering the upper thoracic spinal cord segments, the visceral pain produced by ischaemia is commonly referred to those somatic structures with the same nerve supply, i.e. the left upper limb, the precordium and the left neck.

The conducting system of the heart is formed of specialized cardiac muscle cells and initiates, coordinates and regulates the complex pattern of contraction in the cardiac cycle. It consists of the **sinoatrial (SA) node**, the **atrioventricular (AV) node**, the **AV bundle of His**, its right and left branches, and the terminal subendocardial plexus of Purkinje fibres (Fig. 2.15). The **SA node** (known as the pacemaker) is a small area of conducting tissue in the right atrial wall anterior to the superior vena cava opening. Impulses from it are conducted by the muscle of the atrial wall to the **AV node**, a similar nodule lying on the right of the atrial septum close to the entry of the coronary sinus. From it the **AV bundle** descends the interventricular septum and divides into right and left branches, mainly supplying the corresponding ventricle, which ramify as the subendocardial plexus supplying the ventricular walls and papillary muscles.

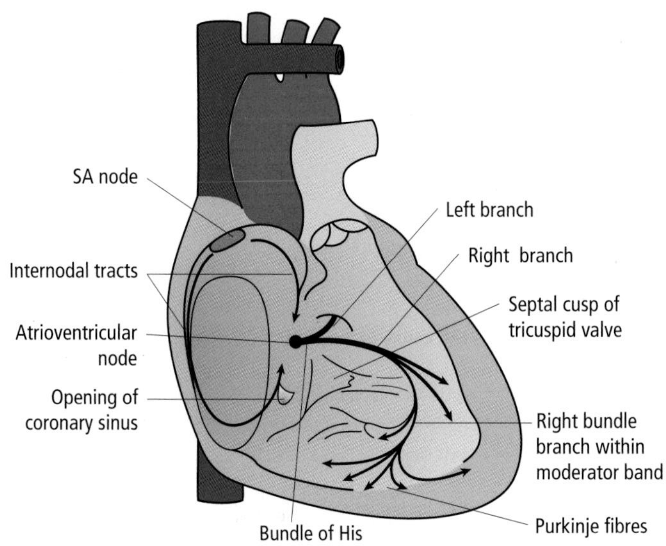

Figure 2.15 Conducting system of the heart – arrows show the anatomical arrangement

THE PERICARDIUM

The pericardium is a fibroserous membrane that surrounds the heart and the adjacent parts of the large vessels entering and leaving it. It consists of an outer fibrous and an inner serous layer, and the latter is divided into two layers, the visceral and parietal, between which is the pericardial sac (Figs 2.17–2.19).

The **serous pericardium** is a closed serous sac, invaginated by the heart and enclosing within its layers a thin pericardial cavity. Visceral pericardium, which covers the outer surface of the heart, is continuous with the parietal pericardium that lines the inside of the fibrous pericardium.

Electrocardiogram (ECG)

The ECG is a record of the electrical potential detected at the body surface. Ten electrodes are placed as shown in Fig. 2.16 – four limb leads on the muscular parts of each forearm and lower leg and six precordial leads, named V_1 – V_6, are placed:

V_1 – right side of sternum, 4th intercostal space
V_2 – left side of sternum, 4th intercostal space
V_3 – midway between V_2 and V_4
V_4 – midclavicular line, 5th intercostal space
V_5 – anterior axillary line horizontal to V_4
V_6 – mid-axillary line horizontal to V_4

The ECG traces measure the electric potential resulting from the heart muscle contraction: each trace corresponds to a specific region of heart muscle, and abnormalities can thus be identified and localized. It is the best way to measure and diagnose abnormalities of heart rhythm caused by abnormalities in the conducting tissue or those caused by electrolyte imbalance. In myocardial infarction it can identify the area of heart muscle damage.

The generation and passage of the impulses from the SA node can be recorded by an ECG and this diagnostic aid is of great importance in detecting cardiac irregularities and the site of cardiac ischaemia. If the AV bundle is damaged, for instance after a coronary artery thrombosis, total heart block may occur, in which the ventricles beat slowly at their own rate independent of the atria, which continue to contract at the rate determined by the SA node. Atheroma may cause ischaemia or myocardial infarction, which may damage the AV node resulting in a delay in impulse propagation (heart block). This is treated by insertion of a cardiac pacemaker whose electrode lies in the right ventricle.

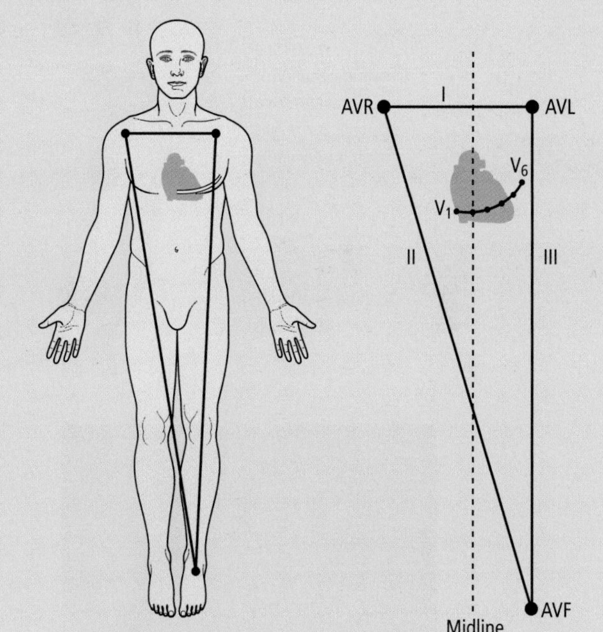

Figure 2.16 The electrocardiogram (ECG) records the electrical activity of the heart. Leads, attached by adhesive pads, are placed on the shoulders, left leg and around the chest (V_1–V_6). Leads I, II and III record voltage between two limb leads; AVR, AVL and AVF, between one limb and the other two; and V_1–V_6 between a point on the chest and an average of the three limb leads. AVR and V_1 are oriented towards the cavity of the heart; II,III and AVF face the inferior surface; I, AVL and V_6 face the lateral wall of the left ventricle; V_1 and V_2 are directed at the right ventricle; V_3 and V_4 at the interventricular septum; and V_5 and V_6 at the left ventricle

Superior vena cava
Aorta
Pulmonary trunk
Right auricle
Left auricle
Right atrium
Right border of the heart
Left border of the heart
Right atrioventricular groove
Anterior interventricular groove
Left ventricle
Inferior vena cava
Inferior border of the heart
Right ventricle
(a)

Aortic opening
Opening of pulmonary trunk (the arrow is passing through the transverse sinus of the pericardium)
Opening of superior vena cava
Openings of right pulmonary veins
Left pulmonary veins
Oblique sinus of the pericardium
Lines of reflection between outer parietal and inner visceral layers of the serous pericardium
Outer layer of serous pericardium
Fibrous pericardium
Opening of inferior vena cava
(b)

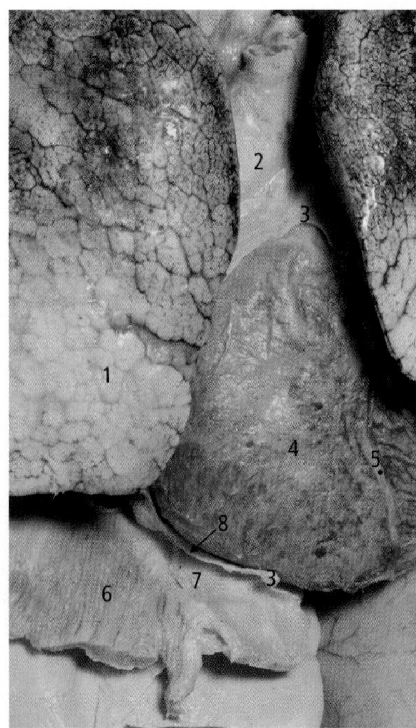

(c)

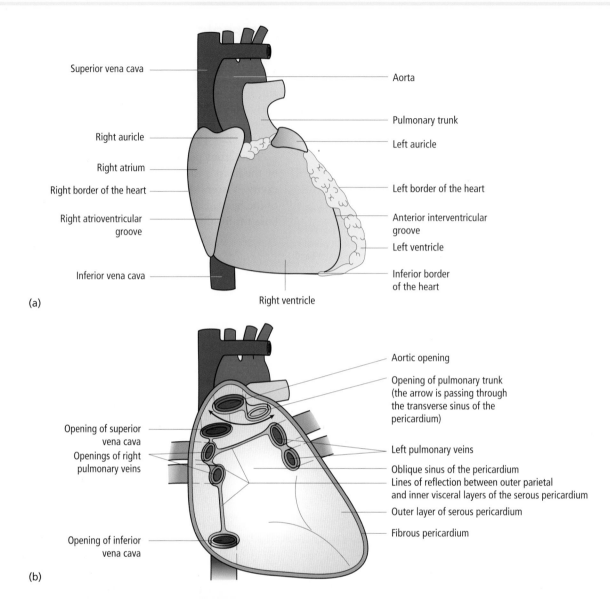

Figure 2.17 (a) Anterior view of heart and great vessels. (b) Pericardial sac after removal of the heart. (c) Anterior thorax revealing opened pericardium *in situ*: 1, lung; 2, pericardium covering the great vessels of superior mediastinum; 3, cut edge of fibrous and serous parietal layers of pericardium; 4, right ventricle; 5, left coronary artery, anterior interventricular branch; 6, diaphragm; 7, fibrous pericardium attachment to central tendon of diaphragm; 8, pericardial cavity

Ascending aorta
Pulmonary trunk (The arrow lies in the transverse sinus of the pericardium)
Superior vena cava
Left pulmonary veins
Right pulmonary veins
Oblique sinus of pericardium
Reflection lines of visceral pericardium
Left atrium
Left ventricle
Inferior vena cava

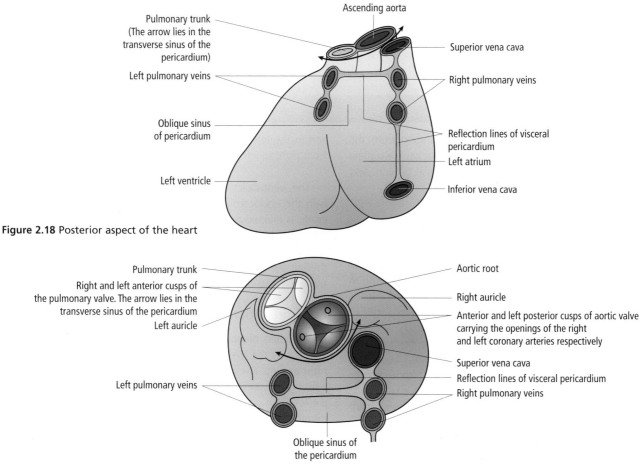

Figure 2.18 Posterior aspect of the heart

Pulmonary trunk
Aortic root
Right and left anterior cusps of the pulmonary valve. The arrow lies in the transverse sinus of the pericardium
Right auricle
Left auricle
Anterior and left posterior cusps of aortic valve carrying the openings of the right and left coronary arteries respectively
Superior vena cava
Reflection lines of visceral pericardium
Left pulmonary veins
Right pulmonary veins
Oblique sinus of the pericardium

Figure 2.19 Superior aspect of the heart showing site of origin of the great vessels and the pericardial reflections and sinuses

Fluid in the pericardium, as the result of trauma or infection (Fig. 2.20), limits the filling and output of the heart (cardiac tamponade). This causes the veins of the face and neck to become congested, and eventually the cardiac output decreases as the pressure of the fluid in the inextensible pericardial sac rises. In these circumstances it is necessary to aspirate the fluid. The pericardial sac is most easily entered by a needle inserted between the xiphoid process and the left costal margin, directed headwards, backwards and medially through the central tendon of the diaphragm (Fig. 2.21).

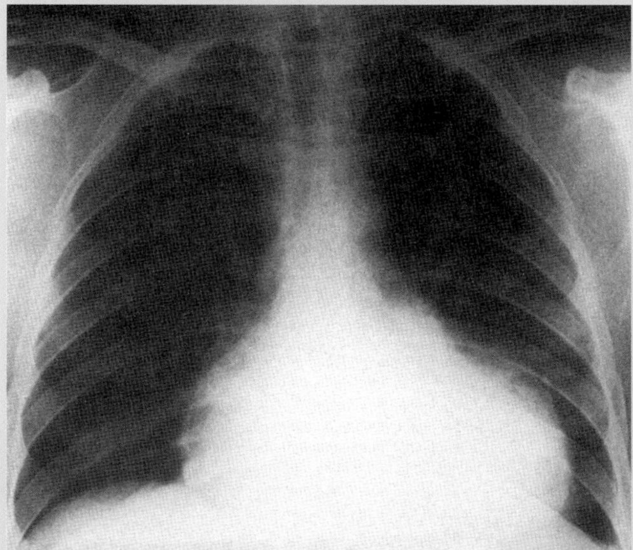

Figure 2.20 Chest X-ray showing pericardial effusion

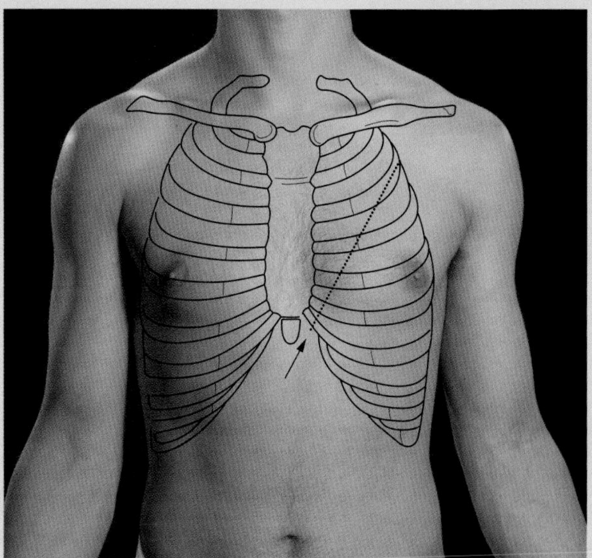

Figure 2.21 Anterior chest wall – arrow and dotted line shows needle direction for pericardial aspiration

The **fibrous pericardium** is a strong flask-shaped sac surrounding the heart and serous pericardium which blends below with the central tendon of the diaphragm and the adventitia of the inferior vena cava, above with the adventitia of the aorta, pulmonary trunk and superior vena cava, and behind with that of the pulmonary veins.

Development of the heart

The heart develops from a vascular tube hanging from the dorsal wall of the pericardial part of the coelomic sac. Two main processes are involved: bending with differential growth, and division into right and left sides.

Bending and differential growth

The heart is suspended from the dorsal wall of the embryo by a mesentery, the dorsal mesocardium. The caudal (venous) end of the heart tube receives vessels, enclosed in a common sheath of pericardium, which become the superior and inferior venae cavae and the pulmonary veins. The cephalic (arterial) end divides to form the aorta and pulmonary artery, similarly enclosed in a single tube of pericardium. The cephalic end elongates and descends in front of the veins, becoming S-shaped. The twisting development of the heart leaves spaces within the pericardial sac – the oblique and transverse sinuses (Fig. 2.17). Four dilatations develop in the primitive heart: the sinus venosus, the atrium, the ventricle and the bulbus cordis. The atrium is continuous with the ventricle via a narrow atrioventricular canal.

Division into right and left sides

Longitudinal partitions divide the atrium, ventricle and bulbus cordis into right and left atria, right and left ventricles, and the pulmonary and aortic trunks, respectively. Two small endocardial cushions unite across the atrioventricular canal to divide it into right and left sides. In the atrial cavity a septum (septum primum) descends to fuse with the endocardial cushions, becoming perforated in its upper part. A septum secundum descends on the right of the septum primum to incompletely overlap the perforation, leaving an oblique communication between the atria, the **foramen ovale** which, by nature of its construction, acts in the fetus in a valve-like manner, allowing blood to flow from right to left atria but not in the reverse direction.

The ventricular cavity is divided by a septum that fuses with the endocardial cushions above; the cavity of the bulbus cordis is divided by a spiral septum to form the pulmonary and aortic trunks. The septa of the ventricles and the bulbus unite so that the right ventricle leads to the pulmonary trunk and the left ventricle to the aorta. The left atrium incorporates the pulmonary veins and the right atrium the sinus venosus.

Fetal circulation

Oxygenated blood from the placenta is carried in the ductus venosus to the liver, and thence to the inferior vena cava and right atrium. The placental blood is then directed by the angle existing between the inferior and superior vena cava through the foramen ovale into the left atrium, thence to the left ventricle into the aorta. Much of this blood is carried to the head and the developing brain. It returns to the heart in the superior vena cava and thence to the right ventricle and the pulmonary artery. It is then shunted by the ductus arteriosus into the aorta, thus bypassing the lungs. It flows to the rest of the body, but the majority passes via the umbilical arteries to the placenta. The venous return from the rest of the body, and the blood from the placenta in the umbilical vein and the ductus venosus, enters the inferior vena cava.

At birth respiration begins and there is a consequent increase in blood flow to the lungs and an increase in venous return in the pulmonary veins. The left atrial pressure therefore rises and results in closure of the foramen ovale. The ductus venosus and ductus arteriosus also close at this time and, in doing so, establish the adult pattern of circulation.

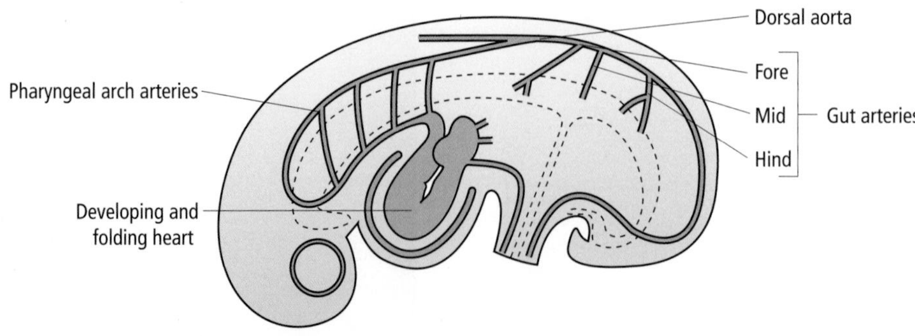

Figure 2.22 The development of the cardiovascular system

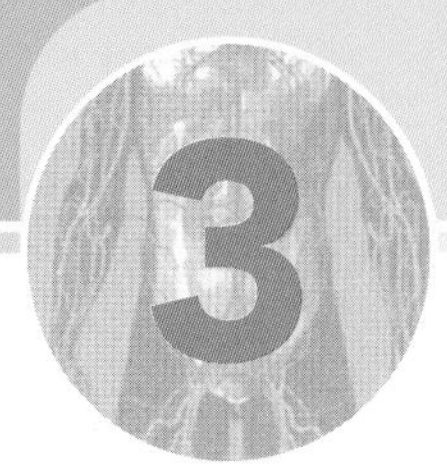

3 The mediastinal structures

THE AORTA

This, the main arterial trunk of the systemic circulation, arises from the left ventricle and ascends briefly before arching backwards over the root of the left lung to descend through the thorax and abdomen. Descriptively it is divided into the ascending part, the arch, a descending thoracic part and an abdominal part.

The ascending aorta

The ascending aorta is a wide vessel some 5 cm long. It begins at the aortic orifice behind the 3rd right costal cartilage below the level of the sternal angle and ascends to the right, around the pulmonary trunk, to the level of the sternal angle. At its base above each of the semilunar valvules of the aortic valve is a dilatation, an aortic sinus.

Relations

The ascending aorta is enclosed in a sheath of serous pericardium common to it and the pulmonary trunk within the fibrous pericardium. Its lower part lies behind the infundibulum of the right ventricle and the origin of the pulmonary trunk, and above this the sternum is anterior. Posterior, from below upwards, are the left atrium, the right pulmonary artery and right main bronchus. On its left lie the left auricle and pulmonary trunk, and to the right the right auricle and superior vena cava.

Branches

The right and left coronary arteries arise from the anterior and left posterior aortic sinuses (p. 37).

Aortic arch

The **arch** of the aorta passes upwards from the sternal angle behind the manubrium to arch backward and to the left over the left lung root, and then descends to the left side of the 4th thoracic vertebra (Fig. 3.1). From the convexity of the arch arise the three arteries supplying the head, neck and upper limbs.

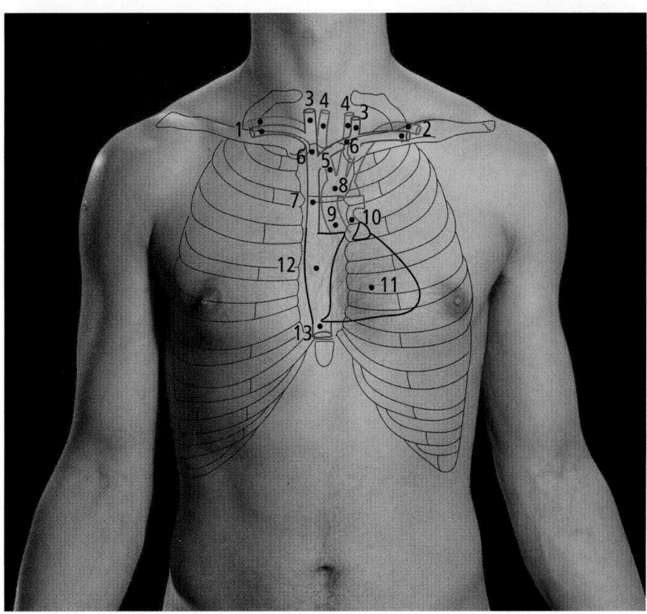

Figure 3.1 Surface markings of the great vessels of the superior mediastinum: 1, right subclavian vessels; 2, left subclavian vessels; 3, internal jugular veins; 4, common carotid arteries; 5, brachiocephalic artery; 6, brachiocephalic veins; 7, superior vena cava; 8, aortic arch; 9, ascending aorta; 10, pulmonary trunk; 11, ventricles; 12, right atrium; 13, inferior vena cava

Relations

To its left lie the mediastinal pleura and lung, the left phrenic nerve and the left vagus. To its right lie the superior vena cava, the trachea and left recurrent laryngeal nerve, the oesophagus and thoracic duct and, finally, the 4th thoracic vertebra. Inferiorly it crosses the bifurcation of the pulmonary trunk, the ligamentum arteriosum and the left main bronchus. Superiorly are its three branches (Fig. 3.2). The arch is connected inferiorly to the left pulmonary artery by the ligamentum arteriosum, a fibrous remnant of the ductus arteriosus. The left recurrent laryngeal nerve passes posteriorly around the ligamentum and the arch. The cardiac plexus is closely related to the ligamentum. Remnants of the thymus gland may be found in front of the arch.

Branches

The first branch, the brachiocephalic artery, arises behind the manubrium and ascends as far as the right sternoclavicular joint, there to divide into two terminal branches, the right subclavian and right common carotid arteries (Fig. 3.3). Anteriorly the left brachiocephalic vein and thymus separate it from the manubrium; posteriorly lies the trachea. To its right lie the right brachiocephalic vein and superior vena cava, and to its left is the left common carotid artery. The left common carotid artery arises from the arch just behind the brachiocephalic artery and passes upwards alongside the left side of the trachea into the neck. The left subclavian artery arises behind the left common carotid artery and arches to the left over the dome of the left pleura behind the left sternoclavicular joint and over the first rib (Fig 3.3).

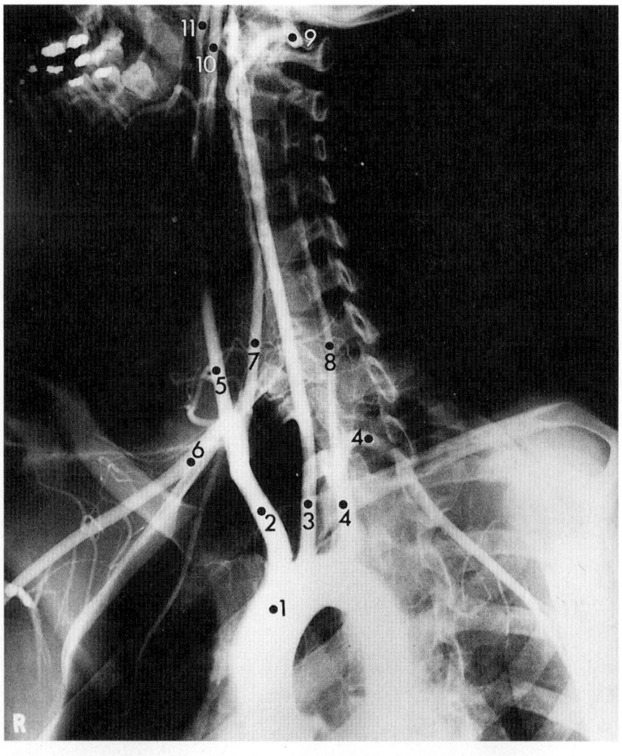

Figure 3.2 Arteriogram of the aortic arch and its main branches: 1, aortic arch; 2, brachiocephalic artery; 3, left common carotid artery; 4, left subclavian artery; 5, right common carotid artery; 6 right subclavian artery; 7, right vertebral artery; 8, left vertebral artery; 9, loop of left vertebral artery as it passes around the lateral mass of the atlas; 10, right internal carotid artery; 11, right external carotid artery

The descending aorta

The descending aorta descends from the left of the 4th thoracic vertebra, inclining medially to the front of the 12th, where it passes through the diaphragm to become the abdominal aorta (Fig. 3.3).

Relations

Anteriorly, from above downwards, are the left lung root, the left atrium, covered by pericardium, the oesophagus and the diaphragm. Posteriorly are the 4th to the 12th thoracic vertebrae. Its left side is in contact with left pleura and lung, and its right side with the oesophagus above and the right lung and pleura below. The thoracic duct and azygos vein are also on its right side.

Branches

These are the 3rd to 11th posterior intercostal arteries, a pair of subcostal arteries, two or three small bronchial arteries, several small oesophageal arteries and arteries to the diaphragm.

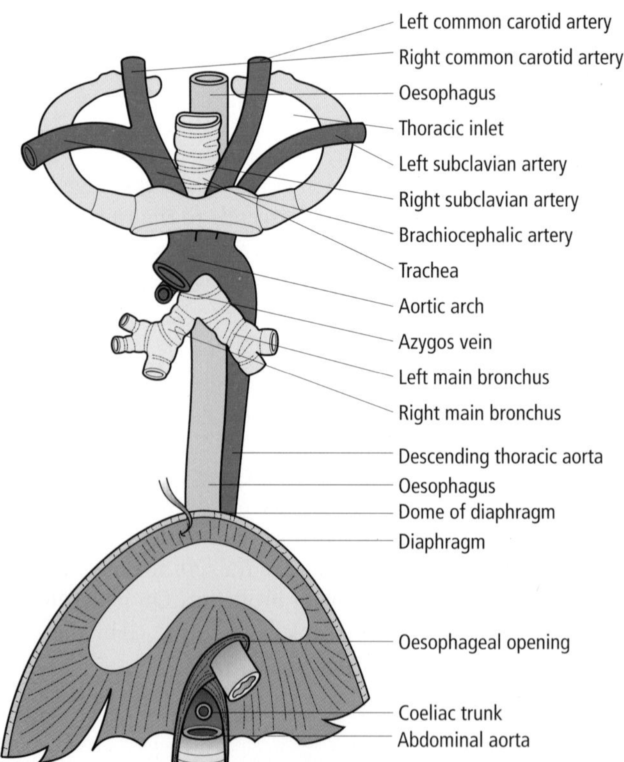

Figure 3.3 Diagram showing thoracic inlet and the structures in the superior and posterior aspect of the mediastinum

THE PULMONARY TRUNK

This wide vessel, about 5 cm long, originates at the pulmonary orifice and ascends posteriorly to the left of the aorta to end at its bifurcation into right and left pulmonary arteries under the concavity of the aortic arch (Figs 3.4 and 3.5). It is contained within a common sleeve of serous pericardium with the ascending aorta and lies in front of the transverse sinus of the pericardium. The two auricles and both coronary arteries surround its base. These mediastinal structures can be conveniently studied by radiological techniques (Fig. 3.6a–i).

Branches

The right pulmonary artery passes to the right lung hilus behind the ascending aorta and superior vena cava, and in front of the oesophagus and right main bronchus. The left pulmonary artery passes in front of the left bronchus and descending aorta to its lung hilus. It is connected by the ligamentum arteriosum to the lower aspect of the aortic arch. Branches of the pulmonary arteries accompany the bronchi and bronchioles.

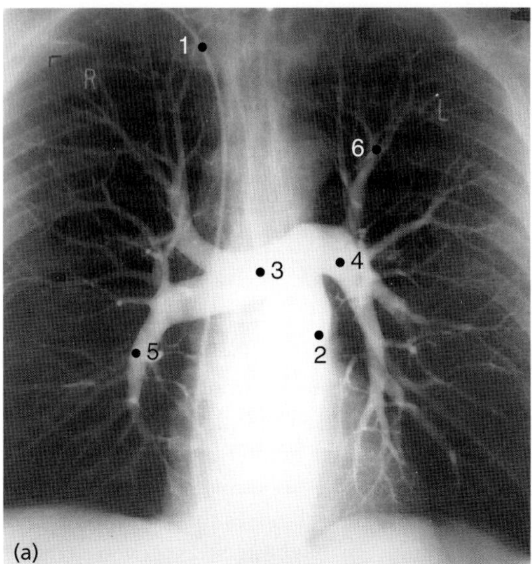

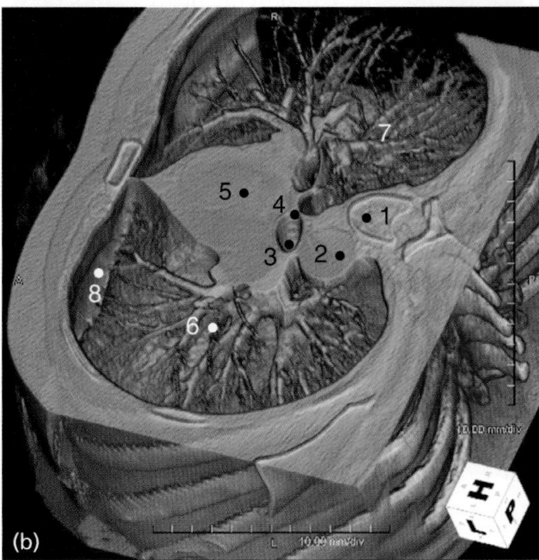

Figure 3.4 (a) Pulmonary arteriogram – performed by passing a catheter, 1, through the venous system, the right atrium, right ventricle and onwards into, 2, the pulmonary trunk. The contrast medium is then injected to outline anatomical features: 3, right pulmonary artery; 4, left pulmonary artery; 5, right basal segmental arteries; 6, left superior lobe segmental arteries. (b) Electron beam CT of thorax showing three-dimensional anatomy. This is part of a video sequence that rotates the whole chest for detailed examination, having only taken a few minutes to acquire the data: 1, vertebral body; 2, desending thoracic aorta; 3, left main bronchus; 4, carina; 5, heart chamber; 6, pulmonary segmental vessels; 7, segmental bronchial 'tree'; 8, diaphragm – left dome

THE GREAT VEINS

The pulmonary veins are paired short wide vessels lying in the hilus of each lung, anterior and inferior to the artery (Fig. 3.6).

Brachiocephalic veins

The brachiocephalic veins (Fig. 3.6) form behind the sternoclavicular joint by the union of the internal jugular and subclavian veins of each side and, after a short course, unite to form the superior vena cava behind the right side of the manubrium. The right brachiocephalic vein is some 3 cm long, with the right phrenic nerve lateral to it, descending behind the right margin of the manubrium anterolateral to the brachiocephalic artery. The longer left brachiocephalic vein descends obliquely behind the manubrium, above the arch of the aorta, and anterior to its three large branches and the trachea.

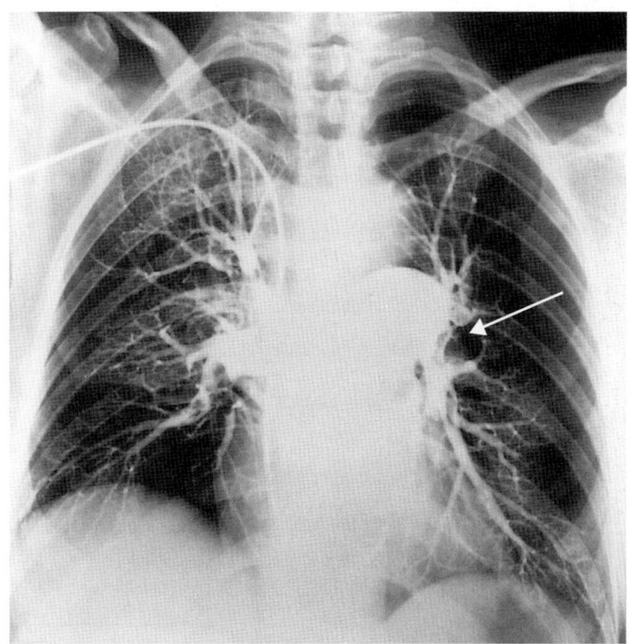

Figure 3.5 Pulmonary arteriogram showing filling defect in arteries (arrow) due to an embolus arising from a thrombus in the deep veins of the leg (p. 220)

Tributaries

These are the vertebral veins draining the neck muscles, the inferior thyroid veins which unite in front of the trachea and drain into the left brachiocephalic vein, and the internal thoracic vein draining the anterior chest wall. The thoracic duct drains into the left brachiocephalic vein and the smaller right lymph duct drains into the right brachiocephalic vein) (Fig. 4.16, p. 67).

Superior vena cava

The superior vena cava, 1.5 cm wide and about 7 cm long, is formed by the union of the two brachiocephalic veins behind the right border of the manubrium and descends behind the body of the sternum to enter the right atrium at the level of the 3rd costal cartilage. It has no valves.

Relations

Its lower half, covered by fibrous and serous pericardium, lies behind the right lung, pleura and manubrium, and anterior to the right lung root. The ascending aorta and right brachiocephalic artery are medial to it; the pleura and right lung are lateral. Its only tributary, the azygos vein, enters posteriorly.

Determination of **right atrial pressure** is important in the management of the critically ill patient, and can be measured by a catheter introduced into the internal jugular or subclavian vein via the superior vena cava into the right atrium (central venous pressure line, p. 361). **Obstruction of the superior vena cava** by tumour leads to diversion of its venous blood into subcutaneous veins of the chest wall and, via them, into veins of the anterior abdominal wall. From there the diverted blood drains into the IVC and azygos system of veins.

Azygos vein

The azygos vein is formed in the abdomen in front of the 2nd lumbar vertebra and passes into the chest via the aortic opening in the diaphragm, lying to the right of the aorta. It ascends the posterior mediastinum on the vertebral bodies. At the level of the 4th thoracic vertebra it arches over the right lung root anteriorly to enter the superior vena cava (Fig. 3.6d,e).

Tributaries

It and the smaller left-sided hemiazygos vein drain the intercostal spaces and the right bronchial veins.

The inferior vena cava has a very short intrathoracic course. It pierces the central tendon of the diaphragm and directly enters the right atrium.

NERVES

The phrenic nerves

The phrenic nerves arise from the ventral rami of C3, 4 and 5 and descend from the neck through the thorax in front of each lung root (Fig. 3.6g). The right phrenic nerve enters the thorax lateral to the right brachiocephalic vein, descends on the pericardium over the superior vena cava, right atrium and inferior vena cava, and passes through the caval opening of the diaphragm. Throughout it is covered laterally by mediastinal pleura. The left phrenic nerve enters between the left subclavian artery and left brachiocephalic vein, descending across the aortic arch and pericardium over the left ventricle to reach and pierce the left diaphragm. It is covered laterally by mediastinal pleura.

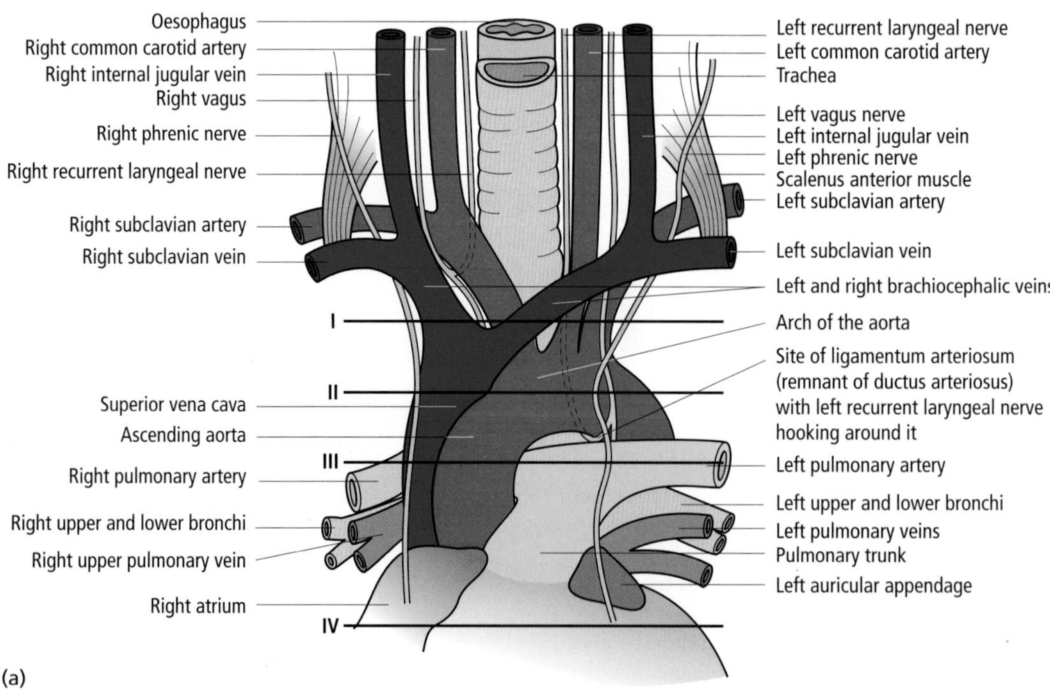

Figure 3.6 (a) Anterior aspect of the thorax showing mediastinal structures: I, II, III and IV are axial planes as shown in parts (b)–(i) opposite

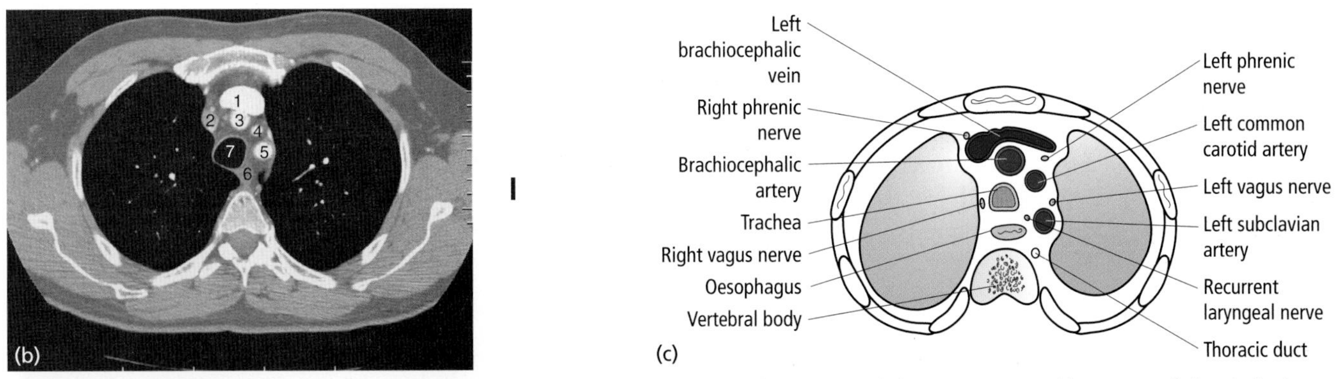

(b) 1, Left brachiocephalic vein; 2, right brachiocephalic vein; 3, brachiocephalic artery; 4, left common carotid artery; 5, left subclavian artery; 6, oesophagus; 7, trachea

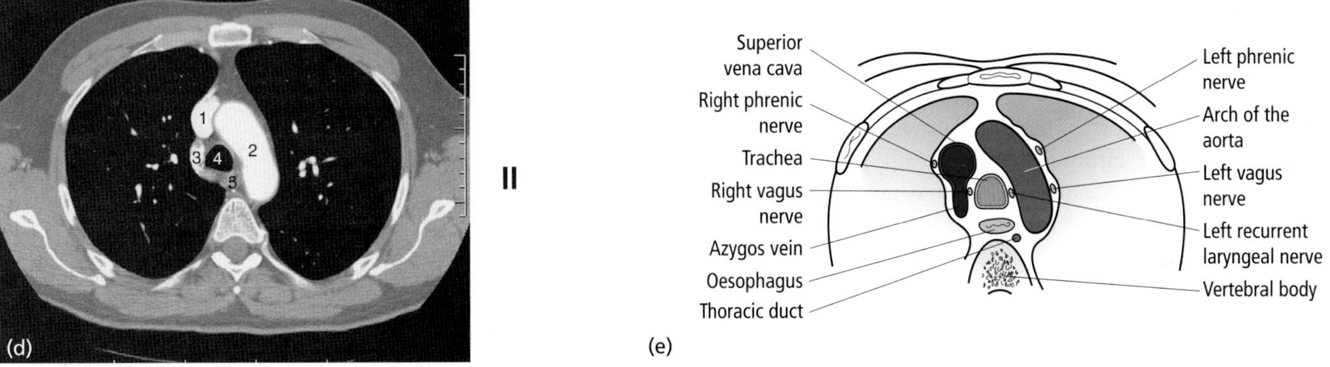

(d) 1, Superior vena cava; 2, arch of aorta; 3, azygos vein; 4, trachea; 5, oesophagus

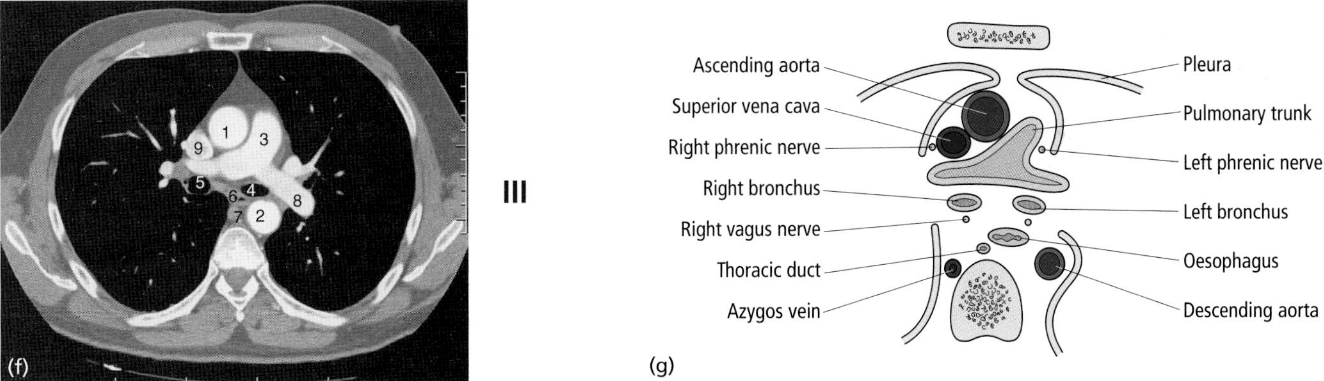

(f) 1, Ascending aorta; 2, descending aorta; 3, pulmonary trunk (artery); 4, left bronchus; 5, right bronchus; 6, oesophagus; 7, azygos vein; 8, left pulmonary artery; 9, superior vena cava

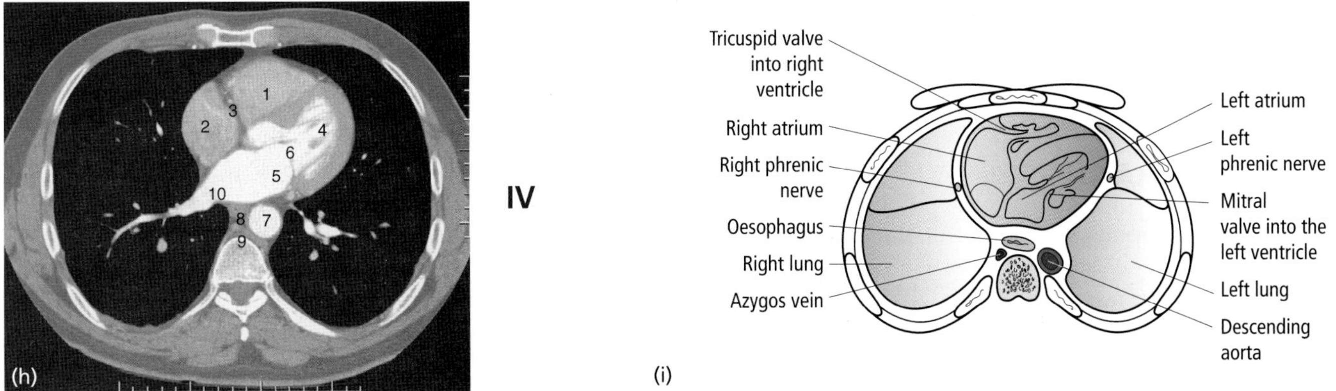

(h) 1, Right ventricle; 2, right atrium; 3, tricuspid valve; 4, left ventricle; 5, left atrium; 6, mitral valve; 7, descending aorta; 8, oesophagus; 9, azygos vein; 10, right pulmonary vein.

Figure 3.6 (*continued*) (b)-(i) transverse sections (CT scans and accompanying diagrams) at levels I–IV (shown on Fig. 3.6a) through the mediastinum

Both nerves are motor to the diaphragm and supply sensory branches to the mediastinal and diaphragmatic pleura, the pericardium and the peritoneum.

Pain arising from inflammation of the diaphragmatic pleura is classically referred to skin over the shoulder tip, which is supplied by nerves derived, like the phrenic nerve, from the C4 spinal segment.

The vagus nerves

The right vagus enters the thorax posterolateral to the right brachiocephalic artery and descends lateral to the trachea under the mediastinal pleura to the back of the right main bronchus, where it gives branches, first to the pulmonary plexus and then to the oesophageal plexus. The left vagus enters the thorax between the left common carotid and subclavian arteries and descends across the left of the aortic arch, where it gives off its recurrent laryngeal branch, before passing behind the left lung root to the oesophagus. The two vagi form the oesophageal plexus, from which emerge anterior and posterior gastric nerves (anterior and posterior vagal trunks) containing fibres of both vagi and sympathetic nerves, which descend to pass through the oesophageal opening of the diaphragm. The nerves supply the stomach, duodenum, pancreas and liver, and contribute branches via the coeliac plexus to other viscera (see pp. 67–9).

Branches

The left recurrent laryngeal nerve winds around the ligamentum arteriosum and aortic arch and ascends between the trachea and oesophagus into the neck (Fig. 3.6a), providing cardiac branches to the cardiac plexus (p. 67) and branches to the pulmonary and oesophageal plexuses (Fig. 2.2, p. 36).

THE THYMUS

The thymus, a bilobed mass of lymphoid tissue, lies in front of the trachea, extending downwards posterior to the manubrium. It may enlarge into the lower neck and upper thorax. Larger at birth, it atrophies after puberty, but is variable in size and so may extend down below the aortic arch to the anterior mediastinum (Fig. 3.7).

Occasionally the **thymus** may develop a tumour – a thymoma – which may be associated with myasthenia gravis and require surgical removal.

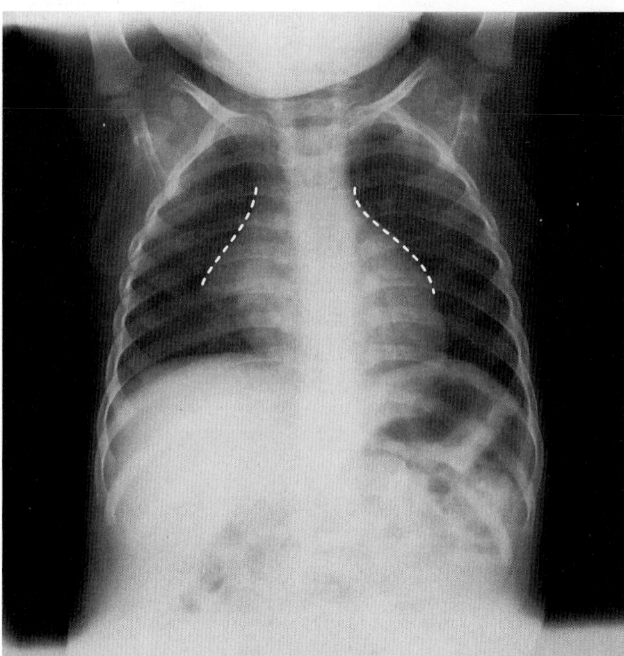

Figure 3.7 Chest X-ray of child, showing normal variant of a relatively large thymus (dashed lines)

THE OESOPHAGUS

The oesophagus begins at the level of the cricoid cartilage (Figs 3.3 and 3.6b–i). Its cervical portion lies in the midline on the prevertebral fascia (see also p. 345) then it descends through the thorax mainly to the left of the midline. Initially close to the vertebral column, it curves forward in its lower part and pierces the diaphragm surrounded by fibres of its right crus at the level of the 10th thoracic vertebra. Its intra-abdominal portion is about 2 cm long and the overall length is 25 cm.

Relations

In the upper mediastinum it lies between the vertebral column posteriorly and the trachea anteriorly, the left recurrent laryngeal nerve lying in the groove between it and the trachea. Below it is separated from the vertebral column by the thoracic duct, the azygos and hemiazygos veins and the aorta. Anteriorly, below the trachea it is crossed by the left bronchus, and below this it is separated from the left atrium by the pericardium. On the right it is covered by mediastinal pleura and the azygos vein; on the left, from above, the aortic arch, the subclavian artery and the descending aorta separate it from mediastinal pleura. Its lower part is in contact with the pleura.

Lymphatic drainage

The cervical oesophagus drains to the deep cervical lymph nodes, the thoracic portion drains to the tracheobronchial and posterior mediastinal nodes and its abdominal portion to the left gastric nodes.

Radiological examination of the oesophagus is achieved by having the patient swallow barium (Fig. 2.5, p. 37). It usually reveals slight constrictions where it is crossed by the aortic arch and the left bronchus and as it passes through the diaphragm. In patients with heart failure the oesophagus will be seen to be compressed by the enlarged left atrium. More direct examination of its luminal surface is obtained by endoscopy (Fig. 6.2, p. 90). **Oesophagoscopy**, whether performed with a rigid or a flexible oesophagoscope, is facilitated by knowledge that, in the adult, its origin is 15 cm from the incisor teeth, and the oesophagogastric junction is usually 40 cm from that point.

THE THORACIC TRACHEA AND BRONCHI

The trachea commences in the neck just below the cricoid cartilage; it lies in the midline and descends into the superior mediastinum, bifurcating into two main bronchi at the upper border of the 5th thoracic vertebra. Its cervical portion is described on page 351. In the chest the left recurrent laryngeal nerve lies in the groove between it and the oesophagus. Its walls, like those of the main bronchi, are strengthened by U-shaped incomplete rings of cartilage. Anteriorly the brachiocephalic artery and the left brachiocephalic vein cross it; on its left lie the common carotid and subclavian arteries, and below them the aortic arch; on the right the right vagus nerve and azygos vein separate it from the pleura.

The tracheal bifurcation (carina) lies at the level of the sternal angle and the lower border of the 4th thoracic vertebra, anterior to the oesophagus and to the right of the pulmonary trunk bifurcation (Fig. 3.6a,g).

The extrapulmonary bronchi

The right and left main bronchi arise at the bifurcation and descend laterally to enter the hilus of the lung, where they divide to form the intrapulmonary bronchial tree. The right bronchus, 3 cm long, is wider and more vertical than the left. The right upper lobe bronchus arises before it enters the hilus.

Relations

Anteriorly, the left pulmonary artery separates the carina from the left atrium; the aortic arch lies above it, and posteriorly lie the oesophagus and descending thoracic aorta.

Because the **trachea** contains air it is recognized on chest X-rays as a radiolucent (dark) structure descending backwards and slightly to the right in the upper mediastinum. It may be compressed or displaced by enlargement of the thyroid gland. Widening or distortion of the carina may result from enlargement of the tracheobronchial lymph nodes or secondary spread of lung cancer. Inhaled foreign bodies tend to pass more frequently to the wider, more vertical right bronchus (Fig. 3.8). Direct viewing of the trachea and proximal bronchi is possible endoscopically. Instillation of a radio-opaque medium, e.g. lipiodol, into the bronchi, permits a radiograph of the bronchial tree to be obtained (Figs 4.9 and 4.10, p. 63). Bronchial cancer commonly produces symptoms of ulceration and bleeding, obstruction of the bronchi and production of blood-stained sputum.

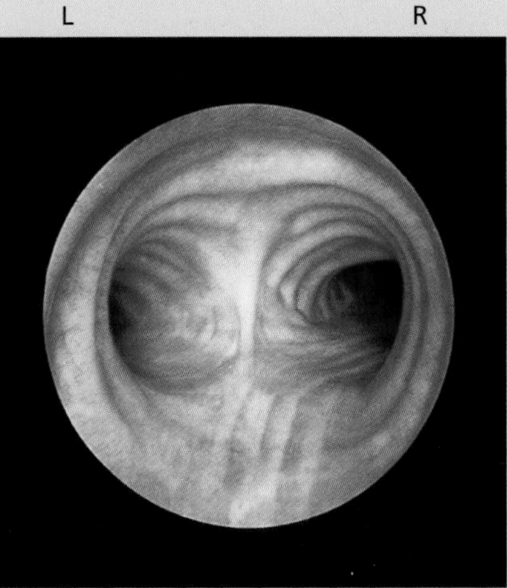

Figure 3.8 The cartilaginous rings indent the mucosa of trachea and carina as seen down the endoscope. Note the wider right bronchus lies more vertically and thus descends more directly and less obliquely. It is into this bronchus that inhaled foreign bodies get lodged

MCQs

1. The left phrenic nerve: **T/F**

- **a** arises from the dorsal rami of C3,4 and C5 cervical nerves (___)
- **b** descends through the thorax in the left pleural cavity (___)
- **c** conveys sensory fibres from the mediastinal and diaphragmatic pleura and from the diaphragmatic peritoneum (___)
- **d** leaves the abdomen through the caval opening of the diaphragm (___)
- **e** descends the thorax posterior to the root of the lung (___)

Answers

1.

- ***a*** ***F*** – *It arises from the ventral rami of these nerves.*
- ***b*** ***F*** – *It descends within the mediastinum covered by the left mediastinal pleura.*
- ***c*** ***T*** – *It also supplies motor branches to the diaphragm.*
- ***d*** ***F*** – *The left phrenic nerve pierces the dome of the diaphragm, giving branches to its undersurface. It is the right phrenic nerve that passes through the caval opening of the diaphragm.*
- ***e*** ***F*** – *Both phrenic nerves pass anterior to the root of the lung.*

---

2. The pulmonary trunk: **T/F**

- **a** lies anterior to the aortic root (___)
- **b** is contained with the ascending aorta (___) in a common sleeve of serous pericardium
- **c** bifurcates anterior to the aortic arch (___)
- **d** is in contact with the left pleura (___)
- **e** is closely related to both right and left coronary arteries (___)

Answers

2.

- ***a*** ***T*** – *It then ascends posteriorly and to the left …*
- ***b*** ***T*** – *… and both are also within the fibrous pericardium.*
- ***c*** ***F*** – *It lies within the concavity of the aortic arch and hence posterior and to the left of the ascending aorta.*
- ***d*** ***T*** – *Both its anterior and left surfaces are covered, with the left pleura covering the lung.*
- ***e*** ***T*** – *Both vessels surround its base.*

---

3. The thoracic oesophagus: **T/F**

- **a** is posterior to the trachea (___)
- **b** is directly related to the vertebral column throughout its course (___)
- **c** is related to the left atrium (___)
- **d** pierces the central tendon of the diaphragm at the level of the 8th thoracic vertebra (___)
- **e** is crossed anteriorly by the left bronchus (___)

Answers

3.

- ***a*** ***T*** – *With the left recurrent laryngeal and right vagus nerves lying between it and the trachea.*
- ***b*** ***F*** – *It is so related in its upper part, but inferiorly it is separated from the vertebral column by the thoracic duct, the azygos and hemiazygos veins and the thoracic aorta.*
- ***c*** ***T*** – *Only separated from it by the pericardium.*
- ***d*** ***F*** – *The oesophagus pierces the right crus of the diaphragm to the left of the midline at the level of the 10th thoracic vertebra.*
- ***e*** ***T*** – *The left bronchus crosses the middle of the oesophagus anteriorly.*

EMQs

Each question has an anatomical theme linked to the chapter, and a list of 10 related items (A–J) placed in alphabetical order: these are followed by five statements (1–5). Match **one or more** of the items A–J to each of the five statements.

Mediastinal structures

A. Aortic arch
B. Ascending aorta
C. Brachiocephalic artery
D. Descending thoracic aorta
E. Left brachiocephalic vein
F. Left carotid artery
G. Left vagus nerve
H. Right phrenic nerve
I. Right subclavian artery
J. Superior vena cava

Match the following statements with the appropriate item(s) from the above list.

1. Related to the medial side of the superior vena cava
2. Related to the left side of the trachea
3. Lies to the left of the oesophagus
4. Lies posterior to the oesophagus
5. Posterior to the left brachiocephalic vein

Answers

1 AB; 2 AFG; 3 DG; 4 D; 5 CF

APPLIED QUESTIONS

1. During a barium swallow what anatomical structures, in their normal or pathological states, may cause indentation of the oesophagus on an oblique view?

1. Oblique X-rays of a barium swallow may reveal three normal impressions on the oesophageal silhouette, caused by the aortic arch, the left main bronchus and the right crus of the diaphragm. Each impression indicates where swallowed foreign objects may lodge and where a stricture may develop after the accidental or suicidal swallowing of a caustic liquid. Pathological compressions may be observed from a dilated left atrium, an aberrant aortic arch or an aberrant right subclavian artery passing retro-oesophageally.

---

2. Why do the trachea and the main bronchi not collapse during the negative pressure of inspiration?

2. The consistent diameters of the trachea and main bronchi are due to the strengthening cartilaginous bands and incomplete rings, which maintain their shape even during inspiration. The walls of the trachea are supported by 15–20 U-shaped bands of hyaline cartilage.

---

3. A young boy throws a peanut in the air and, in attempting to catch it in his mouth, inhales it. Into which bronchus is it likely to pass?

3. It is most likely to be inhaled into the right main bronchus, which is shorter, wider and nearly in the same line as the trachea. Once inhaled, material such as peanuts, pins or even gastric contents, tend to pass into the right middle or lower lobes. However, in the unconscious patient lying on his right side, inhaled material frequently collects in the posterior segment of the right upper lobe.

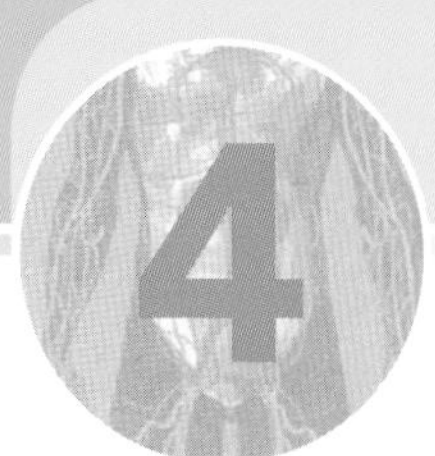

The pleura and lungs

THE PLEURA

The pleura is a fibroelastic serous membrane lined by squamous epithelium forming a sac on each side of the chest. Each pleural sac is a closed cavity invaginated by a lung. Parietal pleura lines the chest wall and visceral (pulmonary) pleura covers the lungs. These two pleural layers are continuous around the root of the lung and are separated by a thin film of serous fluid, permitting them to glide easily on each other. The layers are prevented from separating by the fluid's surface tension and the negative pressure in the thoracic cavity. Thus when the thoracic cage expands the lung also must expand, and air is inhaled.

Parietal pleura lines the ribs, costal cartilages, intercostal spaces, the lateral surface of the mediastinum and the diaphragm's upper surface. Superiorly it extends above the thoracic inlet into the neck as the cervical dome of pleura; inferiorly, around the margin of the diaphragm, it forms a narrow gutter, the **costodiaphragmatic recess;** anteriorly, the left costal and mediastinal surfaces are in contact extending in front of the heart to form the **costomediastinal recess.** Mediastinal pleura invests the main bronchi and pulmonary vessels and passes on to the surface of the lung to become visceral pleura, which covers the lung and extends into its interlobar fissures.

The **surface markings** of the pleural sacs should be noted (Figs 4.1 and 4.2). On both sides the upper limit lies about 3 cm above the medial third of the clavicle. From here the lines of pleural reflections descend behind the sternoclavicular joints to almost meet in the midline at the level of the 2nd costal cartilage. At the 4th costal cartilage, whereas the left pleura deviates laterally and descends along the lateral border of the sternum to the 6th costal cartilage, the right pleural reflection continues down, near to the midline, to the 6th costal cartilage. At this point, on both sides, the pleural reflections pass laterally behind the costal margin to reach the 8th rib in the midclavicular line, the 10th rib in the midaxillary line, and along the 12th rib and the paravertebral line (lying over the tips of the transverse processes, about 3 cm from the midline).

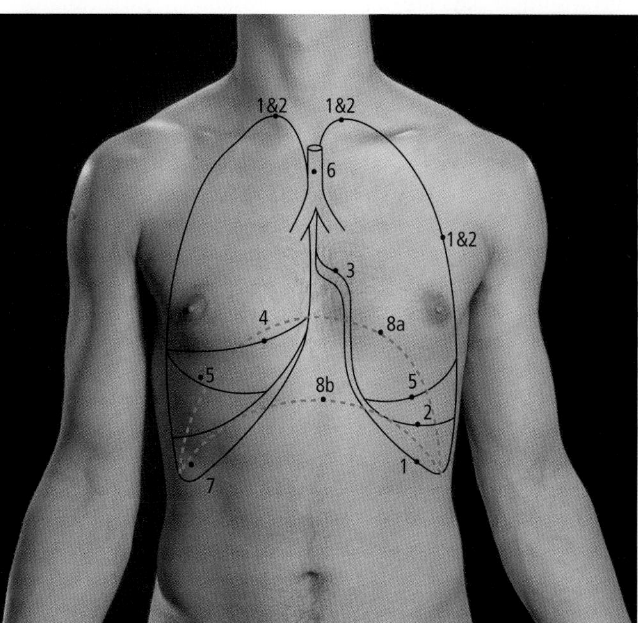

Figure 4.1 Surface markings of pleura and lungs, anterior aspect: 1, pleural markings; 2, lung markings; 3, cardiac notch; 4, horizontal fissure; 5, oblique fissure; 6, trachea; 7, costodiaphragmatic recess; 8, diaphragm, (a) inspiration, (b) expiration

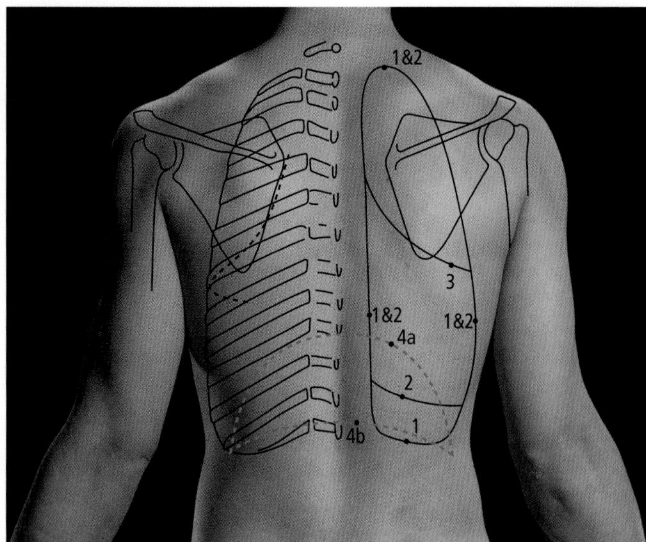

Figure 4.2 Surface markings of pleura and lungs, posterior aspect: 1, pleural markings; 2, lung markings; 3, oblique fissure; 4, diaphragm, (a) inspiration, (b) expiration. Dotted line shows incision for opening chest through 5th intercostal space

Visceral pleura has no pain fibres but the parietal pleura is richly supplied by branches of the somatic intercostal and phrenic nerves. Lymph from the pulmonary pleura passes to a superficial plexus in the lung and then to the hilar nodes. Parietal pleura drains to the parasternal, diaphragmatic and posterior mediastinal nodes.

The pleural sac is a potential space which in pathological conditions can fill with fluid or air; with blood after intrathoracic haemorrhage (**haemothorax**); inflammatory exudate (pleural **effusion**) or pus (**pyothorax**) (Fig. 4.3); or with air (**pneumothorax**) (Fig. 1.6, p. 26) after chest wall trauma that has torn the lung or the rupture of a lung bulla which has burst the visceral pleura. A distended pleural cavity may interfere with lung expansion. Fluid may be drained from the pleural cavity by insertion of a needle or tube attached to an underwater seal, into the 7th intercostal space in the midaxillary line (Figs 1.7a and 1.9, p. 27). Insertion below this level runs the risk of the needle penetrating the diaphragm and the underlying liver or spleen. To avoid danger to the neurovascular bundle it is best to insert the needle along the top of the rib, which avoids the vessels lying in the subcostal groove. Emergency aspiration of air is most safely achieved by inserting a needle, attached to an underwater seal or flutter valve, into the 2nd or 3rd intercostal space in the midclavicular line.

Punch biopsy needles inserted through the intercostal space allow specimens of pleura to be obtained for histological examination. **Pleurisy** – inflammation of the pleura – causes pain that is magnified by respiratory movements. The pain is referred by sensory fibres within the parietal pleura to the cutaneous distribution of the nerve supplying it. Thus costal inflammation is referred to the chest wall or, in the case of lower nerves, to the upper abdominal wall, and inflammation of the diaphragmatic pleura is referred to the area supplied by the nerve root (C4) from which originates the phrenic nerve, i.e. the tip of the shoulder.

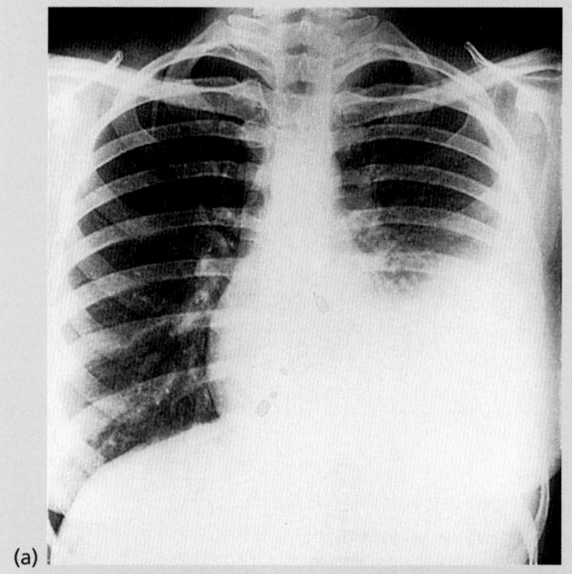

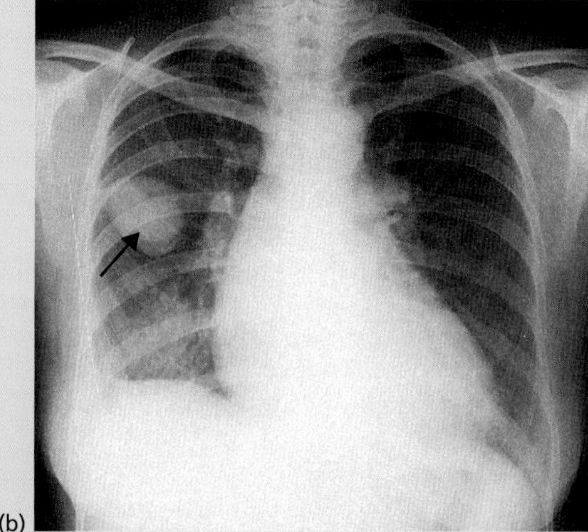

Figure 4.3 (a) Left pleural effusion obliterating much of the lower lung markings; (b) localized interlobar fluid collection (arrow)

THE LUNGS

These paired organs lie in separate pleural sacs attached to the mediastinum at the hila (Figs 4.1, 4.6 and 4.7). Spongy and elastic in composition, they conform to the contours of the thoracic cavity. The right lung weighs about 620 g and the left about 560 g. They have a characteristic mottled appearance on radiographs – lung tissue is clear; denser shadows at the hilus are caused by hilar lymph nodes, and radiating shadows by blood vessels. A PA chest X-ray will also reveal the normal aortic arch (knuckle), the inferior vena cava and the outline of the heart. A lateral view reveals details of the mediastinal structures (Figs 4.4 and 4.5).

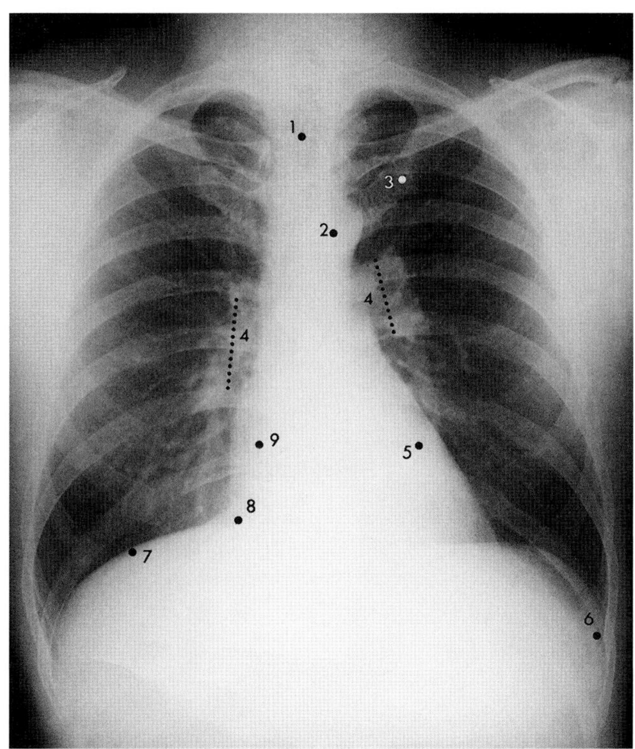

Figure 4.4 Radiograph of chest: 1, trachea; 2, aortic knuckle; 3, 1st costochondral junction; 4, hilar shadows; 5, left ventricle; 6, left costodiaphragmatic recess; 7, right dome of diaphragm; 8, inferior vena cava; 9, right atrium

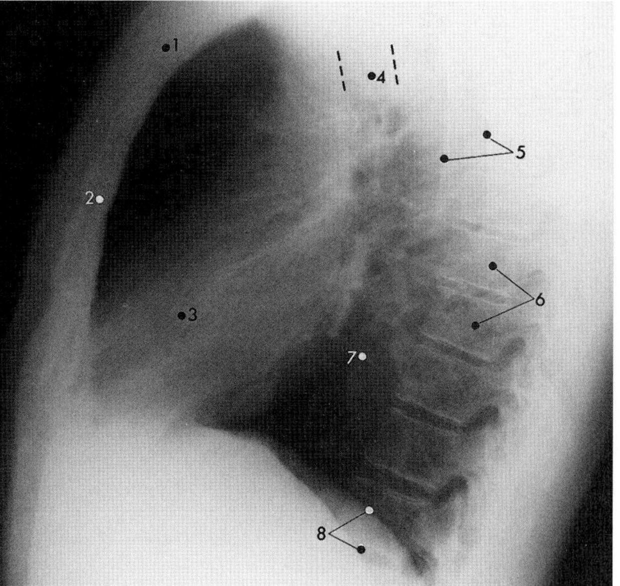

Figure 4.5 Lateral chest X-ray showing mediastinal structures: 1, manubriosternal joint; 2, sternum; 3, cardiac shadow; 4, trachea; 5, border of scapula; 6, vertebral bodies; 7, retrocardiac space; 8, domes of diaphragm

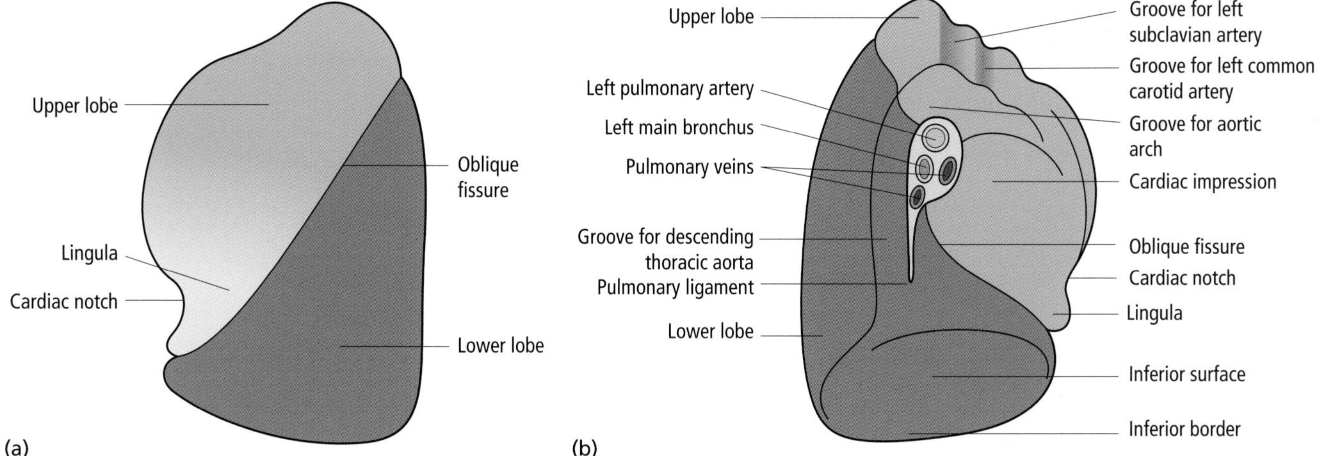

Figure 4.6 Left lung: (a) lateral surface; (b) medial surface

Each lung has an apex in the root of the neck and a base resting on the diaphragm. The base is separated by a sharp inferior border from a lateral convex costal surface and a medial concave mediastinal surface, in the centre of which are the structures of the lung root surrounded by a cuff of pleura (Figs 4.6 and 4.7). The deeper concavity of the left lung accommodates the heart's left ventricle. The left lung's anterior border is deeply indented by the heart to form the cardiac notch; the rounded posterior border of each lung lies in the paravertebral sulcus.

The lungs are each divided by fissures extending deeply into their substance. An **oblique fissure** divides the left lung into an upper and lower lobe (Fig. 4.6); **oblique and horizontal fissures** divide the right lung into upper, middle and lower lobes (Fig. 4.7). The oblique fissure on each side can be marked by a line around the chest wall from the spine of the 3rd thoracic vertebra to the 6th costochondral junction. The horizontal fissure is marked by a horizontal line passing from the 4th right costal cartilage to the oblique line previously drawn (Figs 4.1 and 4.2). The **lower lobes** of both lungs lie

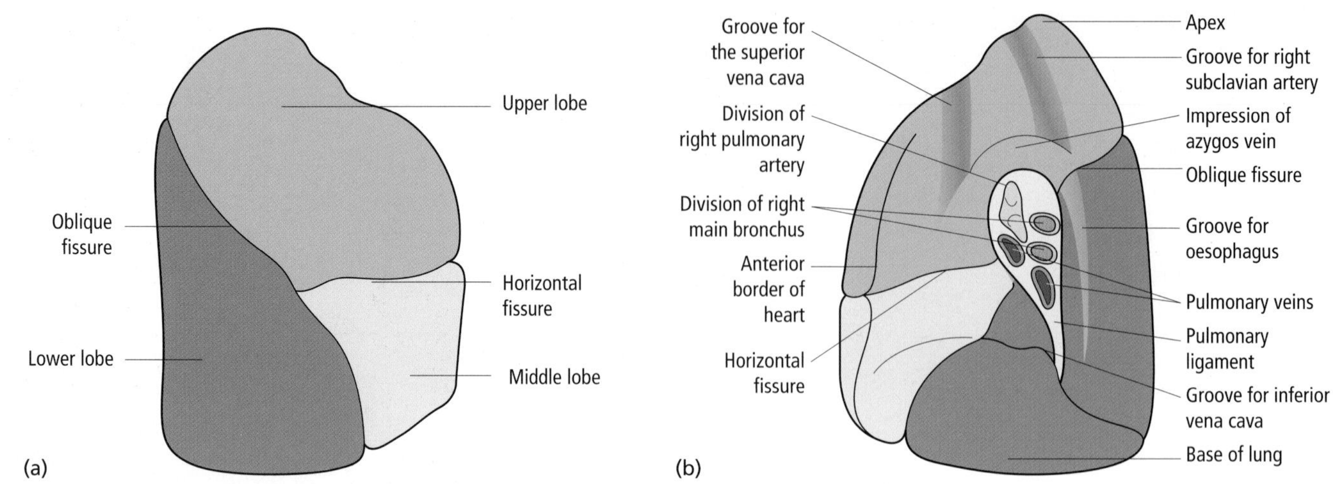

Figure 4.7 Right lung: (a) lateral surface; (b) medial surface

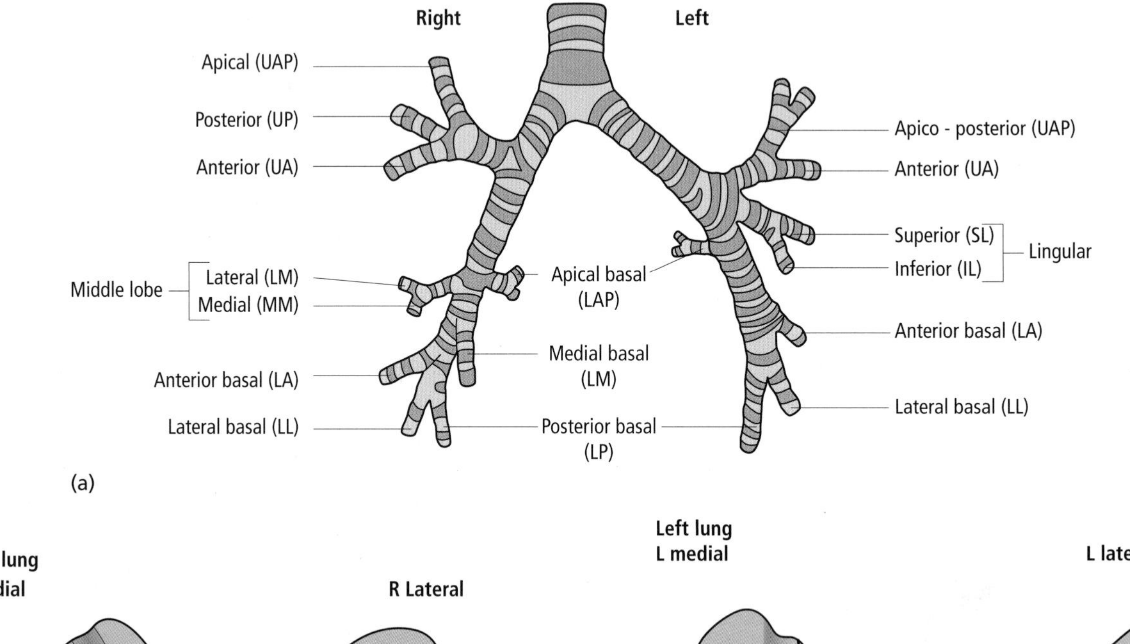

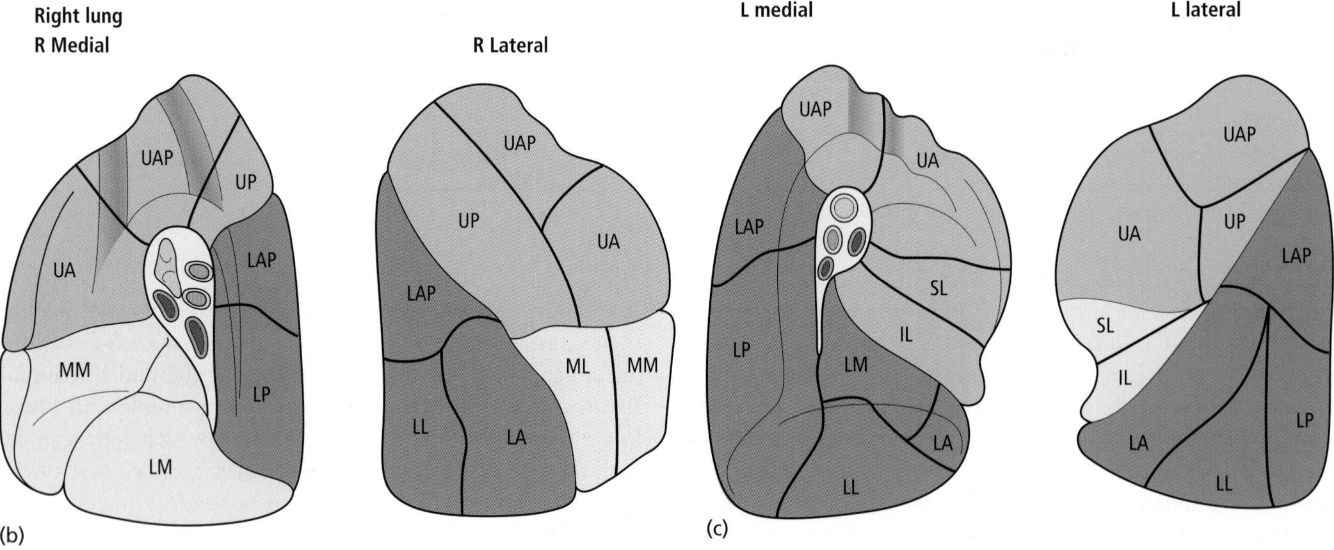

Figure 4.8 (a) Bronchial tree. (b) and (c) Bronchopulmonary segments; (b) right lung – mediastinal and costovertebral surfaces; (c) left lung – medial and lateral surfaces

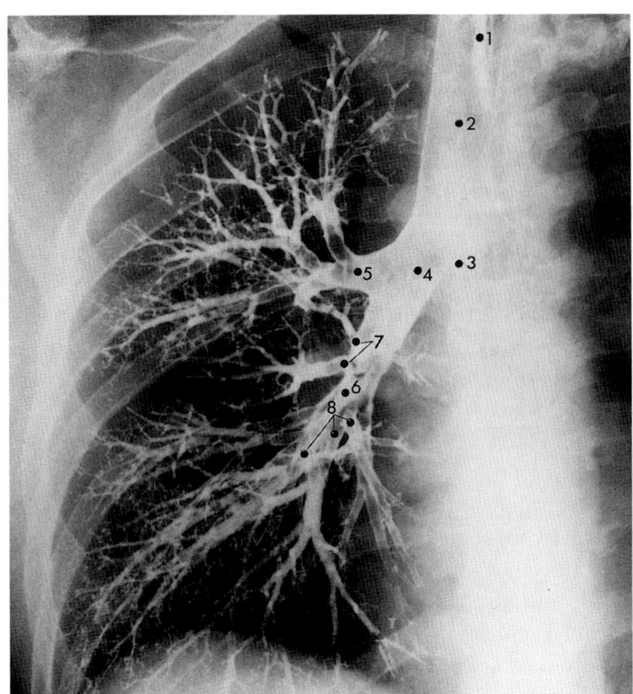

Figure 4.9 Bronchogram of right lung, anteroposterior view: 1, intubation catheter; 2, trachea, 3, carina; 4, right main bronchus; 5, right upper lobe bronchus; 6, right middle lobe bronchus; 7, right apical lower lobe bronchi; 8, right basal lower lobe bronchi

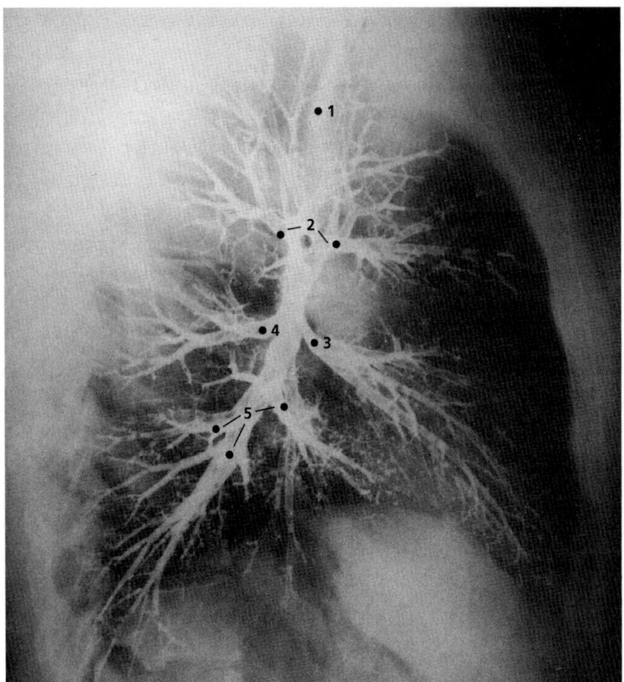

Figure 4.10 Bronchogram of right lung, lateral view: 1, trachea; 2, right upper lobe bronchi; 3, right middle lobe bronchus; 4, right apical lower lobe bronchus; 5, right basal lower lobe bronchi

below and behind the oblique fissure and comprise most of the posterior and inferior borders. The **upper lobe** of the left lung is above and anterior to the oblique fissure and includes the apex and most of the mediastinal and costal surfaces. The equivalent part of the right lung is divided by the horizontal fissure into a large upper lobe and a smaller, anterior, wedge-shaped **middle lobe,** which lies deep to the right breast. A thin anteroinferior part of the left upper lobe, adjacent to the cardiac notch, is known as the **lingula** and is the left-sided equivalent of the middle lobe. Fissures may be incomplete or absent, and occasionally additional lobes are present.

The **hilum** or root of each lung contains a main bronchus, a pulmonary artery, two pulmonary veins, the pulmonary nerve plexus and lymph nodes, all enveloped by the pleural cuff; an inferior narrow extension of the cuff is known as the pulmonary ligament (Figs 4.6 and 4.7). The bronchus lies behind the pulmonary artery and the two veins are below and anterior.

The intrapulmonary bronchi and bronchopulmonary segments

Each main bronchus descends to enter the hilum of the lung: that of the right side is shorter, wider and more vertical than the left with the result that aspiration of foreign bodies is more common on the right side. Each main bronchus divides into **lobar bronchi,** which further divide into **segmental bronchi,** each supplying **bronchopulmonary segments.** Each lung contains ten such segments. The right upper lobe bronchus arises from the right main bronchus before the hilum and, after entering the lung substance, divides into apical, anterior and posterior segmental bronchi (Fig. 4.8a–c). The middle lobe bronchus arises beyond this and divides into medial and lateral segmental bronchi. The continuation of the right main bronchus passes to the lower lobe and divides into apical, anterior, medial, lateral and posterior basal segmental bronchi. The left upper lobe bronchus arises from the main bronchus within the lung and divides into five segmental bronchi, the anterior and inferior passing to the lingula. The continuation of the left bronchus passes to the lower lobe and also, similar to the right side, divides into five segmental bronchi. Each segmental bronchus is divided into a functionally independent unit of lung tissue with its own vascular supply – a **bronchopulmonary segment** (Figs 4.8–4.10). The walls of the bronchi are lined with smooth muscle and hyaline cartilage, and lined by pseudostratified columnar epithelium and mucous glands. Their thin terminal branches, the bronchioles, contain no cartilage and are lined by non-ciliated columnar epithelium.

The comatose or anaesthetized patient is subject to a particular risk of aspiration and such material will gravitate to the most dependent, posterior part of the lung. The apical segment of the lower lobe is supplied by the highest, most posterior of the segmental bronchi and it is, therefore, this segment (particularly the right) that is the commonest site for aspiration pneumonia in these patients.

Relations

The lung borders closely follow the lines of pleural reflection on the chest wall, except inferiorly, where the lower border of the lung lies about two intercostal spaces above the pleural reflection (costodiaphragmatic recess), and in front where, near to the cardiac notch, the anterior border of the left lung lies some 3 cm lateral to the pleural reflection (costomediastinal recess) (Figs 4.1 and 4.2). The costal surfaces are related to the thoracic wall; the base is separated by the diaphragm from the right lobe of the liver on the right, and the liver, stomach and spleen on the left. The apex, covered by the dome of the pleura, lies under the suprapleural membrane, a fibrous sheet extending from the transverse process of the 7th cervical vertebra to the inner border of the 1st rib. The subclavian vessels arch over the membrane. Posteriorly lie the anterior primary ramus of the first thoracic nerve, passing to the brachial plexus, and the sympathetic trunk, both lying on the neck of the 1st rib.

The **medial** relations differ on each side. On the left (Figs 4.6b and 4.11) a large concavity for the left ventricle continues superiorly with a groove for the aortic arch, which passes in front of the hilum. Above the arch the lung is in contact, from before backwards, with the left brachiocephalic vein, left common carotid artery, left subclavian artery and oesophagus. On the right (Figs 4.7b and 4.12) a shallow concavity in front of the hilum for the right atrium is continuous above with a groove for the superior vena cava, and below with a shorter groove for the inferior vena cava. The azygos vein grooves the lung as it arches forwards above the hilum. The oesophagus is in contact throughout its length near to the posterior border, except where the azygos vein separates it from the lung. The oesophagus lies between the superior vena cava and the trachea.

Blood supply

Lung tissue is supplied by the bronchial arteries – branches of the descending aorta – and some of this blood returns to the heart via the pulmonary veins. Other bronchial veins drain to the azygos or hemiazygos veins. The pulmonary artery conveys poorly oxygenated blood to the alveoli by branches that accompany the bronchial tree. From the alveolar capillary network arise veins which accompany the bronchi to form the upper and lower pulmonary veins.

Pulmonary embolism may be a fatal condition. It is caused by large blood clots (thrombi) that originate in the deep veins of the legs or pelvis becoming dislodged and then conveyed through the right side of the heart to rest in and occlude large or segmental pulmonary arteries (Figs 3.5, p. 51, and Fig. 4.13), or worse, the pulmonary trunk. The result is partial or complete obstruction to the arterial supply to a segment or lobe of the lung which, although ventilated, is no longer perfused with blood. If the embolus blocks the main pulmonary artery acute respiratory distress and cyanosis results and death often follows within a few minutes. Segmental emboli cause death of lung tissue, a pulmonary infarct which, if small, resolves over a few weeks.

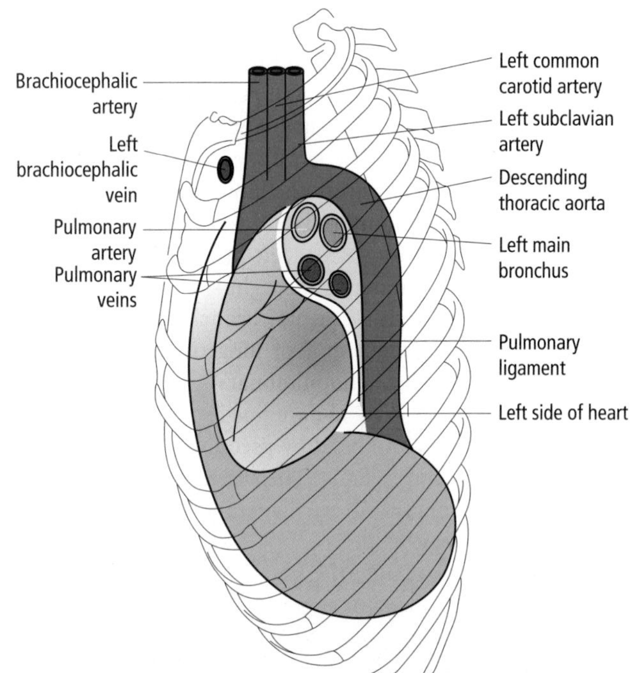

Figure 4.11 Medial relations of the left lung

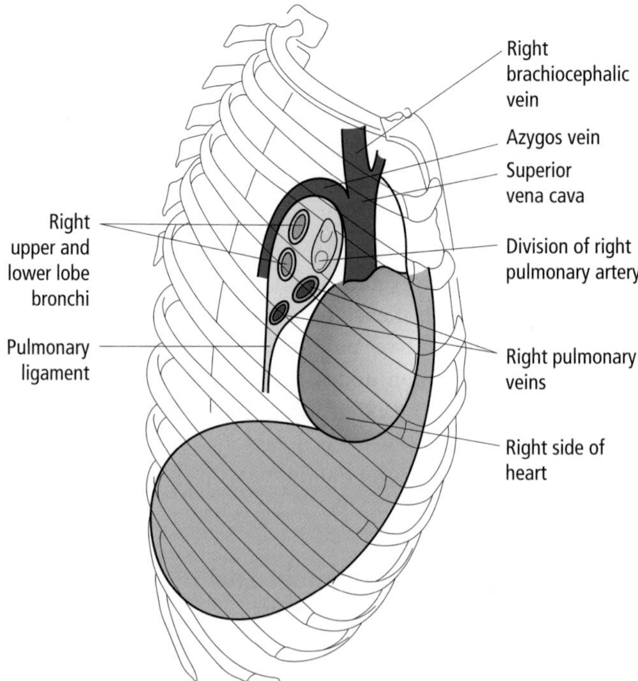

Figure 4.12 Medial relations of the right lung

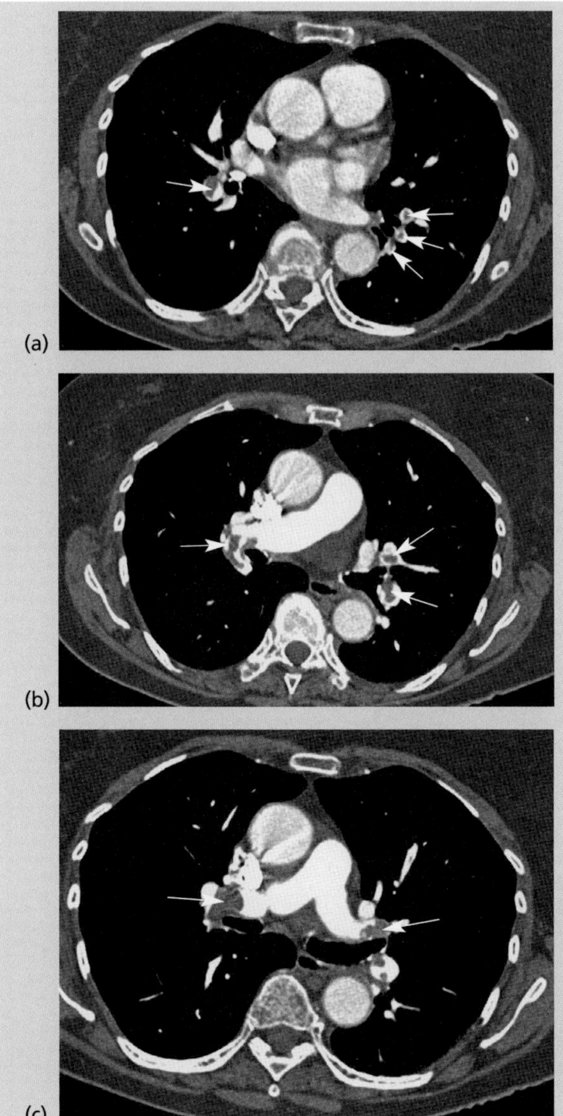

Figure 4.13 These three axial CT images show various cases of pulmonary emboli (arrowed). This is when a blood clot, often from the lower leg or pelvis, detaches and rushes through the venous side of the heart before lodging within the lungs. If as in the case of (c) it is a recently dislodged 'saddle' embolus in both pulmonary arteries – it may be fatal: (a) multiple emboli appear as darker areas within the small peripheral arteries (arrows); (b) a bilateral clot in the main pulmonary arteries; (c) bilateral large clots in both right and left pulmonary arteries

Lymphatic drainage

This is by a superficial subpleural lymph plexus and by a deep plexus of vessels accompanying the bronchi. Both groups drain through hilar (bronchopulmonary) nodes to tracheobronchial nodes around the tracheal bifurcation (carina) and thence to mediastinal lymph trunks.

Nerve supply

The lungs are supplied by sympathetic (bronchodilator) fibres from the upper thoracic segments and parasympathetic (bronchoconstrictor) fibres from the vagus. The latter provide afferent fibres for the cough reflex which is so important for clearing mucus and inhaled material. Both supply the lungs via the pulmonary plexuses (p. 67).

Radiographs of the chest allow accurate localization of disease in the lung and may also define abnormal collections of air or fluid in the pleural space (Fig. 1.6, p. 26). CT and MRI scans can improve the definition of pulmonary lesions and can be used to guide fine biopsy needles inserted percutaneously towards suspect lesions (Fig. 4.14). Radio-opaque contrast media can outline the bronchial tree (Figs 4.9 and 4.10), and radioisotopes assist in the assessment of ventilation and perfusion of lung tissue. Excision of pulmonary segments for localized disease is directly assisted by knowledge of the anatomy of the bronchopulmonary segments. This knowledge is also used to employ effective physiotherapy for the drainage of infected lung segments (Fig. 4.15a–d).

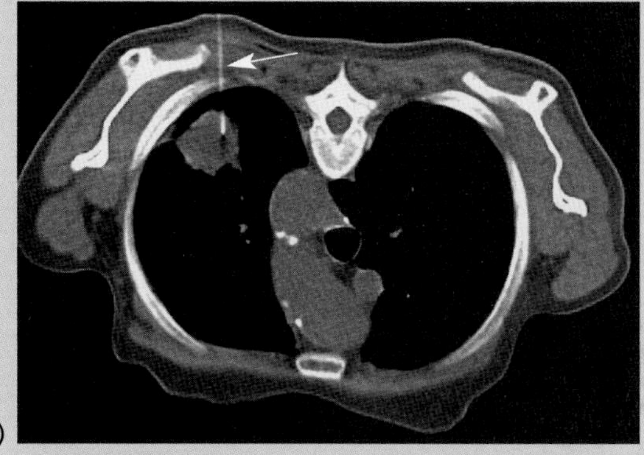

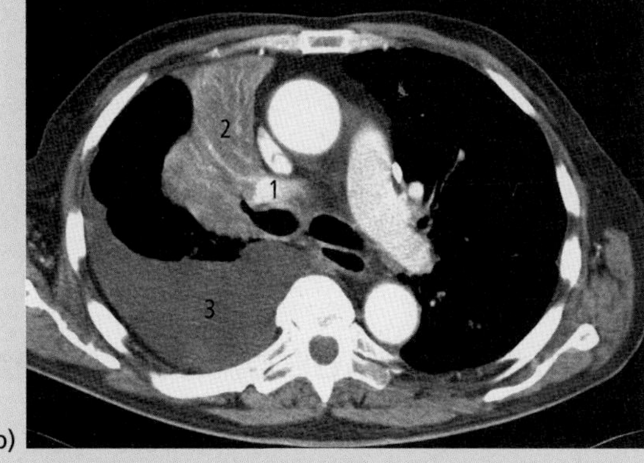

Figure 4.14 (a) Axial CT of lung biopsy into a carcinoma of an apical segment of the lower lobe, patient lying prone (arrow indicates needle). (b) CT taken at the level of the pulmonary arteries, patient lying supine. The left lung field is normal but the right contains an upper lobe carcinoma (1) just posterior to the collapsed lung (2): the posterior part of the pleural cavity is filled with a large malignant pleural effusion (3)

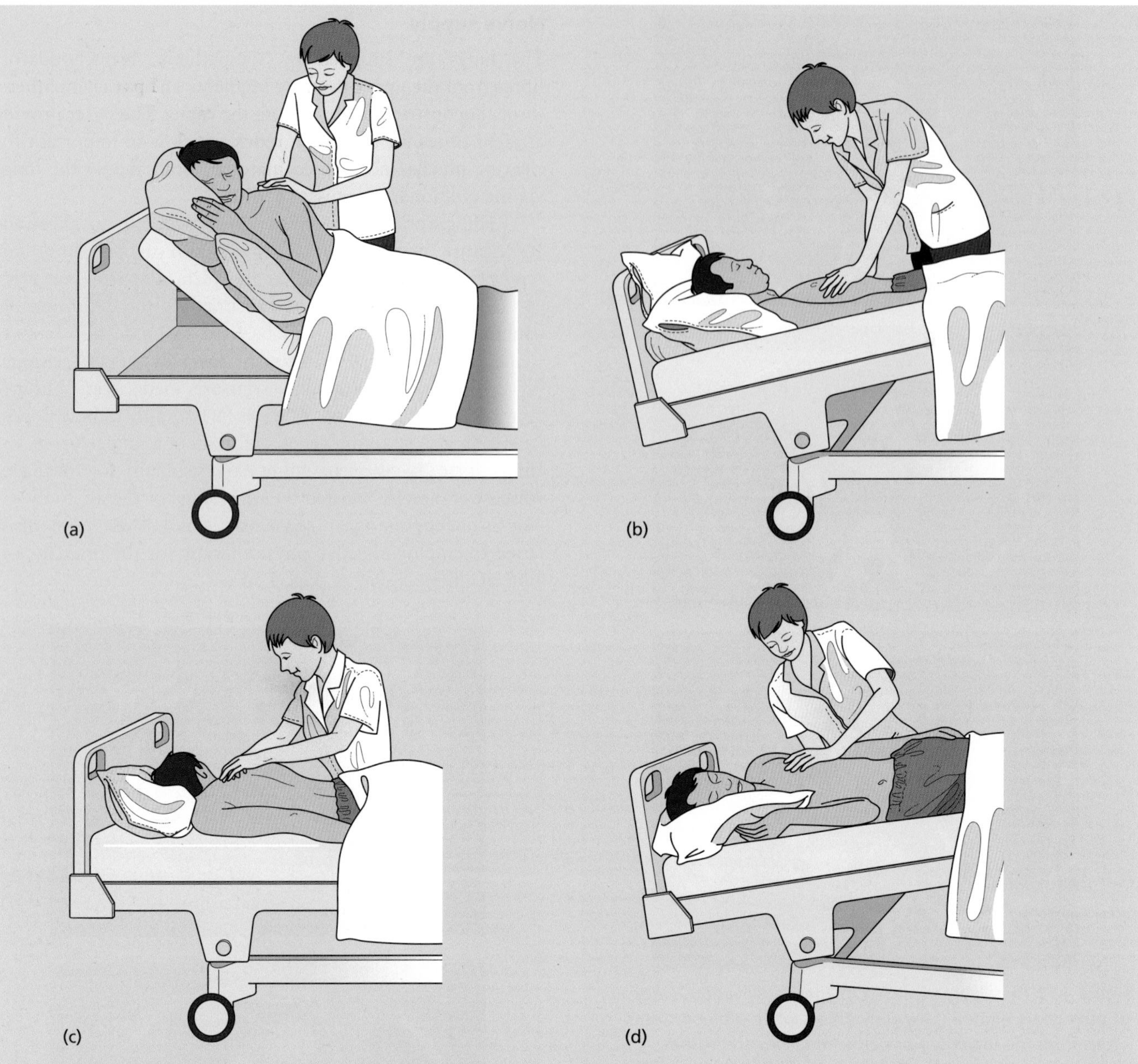

Figure 4.15 Postural drainage positions: (a) Posterior segment, left upper lobe; (b) anterior basal segments, lower lobes; (c) posterior segment, right upper lobe; (d) lingula segment, left upper lobe

LYMPHATIC DRAINAGE OF THE THORAX

There are two groups of lymph vessels in the thorax: those draining the chest wall and those of the thoracic viscera (Fig. 4.16).

The **chest wall** drains by superficial and deep systems. The superficial vessels, like those of the breast, drain to the pectoral and central groups of axillary lymph nodes. There is some communication with vessels of the opposite side.

The vessels draining the deeper chest wall drain to the:

- **Parasternal nodes** alongside the internal thoracic artery, whose efferents drain to the bronchomediastinal lymph trunk.
- **Intercostal nodes** lying at the back of the intercostal spaces, whose efferents drain to the right lymph duct and the thoracic duct.
- **Diaphragmatic nodes** on the upper surface of the diaphragm, whose efferents drain to parasternal and posterior mediastinal nodes and, through the diaphragm, to communicate with those draining the upper surface of the liver.

The **thoracic viscera** drain to the:

- **Anterior mediastinal nodes** in front of the brachiocephalic veins and drain the anterior mediastinum. Their efferents join those of the tracheobronchial nodes.

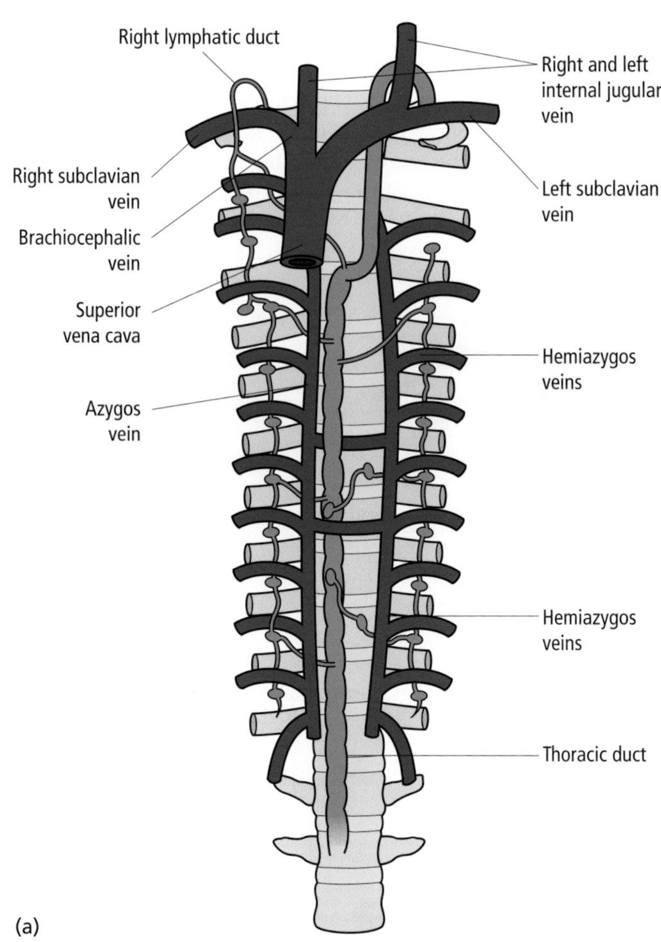

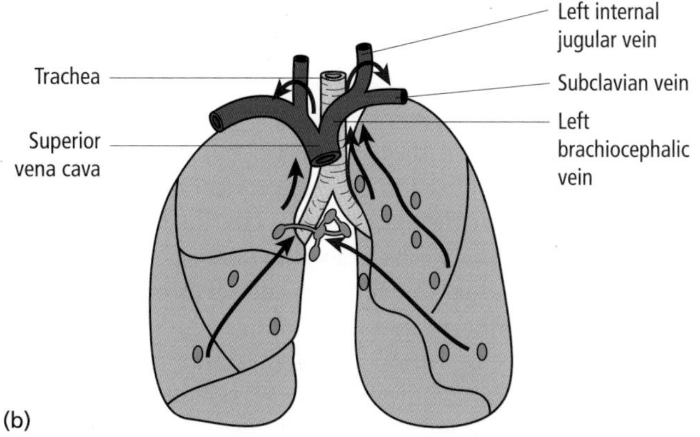

Figure 4.16 Lymphatic and venous drainage of the chest: (a) azygos system and thoracic lymphatics; (b) lymphatic and venous drainage of the lungs. Lymph nodes are situated along the course of the bronchial tree and drain to the hilar nodes and around the carina and tracheal bifurcation. Lymph from the right lung and the left lower lobe tends to follow the nodes on the right side of the trachea and from thence pass in the right mediastinal lymph duct into the right subclavian vein. Lymph from the left upper lobe follows the left side of the trachea and passes into the thoracic duct thence draining into the left subclavian vein as indicated by the arrows

- **Tracheobronchial nodes,** alongside the trachea and main bronchi, which drain the lungs, trachea and heart. Their efferents join those of the anterior mediastinal nodes to form the **bronchomediastinal trunk** which, on the right side, joins the right lymph duct, and on the left the thoracic duct.
- **Posterior mediastinal nodes,** alongside the oesophagus. Their efferents pass into the thoracic duct.

The **thoracic duct** and the smaller right lymph duct return lymph to the bloodstream.

The thoracic duct, about 45cm long, arises in the abdomen as a continuation of the cisterna chyli (Fig. 10.10a, p. 144) and enters the thorax on the right of the aorta through the aortic opening of the diaphragm. It ascends, behind and on the right of the oesophagus, with the azygos vein, passing to the left in front of the 5th thoracic vertebra. At the level of the 7th cervical vertebra it arches laterally behind the carotid sheath and then forwards to enter the origin of the left brachiocephalic vein. It conveys lymph from below the diaphragm and the left half of the thorax; also from the head and neck, via the left jugular and subclavian lymph trunks and the left bronchomediastinal lymph trunk that joins it.

The **right lymph duct** is a short vessel, formed in the neck by the union of the right jugular, subclavian and bronchomediastinal lymph trunks. It enters the origin of the right brachiocephalic vein, conveying lymph from the right side of the head and neck and thorax.

A chylothorax is the abnormal collection of lymph within the pleural cavity. This is most commonly the result of surgical damage, from either surgery at the root of the neck, a left-sided subclavian venous puncture, or extensive surgery in the posterior mediastinum. More rarely a chylothorax may result from a malignant infiltration or a filarial parasitic infection blocking the thoracic duct.

AUTONOMIC NERVOUS SYSTEM

The autonomic nerve supply of the thoracic viscera is via the cardiac, pulmonary and oesophageal plexuses, which each receive sympathetic and parasympathetic contributions.

The **cardiac plexus** lies partly on the ligamentum arteriosum and partly on the tracheal bifurcation. The parts communicate and are a single functional unit. They receive branches from each of the cervical and upper thoracic sympathetic ganglia and parasympathetic branches from both vagi. Branches of the plexus are distributed with the coronary arteries to the heart and its conducting system. The cardiac plexus also sends branches to the pulmonary plexus.

A **pulmonary plexus** lies around the root of each lung; it receives branches from the upper four cervical ganglia and from both vagi, and supplies the lung substance.

The **oesophageal plexus** is a network surrounding the lower oesophagus. It receives branches from the upper cervical ganglia and both vagi. It supplies the oesophagus and over the lower oesophagus the right and left vagal trunks emerge from it and descend with the oesophagus to enter the abdomen as the anterior and posterior gastric nerves (p. 146).

Each thoracic sympathetic trunk (Fig. 4.17a,b) lies alongside the vertebral column behind the parietal pleura. It is continuous above with the cervical trunk and below with the lumbar sympathetic trunk. It usually possesses 12 ganglia, each contributed by a thoracic nerve, but half of the first thoracic ganglion is fused to the 7th cervical to form a larger stellate ganglion on the neck of the 1st rib. Each ganglion receives preganglionic fibres in a white ramus communicantes from its corresponding spinal nerve, and sends postganglionic fibres back to that nerve as a grey ramus communicantes.

Sympathetic denervation (sympathectomy) of the upper limb is employed to dilate cutaneous blood vessels or inhibit sweating. It is achieved by surgically removing the second and third thoracic ganglia. The 1st ganglion is left intact to preserve sympathetic innervation to the head and neck and prevent the development of Horner's syndrome (Fig. 4.18). The features of the syndrome are unilateral ptosis, flushed and dry skin on the same side of the face, enophthalmos and a small pupil (meiosis). The syndrome is due to damage to the upper cervical trunk. It is often caused by cancerous infiltration from the apex of the lung (Fig. 4.19), but may also be caused by surgical removal of the stellate ganglion or a stellate ganglion block.

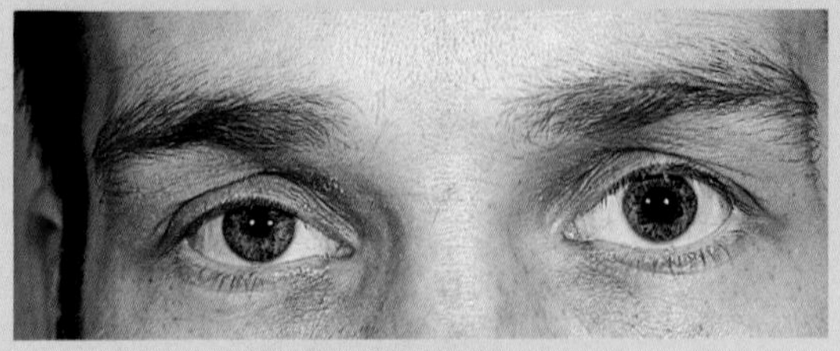

Figure 4.18 Right Horner's syndrome

Cervical sympathetic chain
Right recurrent laryngeal nerve
Right subclavian artery
Right vagus
Trachea
Transected arch of the aorta
Greater splanchnic nerves
Thoracic sympathetic chain
Splanchnic nerves piercing diaphragm
Right common carotid artrey
Cervical oesophagus
Left recurrent laryngeal nerve
Left common carotid artery
Left subclavian artery
Left recurrent laryngeal nerve passing around the aorta
Left vagus
Descending thoracic aorta
Thoracic oesophagus
(a)

Sympathetic chain
White ramus communicantes (preganglionic)
Thoracic spinal nerve
Grey ramus communicantes (postganglionic)
Thoracic sympathetic ganglion
(b)

(c)

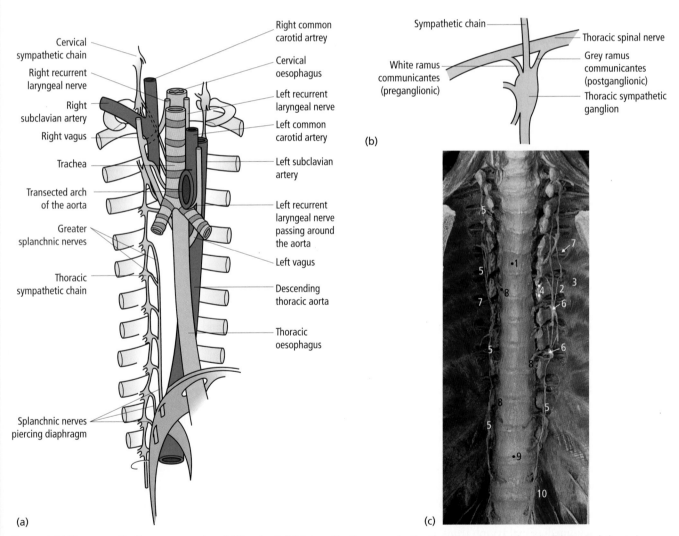

Figure 4.17 The sympathetic nervous system in the chest. (a) Sympathetic nerves in the thorax and root of neck. (b) Typical thoracic sympathetic ganglion. (c) Posterior thoracic wall after removal of organs to show vertebral bodies and sympathetic chains: 1, vertebral bodies; 2, rib; 3, internal intercostal muscles; 4, disarticulated heads of ribs to show demi-facets; 5, sympathetic chain; 6, sympathetic ganglia; 7, intercostal, segmental neurovascular bundles; 8, posterior intercostal arteries; 9, intervertebral discs; 10, psoas major muscle

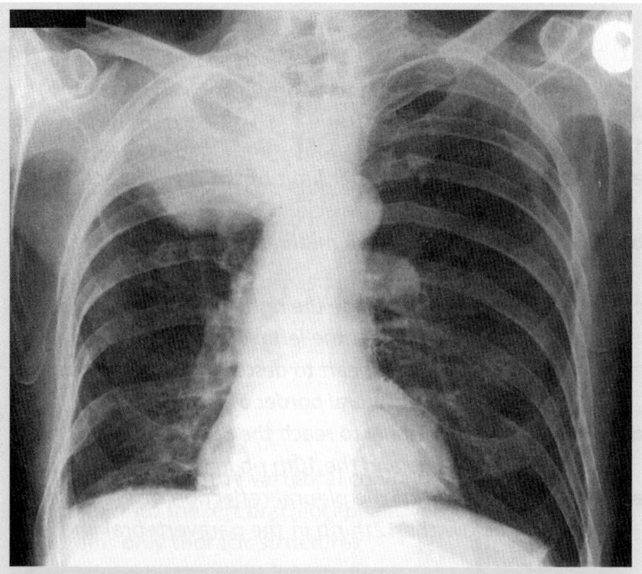
(a)

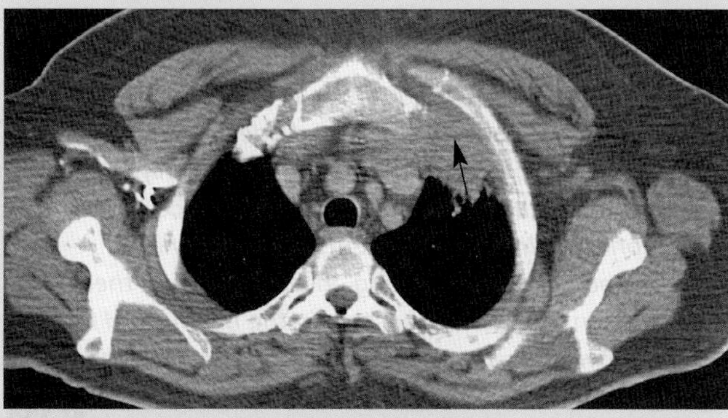
(b)

Figure 4.19 Apical cancer of the lung (Pancoast's syndrome): (a) chest X-ray, right-sided lesion; (b) CT scan (arrow), left-sided lesion

The sympathetic trunk supplies:

- rami communicantes to each of its spinal nerves;
- branches to the cardiac, pulmonary and oesophageal plexuses from the upper four ganglia;
- branches to form the **greater, lesser and least splanchnic nerves** (Figs 4.17 and 10.13, p. 146). These descend medial to the sympathetic chain and enter the abdomen by piercing the diaphragmatic crura. They contribute branches to the coeliac and other preaortic ganglia.

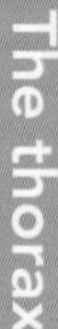

APPLIED QUESTIONS

1. You are informed that a patient has a pleural effusion. Where is the fluid situated?

1. A pleural effusion is an abnormal collection of fluid in the pleural cavity, which normally contains only a thin film of fluid sufficient for lubrication of the opposing visceral and parietal layers of pleura. The exact position of any abnormal collection is influenced by gravity and the patient's posture. In bedridden patients, therefore, it tends to collect at the base of the pleural cavity posteriorly, where it will be detected by percussion and auscultation.

---

2. How would you drain the pleural cavity of air and through which structures would your needle or catheter pass?

2. A pneumothorax is drained by a needle or, more commonly, a tube attached to an underwater seal apparatus inserted at one of two sites, either the 2nd intercostal space in the midclavicular line or the 7th intercostal space in the midaxillary line. With the upper approach the needle or trocar and cannula pass through skin, superficial fascia, pectoralis major and minor, before the intercostal muscle fibres and, finally, the parietal pleura. The lower approach avoids penetration of the pectoral muscles and produces less discomfort for the patient.

---

3. Your patient has unwanted bronchial secretions in her posterior basal segments. Into which position should she be placed to maximize postural drainage?

3. Effective postural drainage is achieved by positioning the patient so that the lung secretions drain from the diseased segment with the aid of gravity. Basal segments therefore require the patient to be tipped head downwards and, for the posterior basal segment, into a prone position. A physiotherapist helps the drainage by chest wall percussion over the diseased segment.

---

4. Why may a misplaced central venous catheter cause a chylothorax?

4. It is prudent to avoid performing a left subclavian or brachiocephalic puncture because of the presence of the thoracic duct terminating in the angle between the internal jugular and subclavian veins. If the pleura is punctured at the same time as the duct is damaged, a chylothorax may result from leakage of lymph into the pleural cavity.

---

5. Why may an apical carcinoma of the lung cause pain in the little finger and a drooping upper eyelid on the same side?

5. An apical carcinoma often affects structures lying in contact with the suprapleural membrane (Sibson's fascia), namely the sympathetic trunk, the stellate ganglion and the 1st thoracic nerve root. Damage to the sympathetic nerves at this level may produce a Horner's syndrome – a constricted pupil (meiosis), flushed and dry skin on the side of the face, drooping of the upper eyelid (ptosis) and retraction of the eyeball (enophthalmos). The ptosis is caused by partial paralysis of levator palpebrae superioris, whose smooth muscle is innervated by sympathetic fibres. The finger pain may be caused by direct involvement of T1 nerve, whose dermatome lies along the medial border of the forearm and hand. This combination is known as Pancoast's syndrome.

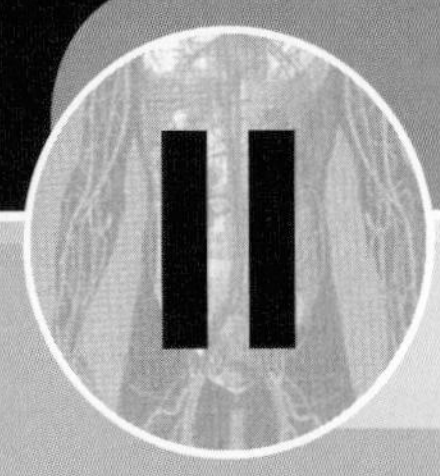

The abdomen

5 The abdominal wall and peritoneum

THE ANTERIOR ABDOMINAL WALL

The anterior abdominal wall is divided, for descriptive and clinical purposes, into nine regions by two horizontal and two vertical planes: horizontal – the **subcostal** (lower costal margin and lower border of the 3rd lumbar vertebra) and the **transtubercular** plane (through the tubercles of the iliac crests); vertical – **the right and left lateral** planes, which are extensions of the midclavicular line down to the midinguinal points. These define nine regions: centrally from above downwards, the epigastric, umbilical and suprapubic, laterally on each side, the hypochondrium, lumbar (lateral) and iliac regions. The **transpyloric plane,** which passes through the first part of the duodenum, is midway between the xiphisternum and the umbilicus at the level of the body of the 1st lumbar vertebra posteriorly (Figs 5.1 and 5.2).

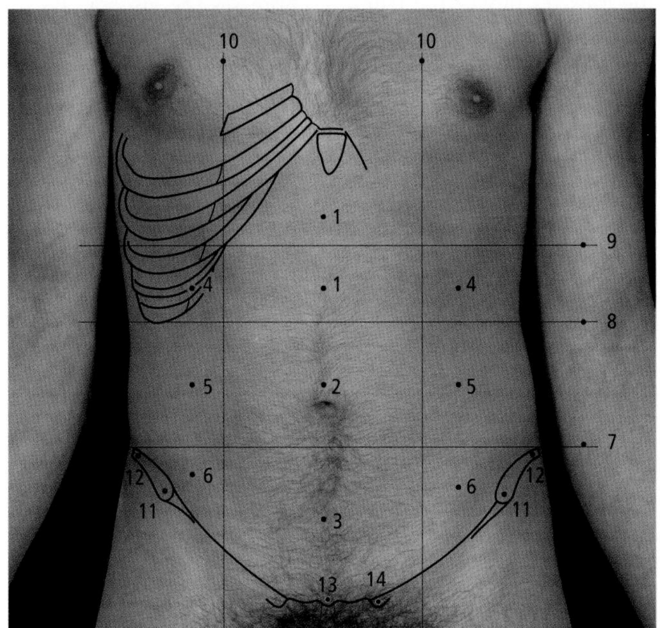

Figure 5.1 Surface anatomy of the abdominal wall, showing abdominal planes and regions: 1, epigastrium; 2, umbilical; 3, suprapubic; 4, L and R hypochondrial; 5, lumbar; 6, iliac; 7, transtubercular plane; 8, subcostal plane; 9, transpyloric plane; 10, midclavicular line; 11, anterior superior iliac spine; 12, iliac tubercle; 13, symphysis pubis; 14, pubic tubercle

The skin of the anterior abdominal wall is supplied by the 6th thoracic to the 1st lumbar nerves in segmental overlapping dermatomes (Figs 1.10 and 1.11, p. 28). T6 innervates the skin of the epigastric region, T10 the umbilical and L1 the groin. The subcutaneous tissues are divided by fascia; the most superficial is fatty and continuous with that of the thorax and thigh, and the deeper layer is membranous and thickened in the lower abdomen where it is attached to the iliac crests, the fascia lata of the thigh and the pubic tubercles. It continues between the tubercles to gain attachment inferiorly to the ischiopubic rami and the posterior border of the perineal membrane (Fig. 9.5a, p. 125).

Muscles

Laterally, the anterior abdominal wall contains three overlapping, flat sheet-like muscles, an outer external oblique, a middle internal oblique and an inner transversus abdominis. Anteriorly these become aponeurotic. The aponeuroses of each side fuse in the midline at the **linea alba** and form the **rectus sheath.** Their attachments, nerve supply and function are summarized in Table 5.1.

- **External oblique** lies superficially and its fibres descend inferomedially. Its origin interdigitates with serratus anterior.
- **Internal oblique** is deep to external oblique and its fibres are at right-angles to it.
- **Transversus abdominis** is deep to internal oblique and its fibres, apart from its lowest, run horizontally.

The pubic crest forms the base of a triangular deficiency in the aponeurosis of external oblique, the **superficial inguinal ring.** Between the **pubic tubercle** and the **anterior superior iliac spine** the thickened lower border of the aponeurosis is known as the **inguinal ligament.** Its free lower border is curved back on itself and gives attachment laterally to internal oblique and transversus abdominis; its medial 2 cm, attached to the pectineal line on the pubis, form the pectineal (lacunar) ligament which, with the inguinal ligament proper, forms the gutter-like floor of the inguinal canal (Fig. 5.5). Below the inguinal ligament the aponeurosis of external oblique is continuous with the fascia lata of the thigh. The fibres of internal oblique arising from the inguinal ligament arch medially over the spermatic cord and unite with the transverse abdominis aponeurosis to form the **conjoint tendon,** attached to the crest and pectineal line of the pubis.

Rectus abdominis, a strap-like muscle, alongside the midline, is enclosed in a **rectus sheath** (Fig. 5.3a–f). It is attached to the sheath's anterior layer by three **tendinous intersections,** situated at the xiphoid process, the umbilicus, and midway between these two points (Fig. 5.3b). The anterior layer of the rectus sheath is formed of the fused aponeuroses of external and internal oblique, and the posterior layer consists of the fused aponeuroses of internal oblique and transversus abdominis. The lowest quarter of the sheath's posterior layer is deficient, revealing its lower crescentic border, the **arcuate line** (Fig. 5.3d). Here the aponeuroses of all three flat muscles pass into the anterior layer (Fig. 8.11, p. 115).

The rectus sheath contains the rectus muscle, the superior and inferior epigastric vessels and the anterior primary rami of T7–T12.

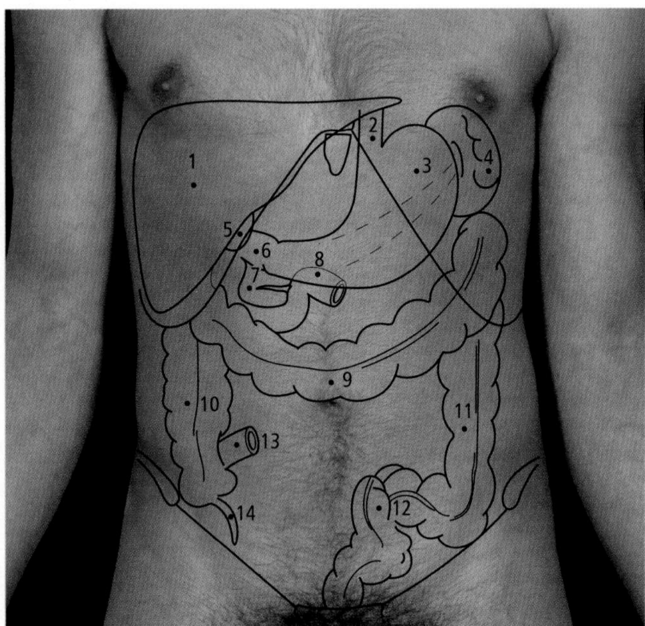

Figure 5.2 Abdominal viscera: 1, liver; 2, oesophagus; 3, stomach; 4, spleen; 5, gallbladder; 6, first part of duodenum; 7, head of pancreas; 8, duodenojejunal flexure; 9, transverse colon; 10, ascending colon; 11, descending colon; 12, sigmoid colon; 13, terminal ileum; 14, appendix

Function

The four muscles of the anterior abdominal wall usually act together and provide a flexible, strong, expandable support and protection for the abdominal contents. Contraction of the muscles moves the trunk, compresses the viscera, assists expiration by depressing the lower ribs, and increases intra-abdominal pressure, thus assisting evacuation, i.e. defecation, micturition and childbirth. Rectus abdominis is the strongest flexor of the trunk.

Blood supply

This consists of the superior and inferior epigastric, the intercostal and subcostal arteries, and branches of the femoral artery. Venous drainage follows the arterial supply.

Table 5.1 Muscles of the abdominal wall

Muscles	Proximal attachment	Distal attachment	Nerve supply	Functions
External oblique	Outer surface of 5th–12th ribs	Linea alba, pubic tubercle, ant. half iliac crest	T6–T12	Support and compression of abdominal contents. Flexion and rotation of trunk
Internal oblique	Thoracolumbar fascia, ant. iliac crest, lat. two-thirds inguinal ligament	External surface 10th–12th ribs, linea alba and pubic crest via conjoint tendon	T6–T12, L1	Support and compression of abdominal contents. Flexion and rotation of trunk
Transversus abdominis	Internal surface of 7th–12th costal cartilages, thoracolumbar fascia, iliac crest and lat. one-third inguinal ligament	Jointly with internal oblique into linea alba and pubic crest via conjoint tendon	T7–T12, L1	Support and compression of abdominal contents
Rectus abdominis	Xiphoid process and 5th, 6th and 7th costal cartilages	Pubic symphysis and pubic crest	T7–T12	Flexion of trunk, compression of abdominal contents

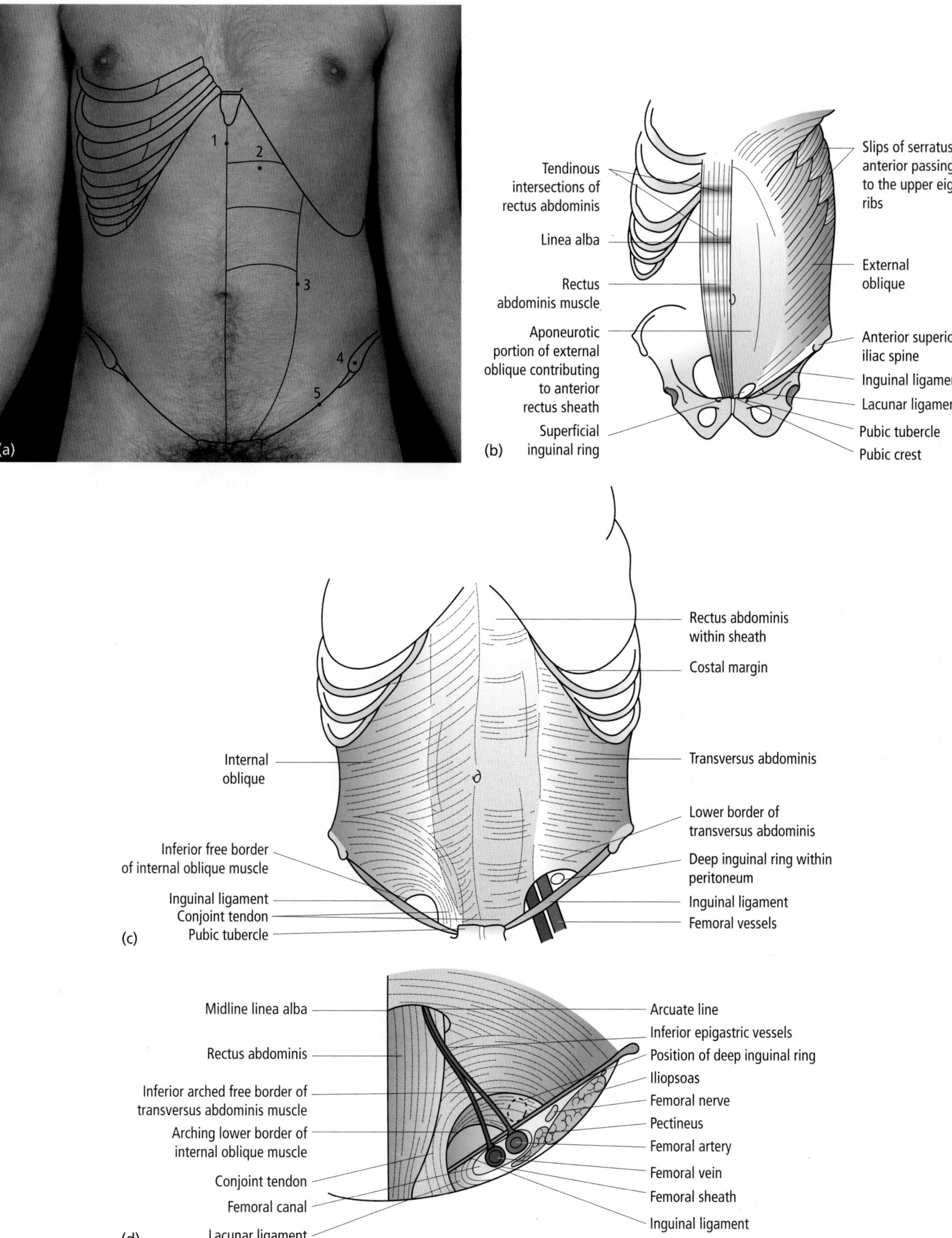

Figure 5.3 Surface anatomy of anterior abdominal wall. (a) Surface anatomy: 1, linea alba; 2, tendinous intersections; 3, linea semilunaris; 4, anterior superior iliac spine; 5, inguinal ligament. (b) Outer musculofascial layer, anterior rectus sheath removed on the right. (c) Deep layer (external oblique on right and internal oblique on left muscles removed). (d) Inguinal region viewed from within the abdomen (*continued*)

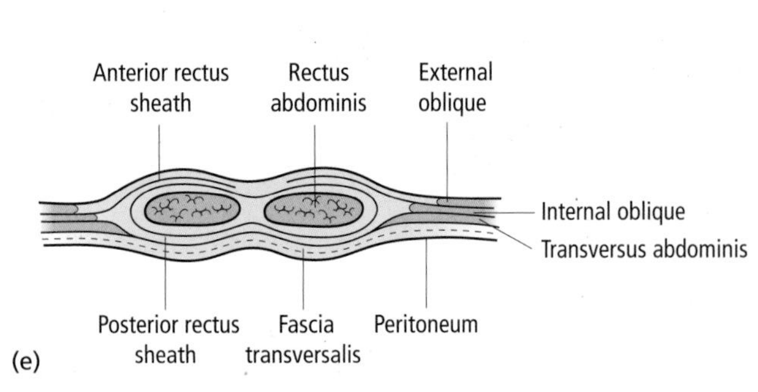

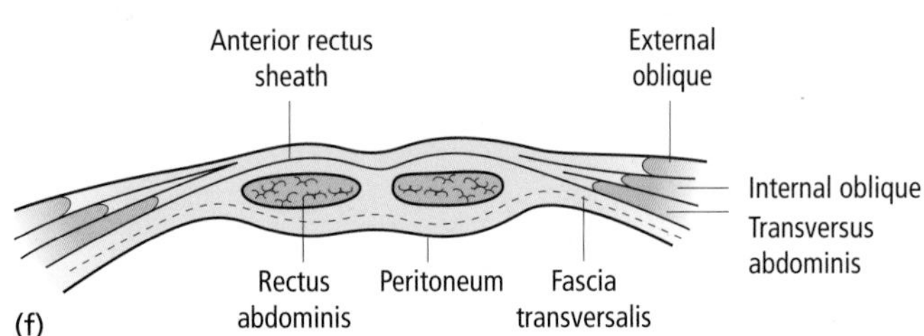

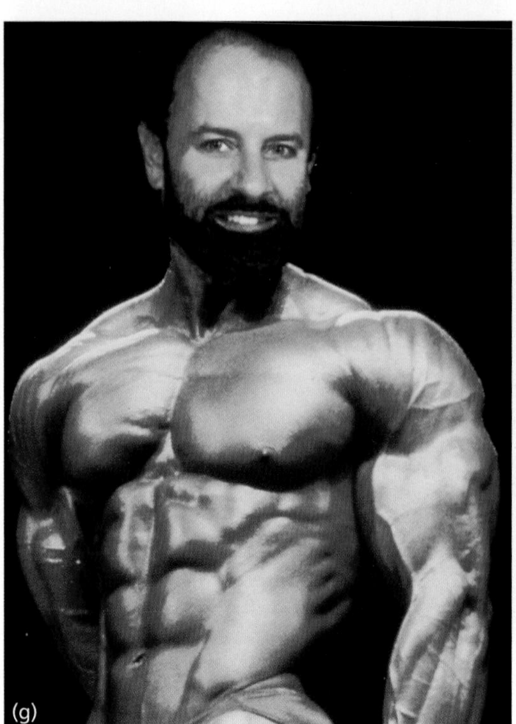

Figure 5.3 (*continued*) (e) Transverse section at the supraumbilical level. (f) Transverse section below the level of the arcuate line. (g) Contraction of rectus abdominis emphasizes the '6-pack' produced by the tendinous intersections

Surgical access to the abdomen is gained by a variety of incisions. The nerve supply of the abdominal wall is a dense network of rich communications, and so surgical division of a few of the terminal branches of the cutaneous nerves produces little or no consequence. Surgical exposure of the stomach, duodenum, transverse colon or aorta is frequently by a midline or paramedian incision (Fig. 5.4); that of the gallbladder or spleen by a subcostal or transverse incision. A short oblique gridiron incision in the right iliac fossa is usually sufficient for an appendectomy; longer ones allow access to the caecum and right colon and, on the left side, the sigmoid colon and rectum. Lower midline incisions may also be used. Pelvic organs and the uterus can be gained by low transverse incisions and lateral retraction of the recti.

Figure 5.4 Abdominal incisions: 1, upper midline; 2, right paramedian; 3, transverse; 4, nephrectomy; 5, cholecystectomy; 6, appendectomy; 7, left iliac; 8, lower midline; 9, suprapubic; 10, laparoscopic ports

The inguinal canal

The **inguinal canal** (Fig. 5.5a–e) is an oblique pathway through the anterior abdominal wall extending from the deep (internal) inguinal ring, a deficiency in transversalis fascia just above the midpoint of the inguinal ligament, to the superficial (external) inguinal ring, a deficiency in the external oblique aponeurosis above, medial to the pubic tubercle. The canal is about 4 cm long with a floor, roof, and anterior and posterior walls:

- **Anterior wall** – formed throughout by the external oblique aponeurosis, reinforced laterally by internal oblique.
- **Posterior wall** – formed by transversalis fascia throughout, reinforced by the conjoint tendon medially. The inferior epigastric artery lies medial to the deep ring.
- The **floor** is the recurved edge of the inguinal ligament and its medial (pectineal) part.
- The **roof** is formed by the arching fibres of transversus abdominis and internal oblique, which become the conjoint tendon medially.

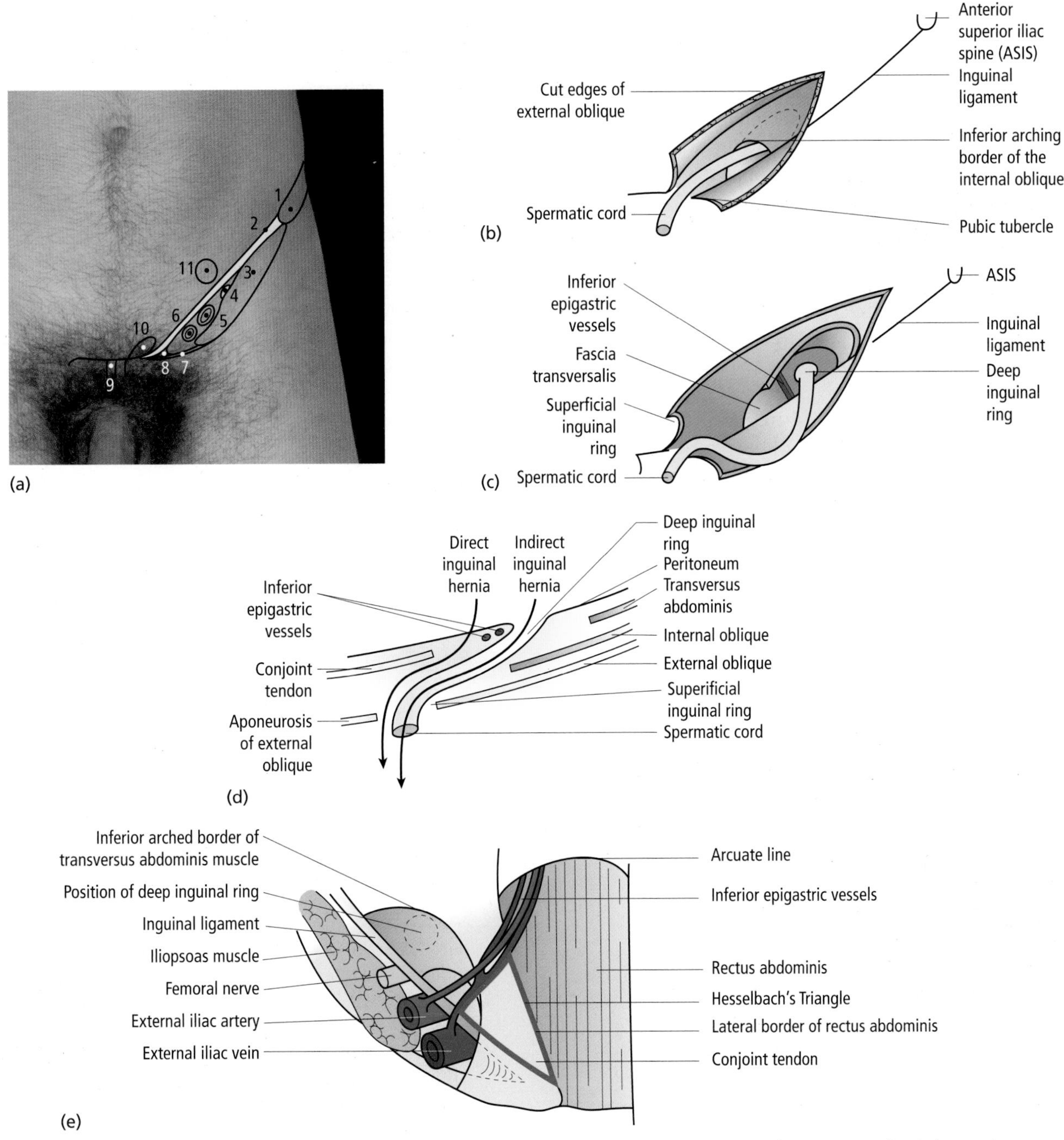

Figure 5.5 Inguinal canal. (a) Surface anatomy: 1, anterior superior iliac spine; 2, inguinal ligament; 3, iliopsoas muscle; 4, femoral nerve; 5, femoral artery passing beneath mid-inguinal point; 6, femoral vein; 7, origin of pectineus muscle; 8, reflected part of the inguinal ligament (pectineal [lacunar] ligament); 9, symphysis pubis; 10, superficial inguinal ring; 11, position of deep inguinal ring above midpoint of the inguinal ligament. (b) Anatomy of the inguinal region, external oblique being divided to demonstrate the course of the inguinal canal. (c) Deeper dissection through internal oblique. (d) Diagram of horizontal section through the inguinal canal. (e) Posterior aspect, as viewed laparoscopically, of inguinal region showing inguinal (Hesselbach's) triangle (thick red lines)

In the male the inguinal canal contains the spermatic cord and, in the female, the round ligament of the uterus.

The **spermatic cord** is formed when the testis, in late fetal life, descends the inguinal canal to reach the scrotum, carrying with it its ductus (vas) deferens, vessels and nerves. The **processus vaginalis,** a prolongation of peritoneum, connecting it with the tunica vaginalis of the testis, is usually obliterated at birth but, when patent, forms the sac of an indirect inguinal hernia (see below).

The cord gains three fascial coverings from the layers through which it passes and contains three nerves, three arteries, three other structures and lymph vessels:

Hernias, defined as protrusions of the contents of a body cavity through the wall of that cavity, are common in the inguinal region. They are especially common in males, because during development the testis carries with it, during its descent into the scrotum, a tongue of peritoneum, the processus vaginalis. Normally, part of the processus forms the tunica vaginalis of the testis and the remainder of the tube is obliterated at birth. When the processus remains patent there remains a hernial sac of peritoneum lying in the inguinal canal, a congenital defect which forms an **indirect inguinal hernia** (so-called because of its oblique emergence from the abdomen – see Figs 5.6 and 5.7). This may appear at the superficial ring and become symptomatic at any age from birth onwards. It can be felt above and medial to the pubic tubercle. The superficial ring can be palpated superolateral to the pubic tubercle and this is most easily done by invaginating the neck of the scrotum with the index finger and gently sliding the finger superiorly along the spermatic cord.

Middle-aged adults may develop a **direct inguinal hernia** due to a weakness in the posterior wall of the inguinal canal, the transversalis fascia. Such hernias are covered by the weakened conjoint tendon. **Femoral hernias**, which are less common, result from protrusions through the femoral ring. They can be palpated below the inguinal ligament (p. 233).

Congenital **umbilical hernias** present in infants through a weakened umbilical scar. Adults are susceptible to hernias in this region, but these occur usually through a weakened linea alba, just above the umbilicus (Fig. 5.8), and, because of their situation, are known as paraumbilical hernias. Less frequently adults present with small **epigastric hernias** in the midline through the linea alba, midway between the umbilicus and the xiphoid process (Fig. 5.9).

Surgical repair of hernias is advisable in the young because all hernias tend to enlarge as time passes, and the possibility of abdominal contents becoming trapped within the sac increases. Hernia repair usually involves the removal of the peritoneal sac together with repair of the abdominal wall defect.

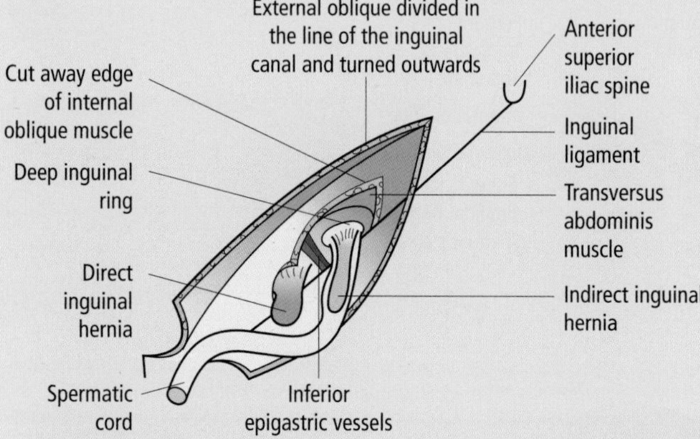

Figure 5.6 Inguinal hernia

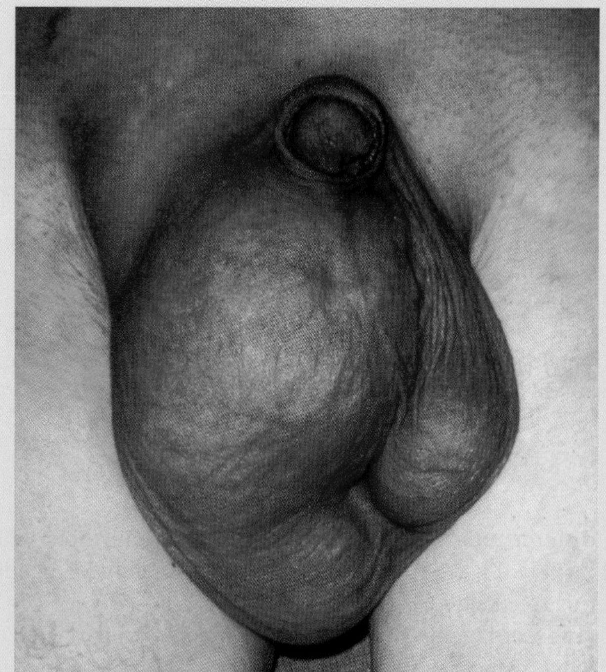

Figure 5.7 Right indirect inguinal hernia extending into the scrotum

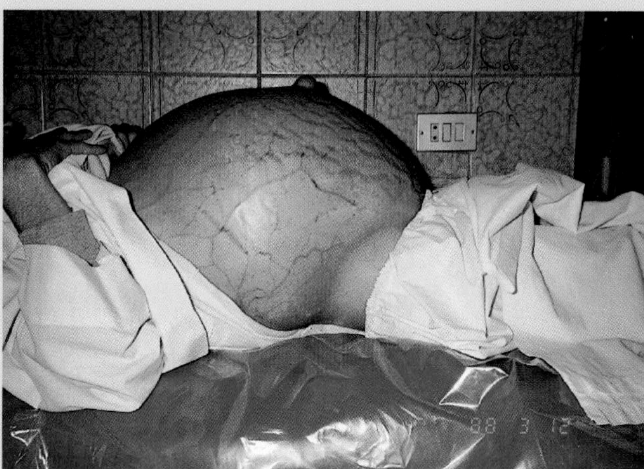

Figure 5.8 Umbilical hernia protruding from a grossly distended abdomen, due to ascites

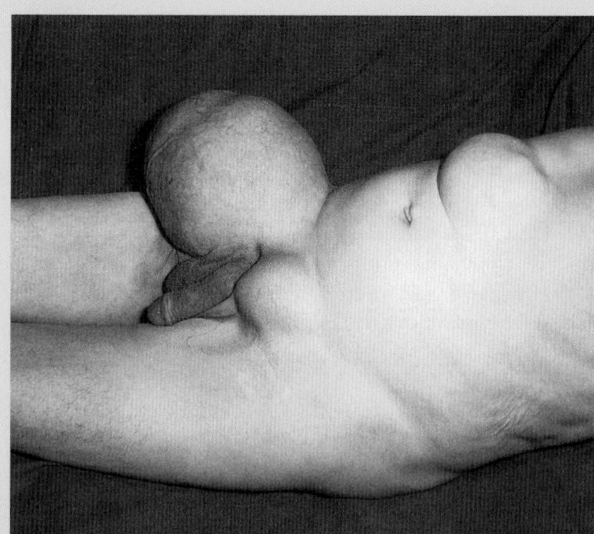

Figure 5.9 Epigastric hernia accompanying bilateral direct inguinal hernias. These are recognized as direct inguinal hernias because they do not descend into the scrotum

- **Fascial coverings** – the innermost layer, the internal spermatic fascia, derived from transversalis fascia; the middle layer, the cremasteric muscle and fascia, derived from internal oblique and transversalis muscles; and the outer external spermatic fascia, derived from external oblique fascia as the cord passes through the external ring.
- **Nerves** – genital branch of the genitofemoral, ilioinguinal and autonomic nerves.
- **Arteries** – testicular (from the aorta), cremasteric and artery to the ductus deferens.
- **Structures** – the pampiniform plexus of veins, the ductus (vas) deferens and remains of the processus vaginalis.
- The **lymphatics** drain to the para-aortic nodes.

THE TESTIS AND EPIDIDYMIS

The two testes are oval, about 4 × 2.5 cm, and suspended in the scrotum by the spermatic cord (Fig. 5.10). Each is separated from its fellow by the midline scrotal septum. Vessels and nerves enter the testis at its lower pole (Fig. 5.11). The epididymis and ductus deferens lie posterolaterally and, with the testis, are covered by the inner layer of a closed serous sac, the **tunica vaginalis.** The testis, spermatic cord and epididymis are accessible to clinical examination, the epididymis being palpable posterior to the testis. The tunica and its contents are in turn covered with extensions of the coverings of the spermatic cord – the internal spermatic fascia, the cremaster muscle and fascia, external spermatic fascia, superficial fascia and dartos muscle, and scrotal skin.

The **epididymis,** a tightly coiled tube, about 6 cm long, applied to the posterolateral surface of the testis, consists of a widened head, a body and a thinner tail. The head, attached to the upper pole of the testis by the efferent ducts, connects via the body to the ductus deferens below.

Blood supply

This is by the testicular artery and, in part, the artery to the ductus. Venous blood drains via a mass of veins, the pampiniform plexus, which forms around the spermatic cord to drain, asymmetrically by the right testicular vein, into the inferior vena cava, and by the left into the left renal vein.

Nerve supply

Sympathetic fibres, originating from T10, pass to the gland; afferent fibres are conveyed by the genitofemoral and ilio-inguinal nerves to the spinal cord.

Lymphatic drainage

Vessels pass along the testicular arteries to para-aortic lymph nodes. There is no lymphatic drainage to the inguinal nodes.

Development

The testis develops in the mesothelium of the posterior abdominal wall. It is attached by its lower pole to that part of the fetal abdominal wall that will become the scrotum by a mesodermal mass, the gubernaculum. Drawn downwards by the gubernaculum the testis descends the posterior abdominal wall and passes through the inguinal canal. At birth, or within 2 weeks of birth, it lies in the scrotum. In the female the gubernaculum forms the round ligament of the uterus and the ligament of the ovary.

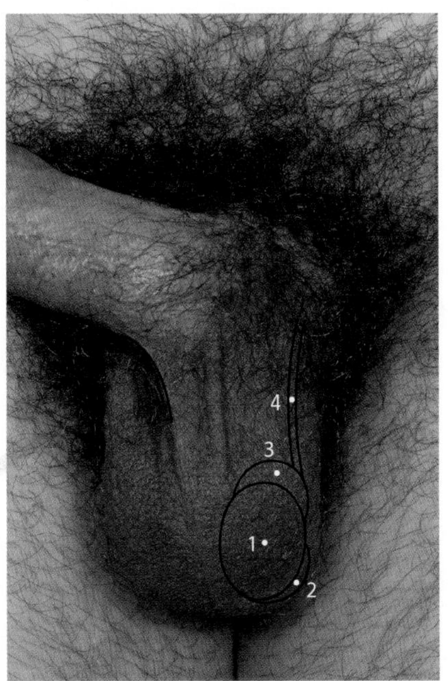

Figure 5.10 Surface anatomy of testis and spermatic cord: 1, testis; 2, inferior and 3, superior pole of epididymis; 4, ductus deferens

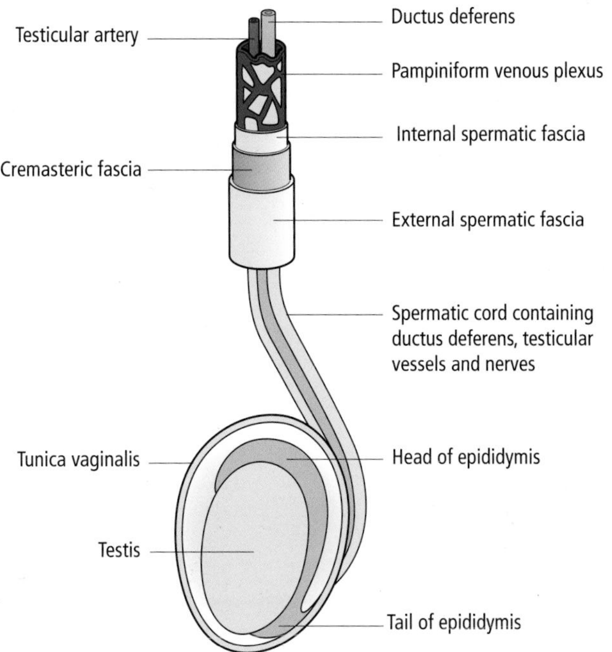

Figure 5.11 Testis, spermatic cord and their coverings

Testicular descent may occasionally be retarded or impeded (**cryptorchidism,** Fig. 5.12). It may descend through the inguinal canal but fail to enter the scrotum, and remains over the pubis in an ectopic position. Surgical correction of the abnormal position is desirable to ensure normal development of the testis and production of testicular hormones.

Fluid may accumulate within the tunica (**hydrocoele**) as the result of infection or trauma. A chronic hydrocoele (Fig. 5.13) may be drained by a needle, but this rarely produces a permanent cure. A surgical operation may be required to excise the parietal surface of the tunica. Cysts may develop in the epididymis. If this occurs once spermatogenesis has started the cyst will contain sperm and is known as a spermatocoele. The pampiniform plexus of veins may distend and dilate to form a varicocoele; this is more common on the left side where the vein drains into the left renal vein (Fig. 5.14). The majority are left-sided and are idiopathic, but occasionally they may be a presenting sign of a left renal cancer which has blocked the left renal vein and, with it, the left testicular vein.

The testis is prone to **torsion** because of the nature of its suspension within the scrotum, and the twisting occludes the organ's arterial supply, rendering the ischaemic testis tender and painful (Fig. 5.15). This, however, rarely occurs outside the 10- to 20-year age group. Unless surgical correction of the torsion is achieved within 8–12 hours then the impairment of the blood supply results in death of the testis.

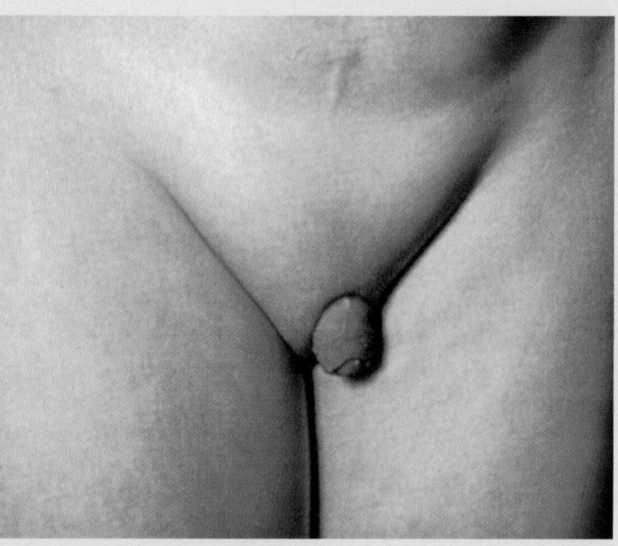

Figure 5.12 Left-sided cryptorchidism showing poorly developed scrotum and swellings over external inguinal rings

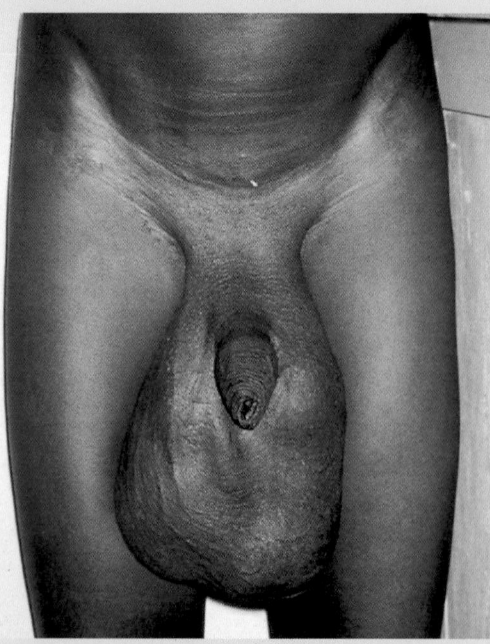

Figure 5.13 Chronic bilateral hydrocoele with scrotal enlargement

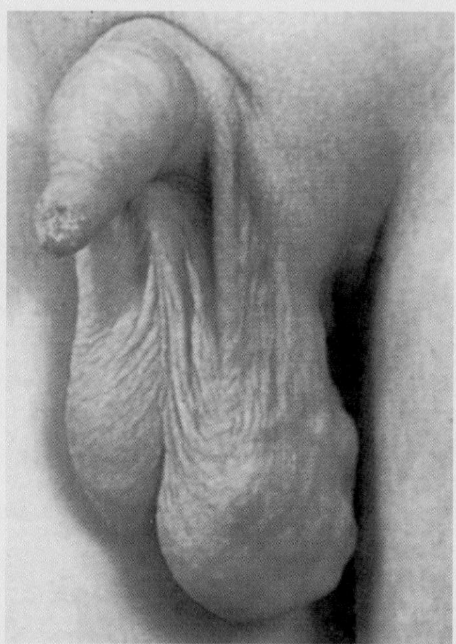

Figure 5.14 Left varicocoele revealing nodular soft swelling around upper pole of testis and spermatic cord

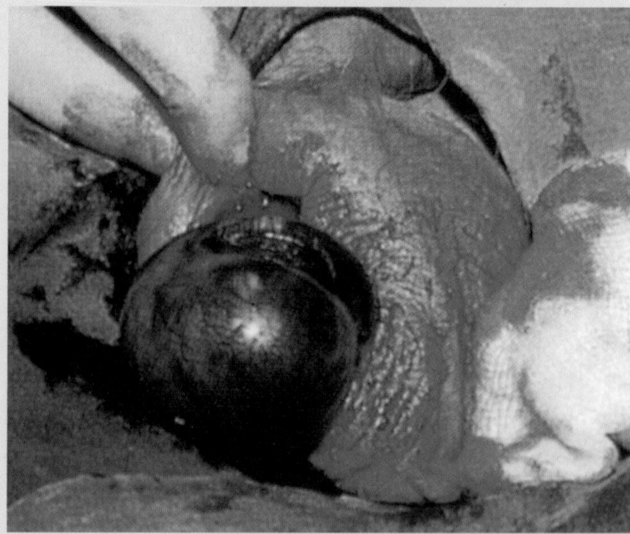

Figure 5.15 Surgical exposure shows torsion of the testis. The tense, dark vascular congestion probably indicates testicular death

THE PERITONEUM

The peritoneum lines the abdominal cavity. It is a thin membrane folded into a serous sac enclosing the peritoneal cavity. The part lining the abdominal wall is known as the parietal layer and this, in places, leaves the abdominal wall, the diaphragm or the pelvic floor to partially or completely invest the viscera. This layer is known as the visceral layer. The parietal and visceral peritoneum are separated by a small amount of serous fluid. Some of the viscera are almost completely invested by peritoneum and are attached to the abdominal wall or adjacent structures by double layers of peritoneum known variously as mesenteries, ligaments, folds or omenta (Fig. 5.16a–d). Others, incompletely invested, have bare areas in contact with the posterior abdominal wall and diaphragm (Fig. 5.17). This invagination increases the complexity of the peritoneal cavity.

To study the complexities of the peritoneum it is best to trace it from one point travelling around the abdominal cavity to return to that point. Beginning on the upper anterior abdominal wall and diaphragm: between the umbilicus and the liver there is a double layer of peritoneum, known as the falciform ligament, that passes back and separates to enclose the liver. Superiorly the right layer reflects from the diaphragm, forming the coronary and right triangular ligaments and enclosing the bare area of the liver (Fig. 7.2, p. 101). The left layer forms the left triangular ligament. On the undersurface of the liver the two layers reunite along the porta hepatitis (Fig. 7.2, p. 101) to form the **lesser omentum,** whose two layers descend to the oesophagus and stomach before separating again to enclose them (Figs 5.18 and 5.19). Rejoining along the greater curvature of the stomach, the two, often fat-laden, peritoneal layers descend in a lax fold, the **greater omentum,** before ascending anterior to the transverse colon and its mesentery.

The **mesocolon,** which suspends the transverse colon from the posterior abdominal wall forms an attachment that runs across the anterior surface of the pancreas (Fig 5.17). The upper peritoneal layer covers the posterior wall of the abdomen and the undersurface of the diaphragm as far as the oesophageal opening. Over the anterior surface of the left kidney two layers of the peritoneum split to enclose the spleen before joining again to extend to the stomach; the spleen is thus suspended by two peritoneal ligaments, the **gastrosplenic** and the **lienorenal.**

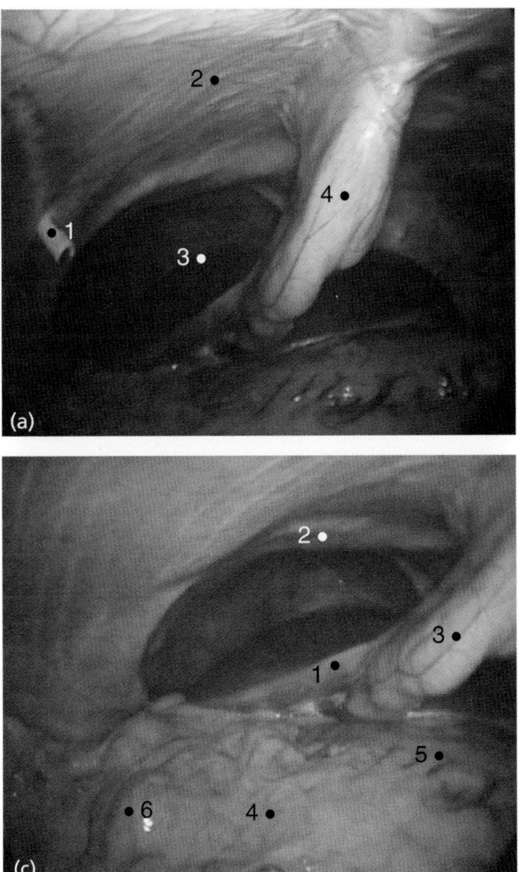

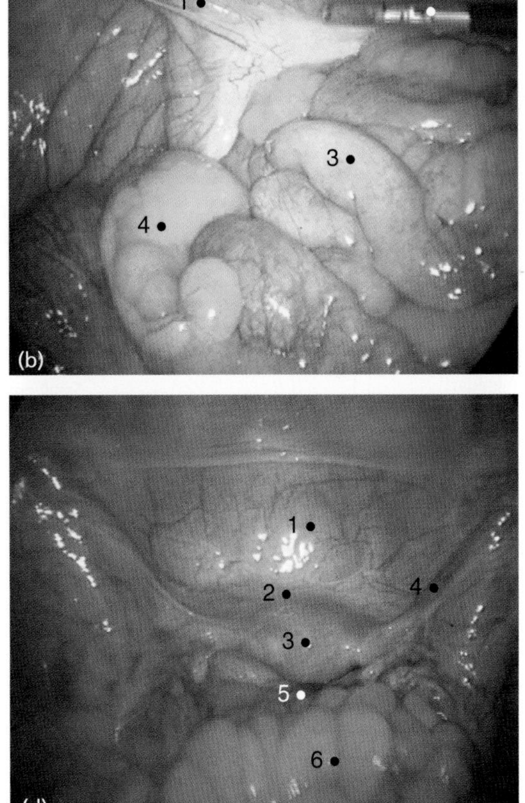

Figure 5.16 Laparoscopic views of intra-abdominal peritoneum. (a) Right upper quadrant: 1, porthole for instruments; 2, anterior abdominal wall; 3, liver; 4, falciform ligament covered in fat. (b) Intestinal folds covered in shiny visceral peritoneum: 1, bowel adhesion; 2, instrument; 3, small intestine; 4, fat overlying large intestine. (c) View from umbilicus on right hand side: 1, right lobe of liver; 2, diaphragm; 3, falciform ligament; 4, greater omentum; 5, greater curvature of stomach; 6, transverse colon. (d) Pelvic peritoneum: 1, bladder; 2, uterovesical pouch: 3, fundus of uterus; 4, round ligament of uterus covered in broad ligament peritoneum; 5, rectouterine pouch (Douglas); 6, loops of fat-covered bowel

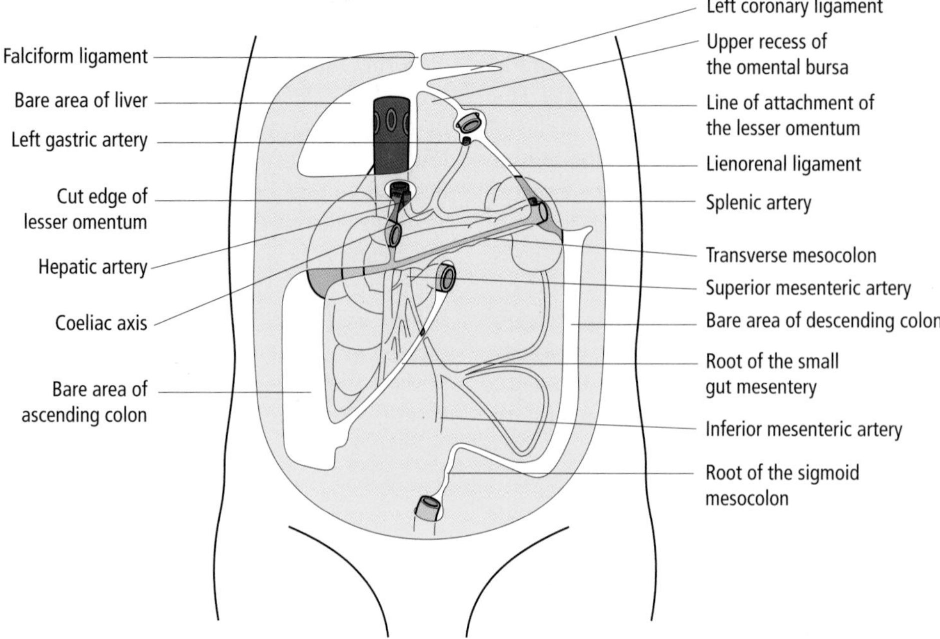

Figure 5.17 Posterior abdominal wall showing peritoneal reflections

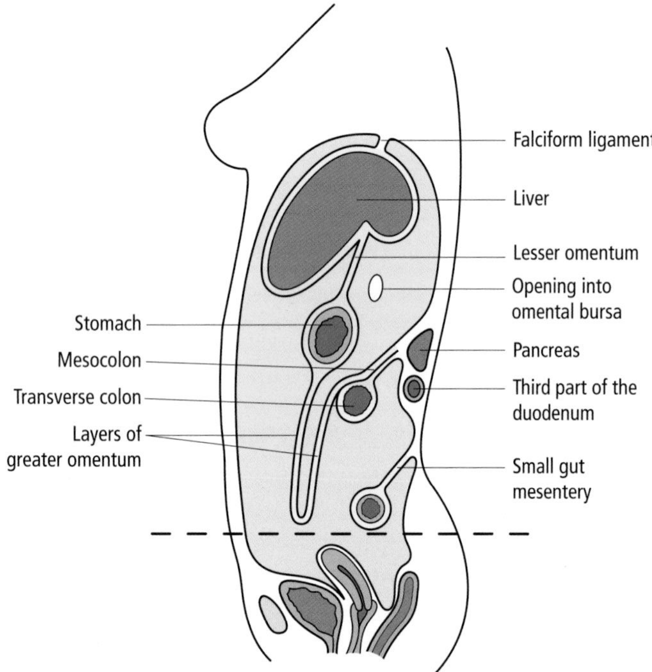

Figure 5.18 Parasagittal section through the abdomen to show peritoneal reflections. Below dotted line mid-sagittal section through female pelvis

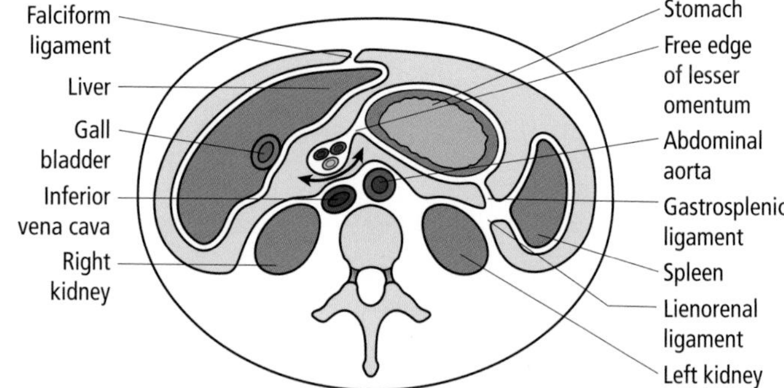

Figure 5.19 Transverse section through the abdomen showing peritoneal reflections, viewed from below. The arrow indicates the opening into the omental bursa, sited at this level

The peritoneum covering the posterior abdominal wall below the mesocolon descends, covering the third part of the duodenum and anterior surfaces of the ascending and descending colon, but it forms a mesentery for the sigmoid colon which is attached along the inverted 'v'-shaped line over the left sacroiliac joint (Fig. 5.17). **The small bowel mesentery** – the posterior parietal peritoneum – also forms a mesentery for the whole jejunum and ileum; this is attached along an oblique line (Fig. 5.17). **The lesser sac** of peritoneum is a diverticulum of the peritoneal cavity lying between the stomach and the posterior abdominal wall, with its opening, the epiploic foramen, lying to the right bounded by the liver above, the inferior vena cava posteriorly, the duodenum inferiorly and the free edge of the omentum (Figs 5.18 and 5.19). In the free edge of the lesser omentum lie the portal vein, the common bile duct and the hepatic artery.

Surgeons employ their knowledge of this anatomy to control haemorrhage from the liver or cystic artery by compressing the hepatic artery between a finger inserted into the epiploic foramen and a thumb applied to its anterior wall.

The anterior abdominal peritoneum descends into the pelvis to cover the pelvic walls and the upper surfaces of the pelvic viscera. In the male it spreads from the bladder to the seminal vesicles to descend into the rectovesical fossa before ascending to cover the front of the rectum. In the female it covers the body of the uterus and uterine tubes. Between the rectum and uterus there is a pouch of peritoneum known as the recto-uterine **pouch of Douglas.** The peritoneal folds over each uterine tube extend to the lateral pelvic wall as the **broad ligament** of the uterus (Fig. 5.16d).

Nerve supply

The parietal peritoneum is supplied segmentally by the somatic nerves supplying the overlying muscles: the diaphragm in its central portion by the phrenic nerve; the peripheral part of the diaphragm and the parietal peritoneum of the abdominal wall by intercostal and lumbar nerves; and the pelvic peritoneum largely by the obturator nerve. The visceral peritoneum is innervated by autonomic nerves that are sensitive only to stretch and pressure, and produce only a dull and generalized abdominal ache. Parietal peritoneum is sensitive to pain and therefore, when it is inflamed, pain is felt over the area of the dermatome supplying the affected part. The central portion of the diaphragm supplied by the phrenic nerve, when inflamed, produces pain referred to the tip of the shoulder. The greater omentum has considerable mobility and the potential to wrap itself around any infected focus. Thus an inflamed appendix or small perforated duodenal ulcer is frequently found, at operation, to be 'walled off' and its infection partially localized.

Peritoneal anatomy and gravity ensure that fluid or pus tends to collect in certain locations. The right and left **subphrenic** spaces lie between the diaphragm and liver, separated by the falciform ligament. In each space infected peritoneal fluid can accumulate to form subphrenic abscesses. Below the liver is the **right subhepatic space** (the **hepatorenal pouch of Morrison**), the most dependent part of the peritoneal cavity in a patient lying on his back and hence this too is a frequent site for a peritoneal abscess. To the lateral side of the ascending colon is the **right paracolic gutter,** a potential route for the transmission of infection from the pelvis or appendix to the subhepatic space. The **lesser sac** (omental bursa) may contain inflammatory fluid arising from pancreatitis or infection from a posterior perforation of the stomach. The pouch of Douglas (Fig. 5.16d), low in the pelvis, frequently contains localized peritoneal abscesses which have gravitated there from higher in the peritoneal cavity. They can be palpated by rectal or vaginal examination. Drainage of intra-abdominal abscesses can be achieved by ultrasonically guided needle aspiration or surgical procedures.

An abnormal collection of fluid in the peritoneum (**ascites;** Fig. 5.20) may be the result of heart, liver or renal failure, low-grade infection or malignancy. It can be drained from the abdomen or samples obtained for diagnostic purposes by the insertion of a cannula into the peritoneal cavity through the anterior abdominal wall below the umbilicus. In order to avoid puncturing the inferior epigastric vessels the puncture site should be in the midline or lateral to the rectus muscle. The same site may be used for peritoneal cavity lavage – the washing out of peritoneal fluid with saline – or for aspiration as a diagnostic test for the presence of intraperitoneal bleeding after abdominal trauma.

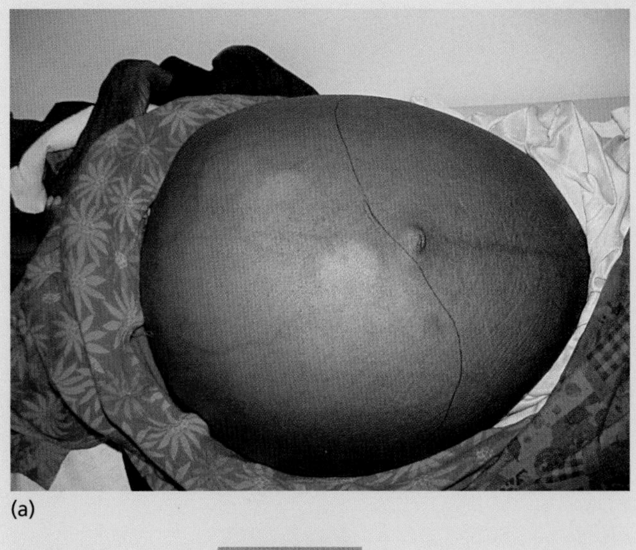
(a)

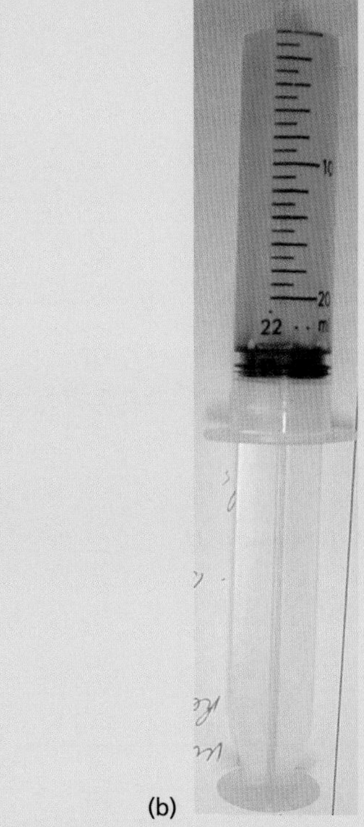

(b)

Figure 5.20 (a) Gross ascites due to haematoma pre-paracentesis. Liver edge is marked with abdominal line. (b) Paracentesis ascites fluid showing typical colour

MCQs

1. The inguinal canal: T/F

a transmits the ilioinguinal nerve in men only (___)
b transmits the genital branch of the genitofemoral nerve in both sexes (___)
c is more oblique in the newborn than in the adult (___)
d has fascia transversalis and conjoint tendon along its posterior wall (___)
e has the external oblique as its roof (___)

Answers

1.

a *F – The ilioinguinal nerve (L1) is transmitted in both sexes. In the male the contents of the spermatic cord are also transmitted, whereas in the female the ilioinguinal nerve, the genital branch of the genitofemoral nerve and the round ligament of the uterus pass along the canal.*

b *T – In the male the genital branch of this nerve is involved in the cremasteric reflex. Although the female has no such muscle, the nerve passes along the canal to supply the labia majora.*

c *F – In the newborn the deep ring lies almost directly behind the superficial ring, and so the canal is shorter and less oblique than in the adult.*

d *T – The inguinal canal has the fascia transversalis along its whole posterior wall and this is reinforced in its medial third by the conjoint tendon. This strong tendon attached to the pubic crest and pectineal line forms a tough posterior wall behind the superficial inguinal ring.*

e *F – The roof of the canal is formed by the arching fibres of internal oblique and transversus muscles. The external oblique aponeurosis forms the entire anterior wall.*

---

2. The porta hepatis: T/F

a is enclosed by the lesser omentum (___)
b contains the hepatic veins (___)
c contains the portal vein anterior to the hepatic artery (___)
d contains the whole of the cystic duct (___)
e contains lymph nodes (___)

Answers

2.

a *T*

b *F – The hepatic veins pass from the liver's posterior surface to drain to the inferior vena cava.*

c *F – The portal vein lies posterior to the hepatic artery and common bile duct.*

d *F – Only the distal end of the cystic duct lies in the porta hepatis.*

e *T – These drain the gallbladder and its bed.*

---

3. The lesser omentum: T/F

a is attached superiorly to the porta hepatis (___)
b extends inferiorly to the transverse colon (___)
c separates the lesser and greater sacs of peritoneum (___)
d forms part of the boundary of the foramen of the lesser omentum (___)
e contains the portal vein (___)

Answers

3.

a *T – Its two layers are formed from the left and right sacs of peritoneum, which meet at this point.*

b *F – Inferiorly it meets to enclose the oesophagus and stomach.*

c *T – The lesser sac lies behind the stomach and lesser omentum and communicates with the greater sac only via the foramen of the lesser sac.*

d *T – The foramen is bounded by the free edge of the lesser omentum anteriorly, the liver superiorly, the inferior vena cava posteriorly and the duodenum inferiorly.*

e *T – The free edge of the lesser omentum contains the common bile duct, the hepatic artery and the portal vein.*

EMQs

Each question has an anatomical theme linked to the chapter, and a list of 10 related items (A–J) placed in alphabetical order: these are followed by five statements (1–5). Match **one or more** of the items A–J to each of the five statements.

Inguinal region

A. Conjoint tendon
B. Deep inguinal ligament
C. External oblique muscle aponeurosis
D. Inferior epigastric artery
E. Inguinal ligament
F. Mid-inguinal point
G. Mid-point of the inguinal ligament
H. Reflected part of the inguinal ligament
I. Superficial inguinal ring
J. Transversalis fascia

Match the following statements with the appropriate item(s) from the above list.

1. Posterior relationship to the medial end of the inguinal canal
2. Forms the superficial inguinal ring
3. Forms the deep inguinal ring
4. Lies between the deep and superficial inguinal rings
5. Surface marking of the femoral artery

Answers

1 A; 2 C; 3 J; 4 D; 5 F

APPLIED QUESTIONS

1. Why might a patient, after an inguinal hernia repair, complain of a pain in his scrotum?

1. The patient was unfortunate enough to have his ilioinguinal nerve trapped in the hernia repair and now suffers pain in the L1 dermatome, which includes the scrotum. There may also be haemorrhage from the surgical site, which has produced a haematoma in the scrotum.

2. Where does a kick in the testes produce pain?

2. The testis is an internal organ innervated by the T10 dermatome. Therefore, pain arising in the testis is felt as dull pain in the umbilical region.

3. What structures develop from the gubernaculum in the female?

3. The gubernaculum of the ovary becomes both the ligament of the ovary and the round ligament of the uterus in the adult. These are continuous and attached to the uterus just below the uterine tube, and take a course similar to that in the male, passing along the inguinal canal to end in the female scrotal homologue, the labia majora.

4. What are the subphrenic spaces and why are they important?

4. The subphrenic spaces are potential spaces within the peritoneal cavity which may become filled with pus or fluid and form subphrenic abscesses. The right and left subphrenic spaces lie between the diaphragm and the liver but are separated by the falciform ligament. Both spaces are limited anteriorly by the anterior abdominal wall and superiorly by the diaphragm. The posterior border on the right is the coronary ligament, and on the left the left triangular ligament. Abscesses more commonly accumulate in the right subphrenic space.

6 The abdominal alimentary tract

Figure 6.1 shows the approximate surface markings of the major abdominal viscera.

THE OESOPHAGUS

The **abdominal oesophagus,** about 3 cm long, enters the abdomen to the left of the midline through the right crus of the diaphragm to join the stomach at the cardiac orifice (Fig. 6.2). The fibres of the right crus form a sling around the oesophagus. At the gastro-oesophageal junction (cardia) or just above it the oesophageal lining of stratified squamous epithelium changes to columnar epithelium, and this lines the whole of the remainder of the gastro-intestinal tract. The junction between the two different epithelial linings is normally 40 cm from the incisors, and is readily recognizable endoscopically (Fig. 6.2). The oesophagus lies between the diaphragm posteriorly and the liver anteriorly, covered anterolaterally by peritoneum. Gastric vessels and nerves lie in its walls. Reflux of gastric contents is normally prevented by the lower oesophageal sphincter and the oblique angle of entry of the oesophagus into the stomach, and the positive abdominal pressure that compresses the walls of the intra-abdominal oesophagus.

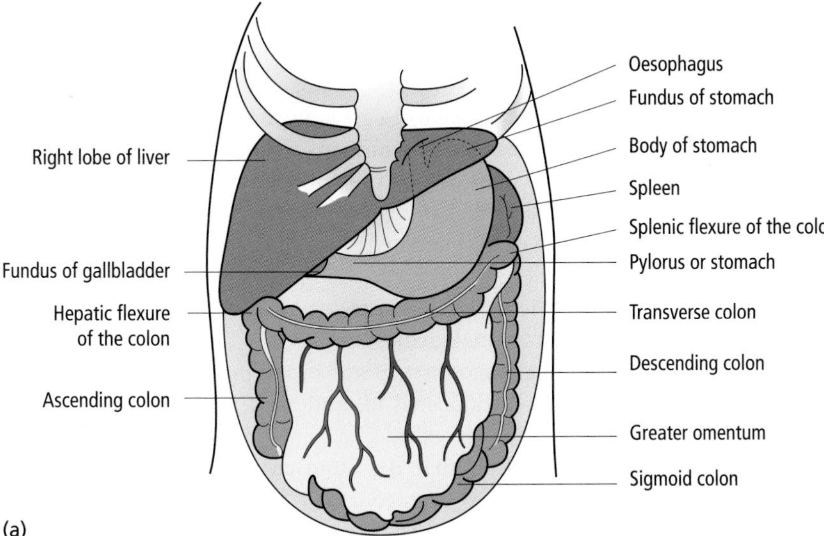

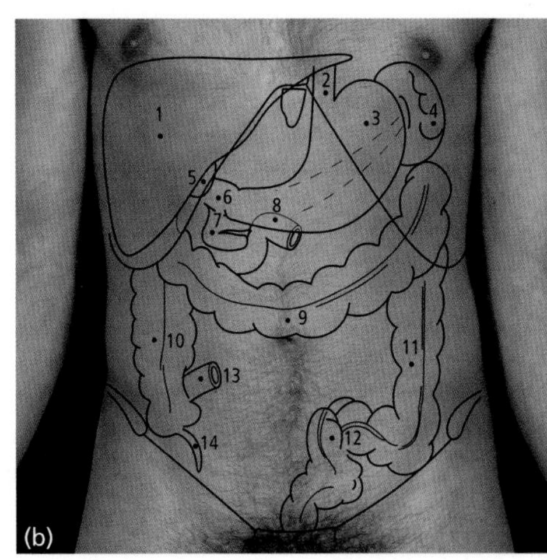

Figure 6.1 (a) Abdominal cavity showing the positions of the viscera. (b) Abdominal viscera: 1, liver; 2, oesophagus; 3, stomach; 4, spleen; 5, gallbladder; 6, first part of duodenum; 7, head of pancreas; 8, duodenojejunal flexure; 9, transverse colon; 10, ascending colon; 11, descending colon; 12, sigmoid colon; 13, terminal ileum; 14, appendix

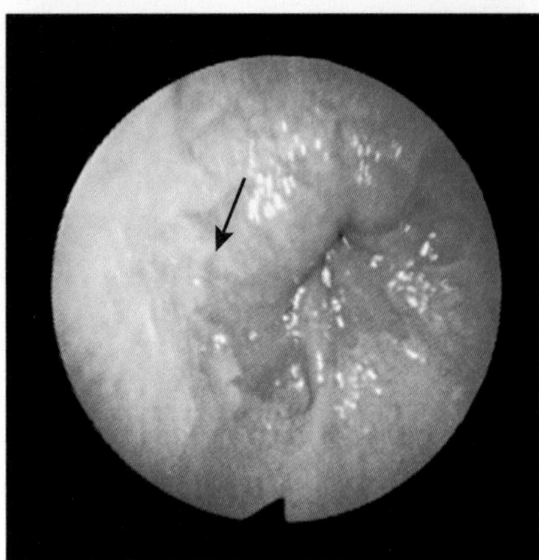

Figure 6.2 Endoscopic view of normal gastro-oesophageal junction: note the junction of the pale pink squamous epithelium of the oesophagus on the left with the redder stomach mucosa (arrowed)

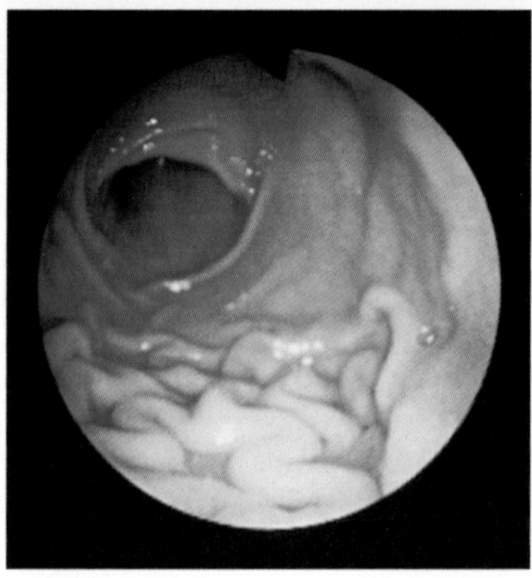

Figure 6.3 Gastric body and antrum: endoscopic view showing normal rugal folds in the body of the stomach – the distal antrum is smooth

If reflux does occur, inflammation, spasm and stricture of the lower oesophagus may follow. In later life the oesophageal opening in the diaphragm may become more lax and allow part of the upper stomach to slide into the mediastinum. This condition (**hiatus hernia**) also predisposes to reflux of gastric contents.

THE STOMACH

The **stomach,** although variable in size, shape and position, is usually J-shaped. It is situated in the left hypochondrium and epigastrium, its lower part extending to the umbilicus.

The stomach is divided into a fundus, a body and a pyloric part (Figs 6.3 and 6.5). It possesses anterior and posterior surfaces, both covered by peritoneum, and lesser (right) and greater (left) curvatures. The **fundus** is that part above the oesophageal opening; the **body** extends from the fundus to the **angular notch,** which is the most dependent part of the lesser curvature. The **pyloric portion** extends from the notch to the pyloric sphincter (pylorus), which separates the stomach and duodenum. The pyloric part possesses a proximal dilated **pyloric antrum** and a distal tubular **pyloric canal.** The pyloric sphincter, a thickening of the stomach's circular muscle, lies at the level of the 1st lumbar vertebra. It regulates the flow of stomach contents into the duodenum. The **lesser curvature** extends from the oesophagus to the pylorus; attached to it is the lesser omentum. The **greater curvature** extends from the left of the oesophagus, over the fundus to the pylorus, and gives attachment to the gastrosplenic ligament and the greater omentum.

Relations

Anterior – the left lobe of the liver, diaphragm and anterior abdominal wall; *posterior* – the lesser sac separates it from a group of structures known collectively as the stomach bed: the diaphragm above and below the splenic vessels, pancreas, left kidney and suprarenal gland and spleen. Below these are the transverse mesocolon and the splenic flexure of the colon (Fig. 6.4a).

Blood supply

The left and right gastric arteries supply the lesser curvature and nearby gastric wall; the left and right gastroepiploic arteries supply the greater curvature and nearby, and the short gastric branches of the splenic artery supply the fundus gastric wall (Fig. 6.4b). Veins from the stomach pass to the portal vein either directly or via the splenic or superior mesenteric veins (Fig. 6.4c).

Nerves

Anterior and posterior vagal trunks enter the abdomen through the oesophageal hiatus; the anterior trunk is in contact with the oesophagus, the posterior lies in areolar tissue to the right of the oesophagus. The anterior trunk supplies a branch to the liver and each trunk supplies many branches to the stomach. The posterior trunk supplies the coeliac plexus and via that plexus, the pancreas, small intestine and right half of the colon. The vagi provide motor and secretomotor nerves to the stomach.

Differences in the size, shape, motility and rate of emptying of the stomach can be demonstrated by radiographs taken after a barium meal. The mucosal pattern and its irregularities can also be seen. The contours of the fundus can usually be seen outlined by air in a radiograph. The diagnosis of all gastric and duodenal disease is aided by barium meals and by fibreoptic **gastroduodenoscopy**. The oesophagus, stomach and duodenum can be directly inspected by a gastroscope and biopsies taken of suspected abnormalities. Benign gastric ulcers are usually situated along the lesser curve, particularly near to the angular notch. Malignancies may be found in any part of the stomach. Gastrectomy (partial or total) may be indicated for malignancy.

Surgical vagotomy is still occasionally employed in the treatment of duodenal ulceration. It abolishes gastric acid secretion but is always accompanied by gastric atony, with the result that the stomach empties with difficulty unless drainage is encouraged by widening the pylorus (pyloroplasty) or by a gastrojejunostomy (anastomosis of the stomach and proximal small intestine). It is performed less frequently now, since the development of effective drugs that block gastric acid output, such as proton-pump inhibitors.

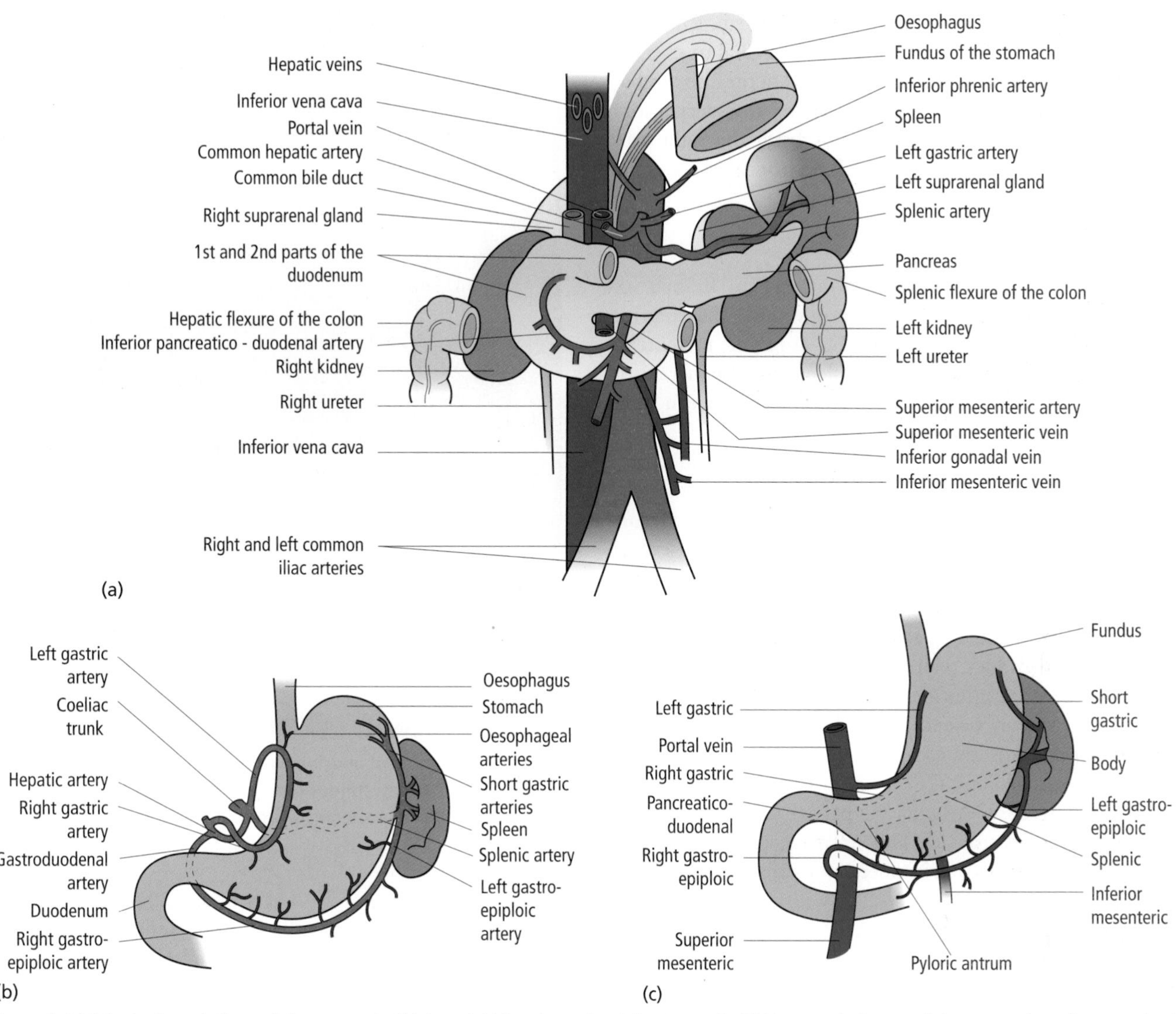

Figure 6.4 (a) Posterior relations of the stomach. (b) Arterial blood supply of the stomach. (c) Venous drainage of the stomach to the portal vein

Lymph drainage

This is to the coeliac group of preaortic nodes, via nodes along the left gastric artery, nodes in the porta hepatis, and nodes around the splenic artery and the greater curvature.

Occasionally a gastric cancer may spread via the left thoracic duct to involve and produce palpable enlargement of the left supraclavicular node (Troisier's sign).

THE DUODENUM

The **duodenum** lies on the posterior abdominal wall. About 25 cm long, it extends from the pylorus to the duodenojejunal flexure, embracing the head of the pancreas in a C-shaped curve open to the left. The duodenum is retroperitoneal apart from the first part of duodenum and duodojejunal flexure; for descriptive purposes it is divided into four parts.

The first part, 5 cm long, ascends to the right from the pylorus and turns down to form the second part (8 cm long), which descends to the right of the 3rd lumbar vertebra. The third part (10 cm long) passes left across the posterior abdominal wall to turn upwards as the fourth part on the left of the 2nd lumbar vertebra.

Relations

The **first part** is covered with peritoneum; posteriorly it lies on the portal vein, the common bile duct and the gastroduodenal artery (Fig. 6.4a,b); anteriorly it is in contact with the liver and gallbladder. The **second part** lies on the right kidney and ureter; it is crossed by the attachment of the transverse mesocolon, above which it is in contact with the liver and below with coils of small intestine. On its left lies the head of the pancreas and common bile duct and the duodenal papilla; the common opening of the pancreatic and bile ducts opens into its lumen halfway down its posteromedial border (see Figs 7.9 and 7.10, p. 104). The **third part** lies below the head and uncinate process of the pancreas and crosses, from the left, the right ureter, the inferior vena cava, the inferior mesenteric artery and the aorta. It is crossed anteriorly by the superior mesenteric vessels and the root of the small bowel mesentery. The **fourth part** lies on the left psoas muscle to the left of the vertebral column, with the inferior mesenteric vein, left ureter and left kidney on its left. The pancreas lies medial to it.

The **duodenojejunal flexure** lies to the left of the 2nd lumbar vertebra. A well-marked peritoneal fold, the suspensory ligament (ligament of Treitz), descends from the right crus of the diaphragm to the flexure. Small peritoneal recesses are occasionally found to the left of the flexure.

Blood supply

The superior pancreaticoduodenal artery, a branch of the gastroduodenal artery, anastomoses with the inferior pancreaticoduodenal artery from the superior mesenteric artery in the groove between the duodenum and pancreas to supply both structures. This is an anastomosis between fore- and midgut arteries.

Duodenal ulcers are common and the majority occur in the superior part of the first part of the duodenum. Posterior ulcers may penetrate and cause bleeding from the gastroduodenal artery or erosion into the pancreas, which results in severe back pain. Anterior ulcers may be complicated by perforation into the peritoneal cavity or, sometimes, by penetration into the adjacent gallbladder. **Gallstones** may ulcerate through an infected gallbladder wall into the duodenum and then pass down the small intestine to impact and cause intestinal obstruction in the narrower ileum (gallstone ileus). Treatment of duodenal ulcers is aimed at reducing the stomach's acid output by pharmacological means, but removal of the acid-producing part of the stomach (partial gastrectomy) or denervation of the stomach and drainage (vagotomy and pyloroplasty) are employed in emergency situations.

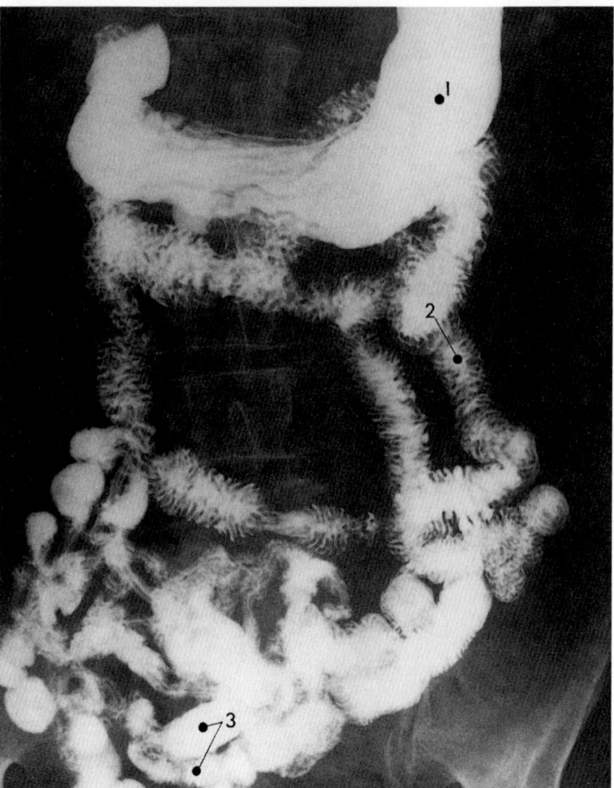

Figure 6.5 Barium meal and follow-through, demonstrating stomach and small intestine showing circular folds of duodenal mucosa and featureless ileum: 1, stomach; 2, jejunum; 3, loops of ileum

THE SMALL INTESTINE

The **small intestine** comprises the jejunum and ileum, with a total length which varies between 4 and 7 m. It lies in the central abdomen, below the transverse colon, suspended from the posterior abdominal wall by a mesentery which conveys blood and lymph vessels and nerves to it. The **jejunum** is wider and thicker walled than the **ileum**; its mucous membrane is thrown into circular folds, which give it a characteristic appearance in radiographic contrast studies (Fig. 6.5), and it has less fat in its mesentery, which allows the surgeon to distinguish it from the ileum at operation.

Relations

The shorter jejunum lies above and to the left of the ileum. The root of the mesentery, some 15 cm long, passes obliquely down from the left of the 2nd lumbar vertebra to the right sacroiliac joint, crossing the left psoas, aorta, inferior vena cava and right psoas (Fig. 5.17, p. 84).

Blood and nerve supply

The superior mesenteric artery supplies almost the whole small intestine by numerous jejunal and ileal branches, anastomosing with the right colic artery in the terminal ileum. Its venous drainage is by branches of the superior mesenteric vein and thence to the portal vein. Vagal branches convey a parasympathetic supply and stimulate both motor and secretory activity; the sympathetic supply inhibits both motor and secretory activity. Pain is conveyed by afferents of the sympathetic system, these cells lie in T9 and T10 segments. Hence pain arising from the small intestine is felt in the central para-umbilical region of the abdomen.

THE LARGE INTESTINE

This extends from the ileocaecal junction to the anus and is about 1.5 m long. It comprises the caecum, appendix, ascending, transverse, descending and sigmoid colon, rectum and anal canal. The longitudinal muscle of the colon, lying outside a continuous circular muscle coat, is confined to three bands, the **taeniae coli,** which are shorter than the rest of the colonic wall and cause it to be sacculated (Fig. 6.6). Fatty tags, the **appendices epiploicae,** project outwards from the wall. It is commonly investigated by radiographic contrast studies; barium and gas, injected per anum, are manipulated to coat the mucosa of the whole colon and rectum (Fig. 6.6).

The **caecum** is a blind sac, about 8 cm in diameter and invested in peritoneum, and is continuous with the ascending colon. It lies in the right iliac fossa on the iliacus and psoas muscles. Its taeniae coli converge on the appendix, attached to its posteromedial wall. The **ileocaecal orifice,** an oval slit on its medial wall, allows the onward progression of small bowel contents into the caecum.

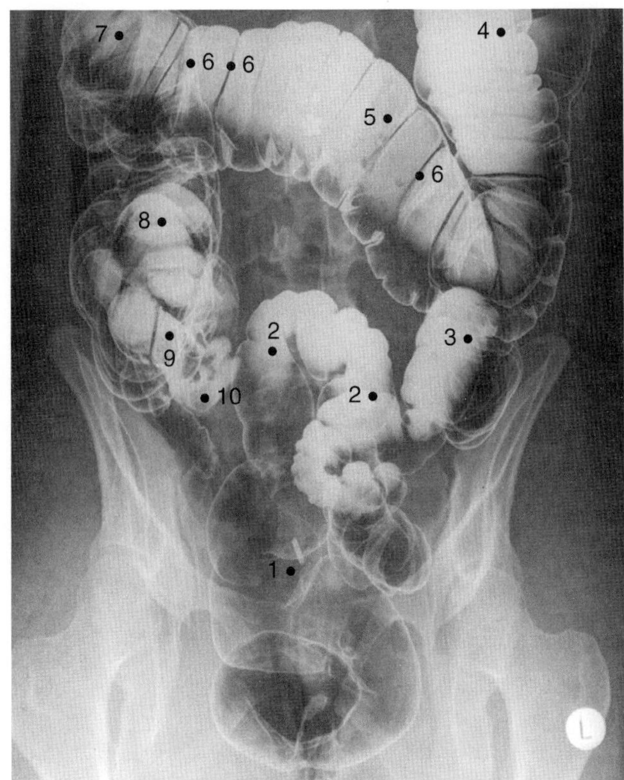

Figure 6.6 Double contrast enema of large bowel. The two contrast media used are barium and air which are inserted in that order via the anus and the patient tilted so that all regions are outlined: 1, rectum; 2, sigmoid colon; 3, descending colon; 4, splenic flexure; 5, transverse colon; 6, haustrations; 7, hepatic flexure; 8, ascending colon; 9, caecum; 10, terminal ileum. Note the twisting, angulated sigmoid colon, which has a long mesentery

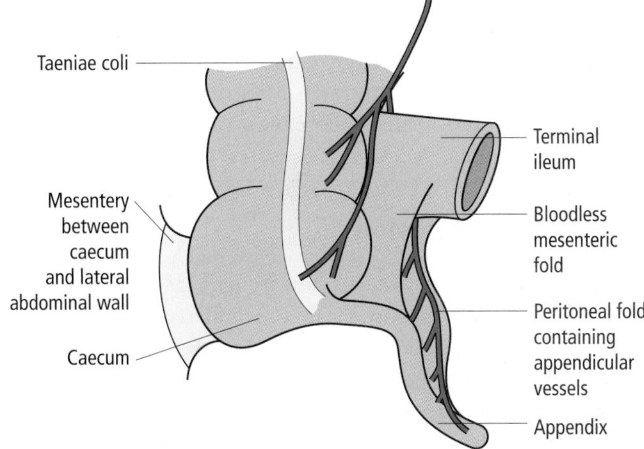

Figure 6.7 Diagram of appendix fold, its blood supply and the ileocaecal junction

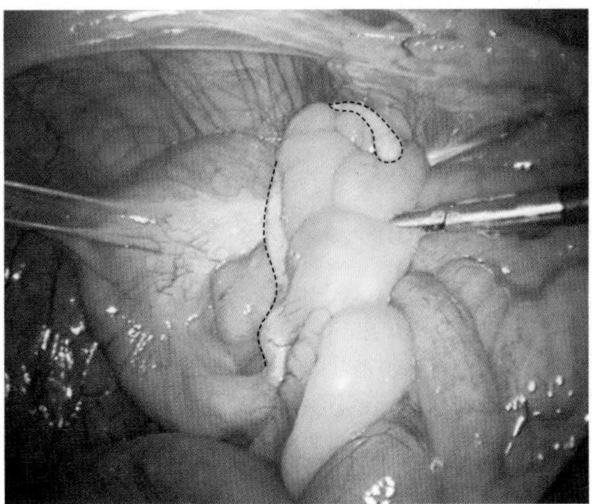

Figure 6.8 Laparoscopic view of normal appendix (outlined), elevated from a pelvic position

The **appendix,** a narrow diverticulum of variable length but usually about 8 cm long, arises from the posteromedial wall of the caecum below the ileocaecal orifice (Fig. 6.7). It is covered with peritoneum and connected by a mesentery – the mesoappendix, which contains the appendicular artery – to the terminal ileum. Much lymphoid tissue is found in its wall. It is very mobile and therefore its relations are variable; most commonly it lies in a retrocaecal position, but not infrequently it is in the pelvis (Fig. 6.8).

Appendicitis – inflammation of the appendix – is usually a consequence of obstruction of its lumen by faeces. Because the lumen is wider in infancy and often non-existent in the elderly, appendicitis is uncommon in these age groups. Appendicitis causes tense swelling of the organ and this may be severe enough to impair flow in the appendicular artery, an end artery, which is followed by gangrene of the appendicular wall and perforation, with the development of generalized peritonitis. Distension of the organ in early appendicitis produces vague colicky pain in the central abdomen, but later, when local inflammation develops in the parietal peritoneum of the right iliac fossa, the pain changes in character, becoming localized to the right iliac fossa, continuous, and exacerbated by movement.

The ascending colon

The **ascending colon** lies in the right lateral region, extending from the caecum to the **hepatic flexure** of the colon under the right lobe of the liver. It is about 15 cm long and peritoneum covers it anteriorly and on both sides, fixing it to the posterior abdominal wall. There is a **right paracolic gutter** of peritoneum along its right side which leads to the right subphrenic space.

Relations

It lies on the iliacus, the quadratus lumborum and the lower pole of the right kidney. It is covered anteriorly by coils of small intestine.

The transverse colon

The transverse colon extends from the hepatic flexure to the **splenic flexure** across the abdomen, suspended by the transverse mesocolon. It is about 50 cm long.

Relations

Initially it lies directly on the second part of the duodenum and the head of the pancreas, but subsequently it is attached by its long mesentery to the body of the pancreas. Above it is in contact with the liver, gallbladder, stomach, greater omentum and spleen; posteriorly it lies on the second part of the duodenum and head of the pancreas, the small intestine and the left kidney.

The descending colon

The descending colon, the narrowest part of the colon and about 30 cm long, lies in the left lateral region, extending from the left colic flexure to the brim of the pelvis, where it becomes the sigmoid colon. Peritoneum covers it anteriorly and on both sides, fixing it to the posterior abdominal wall; to its left lies the paracolic gutter (of peritoneum). The left colic flexure lies higher than the right and is attached to the diaphragm by a peritoneal fold, the phrenocolic ligament.

Relations

Posteriorly it lies on the lower pole of the left kidney, quadratus lumborum, iliacus and psoas. Anteriorly it is in contact with coils of small intestine.

The sigmoid colon

The sigmoid colon, about 40 cm long, lies in the left iliac region extending from the pelvic brim to the front of the 3rd sacral vertebra, where it becomes the rectum. It is attached to the pelvic wall by an inverted 'v'-shaped mesentery, the sigmoid mesocolon (Fig. 5.17, p. 84). The apex of the inverted 'v'-shaped mesentery overlies the left ureter, the bifurcation of the left common iliac artery and the left sacroiliac joint.

Relations

It lies on the left ureter and common iliac vessels; above it is covered by coils of small intestine, and inferiorly lie the bladder and, in the female, the uterus.

The advances in fibreoptic technology over the last two decades have permitted **colonoscopy** – the passage of a flexible light and lens system – to become a most useful method of visualizing the whole of the large bowel (Fig. 6.9). It is particularly useful in looking for tumours and ulcerations. The bowel may be obstructed anywhere by narrowing due to inflammation or malignancy. **Chronic colonic obstruction** often presents with a change in bowel habit. More acute obstruction causes colicky lower abdominal pain, swelling of the abdomen and high-pitched bowel sounds may be noted. **Cancer** of the large intestine (Fig. 6.10) arises from mucosal epithelial cells and spreads to invade the deeper layers of the wall and, eventually, the peritoneum. It may spread via the lymphatics to the nodes in the mesentery and para-aortic region, and by blood vessels to the liver. Peritoneal involvement may result in cancer seeding throughout the peritoneal cavity and lead to an increase in peritoneal fluid (ascites). Surgical resection of cancers in the left colon or rectum is frequently accompanied by the formation of a colostomy, the establishment of a temporary or permanent abdominal wall exit for the colon which allows the faeces to be collected into an abdominal wall bag (Fig. 6.11). Colostomies are also used in the temporary surgical relief of large bowel obstruction.

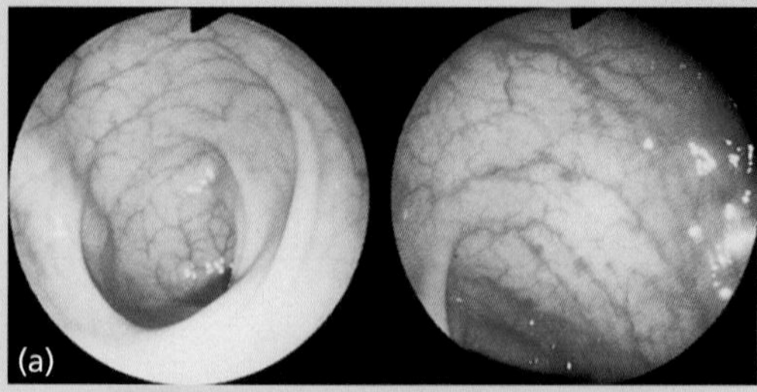

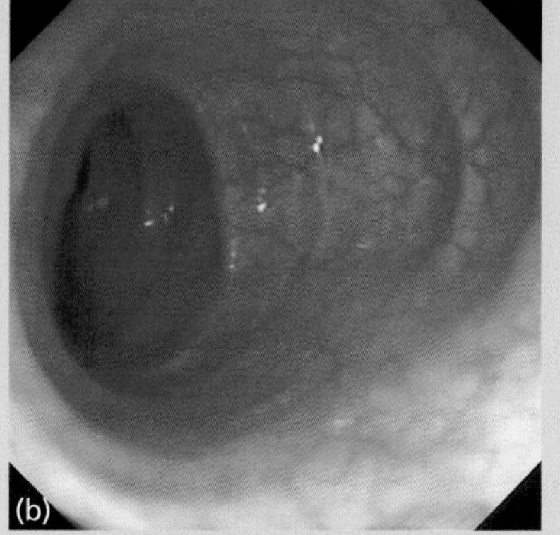

Figure 6.9 (a) and (b) Colonoscopic view of left colon. The mucosa is indented by contracting circular muscle

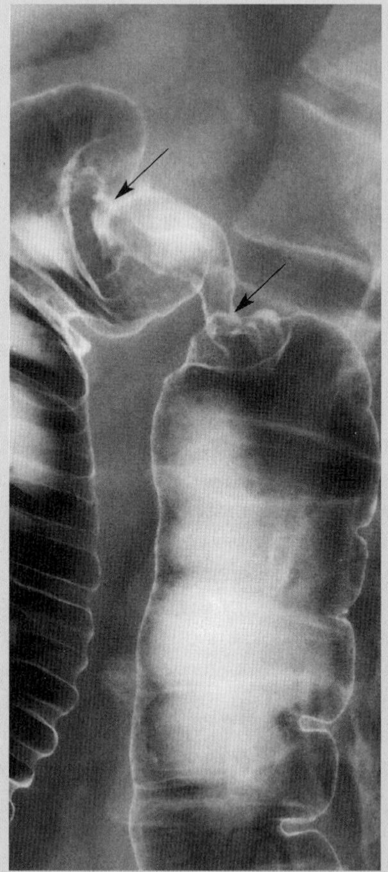

Figure 6.10 Barium enema showing carcinoma of the large bowel producing an 'apple core'-shaped narrowing of the colon (arrowed)

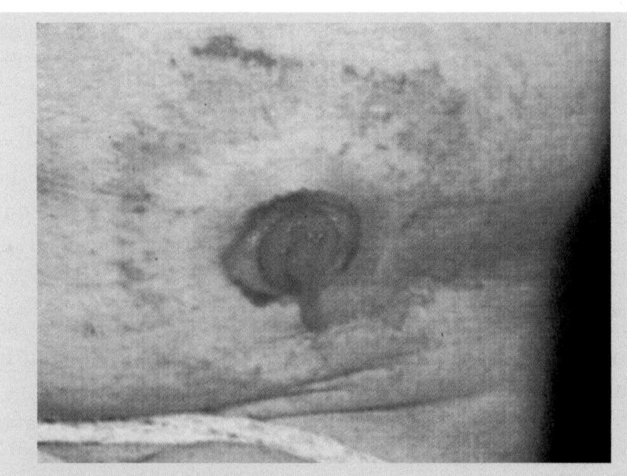

Figure 6.11 End colostomy

ARTERIAL SUPPLY OF THE GASTROINTESTINAL TRACT

Three arteries arising from the front of the aorta, the coeliac, superior and inferior mesenteric arteries, supply, respectively, the foregut, midgut, hindgut and their derivatives (Figs 6.12–6.14).

The **coeliac artery** arises just above the pancreas and soon divides into the left gastric, common hepatic and splenic arteries (Figs 6.4a and 7.17, p. 107). The **left gastric artery** passes upwards and left to the oesophagus, where it turns down into the lesser omentum. Branches anastomose with those of the right gastric artery, and it supplies the lower oesophagus and the stomach. The **common hepatic artery** passes above the first part of the duodenum to enter the lesser omentum, in whose free edge it ascends in front of the portal vein. It branches to form:

- The **right gastric artery,** which runs along the lesser curvature to anastomose with the left gastric in the lesser omentum.
- The **gastroduodenal artery,** which descends behind the duodenum to divide into the right gastroepiploic and superior pancreaticoduodenal arteries. The former passes along the greater curvature to anastomose with the left gastroepiploic; the latter descends between the duodenum and pancreas to supply both structures.
- The **right and left hepatic arteries,** which both ramify in the liver. The right gives a small cystic artery to the gallbladder. Knowledge of the variations in the pattern of these vessels is important in gallbladder surgery.

The **splenic artery** runs a tortuous course to the left along the upper border of the pancreas and passes in the lienorenal ligament to the splenic hilum, before dividing into many terminal branches. It branches to form the:

- **Pancreatic vessels,** several.
- **Short gastric arteries,** several of which pass in the gastrosplenic ligament to the fundus of the stomach.

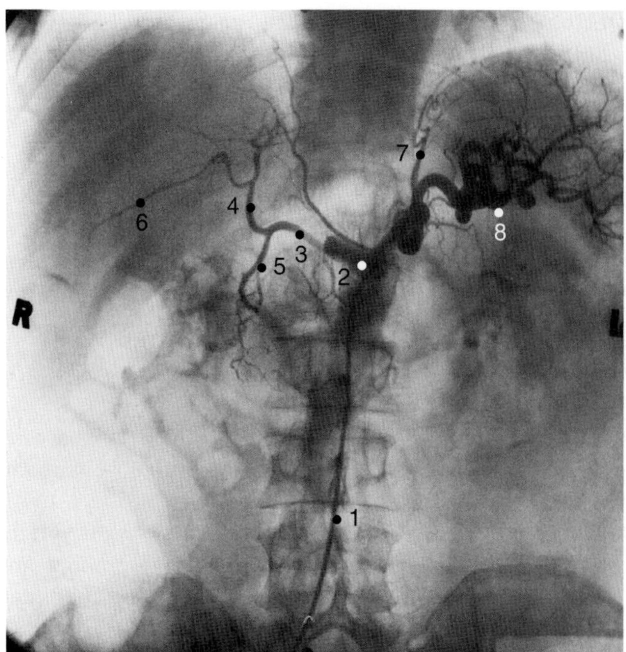

Figure 6.12 Selective coeliac angiogram. The catheter is introduced percutaneously via the femoral and iliac arteries and passes along the aorta to the coeliac trunk at level of the first lumbar vertebra. A computer technique 'removes' other tissues to highlight the arteries (subtraction): 1, catheter in aorta; 2, coeliac trunk; 3, common hepatic artery; 4, proper hepatic artery; 5, gastroduodenal artery; 6, cystic artery; 7, left gastric; 8, splenic artery – note its convolutions

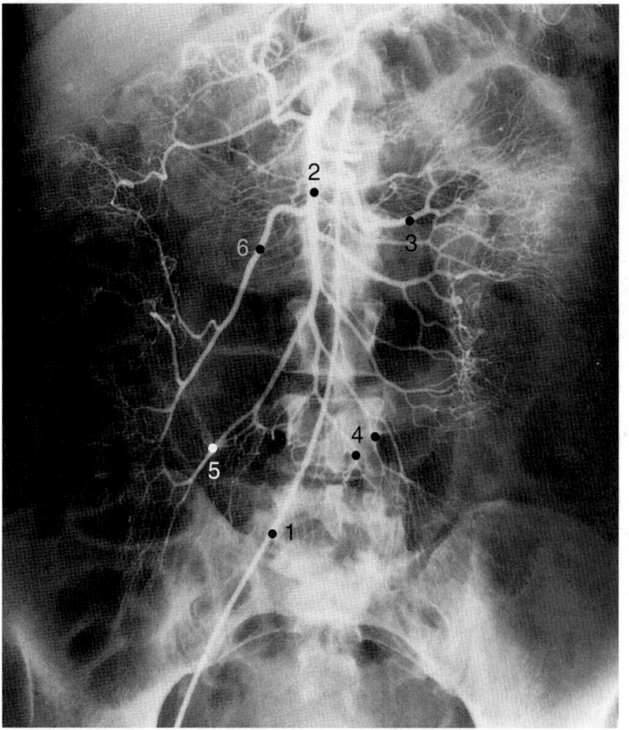

Figure 6.13 Selective superior mesenteric angiogram showing multiple jejunal, ileal, ileocolic and colic branches: 1, catheter; 2, superior mesenteric artery; 3, jejunal branches; 4, ileal branches; 5, ileocolic artery; 6, right colic artery

- **Left gastroepiploic artery,** which runs in the gastrosplenic ligament to the greater curvature, supplying the stomach and greater omentum to anastomose with the right gastroepiploic artery.

The **superior mesenteric artery** (Fig. 6.13) arises below the coeliac artery, descends behind the body of the pancreas, anterior to its uncinate process, and crosses the third part of the duodenum to enter the root of the mesentery of the small intestine. It supplies the small intestine and ends by dividing into the ileocolic, middle and right colic arteries (Fig. 6.15). Within the mesentery it is accompanied by veins, lymph vessels and nerves. It branches to form the:

- **Inferior pancreaticoduodenal artery,** which runs between the pancreas and the duodenum to anastomose with the superior pancreaticoduodenal artery.
- **Right colic artery,** which descends to the right on the posterior abdominal wall to divide into ascending and descending branches. It supplies the ascending colon and anastomoses with the ileocolic and middle colic arteries.
- **Middle colic artery,** which passes upwards on the body of the pancreas to the mesocolon, within which its branches supply the right two-thirds of the transverse colon.
- **Jejunal and ileal arteries,** 15–20 in number, arising from the left of the artery within the small bowel mesentery. There are many side-to-side anastomoses between these branches, and tiers of arterial arcades are formed.
- **Ileocolic artery,** which descends to the right, dividing to supply the caecum, appendix and lower ascending colon.

The **inferior mesenteric artery** (Figs 6.14 and 6.16) arises behind the duodenum and descends behind the peritoneum to the left, continuing beyond the pelvic brim as the superior rectal artery. Its branches form the:

- **Left colic artery,** which ascends to the left to the left colic flexure to supply the transverse and descending colon. It anastomoses with the middle colic and sigmoid arteries.
- **Sigmoid arteries,** which enter the sigmoid mesocolon and supply the sigmoid and lower descending colon.
- **Superior rectal artery,** which is the continuation of the inferior mesenteric artery, descends in the sigmoid mesocolon to reach the back of the rectum. It supplies the rectum and upper anal canal.

The terminal arteries supplying the gut form a continuous anastomotic arcade known as the 'marginal' artery, along the mesenteric border of the colon.

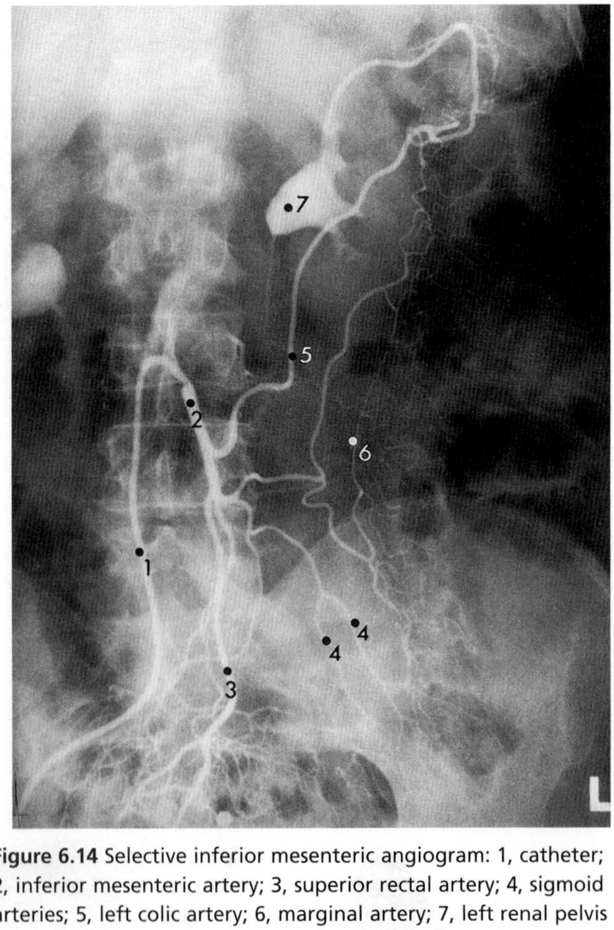

Figure 6.14 Selective inferior mesenteric angiogram: 1, catheter; 2, inferior mesenteric artery; 3, superior rectal artery; 4, sigmoid arteries; 5, left colic artery; 6, marginal artery; 7, left renal pelvis (outlined by contrast medium being excreted by the kidney)

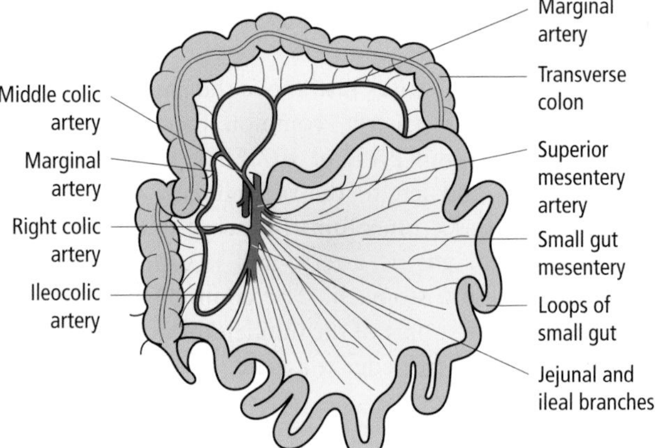

Figure 6.15 Superior mesenteric artery and its branches

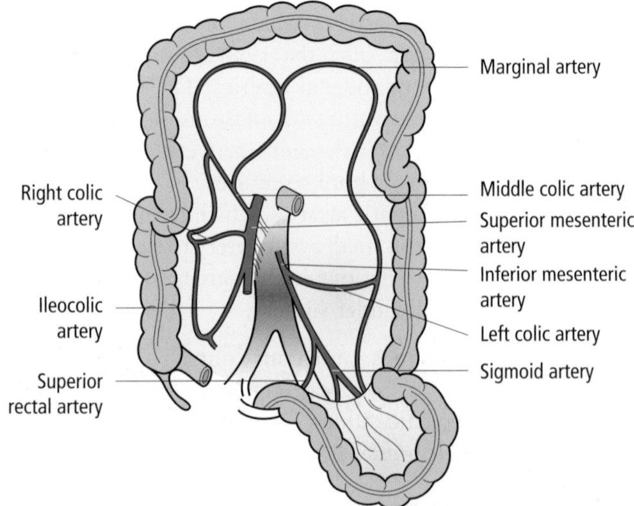

Figure 6.16 Superior and inferior mesenteric arterial supply of the large intestine – small bowel removed for clarity

Bowel ischaemia is most commonly the result of torsion (twisting) of the bowel or the entrapment of the bowel in a hernial sac (Fig. 6.17). **Volvulus**, the twisting of the bowel on its mesentery, may occur in the sigmoid colon and the caecum. Bowel ischaemia in the elderly may also be the result of arterial disease and inadequate blood flow, which threatens the viability of the colon in the region where its blood supply is the lowest, the so-called 'marginal' area in the region of the splenic flexure.

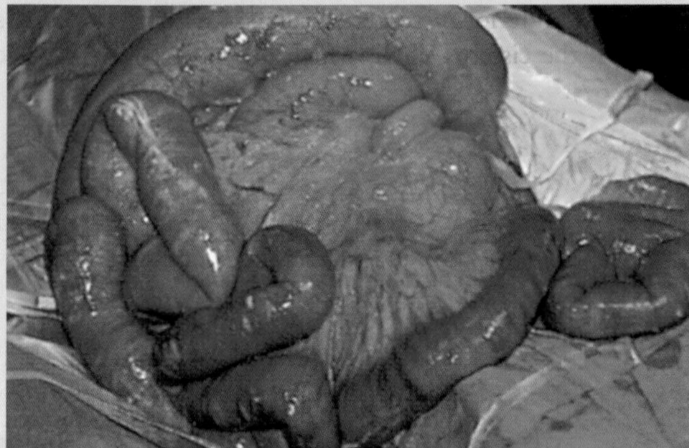

Figure 6.17 Acute mesenteric ischaemia – discoloured loops of small intestine

VENOUS DRAINAGE OF THE GASTROINTESTINAL TRACT – THE PORTAL VENOUS SYSTEM

From the lower end of the oesophagus to the upper end of the anal canal, blood from the gastrointestinal tract drains into the liver (Fig. 6.18). The distal tributaries correspond to the arterial branches described above, but more proximally the venous anatomy differs: the superior mesenteric vein joins the splenic vein behind the pancreas to form the portal vein; the inferior mesenteric vein enters the splenic vein to the left of this (Fig. 6.18). The **portal vein** ascends behind the pancreas and first part of the duodenum to the free edge of the lesser omentum, and thence to the porta hepatis, where it divides into right and left branches. It is 8 cm long and receives branches from right and left gastric veins and the superior pancreaticoduodenal vein. This pattern, as with all veins, is variable. Injection of contrast into the spleen permits radiological demonstration of the portal venous system (Fig. 6.19).

Relations

In the lesser omentum the portal vein lies behind the common hepatic artery and the common bile duct, and is separated from the inferior vena cava by the opening into the lesser sac (epiploic foramen).

Tributaries of the portal vein divide to supply all the liver cells, and from them blood is conveyed into the systemic venous system, i.e. the inferior vena cava, via the numerous hepatic veins.

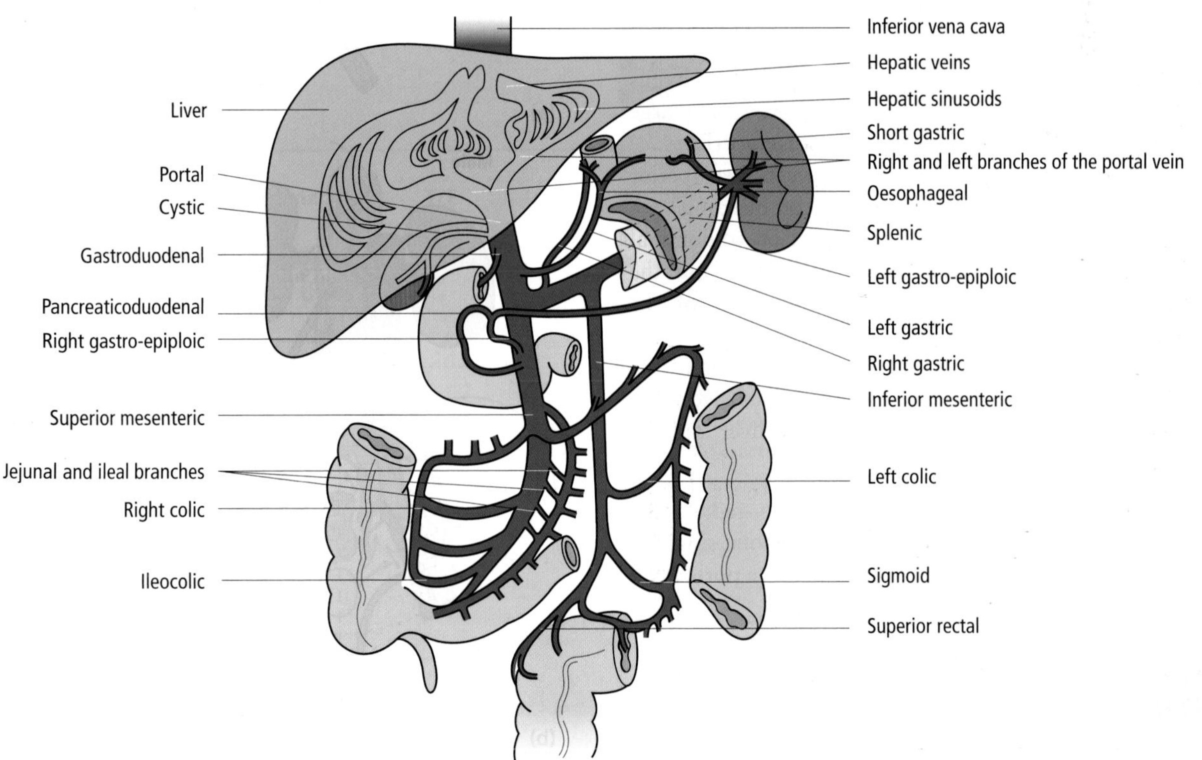

Figure 6.18 Portal venous system showing portal vein and its branches

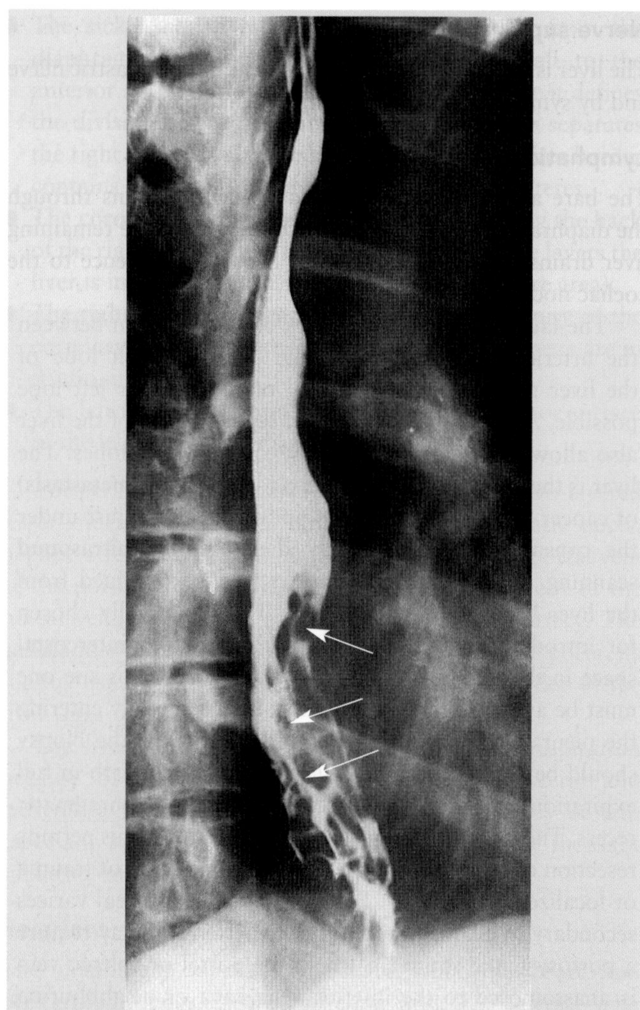

Figure 7.8 Oesophageal varices distorting the barium column in the lower oesophagus (arrows)

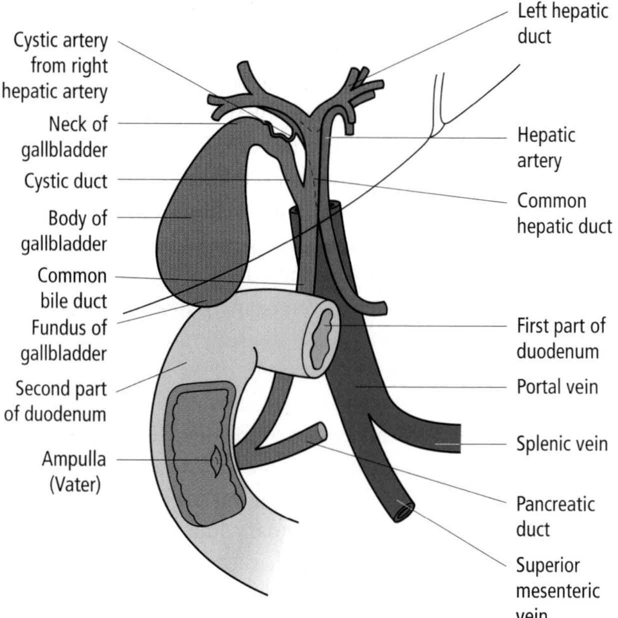

Figure 7.9 Extrahepatic biliary system

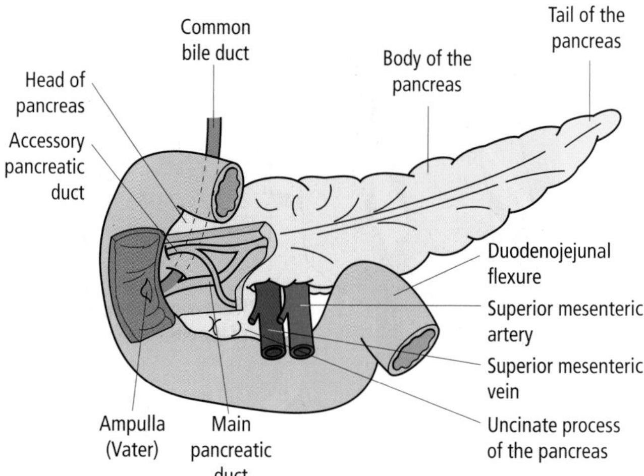

Figure 7.10 Pancreas: part of the head has been removed to show the duct system

THE EXTRAHEPATIC BILIARY SYSTEM

This comprises the right and left hepatic ducts, the common hepatic duct, the gallbladder and cystic duct and the common bile duct (Figs 7.9–7.12). It conveys bile to the duodenum.

The **common hepatic duct**, formed by the union of the **right and left hepatic ducts** in the porta hepatis, descends in the free edge of the lesser omentum to be joined by the cystic duct from the gallbladder to form the bile duct.

The **bile duct,** 8 cm long, descends in the free edge of the lesser omentum behind the first part of the duodenum and the head of the pancreas to enter the duodenum at the duodenal papilla.

Relations

In the lesser omentum, the portal vein lies posterior to the bile duct; the hepatic artery lies to its left. Behind the duodenum, the bile duct is accompanied by the gastroduodenal artery; behind the head of the pancreas and anterior to the inferior vena cava it is joined by the main pancreatic duct, and both open into the ampulla. The **ampulla** opens into the medial wall of the second part of the duodenum at the **duodenal papilla,** 10 cm beyond the pylorus. The papilla contains a sphincter of smooth muscle (Fig. 7.10). A postoperative cholangiogram gives an excellent *in vivo* demonstration of the anatomy (Fig. 7.11).

The gallbladder

The gallbladder concentrates and stores bile. It is a pear-shaped sac lying in the right hypochondrium firmly connected to the visceral surface of the right lobe of the liver by fibrous tissue. It has a fundus, body and neck. Its mucous membrane shows a honeycombed appearance and is thrown into numerous folds.

The neck of the gallbladder is sinuous and contains a constant spiral fold and is continuous with the cystic duct. The fundus and inferior surface of the body are covered with peritoneum.

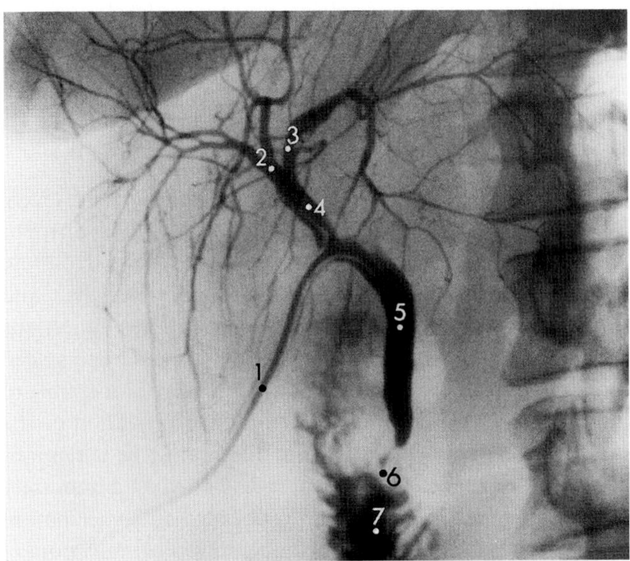

Figure 7.11 Biliary tree, contrast material having been introduced into the common bile duct by a T tube (the gallbladder has been removed): 1, T tube; 2, right hepatic duct; 3, left hepatic duct; 4, common hepatic duct; 5, common bile duct; 6, site of biliary ampulla; 7, duodenum

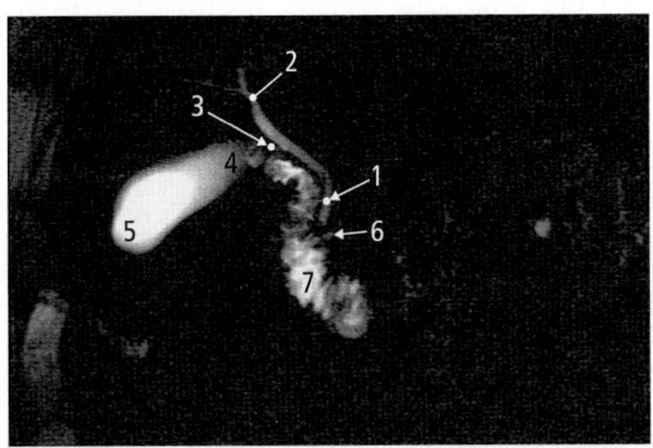

Figure 7.12 Magnetic resonance cholangiopancreatogram (MRCP). 1, common bile duct; 2, common hepatic duct; 3, cystic duct; 4, neck of gallbladder; 5, fundus of gallbladder; 6, pancreatic duct; 7, duodenum, second part

Relations

The fundus lies just below the inferior border of the liver in contact with the anterior abdominal wall deep to the tip of the 9th costal cartilage; the transverse colon is adjacent. The body overlies the second part of the duodenum.

Vessels

The cystic artery, usually a branch of the right hepatic artery, supplies the gallbladder. Lymph drains via nodes in the porta hepatis to the coeliac group of nodes.

Some radio-opaque media are excreted by the liver and concentrated by a normally functioning gallbladder, a feature that is exploited by **cholecystography**, and which can thus explore irregularities of function and the presence of gallstones may be revealed (Fig. 7.13b). Stones formed in the gallbladder may pass into the common bile duct and, occasionally cause obstructive jaundice. Their presence may be confirmed by endoscopic retrograde cannulation of the pancreatic duct (ERCP) via the ampulla of Vater and subsequent injection of contrast. Gallstones that impact in the neck obstruct the gallbladder and cause painful biliary colic; this is felt typically in the epigastrium. If infection of the gallbladder (cholecystitis) follows then tenderness over the area of the ninth right costal cartilage is present and, if the inflammation spreads to the diaphragm, the pain may be referred to the right shoulder region.

Stones in the common bile duct may produce obstructive jaundice. They can usually be removed by opening the common bile duct, although a stone impacted in the ampulla requires an incision in the second part of the duodenum to gain access to the ampulla. Modern duodenoscopes equipped with diathermy allow this to be done endoscopically. Symptomatic gallstones are usually treated by surgical removal of the gallbladder (cholecystectomy, Fig. 7.13a) and exploration and removal of stones (if present) from the bile duct. The biliary tree may be visualized radiographically by cholangiography (Fig. 7.11) or by MRCP (Fig. 7.12).

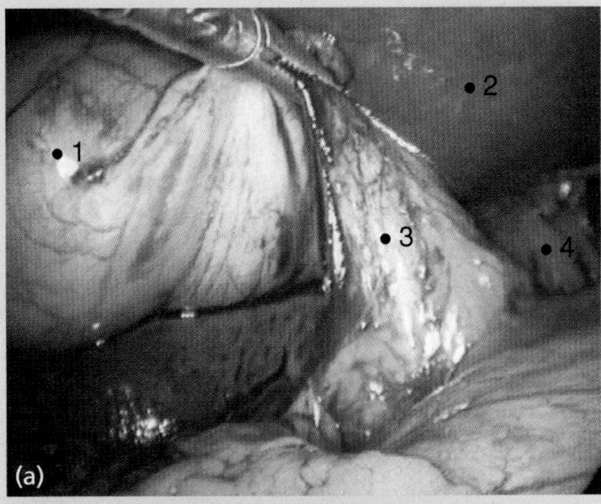

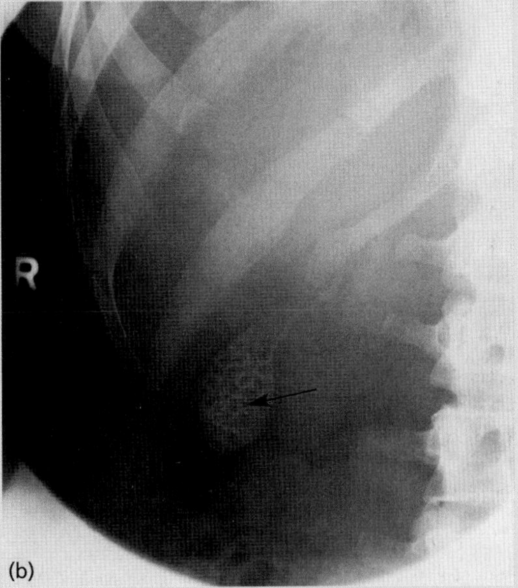

Figure 7.13 (a) Laparoscopic view of gallbladder during cholecystectomy: 1, gallbladder; 2, right lobe of liver; 3, free edge of lesser omentum; 4, lesser omentum. (b) Oral cholecystogram showing multiple gallstones in gallbladder (arrowed)

THE SPLEEN

This large lymphoid organ lies deep in the left hypochondrium, obliquely beneath the 9th, 10th and 11th ribs. In health it is approximately 3 cm thick, 8 cm wide and 13 cm long, and weighs about 200 g. It has anterior and posterior surfaces, inferior, posterior and superior (notched) borders, and a diaphragmatic and a visceral surface that bears the hilum containing the splenic vessels (Fig. 7.14).

Relations

The spleen is invested in peritoneum and suspended at its hilum by two peritoneal folds, the lienorenal and gastrosplenic ligaments, which form the lateral limit of the lesser sac (omental bursa) (Fig. 5.19, p. 84). The diaphragm separates the spleen from the left pleural sac, the left lung and the 9th, 10th and 11th ribs; the visceral surface is in contact with the stomach anteriorly, the left kidney posteriorly and the splenic flexure of the colon inferiorly. The tail of the pancreas, lying in the lienorenal ligament, is close to the hilum (Fig. 7.15). Anteriorly the normal spleen extends no further than the left midaxillary line and its tip may be palpated in the left hypochondrium during deep inspiration (Fig 7.16). If enlarged the spleen extends down towards the right iliac fossa and may be recognized by palpating the notch on its anterior border.

Blood supply

This is by the splenic artery and vein.

Lymphatic drainage

This is to the suprapancreatic and coeliac nodes.

The chest wall gives protection to the spleen, but severe blows over the left lower chest may fracture the ribs and result in contusion or fracture of the splenic tissue. Severe intraperitoneal haemorrhage then usually results, and urgent surgery is required to remove the spleen unless the injury allows conservation of part of it. An enlarged spleen that extends beyond the costal margin is more susceptible to injury. When removing the spleen the close relation of the tail of the pancreas to the splenic hilum must be taken into account. A splenectomized patient has a reduced immunity to infection and prophylactic antibiotics and vaccination are advised, particularly against pneumococcal infections.

THE PANCREAS

The pancreas is both an endocrine and an exocrine gland. It is about 15 cm long and weighs about 80 g. It possesses a head with an uncinate process, a neck, a body and a tail, and lies obliquely across the posterior abdominal wall crossing

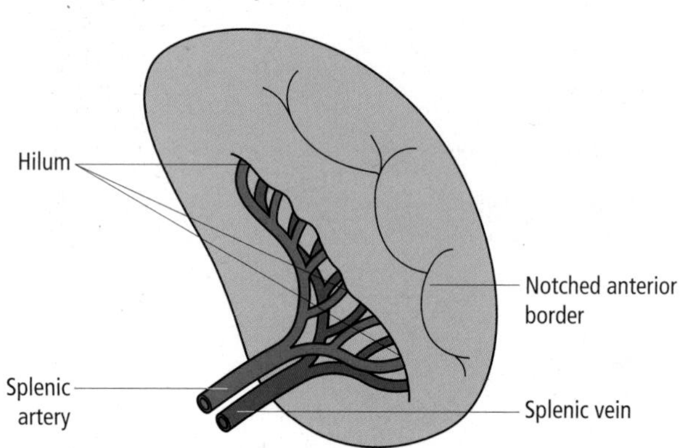

Figure 7.14 Hilum of the spleen

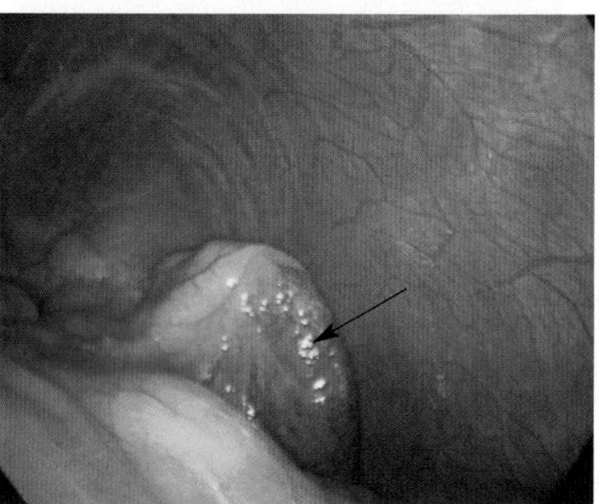

Figure 7.16 Laparoscopic view of spleen – notched anterior border arrowed

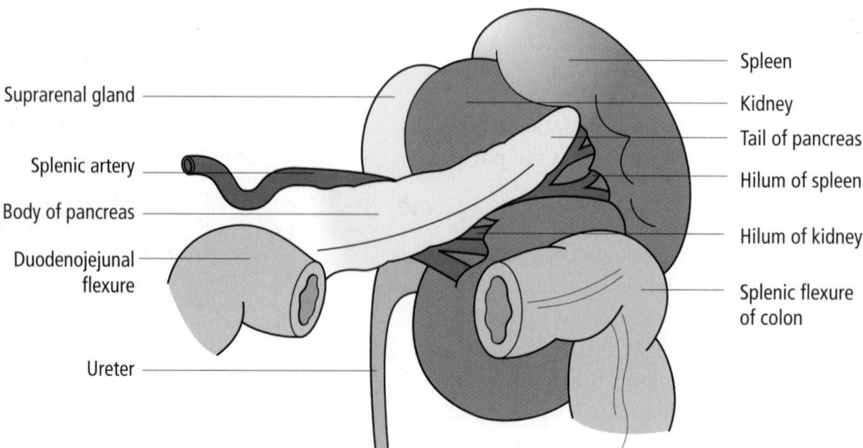

Figure 7.15 Anterior view and relationships of the spleen, tail of the pancreas and left kidney

the first lumbar vertebra and the aorta and inferior vena cava. The head, the expanded right extremity of the gland, bears inferiorly the **uncinate process.** The body, triangular in section, has anterior, inferior and posterior surfaces; the tail is the narrow left extremity and lies in the lienorenal ligament.

Relations

The head lies within the curve of the duodenum. Anteriorly it is covered, from above downwards, by the pylorus, the transverse colon and the small intestine; posteriorly it lies on the inferior vena cava, the right renal vessels and the bile duct (Fig. 7.17). The **uncinate process** lies on the left renal vein and the aorta and is crossed by the superior mesenteric vessels. The **neck** overlies the portal vein and is behind the pylorus and the gastroduodenal artery. Above the **body** is the coeliac artery, and the common hepatic and splenic arteries run along its superior border. Anteriorly lie the stomach and lesser sac. Inferiorly its surface is covered by the peritoneum of the greater sac and it is related to coils of small intestine. The transverse mesocolon is attached by its mesentery to its anterior surface. The body, from right to left, lies on the aorta and superior mesenteric artery, the left crus of the diaphragm, the left renal vessels, and the left kidney, and the splenic vein runs behind it throughout its length, being joined by the inferior mesenteric vein.

The **pancreatic duct** (Figs 7.9 and 7.10) traverses the length of the gland to the head, where it joins the bile duct in the ampulla before opening into the second part of the duodenum. An accessory duct drains the uncinate process and usually drains into the ampulla, but may open separately into the duodenum about 3 cm proximal to the main duct (Fig. 7.10, p. 104).

Blood supply

This is from the splenic and superior and inferior pancreaticoduodenal arteries. The veins drain to the splenic vein and, via the pancreaticoduodenal veins, to the superior mesenteric vein.

Nerve supply

This is from the thoracic splanchnic nerves (p. 69) and the vagi via the coeliac plexus. Pain fibres, whose cell bodies are located in the 6th to 10th thoracic segments, are conveyed with the sympathetic nerves. Pancreatic pain is commonly referred to the back.

Lymphatic drainage

This is via suprapancreatic nodes to the preaortic coeliac nodes.

Embryology

The pancreas develops from the foregut. A ventral bud arises from the duodenum and a dorsal bud arises more proximally. Differential growth and rotation of the duodenum bring the buds together dorsally and fusion occurs.

Rarely the two embryonic buds encircle the duodenum and may cause duodenal obstruction. **Pancreatitis** (inflammation of the gland) is often the result of gallstone impaction in the ampulla or reflux of bile into the pancreatic duct. It causes glandular secretions rich in proteolytic enzymes to escape into the surrounding tissues to produce severe abdominal and back pain, peritonitis and severe systemic upset. The inflammatory fluid produced may accumulate in the lesser sac to form a 'pseudocyst' of the pancreas.

The pancreas is rarely **injured** because of its deep-seated location, but severe crush injuries of the abdomen may result in the pancreas being crushed against the vertebral column, producing ductal tears and leakage of pancreatic secretions into the abdomen. **Cancer of the pancreas** (Fig. 7.18) is usually advanced at the time of diagnosis because of spread to the lymph nodes and curative excision is rarely possible. If the cancer involves the head then obstructive jaundice secondary to bile duct or ampullary obstruction is a likely presentation; if it involves the body then unremitting back pain may result, owing to the invasion of the neighbouring neural plexuses.

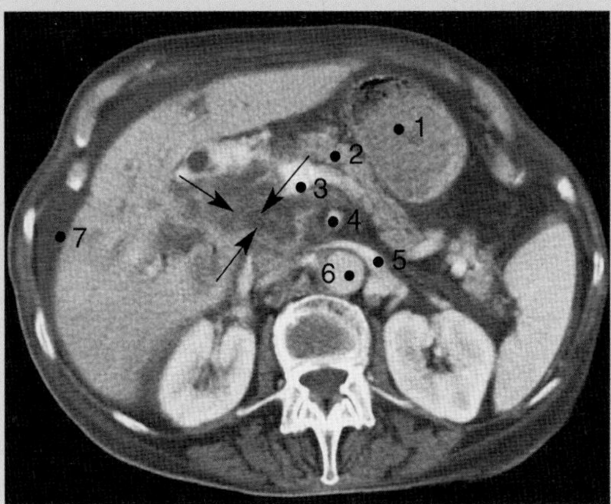

Figure 7.18 CT showing malignant tumour in the head of the pancreas (arrows): 1, stomach; 2, pancreatic body; 3, origin of portal vein; 4, superior mesenteric artery; 5, left renal vein; 6, aorta; 7, ascites (viewed from below)

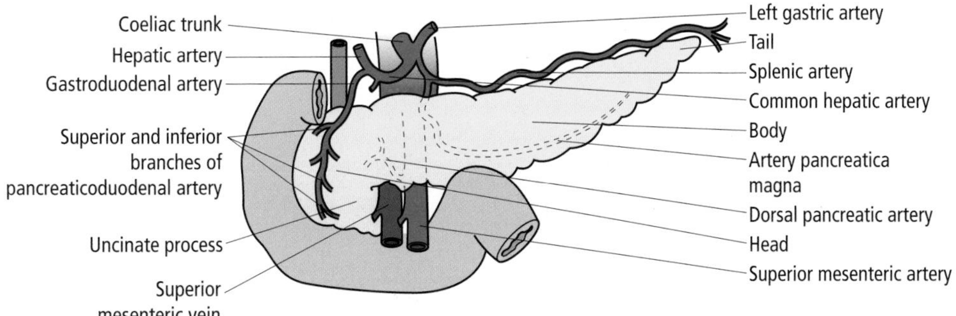

Figure 7.17 Arterial supply of the pancreas

MCQs

1. The pancreas: **T/F**

- **a** is an intraperitonal structure (____)
- **b** usually has two major ducts (____)
- **c** is related to the greater sac of peritoneum (____)
- **d** lies anterior to the right and left renal veins (____)
- **e** is closely related to the hepatic duct (____)

Answers

1.

a ***F*** *– It is only covered by peritoneum anteriorly, the tail lies within the lienorenal ligament.*

b ***T*** *– The main pancreatic duct joins the bile duct in the ampulla and opens about the middle of the medial wall of the descending duodenum. The accessory duct draining the uncinate process may open separately into the duodenum proximal to the duodenal papilla, but frequently joins the main pancreatic duct.*

c ***T*** *– The transverse mesocolon which is attached to the border between the anterior and inferior surfaces to the gland separates these two peritoneal sacs.*

d ***T*** *– Both renal veins join the inferior vena cava behind the head of the pancreas.*

e ***F*** *– The hepatic duct lies superior to the duodenum and pancreas.*

---

2. The spleen: **T/F**

- **a** lies deep to the 9th, 10th and 11th ribs (____)
- **b** is separated by the diaphragm from the chest wall (____)
- **c** is closely related to the stomach (____)
- **d** is separated by the stomach from the tail of the pancreas (____)
- **e** is closely related to the left kidney (____)

Answers

2.

a ***T*** *– It lies posterior to the midaxillary line deep to these ribs …*

b ***T*** *– … being separated from them by the diaphragm and the left pleural sac.*

c ***T*** *– Its anterior surface is directly related to the greater curvature of the stomach.*

d ***F*** *– The tail of the pancreas extends in the lienorenal ligament to the hilum of the spleen.*

e ***T*** *– The posterior surface is closely related to the left kidney and suprarenal gland.*

EMQs

Each question has an anatomical theme linked to the chapter, and a list of 10 related items (A–J) placed in alphabetical order: these are followed by five statements (1–5). Match **one or more** of the items A–J to each of the five statements.

Liver

A. Caudate lobe
B. Caudate process
C. Coronary ligament
D. Falciform ligament
E. Left lobe
F. Left triangular ligament
G. Lesser omentum
H. Porta hepatis
I. Quadrate lobe
J. Right triangular ligament

Match the following statements with the appropriate item(s) from the above list.

1. Lies to the left of the gallbladder
2. Site of exit of the common bile duct from the liver
3. Encloses the bare area of the liver
4. Related posteriorly to the oesophagus
5. An anterior relation to the opening of the lesser sac

Answers

1 I; 2 H; 3 CJ; 4 E; 5 G

APPLIED QUESTIONS

1. What may be the consequences of a boy falling from his bike on his left side? Why may the abdominal injury sustained cause left shoulder tip pain?

1. Severe blows to the left hypochondrium, especially when associated with rib fractures, can tear the splenic capsule and lacerate the soft, pulpy, friable parenchyma of the spleen. Splenectomy often has to be performed to arrest haemorrhage, but repair is preferable because of the spleen's importance in immunity. Left shoulder tip pain is due to irritation of the nearby diaphragm; pain is referred by its nerve supply, the phrenic, to the supraclavicular C4 dermatome, which also supplies the skin of the shoulder region.

---

2. Why must the patient hold his breath during a liver biopsy?

2. When the biopsy needle is in the liver the diaphragm must remain stationary, otherwise the liver moves and can be lacerated by the needle. Diaphragmatic movement may cause the pleura to be punctured and cause a pneumothorax.

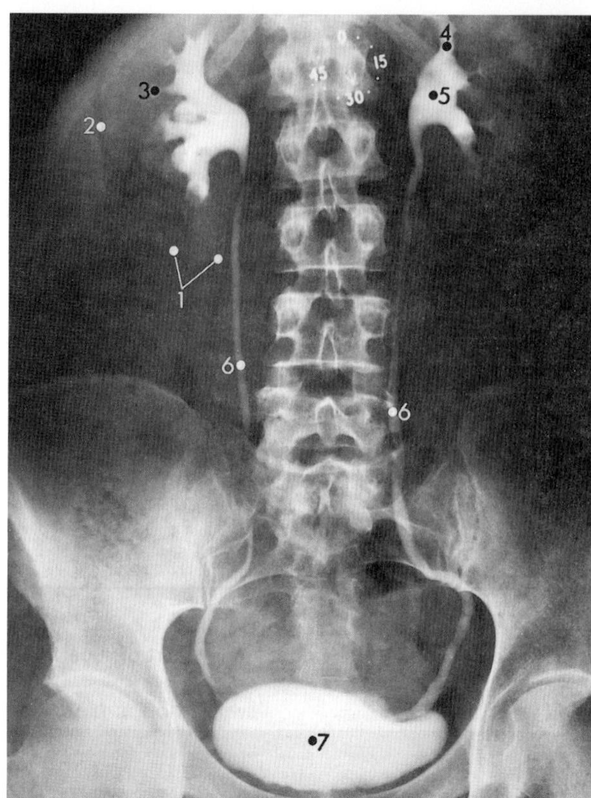

Figure 8.5 Intravenous urogram (IVU): 1, contour of lower pole of right kidney; 2, lateral margin of kidney; 3, minor calyx; 4, major calyx; 5, left renal pelvis; 6, left and right ureters; 7, urinary bladder

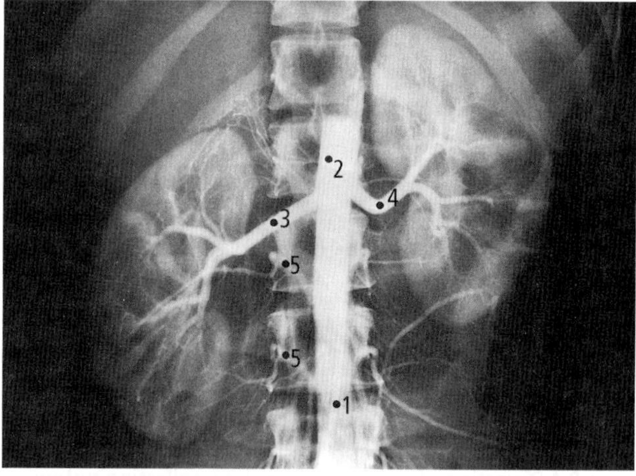

Figure 8.6 Angiogram showing both renal arteries: 1, catheter; 2, aorta; 3, right renal artery; 4, left renal artery; 5, lumbar arteries

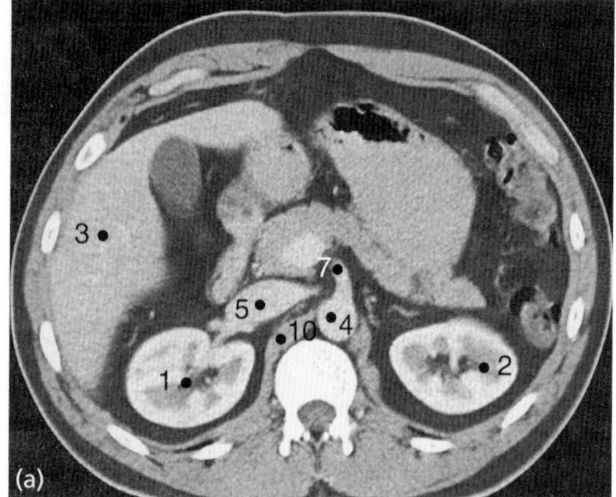

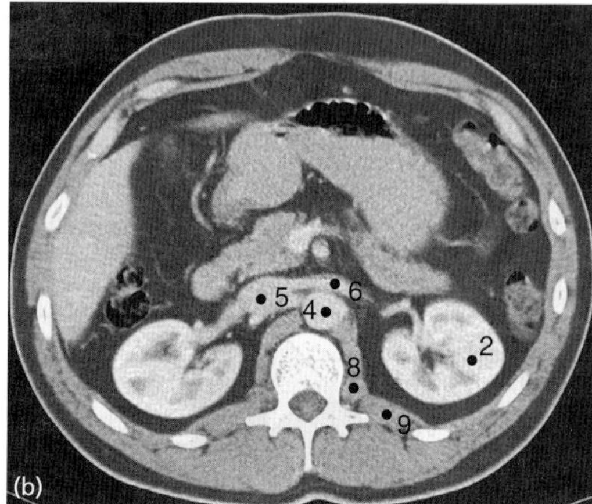

Figure 8.7 (a) and (b) Axial CT scans at the L1/L2 level showing the hila of the kidneys: 1, right kidney; 2, left kidney; 3, liver; 4, aorta; 5, IVC; 6, left renal vein; 7, superior mesenteric artery; 8, psoas muscle; 9, quadratus lumborum muscle; 10, right crus diaphragm

THE URETERS

The ureters are narrow muscular tubes about 25 cm long. Each has a dilated upper end, the pelvis. They are lined with transitional epithelium, as is the bladder. The upper half of each ureter lies on the posterior abdominal wall and the lower half is within the pelvis. There are three narrowings in the ureter: at the pelviureteric junction, at the brim of the pelvis, and on entering the bladder. A stone or blood clot may impact at these sites, causing ureteric obstruction.

Relations

The abdominal course of the ureters is similar in both sexes but their relationships differ on the right and the left sides, whereas in the pelvis, although their courses are different in the two sexes, their relations on both sides are the same.

- **Abdominal part** – the **right ureter** descends on the psoas muscle and is crossed by the second part of the duodenum and vessels supplying the right colon and small bowel. The **left ureter** also descends on psoas but is crossed by the root of the sigmoid colon. Both ureters are covered by and adherent to the peritoneum.
- **Pelvic part** – in the **male,** in front of the sacroiliac joint it crosses the common iliac vessels and descends on the pelvic wall to the ischial spine, where it is crossed by the ductus deferens before turning medially above levator ani. In the **female** it similarly descends to the ischial spine and turns medially, passing under the root of the broad ligament, where it lies adjacent to the vaginal lateral fornix, and is there crossed superiorly by the uterine artery just before it enters the bladder.

Blood supply

This is via anastomoses between the renal, gonadal and inferior vesical arteries. Venous drainage is into renal, gonadal and internal iliac veins.

Lymphatic drainage

This is to the para-aortic and internal iliac nodes.

Embryology

Urinary tissue develops bilaterally from the mesonephros and a more caudal metanephros. Ureters, calyces and collecting ducts arise from the mesonephros and the remaining parts of the kidney from the metanephros.

Abnormalities occasionally occur: for example a double kidney or double ureter on one or both sides; occasionally a 'horseshoe' kidney is present, the caudal ends of each kidney being fused in front of the aorta.

Radiology

The outline of the calyces, pelvis, ureter and bladder can be readily shown (Fig. 8.5) by injection of contrast material intravenously or by retrograde instillation into the ureter. Injection of contrast intra-arterially (Fig. 8.6) may reveal vascular abnormalities or abnormal vascular patterns characteristic of malignant change in the kidney. A plain X-ray of the abdomen may reveal radio-opaque calculi along the course of the ureter, which lies, as seen radiographically, over the tips of the transverse processes of the lumbar vertebrae, in front of the sacroiliac joint, and over the ischial spine prior to passing medially to the bladder (Fig. 8.8b). Obstruction of the ureter by stone or clot produces sharp severe renal colic, felt in the lateral abdomen, the groin and, sometimes, the external genitalia (see above).

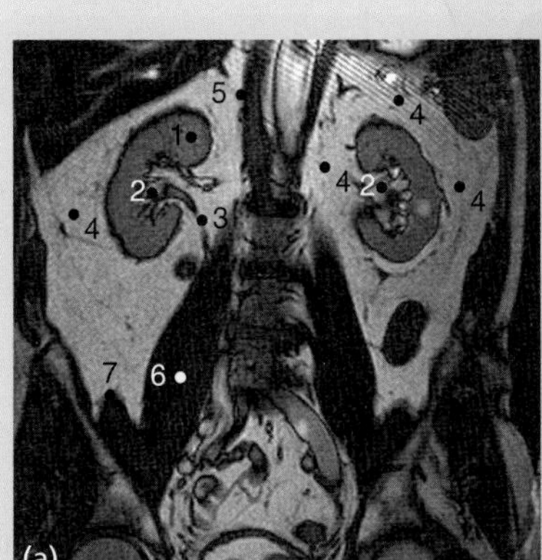

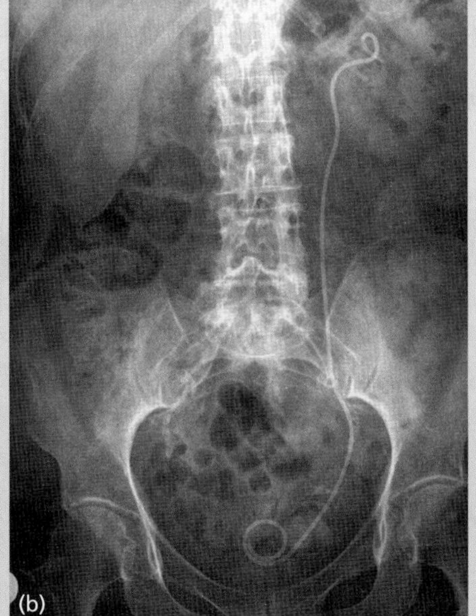

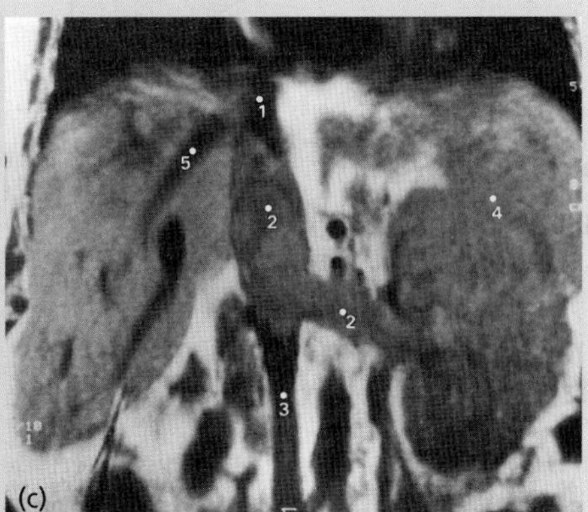

Figure 8.8 (a) Coronal MRI of normal kidneys: 1, upper pole of kidney; 2, hilum of kidney; 3, ureter; 4, perinephric fat (white region); 5, right crus diaphragm; 6, psoas muscle; 7, quadratus lumborum muscle. (b) Plain X-ray of an abdomen showing stent in left ureter. (c) MRI of coronal abdominal section illustrating left renal carcinoma with tumour extending along the renal vein into the inferior vena cava: 1, inferior vena cava above tumour mass; 2, tumour mass in inferior vena cava and left renal vein; 3, inferior vena cava below tumour mass; 4, renal carcinoma; 5, hepatic vein

THE SUPRARENALS

These lie on the upper pole of each kidney, enclosed in a sheath outside but adjacent to the perirenal fascia (Fig. 8.9). Each weighs about 5 g. The **right suprarenal** is pyramidal in shape and lies on the right crus of the diaphragm behind the inferior vena cava (Fig. 8.10a). The **left suprarenal** is crescentic and lies superomedially (Fig. 8.10b), its lower pole reaching the hilum of the kidney. It lies in front of the left crus, behind the pancreas and splenic vessels. Between the two glands is the coeliac plexus, with which they are intimately connected.

Blood supply

This is via suprarenal arteries arising on each side from the phrenic and renal arteries and the aorta. A large vein drains, on the right, to the inferior vena cava and, on the left, to the left renal vein.

Nerve supply

Preganglionic fibres from the thoracic splanchnic nerves, especially the greater splanchnic (Fig. 4.17, p. 68), pass via the coeliac plexus to end by synapsing with cells in the suprarenal medulla.

Nerves of the posterior abdominal wall

These comprise the subcostal nerve and the upper branches of the lumbosacral plexus (Figs 8.13 and 8.14).

The **subcostal nerve,** the ventral ramus of the 12th thoracic nerve, enters the abdomen under the lateral arcuate ligament on quadratus lumborum to cross the muscle obliquely. It supplies the posterior wall muscles and skin and parietal peritoneum in the suprapubic region.

The **lumbar part of the lumbosacral plexus** forms in the substance of psoas from the ventral rami of the first four lumbar nerves.

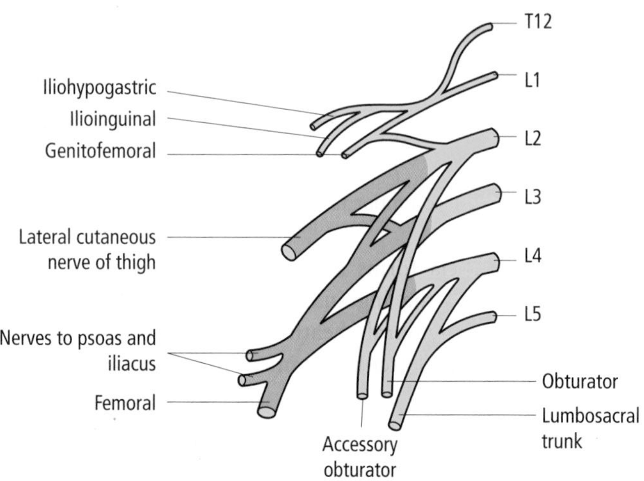

Figure 8.13 Lumbar plexus

Branches

The **iliohypogastric** and **ilioinguinal** nerves pass laterally around the posterior abdominal wall (Fig. 8.14a,b), the latter passing along the inguinal canal. They supply anterior wall muscles and skin over the pubis and external genitalia. The genitofemoral nerve descends on the surface of psoas; the genital branch traverses the inguinal canal to supply the cremasteric muscle and the femoral branch, passing below the inguinal ligament to supply the skin of the femoral triangle. The **lateral femoral cutaneous nerve** descends on iliacus and enters the thigh under the lateral inguinal ligament just below the anterior superior iliac spine, to supply the skin over the upper lateral thigh. The **femoral nerve** (2nd, 3rd and 4th lumbar nerves) descends between iliacus and psoas, passing deep to the inguinal ligament on the lateral side of the femoral artery. In the abdomen it supplies iliacus. Its distribution in the thigh is described on p. 237. The **obturator nerve** (2nd, 3rd and 4th lumbar nerves) descends medial to psoas along the medial pelvic wall to the obturator foramen, through which it passes into the thigh. In the female it lies just lateral to the ovary. It has no branches in the pelvis; its branches in the thigh are described on p. 237. The **lumbosacral trunk** (4th and 5th lumbar nerves) descends medial to psoas over the lateral sacrum to join the sacral part of the lumbosacral plexus (p. 145). The autonomic nerves of the abdomen are described on p. 146.

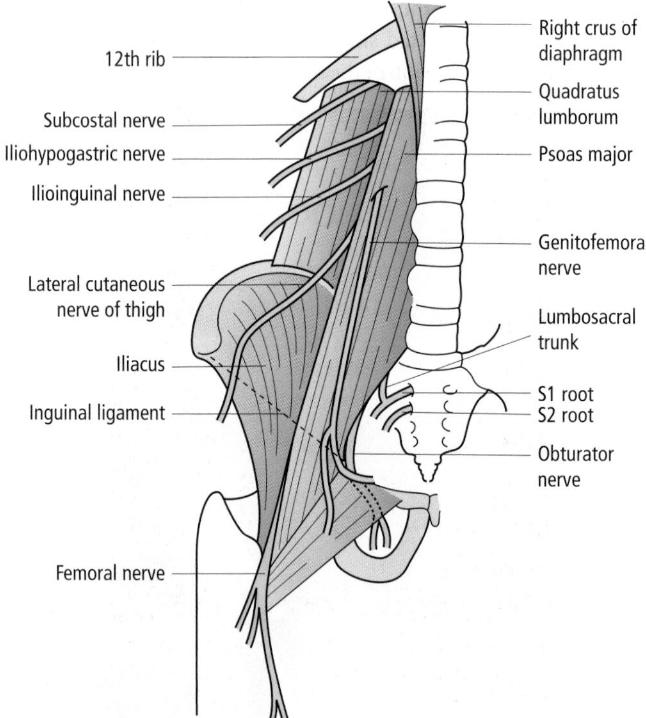

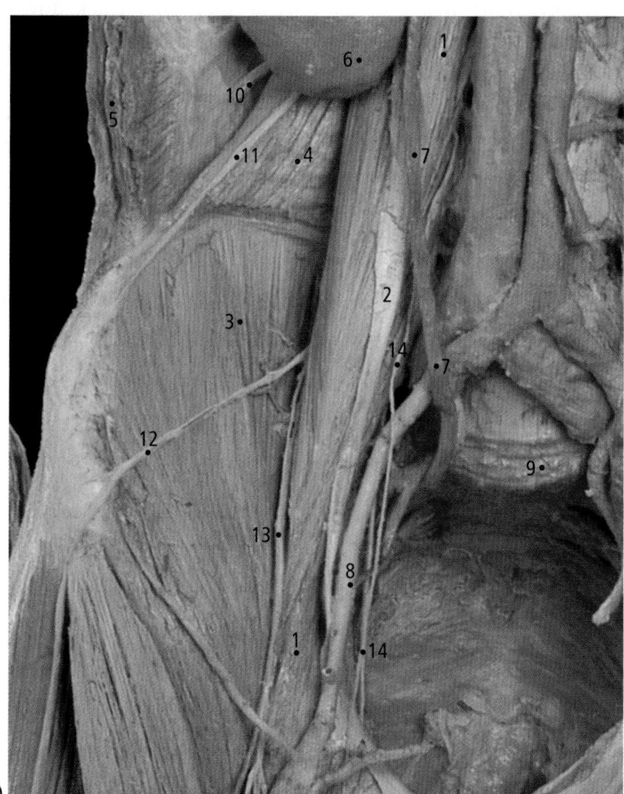

Figure 8.14 (a) Nerves of lumbar plexus on posterior abdominal wall and relationship to psoas muscle. (b) Dissection of posterior abdominal wall with lumbar plexus: 1, psoas major muscle; 2, psoas minor muscle; 3, iliacus muscle; 4, quadratus lumborum muscle; 5, lateral abdominal wall muscles (three layers); 6, kidney; 7, ureter; 8, external iliac artery; 9, sacral promontory; 10, iliohypogastric nerve; 11, ilioinguinal nerve; 12, lateral cutaneous nerve of the thigh; 13, femoral nerve; 14, genitofemoral nerve

Blood supply

1. *Abdominal aorta*

The abdominal aorta, the continuation of the thoracic aorta, enters the abdomen between the two crura of the diaphragm in front of the 12th thoracic vertebra (Fig. 8.9). It descends on the posterior abdominal wall slightly to the left of the midline, and ends on the body of the 4th lumbar vertebra by dividing into the two common iliac arteries (Fig. 8.15).

Relations

The abdominal aorta is surrounded by autonomic nerve plexuses and ganglia, lymph vessels and nodes. The cisterna chyli lies between it and the right crus. It lies on the bodies of the upper four lumbar vertebrae and lumbar veins traverse behind it. On its right is the inferior vena cava and cisterna chyli; on its left lie the left sympathetic trunk and, from above downwards, the left crus, the pancreas, the fourth part of the duodenum and the small intestine. Anteriorly, from above downwards, it is covered by the lesser sac, the pancreas and splenic vein, the left renal vein, the third part of the duodenum and coils of small intestine.

Branches

The abdominal aorta has unpaired and paired branches.

- **Unpaired** – these are the arteries supplying the abdominal alimentary tract, namely the **coeliac, superior and inferior mesenteric arteries** and the **median sacral,** descending to the pelvis to supply the lower rectum.
- **Paired** – the **inferior phrenic arteries** arise as the aorta enters the abdomen to supply the crura and the suprarenal arteries. The **suprarenal arteries** are two or three small short vessels to each gland; the **renal arteries** arise at the level of the 1st lumbar vertebra, pass laterally, and divide into terminal branches in the hilum of each kidney. The shorter left artery crosses the left crus and psoas behind the body of the pancreas; the right artery crosses the right crus and psoas behind the neck of the pancreas and the inferior vena cava. Each supplies the kidney, upper ureter and suprarenal gland.

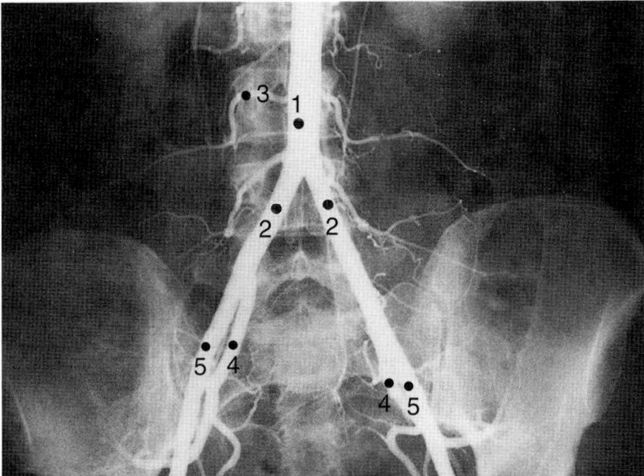

Figure 8.15 Abdominal aortogram: 1, aorta; 2, common iliac arteries; 3, lumbar artery; 4, internal iliac arteries; 5, external iliac arteries

The **testicular arteries** arise at the level of the 2nd lumbar vertebra, descend the posterior abdominal wall obliquely and pass around the pelvic brim to the deep inguinal ring, where each passes in the spermatic cord to supply the testis.

The **ovarian arteries** follow a course similar to the testicular arteries in the abdomen, but at the pelvic brim they cross the external iliac vessels to be conveyed in the suspensory ligaments of the ovary to supply that structure. Each anastomoses with the uterine artery in the broad ligament of the uterus.

There are four pairs of **lumbar arteries,** which each pass back, deep to psoas, to supply the vertebral column, spinal cord and posterior abdominal wall.

Atheroma, a degenerative arterial disease, produces several adverse effects: loss of elasticity of the walls of the larger vessels, luminal narrowing due to subintimal lipid deposits, and loss of smooth muscle of the arterial wall with thinning and loss of strength and consequent dilatation of the artery. The dilatation is known as an **aneurysm** and the abdominal aorta is the artery most commonly affected (Fig. 8.16).

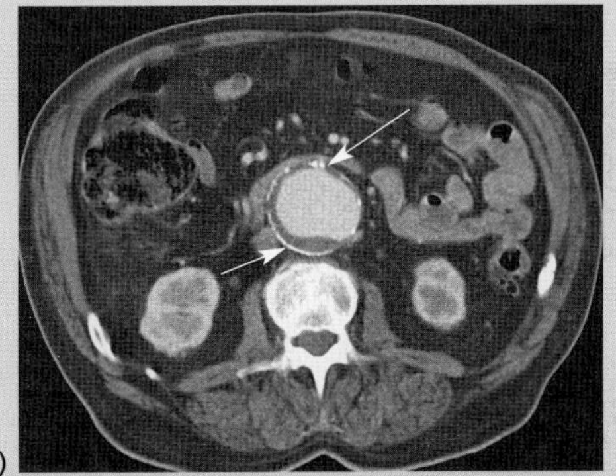

(a)

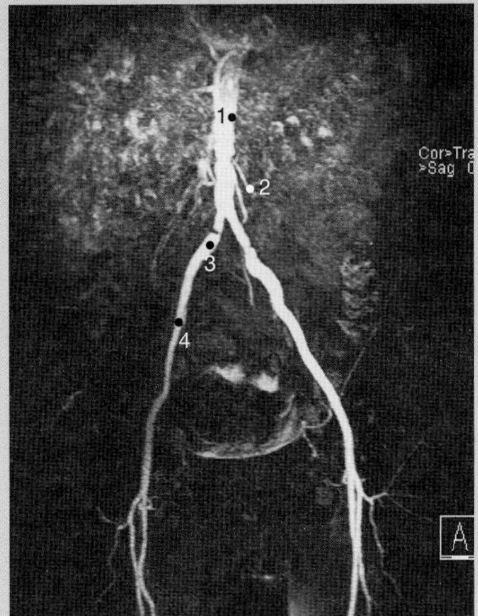

(b)

Figure 8.16 (a) Axial CT scan of the lumbar region shows an enlarged abdominal aortic aneurysm (arrows). Lying immediately anterior to the vertebral body it is about 4–5 cm in diameter and can be seen to have a double or false passage as well as calcification deposits along its outer edge; these are seen as white spots in the aortic wall (arrows). (b) Arteriogram showing arteries with atherosclerotic irregularity, the internal iliac arteries occluded: 1, aorta; 2, lumbar artery; 3, common iliac; 4, external iliac

2. *Inferior vena cava*

The inferior vena cava (Fig. 8.9) is formed in front of the body of the 5th lumbar vertebra by the union of the two common iliac veins and ascends the posterior abdominal wall covered by peritoneum to the right of the midline to the caval opening in the central tendon of the diaphragm. It traverses the diaphragm at the level of the 8th thoracic vertebra and, after a short thoracic course, opens into the right atrium.

Relations

The IVC lies on the right psoas, the sympathetic trunk, the lower two lumbar vertebrae and the right crus, from which it is separated by the right suprarenal gland and right renal artery. Anteriorly it is related, from below upwards, to the right common iliac artery, the root of the small bowel mesentery, the third part of the duodenum, the head of pancreas and common bile duct, the second part of the duodenum, the opening into the lesser sac and the visceral surface of the liver. The aorta is in contact with its left side and the right ureter lies to its right.

Tributaries

- The lower two **lumbar veins.**
- The right **gonadal vein** (the left gonadal vein drains into the left renal vein).
- The **renal veins,** formed in the hilum of the kidney, lie anterior to the renal arteries. The right vein, 3 cm long, lies behind the second part of the duodenum; the left, about 8 cm long, lies behind the body of the pancreas and crosses anterior to the aorta.
- The right **suprarenal vein.**
- **Hepatic veins,** two or three large trunks and a variable number of smaller vessels convey portal and systemic blood from the liver. They have no extrahepatic course.
- The **phrenic veins.**

If the inferior vena cava is obstructed by thrombus or tumour, collateral channels develop to return blood to the heart. For example:

- Within the rectus sheath of the anterior abdominal wall the inferior epigastric veins, branches of the external iliac vein, anastomose with the superior epigastric vein which passes via the internal thoracic veins to the superior vena cava.
- Branches of the saphenous vein, the circumflex iliac and the superficial epigastric vein anastomose in the lateral abdominal wall with branches of the axillary vein, such as the lateral thoracic vein, to carry blood to the superior vena cava. The collateral channels become dilated and tortuous and are visible in these circumstances.

Lymphatic drainage

See p. 98.

MCQs

1. The inferior vena cava: **T/F**

- **a** passes through the diaphragm at the level of the 8th thoracic vertebra (___)
- **b** lies in a deep groove on the posterior aspect of the liver (___)
- **c** is related to the fourth part of the duodenum (___)
- **d** in the abdomen, lies to the left of the aorta (___)
- **e** is formed by the union, in front of the right common iliac artery, of the two common iliac veins (___)

Answers

1.

- ***a*** ***T*** – *Accompanied by the right phrenic nerve.*
- ***b*** ***T*** – *It is embedded in the posterior surface of the liver.*
- ***c*** ***F*** – *It ascends the posterior abdominal wall, passing behind the third part of the duodenum.*
- ***d*** ***F*** – *It lies to the right of the aorta throughout its abdominal course.*
- ***e*** ***F*** – *Despite being formed by the two common iliac veins their union lies posterior to the common iliac artery.*

---

2. The psoas major muscle: **T/F**

- **a** is attached to the middle of the sides of the lumbar vertebral bodies (___)
- **b** is attached to the lesser trochanter of the femur (___)
- **c** receives a nerve supply from all the lumbar nerves (___)
- **d** flexes both the hip joint and the trunk (___)
- **e** gains the thigh by passing below the pubic rami (___)

Answers

2.

- ***a*** ***F*** – *It is attached to fibrous arches which cross the concave sides of the vertebral bodies to the edge of the bodies, the intervertebral discs between them, and to the lumbar transverse processes.*
- ***b*** ***T*** – *As it approaches the femur it is joined by the iliacus muscle on its lateral side.*
- ***c*** ***F*** – *It is supplied by branches of the 1st and 2nd lumbar nerves.*
- ***d*** ***T*** – *Contraction will produce flexion and medial rotation at the hip joint or flexion of the lumbar trunk on the femur.*
- ***e*** ***F*** – *It gains the thigh by passing posterior to the inguinal ligament above the superior pubic ramus.*

---

3. The ureter: **T/F**

- **a** contains circular and longitudinal smooth muscle (___)
- **b** is lined by columnar epithelium (___)
- **c** is innervated by L2, 3 and 4 (___)
- **d** develops from the mesonephric duct (___)
- **e** descends the posterior abdominal wall on a line joining the tips of the transverse processes of the lumbar vertebrae (___)

Answers

3.

- ***a*** ***T*** – *The ureter is a muscular structure and peristalsis occurs.*
- ***b*** ***F*** – *It is lined, as is the bladder, with transitional epithelium.*
- ***c*** ***F*** – *The sensory nerve supply is from the lower thoracic nerves, L1 and L2.*
- ***d*** ***T*** – *The ureter develops from the mesonephric duct; the kidney from the metanephric cap.*
- ***e*** ***T*** – *This radiologically defined relationship is of great clinical use. Radio-opaque calculi within the ureter can be seen overlying this line.*

EMQs

Each question has an anatomical theme linked to the chapter, and a list of 10 related items (A–J) placed in alphabetical order: these are followed by five statements (1–5). Match **one or more** of the items A–J to each of the five statements.

Relationships of the kidney, ureter and adrenal glands

A. Female pelvic ureter
B. Left abdominal ureter
C. Left adrenal gland
D. Left kidney
E. Left renal pelvis
F. Male pelvic ureter
G. Right abdominal ureter
H. Right suprarenal gland
I. Right kidney
J. Right renal pelvis

Match the following statements with the appropriate item(s) from the above list.

1. Crossed by the root of the sigmoid mesentery
2. Turns medially near the spine of the ischium
3. Related to the bare area of the liver
4. Related to the proximal transverse colon
5. Related to the tail of the pancreas

Answers

1 B; 2 AF; 3 H; 4 I; 5 E

APPLIED QUESTIONS

1. Describe the structures pierced by a needle in performing a percutaneous renal biopsy.

1. The needle pierces, in succession, the skin, the superficial fascia and the posterior layer of the lumbar fascia and, usually, the lateral part of quadratus lumborum. It passes through the anterior lumbar fascia and perinephric fascia and fat, then, with the patient holding his breath in inspiration, it is advanced into the kidney. It is advisable to biopsy the lower pole, as parietal pleura covers the upper part of the kidney.

---

2. Discuss the clinical significance of the relations of the iliopsoas muscle.

2. The iliopsoas muscle has important relations to the kidney, ureter, caecum, appendix, sigmoid colon, pancreas and nerves of the posterior abdominal wall. When any of these structures is diseased, especially if they are the site of infection, the muscle goes into spasm – a protective reflex – and any movement of it causes pain. This physical sign often gives important diagnostic clues. A chronic tuberculous abscess in a lumbar vertebra may spread to the psoas and within its sheath, to track down within it and present as a fluctuant swelling in the femoral triangle of the thigh.

MUSCLES AND FASCIAE OF THE PELVIS

The muscles lining the walls of the pelvis, iliacus, obturator internus and piriformis, are covered with pelvic fascia, which, where it overlies the obturator internus, gives attachment to levator ani.

Iliacus

Attachments

Pelvic – upper two-thirds of the iliac fossa and sacroiliac ligament; *distal* – the lesser trochanter of the femur.

Nerve supply

The femoral nerve.

Function

Flexion of the trunk on the thigh; flexion and medial rotation of the femur on the trunk.

Obturator internus

Attachments

Pelvic – pelvic surface of the obturator membrane and adjacent bone. It is covered with the strong obturator internus fascia; *femoral* – the fibres converge on the lesser sciatic foramen and turn laterally to its attachment on the greater trochanter of the femur.

Nerve supply

Nerve to obturator internus, a branch of the sacral plexus.

Function

Lateral rotation of the femur.

Piriformis

Attachments

Sacral – the lateral part of the pelvic surface of the sacrum; *femoral* – it passes laterally through the greater sciatic foramen to the greater trochanter of the femur.

Nerve supply

Direct branches from the sacral plexus.

Function

Lateral rotation of the femur, but it is also an important landmark of the gluteal region.

THE PELVIC FLOOR

This fibromuscular diaphragm, separating the pelvic cavity from the perineum and ischioanal fossae below, is formed by the two levator ani and coccygeal muscles (Fig. 9.5). The **pelvic fascia** has parietal and visceral parts. The parietal part covers the walls and floor of the pelvic cavity. It is thick over obturator internus where levator ani is attached,

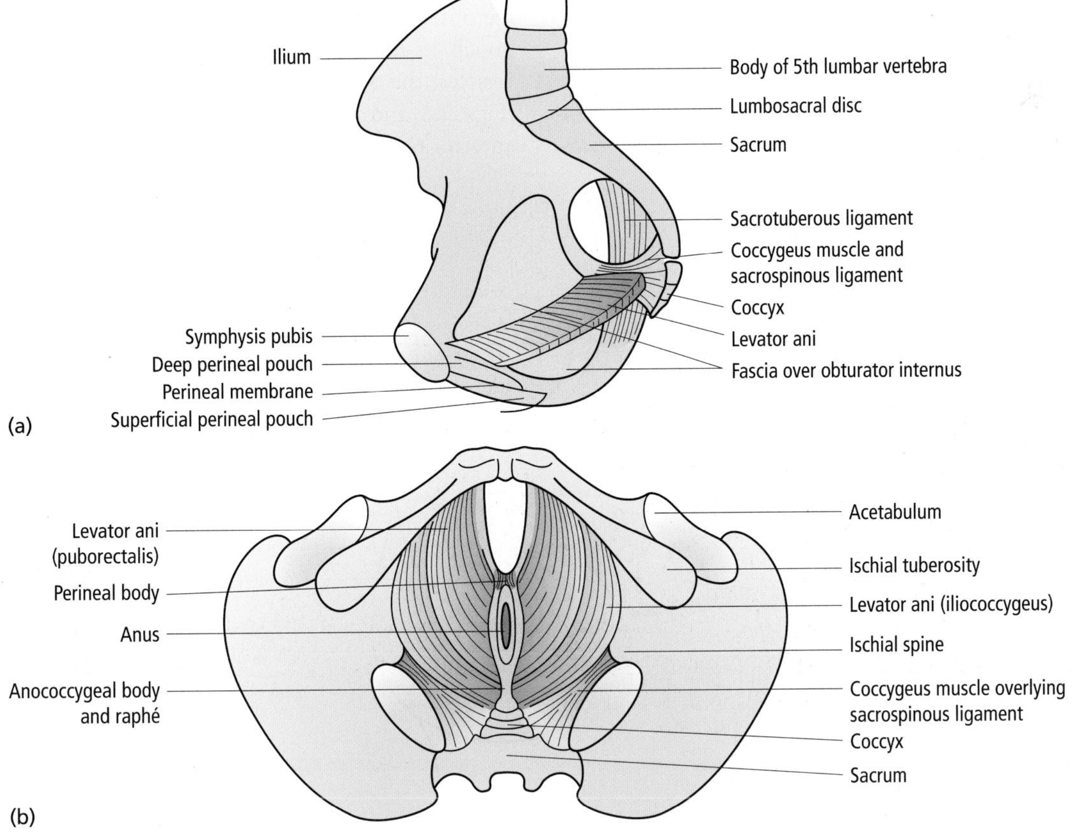

Figure 9.5 (a) Muscles and ligaments of lateral pelvis. (b) Pelvic floor showing parts of levator ani

and continuous superiorly with iliacus and transversalis fascia. It covers levator ani. The vessels of the pelvis lie internal to it and the spinal nerves external to it. The visceral fascia covers the bladder, uterus and rectum. It is thickened over the lower parts of these viscera, forming ligaments that attach and suspend them from the pelvic walls (p. 129).

Levator ani

This is a broad, flat, thin muscle (Fig. 9.5a,b).

Attachments

Lateral – in a continuous line from the back of the body of the pubis, the ischial spine, and fascia over obturator internus between the pubis and ischium. *Medial* – the muscle descends to the midline and there meets its fellow in the midline anococcygeal raphé.

The anterior fibres pass backwards around the prostate or vagina to the fibrous perineal body or central tendon of the perineum; the middle fibres pass backwards and down around the rectum (puborectalis) to the fibrous anococcygeal body. Some of these fibres blend with the anal sphincter. The posterior fibres pass to the coccyx and a midline raphé lying behind the rectum between it and the anococcygeal body.

Coccygeus

This triangular muscle passes from the ischial spine to the sides of the lower sacrum and coccyx.

Functions

Both muscles act together to provide muscular support for the pelvic viscera when intra-abdominal pressure rises during coughing or heavy lifting. They relax during the expulsive efforts of defecation and micturition. They also reinforce the anal and urethral sphincters. The gutter-like arrangement of the two muscles rotates the fetal head into the anteroposterior plane as it descends through the pelvis during birth.

Nerve supply

Both are supplied by the pudendal nerve and direct branches from S3 and S4.

THE RECTUM AND ANAL CANAL

The **rectum** extends from the sigmoid colon to the anal canal. It lies in the posterior pelvis, is about 12 cm long, and begins in front of the 3rd sacral segment, curving forwards with a loop to the left to the tip of the coccyx. Inferiorly it widens – the **rectal ampulla.** It has no mesentery; its upper third is covered by peritoneum on its front and sides, the middle third on its front only, and its lower third lies extraperitoneally, embedded in pelvic fascia.

Relations

Its upper part is in contact laterally with coils of small intestine; below this it is related to levator ani and coccygeus. Posteriorly the superior rectal artery, the 3rd, 4th and 5th sacral nerves, the sympathetic plexus and the sacral vessels separate it from the lower sacrum and coccyx. Anteriorly in both sexes the upper two-thirds form the posterior wall of a peritoneal pouch, the rectovesical in the male and the rectouterine (pouch of Douglas) in the female. Below the pouch in the male, anterior to the rectum, lie the seminal vesicles, the ducta deferentia, the bladder and prostate gland (Figs 9.6 and 9.7); in the female the vagina and uterus lie anterior to the rectum.

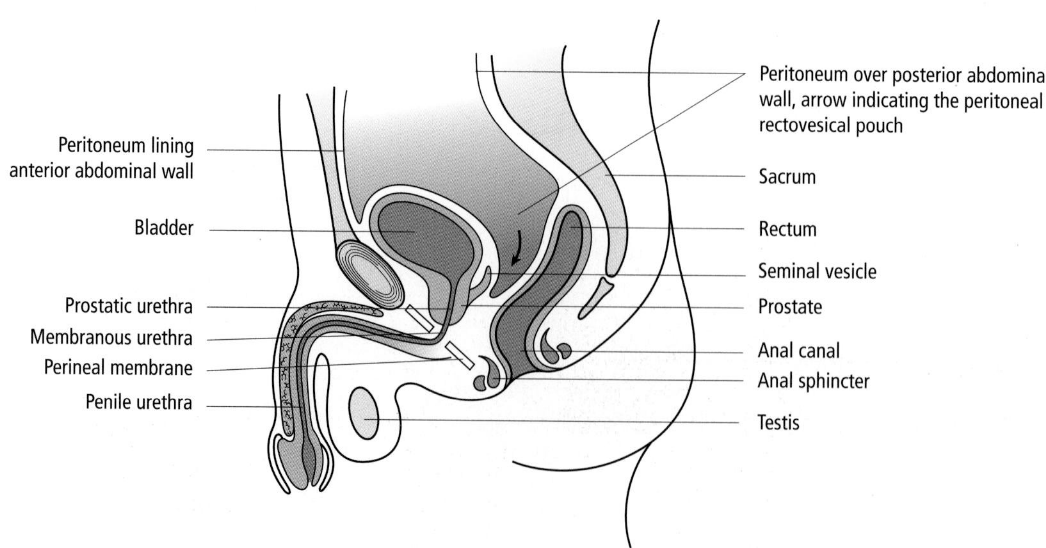

Figure 9.6 Mid-sagittal section of male pelvis showing peritoneal relationships

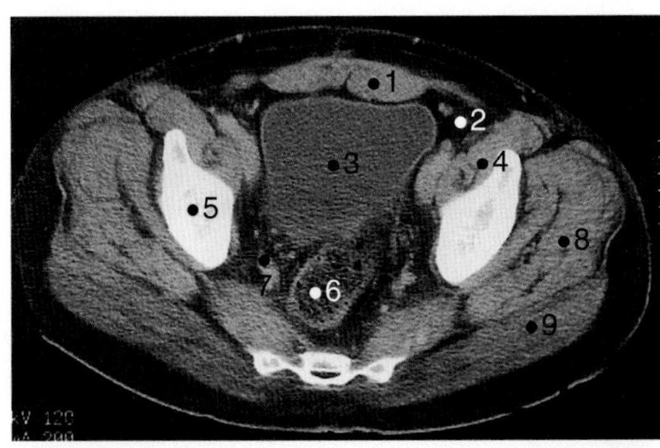

Figure 9.7 MRI of an axial (transverse) section through the male pelvis at the level of the upper bladder: 1, rectus abdominus; 2, external iliac vessels; 3, bladder; 4, iliopsoas; 5, hip bone; 6, rectum; 7, internal iliac vessels; 8, gluteus medius; 9, gluteus maximus

The rectovesical and rectouterine pouches form the lowest part of the peritoneal cavity and are palpable on rectal examination in both sexes. Inflammation of the peritoneum (peritonitis) from, for example, a perforated appendix may result in an abscess collecting in the pouch. Palpation will reveal a tender swelling anterior to the rectal wall. Infection may also be introduced into the pouch by a 'knitting needle' or 'backstreet' abortion in which an unintentional perforation of the uterus or posterior vaginal fornix has occurred.

The anal canal

This, the terminal part of the alimentary tract, is 3–4 cm long (Figs 9.8 and 9.9). It is surrounded by internal and external sphincters that hold it closed except for the occasional passage of flatus and faeces. It descends, turning posteriorly through the pelvic floor at 90° to the rectum, to open externally at the anus. Posteriorly lies the anococcygeal body; laterally levator ani separates it from the ischioanal fossae, and anteriorly the perineal body separates it from, in the female, the lower vagina and, in the male, the bulb of the penis and prostate. The involuntary **internal sphincter,** a continuation of the circular muscle of the rectum, surrounds its upper two-thirds. The voluntary **external sphincter** encircles the lower two-thirds of the anal canal and is arranged in deep, superficial and subcutaneous parts (Fig. 9.8):

- The deep part surrounds the middle anal canal and is reinforced by fibres of levator ani. Damage to this part of the muscle results in faecal incontinence.
- The superficial part surrounds the lower anal canal, attached to the anococcygeal body posteriorly and the perineal body anteriorly.
- The subcutaneous part is a thick ring of muscle surrounding the anal orifice.

The mucous membrane of the upper anal canal reveals 8–10 longitudinal ridges, the anal columns (Fig. 9.8) joined at their distal ends, at the **pectinate line**, by ridges or anal valves into which open the anal glands. Beneath the anal mucosa lie three **anal cushions** one on the left and two on the right, composed of connective tissue and dilated venous tissue. They assist in maintaining continence and closure of the anal canal. The lowest few centimetres of the anal canal is lined by skin.

Embryology

The rectum and upper two-thirds of the anal canal are derived from the cloaca, and the lower third from the wall of an ectodermal pouch, the proctodeum; the line of division of these two parts is marked by the pectinate or dentate line, at which point the anal glands enter into small recesses, the anal sinuses. The membrane that separates the cloaca and proctodeum breaks down before birth, but may persist as an imperforate anus. This dual development accounts for the differences in the blood supply, lymph drainage and nerve supply of these two parts.

Blood supply

This is via the superior, middle and inferior rectal arteries. The veins form submucous plexuses which drain via the superior rectal vein to the portal system, and via middle and inferior rectal veins to the internal iliac vein.

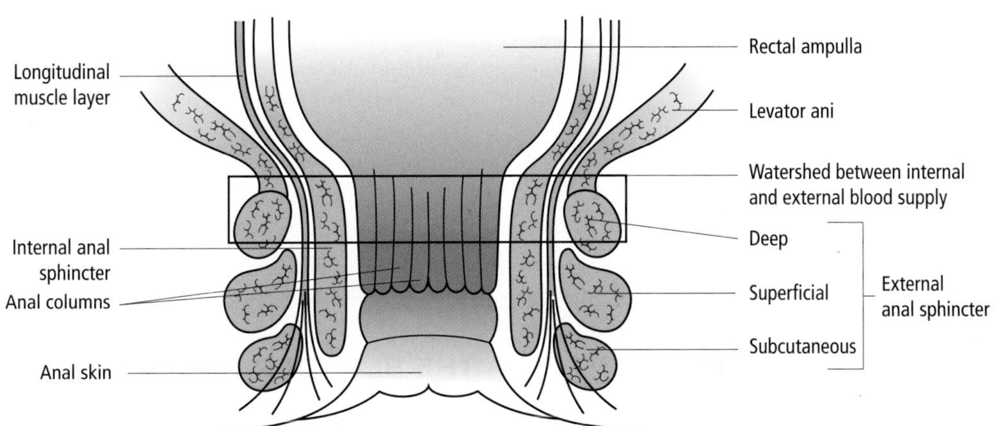

Figure 9.8 Anal sphincter – coronal section

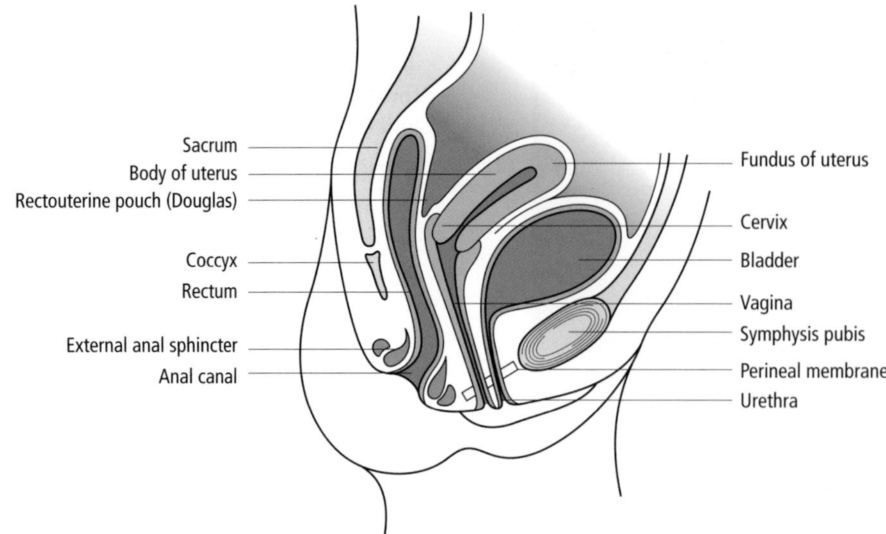

Figure 9.9 Mid-sagittal section of female pelvis showing peritoneal relationships

Haemorrhoids are caused by congestion of the anal cushions, which is usually the result of straining at defecation. They result in prolapsed and congested anal mucosa that may bleed and, occasionally, strangulate. Haemorrhoids are best assessed with a proctoscope. **Perianal abscesses** originate in the anal glands that emerge in the anal valves. They may spread to form subcutaneous abscesses in the perineum or ischioanal space (clinically known as ischiorectal abscesses). Anal fistulae result from the rupture of abscesses through the skin and usually require surgical excision. Anal fissures – tears in the anal mucosa – are common and occur most frequently in the posterior midline.

Lymphatic drainage

The rectum and upper anal canal drain via the inferior mesenteric nodes to the para-aortic nodes, and thence to preaortic nodes. The upper anal canal drains upwards with those lymphatics of the rectum; the lower anal canal drains to the superficial inguinal nodes.

Cancer of the rectum spreads via the lymph vessels, and so surgical attempts at cure must include removal of these nodes. If the whole rectum and anal canal is removed the cut end of the sigmoid colon is brought out and sutured to the anterior abdominal wall to form an artificial anus (colostomy) (see Fig. 6.11, p. 95). **Anal cancer** may present as an enlarged groin lymph gland. Its surgical treatment requires removal of the superficial inguinal lymph nodes, and radiotherapy, to which anal cancer is usually responsive, must include the groin nodes in the treatment fields.

Nerve supply

The rectum and upper anal canal: sympathetic nerves from the pelvic plexuses contract the circular muscle of internal sphincter; parasympathetic nerves from the pelvic splanchnic nerves (S2, 3, 4 relax the internal sphincter). The lower anal canal and the external sphincter are under voluntary control and are supplied by the inferior rectal nerves and the perineal branch of the 4th sacral nerve.

DEFAECATION

Faeces entering the rectum give rise to the desire to defaecate. Defaecation begins with massive peristaltic waves passing through the colon which advance more faeces into the rectum. The rectum then contracts to expel the faeces through a relaxed anal canal. Simultaneous contraction of the diaphragm and anterior abdominal wall helps this expulsion. The anal canal is emptied by levator ani pulling forwards the anorectal angle, squeezing its lumen flat while simultaneous relaxation of the voluntary external sphincter occurs. The anal canal is open only during the passage of faeces or flatus, and continence is maintained by these sphincter muscles.

Faecal continence is maintained by complex mechanisms that are not completely understood. It involves both internal and external anal sphincters, but possibly the most important is the anorectal angle maintained by the puborectalis fibres of levator ani. Normally this is about 90°, but if it is increased to more than 100° then incontinence is likely. Puborectalis, when functioning normally, is palpable rectally as a firm edge posteriorly just above the prostate (the anorectal ring).

On **digital examination** of the rectum the tip of the coccyx and sacrum are felt posteriorly. Anteriorly, in the male, the prostate, and above it the ducta deferentia and seminal vesicles, may be palpable if diseased; in the female the cervix can be felt through the rectal and vaginal walls. This fact is used by midwives, who assess cervical dilatation during labour via a rectal examination. The anal canal and lower rectum are best examined by a **proctoscope,** but a **sigmoidoscope** is required to examine the whole rectum and lower sigmoid colon. Each gives an opportunity for biopsies to be taken.

THE BLADDER

The bladder is a hollow muscular organ lying extraperitoneally in the anterior pelvis, its lower part surrounded by fibrous tissue. Its wall is composed of smooth muscle which is lined with transitional epithelium. Its size and shape vary with the amount of urine it contains: when empty it is pyramidal, with an apex behind the pubic symphysis, a posterior base and a superior and two lateral surfaces. When full it is ovoid and distends up behind the anterior abdominal wall. From the apex the median umbilical ligament, a remnant of the urachus, ascends to the umbilicus. The ureters enter the posterolateral angles of the base and the urethra leaves inferiorly at the narrow neck, surrounded by the bladder sphincter.

Peritoneum covers its superior surface and, in the female, passes backwards over the body of the uterus. Pelvic fascia surrounds the bladder base and is thickened to form ligaments, which attach at the back of the pubis (pubovesical and puboprostatic ligaments), the lateral walls of the pelvis (lateral ligaments of the bladder) and the rectum (posterior ligament). The mucosa of the bladder is thrown into many folds (trabeculations) except over a smooth triangular area, the trigone, between the two ureters and the internal urethral orifice inferiorly.

Relations

The inferolateral surfaces are separated by a fat-filled retropubic space from the pubic bones, levator ani and obturator internus; the superior surface is in contact with the small intestine and, in the female, the uterus. The base is in front of the rectum, separated from it in the female by the vagina, and in the male by the seminal vesicles and ducta deferentia. Inferiorly the base overlies the prostate or, in the female, the urogenital diaphragm (Figs 9.6, 9.9 and 9.15a,b below).

Blood supply

This is by superior and inferior vesical branches of the internal iliac arteries. Venous drainage is via the vesical venous plexus to the internal iliac veins.

Lymphatic drainage

This is to the internal and external iliac nodes.

Nerve supply

These are sympathetic fibres (motor to the vesical sphincter and inhibitory to bladder wall), from the 1st and 2nd lumbar segments via the pelvic plexuses. Parasympathetic fibres (motor to the bladder wall and inhibitory to the sphincter) are derived from the pelvic splanchnic nerves S2, 3 and 4. Bladder sensation is carried with the parasympathetic fibres.

Embryology

The bladder develops mainly from the urogenital sinus of the cloaca; the trigone develops from the mesonephric (Wolffian) ducts. The median umbilical ligament is a remnant of the urachus; rarely its cavity persists from the bladder to the umbilicus, and urine may then drain through the umbilicus after birth.

MICTURITION

A bladder volume of more than about 300 mL in the adult usually provokes the desire to micturate. Micturition begins with slight relaxation of the vesical sphincter, which allows some urine to enter the urethra (or in the female the upper urethra). This initiates a reflex contraction of the bladder wall (detrusor muscle) and relaxation of the vesical and urethral sphincter muscles. Reflexes producing the desire to micturate can be voluntarily inhibited: the urethral sphincter is contracted, tone increases in the vesical sphincter and the detrusor relaxes. Once urine leaks into the urethra, however, micturition becomes inevitable.

The enlarged obstructed bladder, as it distends into the abdomen, strips off its peritoneal covering and hence it is a simple and safe procedure to introduce a needle/catheter in the midline suprapubically, without entering the peritoneum (suprapubic catheterization). The bladder is prone to injury in fractures involving the pubic and ischial rami. If the bladder is distended when this occurs then it is liable to rupture, with extravasation of urine intra- or extraperitoneally. Cystoscopy allows inspection of the bladder, biopsy of its mucosa, and some treatments of small cancers. Advanced cancer of the bladder requires surgical excision.

THE FEMALE INTERNAL GENITAL ORGANS

These comprise the uterus and uterine tubes, the ovaries and the vagina (Figs 9.9–9.11). All are related to the **broad ligament** of the uterus, a bilateral double layer of peritoneum containing fibrous tissue extending from the lateral pelvic wall to the lateral margin of the uterus. The **uterine tubes** lie in the medial two-thirds of the ligament's free upper border; the suspensory ligament of the ovary, containing the ovarian vessels, forms in its lateral third. The ovary is attached to the posterior surface of the ligament by a peritoneal fold, the

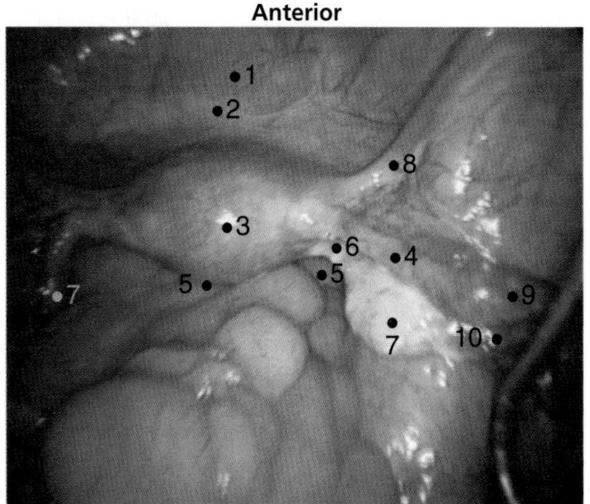

Figure 9.10 Laparoscopic view of female pelvis: 1, bladder; 2, uterovesical pouch of peritoneum; 3, fundus of uterus; 4, uterine tube (Fallopian); 5, rectouterine pouch (Douglas); 6, ligament of ovary; 7, ovary; 8, round ligament of uterus; 9, infundibulum of uterine tube; 10, suspensory ligament of ovary

mesovarium, which contains the **ovarian ligament,** which is continuous with the **round ligament of the uterus.** Within the base of the broad ligament fibrous tissue, the **parametrium** contains ligaments that attach the uterus to pelvic structures. The uterine artery crosses over the ureter lateral to the cervix.

The uterus

The **uterus** is a pear-shaped, thick-walled, hollow muscular organ about 8cm long, 5cm wide and 3cm thick, lying between the bladder and rectum. It provides protection and nourishment for the fetus. Contraction of its muscular walls propels the fetus through the birth canal. It opens into the vagina below and its long axis is usually directed forwards at right-angles to the vagina (anteverted). The upper two-thirds, the **body,** meets the **cervix** at a slight angle which faces forwards (anteflexion) and overhangs the bladder. The uterine tubes join the body at its upper lateral angle. The part of the body above the tubes is known as the **fundus.**

The cylindrical cervix is, because of its attachments, the most fixed part of the uterus. It projects into the upper anterior vaginal wall and is surrounded by a sulcus, the **vaginal fornix;** on the apex of the cervix is the opening of the cervical canal. The larger supravaginal part of the cervix is surrounded by the parametrium and its ligamentous thickenings (see below). Peritoneum covers much of the uterus posteriorly. It covers

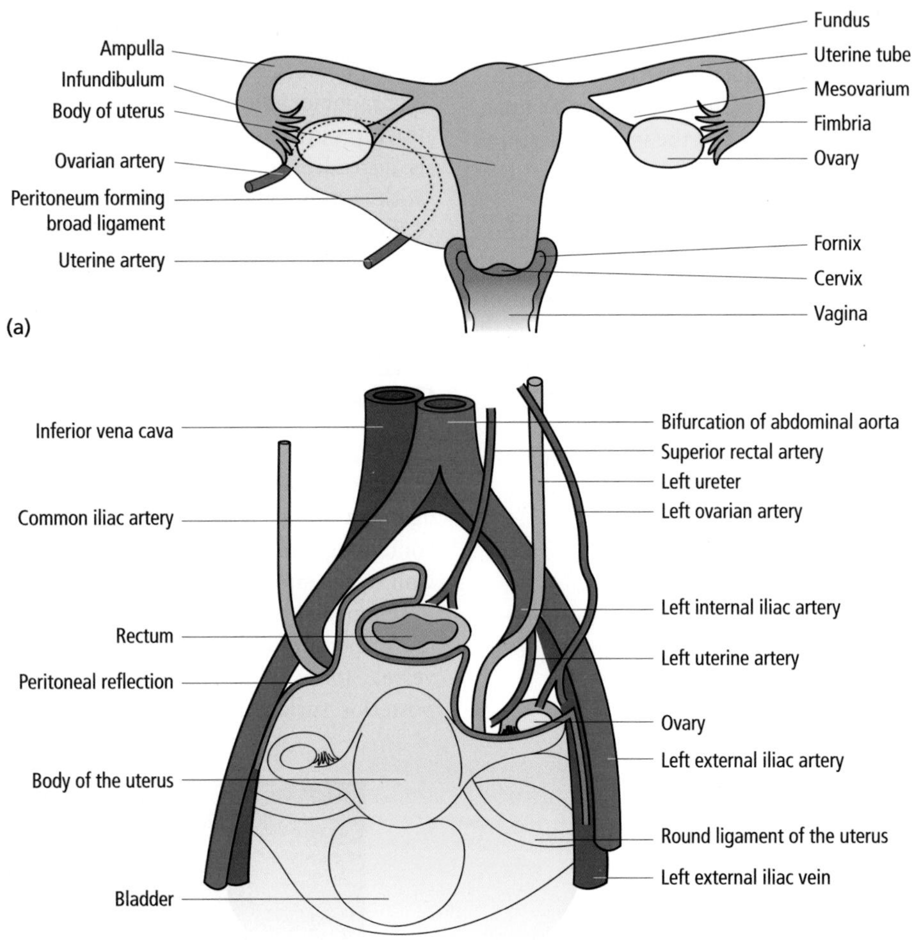

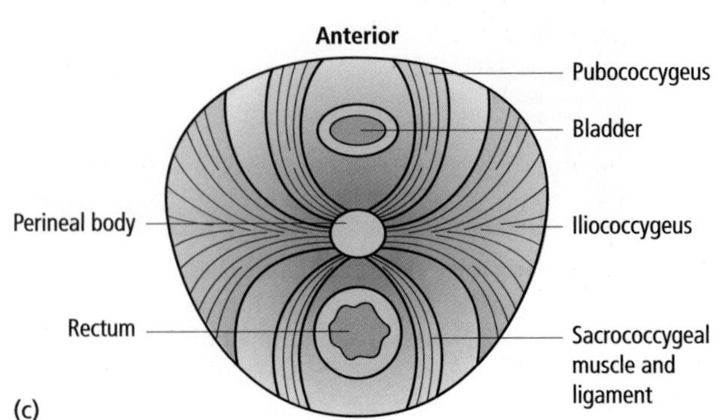

Figure 9.11 (a) Uterus, uterine tubes and ovaries, posterior view. (b) Pelvic viscera and peritoneum. (c) Pelvic floor supports as seen from below. The major supports for the pelvic floor are the pelvic floor muscles, which include the levator ani and its deep portion – puborectalis – which keeps the anorectal angle at approximately 90°. Other important fibres include those from pubo/ilio and sacrococcygeus muscles all of which meet in the midline raphé and especially in the perineal body, a tough fibrous 'knot' of tissue also known as the central tendon of the perineum. Tearing of this structure during childbirth will weaken the floor and may lead to incontinence

the fundus, body, supravaginal cervix and the posterior wall (fornix) of the vagina, and anteriorly it covers the fundus and body, before passing on to the superior surface of the bladder (Fig. 9.9). From both anterior and posterior surfaces the peritoneum passes laterally as the broad ligament on to the lateral pelvic wall.

Intrauterine contraceptive device (IUCD) is a small plastic device, often covered with copper which, placed inside the uterine cavity, will reduce the chance of conception. **Dilatation and curettage (D&C)** is frequently employed in the diagnosis of irregular menstrual bleeding: the neck of the cervix is dilated and scrapings of the uterine mucosa are taken for microscopic study. **Cancer of the cervix** is common; it can be diagnosed at an early stage by vaginal examination, which should include obtaining a specimen of its superficial cells by gentle scraping of the cervix and examining the stained specimen microscopically (Papanicolaou smear). This is the basis of the screening programme for cervical cancer.

Ligaments of the uterus

The **round ligament** is a fibromuscular band passing from the upper lateral angle of the uterus through the broad ligament to the deep inguinal ring, and then through the inguinal canal to end in the labium majus (Fig. 9.11a–c). It is a remnant of the gubernaculum ovarii and carries lymph vessels from the uterus to the superficial inguinal lymph nodes.

The **parametrium** surrounds the supravaginal cervix. It is thickened to form three paired ligaments on the pelvic surface of levator ani:

- The **uterosacral ligaments** – pass posteriorly around the rectum to the sacrum.
- The **lateral cervical (cardinal) ligaments** – pass to the lateral pelvic wall.
- The **pubocervical ligaments** – pass forwards to the body of the pubis.

The uterus is supported and stabilized by these ligaments. The round ligaments may help to maintain the anteverted position. Major support is also given by levator ani.

Stretching and tearing of levator ani during a difficult childbirth may prevent it from supporting and lifting the base of the bladder, and the urethral sphincter then cannot prevent unintended loss of urine from the bladder (stress incontinence) when the intra-abdominal pressure is increased, e.g. during coughing or laughing.

Relations

Posterosuperiorly, coils of small intestine and sigmoid colon separate the uterus from the rectum; anteroinferiorly is the bladder, and on each side are the broad ligaments. The vaginal cervix, surrounded by its fornix and vaginal walls, separate it from the rectum posteriorly and the ureter and uterine artery laterally.

This close relationship of the ureter to the cervix and uterine artery means that it is at risk of injury when the artery is clamped during a hysterectomy. It also explains the frequent obstruction of the ureter in advanced cancer of the cervix or uterus.

Blood supply

This is from the uterine artery, a branch of the internal iliac. The veins drain via the uterine plexus in the lower broad ligament to the uterine and internal iliac veins.

Lymphatic drainage

Drainage is mainly to the external and common iliac nodes, but some drain along the round ligament to the superficial inguinal nodes in the groin.

Nerve supply

There are sympathetic and parasympathetic fibres from the pelvic plexus.

The uterine ligaments are stretched in pregnancy. Failure to regain their original tension may allow the uterus to descend into the vagina (uterine prolapse) and, if associated with laxity in the vaginal wall, would cause the bladder (cystocoele) or rectum (rectocoele) to bulge into the anterior vaginal wall and interfere with normal micturition and defecation. A difficult childbirth may result in partial tearing of levator ani and thereafter the support of the pelvic viscera is similarly weakened, so that the uterus may descend (prolapse) and urinary incontinence result. Thus sudden increases in intra-abdominal pressure, which follows coughing for example, are followed by the involuntary expulsion of a small amount of urine (stress incontinence).

Age changes

Until puberty the cervix and body of the uterus are equal in size, but after puberty the body enlarges. Pregnancy produces a 30-fold increase in the uterine body due to muscle hypertrophy. Atrophy of muscle and endometrium occurs after the menopause.

The uterine tubes

The uterine tubes (Fig. 9.11a,b) are about 10 cm long and lie in the upper borders of the broad ligament. They open into the uterus at its superomedial angle. Each passes laterally to overlap the lateral surface of the ovary, and there opens into the peritoneal cavity. Their function is to convey ova to the uterus. They are described as having, from medial to lateral:

- A uterine part – within the wall of the uterus
- A narrow isthmus
- A dilated and convoluted ampulla
- A funnel-shaped infundibulum
- Several finger-like fimbriae, one of which is attached to the ovary.

Throughout its course the tube is related to coils of small intestine.

Blood supply

The uterine tubes are supplied by the uterine arteries; these anastomose with the ovarian vessels that arise directly from the aorta.

Nerve supply

There are sympathetic fibres from the pelvic plexuses.

Lymphatic drainage

Drainage is to para-aortic and iliac nodes.

Infection can spread directly to the uterine tubes from the vagina and uterus, causing **salpingitis** (infection of the tubes). This occasionally results in a tubal fibrosis and blockage and can be a cause of infertility. **Ectopic pregnancy** is a pregnancy that develops outside the uterine cavity, a consequence of implantation occurring in the uterine tubes and, rarely, in the peritoneum, rather than in the uterine body. In the uterine tubes these pregnancies usually develop for no longer than 6–8 weeks before the tube ruptures to cause an intraperitoneal bleed. The patency of the uterine tube may be assessed radiographically by hysterosalpingography, a procedure that employs the injection of radio-opaque material into the uterine tubes (Fig. 9.12). Ligation of the uterine tubes is used as a method of birth control.

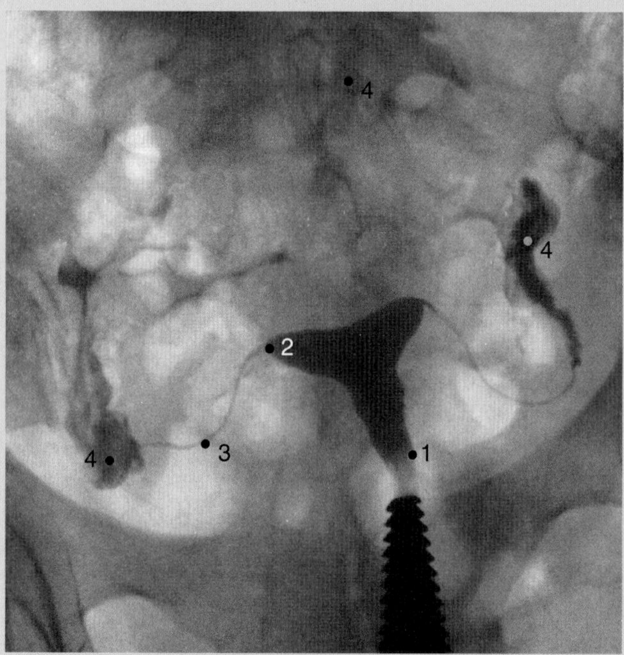

Figure 9.12 Hysterosalpingogram – contrast medium outlining: 1, body of uterus; 2, cornu; 3, uterine tube; 4, ampulla and intraperitoneal leakage (normal)

The ovary

The ovary is an almond-shaped organ about 3 cm long. Its position and mobility vary and it is displaced considerably during pregnancy. It lies on the back of the broad ligament, attached by a double fold of peritoneum, the mesovarium, which covers the ovary (Fig. 9.11a).

Relations

The lateral surface, adjacent to the pelvic wall, occupies the ovarian fossa. This is bounded by the obliterated umbilical ligament anteriorly, by the internal iliac artery superiorly and the ureter posteriorly. Laterally the ovary is clasped by the infundibulum and the fimbriae of the tube; its medial surface lies close to the broad ligament. Its tubal end is attached to the tube by one of the fimbriae and the suspensory ligament of the ovary, which conveys the ovarian vessels.

Blood supply

This is via the ovarian artery and branches of the uterine artery. Venous drainage is via an ovarian pampiniform plexus to the ovarian vein which, on the left, drains to the left renal vein, and usually on the right directly into the inferior vena cava.

Lymphatic drainage

Drainage is to para-aortic nodes.

Nerve supply

There are sympathetic fibres from the 10th thoracic segment via the aortic plexuses.

Embryology

The ovary develops from mesothelium adjacent to the paramesonephric ridge on the posterior abdominal wall. It descends, like the testis, preceded by a gubernaculum, which persists as the round ligament of the uterus and ligament of the ovary.

The ovary is subject to cyst formation and, occasionally, to malignant change. Surgical treatment of the latter requires excision of the ovary and associated lymph nodes. Some women feel their ovulation as pain referred to the paraumbilical region (T10). This occurs about halfway through the menstrual cycle and is known by the German term *mittelschmertz*.

THE MALE INTERNAL GENITAL ORGANS

The prostate

The prostate (Figs 9.13 and 9.14) is a fibromuscular organ containing glandular tissue and lies below the bladder on the urogenital diaphragm (Fig. 9.5b). It resembles a truncated cone some 3 cm in diameter and possesses a base above, an apex below, and anterior, posterior and two lateral surfaces. It is traversed by the urethra and, posteriorly, by the two ejaculatory ducts in its upper half. These, and fibrous septae, divide it into a median and two lateral lobes: the **median lobe** lies between the urethra and ejaculatory ducts; the **lateral lobes** lie below and lateral. Pelvic fascia – the prostatic sheath – invests the organ and its surrounding venous plexus; the fascia is continuous with that surrounding the bladder neck and covering the seminal vesicles; it separates the prostate from the rectum (rectovesical fascia).

Relations

Superiorly – the bladder neck; inferiorly – the urethral sphincter; anterolaterally: the levator ani and posteriorly the rectum and seminal vesicles (Figs 9.7 and 9.15a).

The abdomen

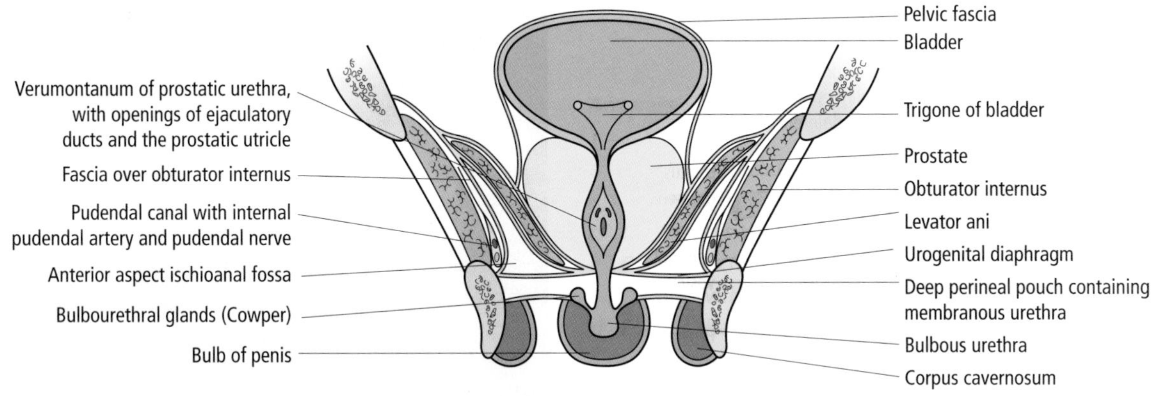

Figure 9.13 Coronal section through male pelvis and perineum; bladder and prostatic urethra

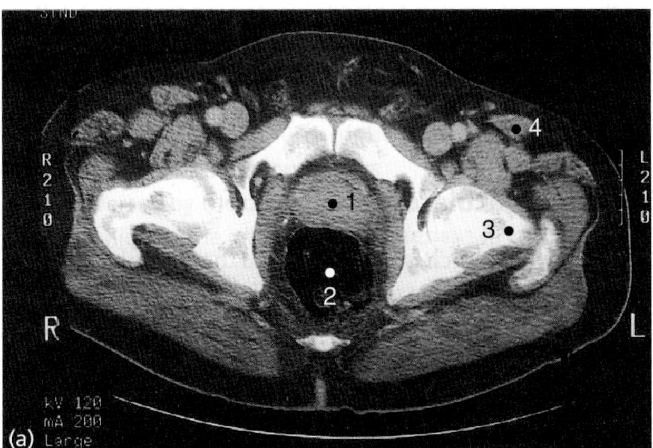

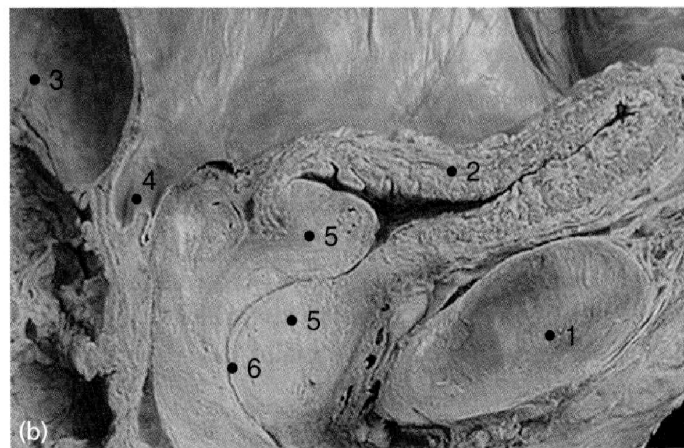

Figure 9.14 (a) Axial CT of low pelvis: 1, prostate gland; 2, rectum; 3, head of femur; 4, sartorius. (b) Sagittal dissection of male pelvis to show enlarged prostate: 1, pubic symphysis; 2, thickened bladder wall; 3, rectum; 4, rectovesical pouch; 5, enlarged prostate; 6, urethra trapped between swollen prostatic lobes

Blood supply

This is by inferior vesical and middle rectal branches of the internal iliac artery. Venous drainage is via the prostatic plexuses to the internal iliac veins and to the vertebral venous plexus.

Lymphatic drainage

This is to the internal iliac nodes.

Nerve supply

There are sympathetic fibres (L1, 2) from the pelvic plexus; parasympathetic from the pelvic splanchnics (S2, 3, 4).

The prostate is readily palpated by rectal examination; the normal gland is felt as a smooth firm mass, possessing a vertical sulcus, under the anterior rectal mucosa. In middle age there is often **hypertrophy** of the glandular tissue, especially that of the median lobe, which enlarges to project upwards, disturbing vesical sphincter action and rendering micturition difficult and incomplete (Fig. 9.14b). Surgical treatment is often employed, although pharmacological methods of reducing prostate size are now being used more frequently. Transurethral resection of the prostate (TURP) is carried out with an operating cystoscope and permits the 'coring out' of the median lobe. Infection in the prostate (**prostatitis**) is very difficult to eradicate because of the prostate's extremely coiled duct system. It is marked by vague perineal pain, and a swollen tender prostate may be felt rectally. **Cancer of the prostate** most commonly first affects the lateral lobes and may be diagnosed by a hard irregular mass on rectal examination. Secondary spread of the cancer is frequently to the vertebral column, the cancer cells being carried there in the vertebral venous plexus.

Ductus (vas) deferens

Each ductus is a narrow muscular tube about 45 cm long, a continuation of the canal of the epididymis. It extends from the tail of the epididymis through the scrotum, inguinal canal and pelvis to the ejaculatory duct.

Relations

In the scrotum, where it is palpable as a firm 4-mm diameter cord, and the inguinal canal it lies within the spermatic cord. It enters the pelvis at the deep inguinal

EMQs

Each question has an anatomical theme linked to the chapter, and a list of 10 related items (A–J) placed in alphabetical order: these are followed by five statements (1–5). Match **one or more** of the items A–J to each of the five statements.

Pelvic viscera

A. Broad ligament
B. Greater sciatic notch
C. Lesser sciatic notch
D. Membranous urethra
E. Obturator internus
F. Ovary
G. Penile urethra
H. Piriformis
I. Prostatic urethra
J. Vas deferens

Match the following statements with the appropriate item(s) from the above list.

1. Transmits the inferior gluteal nerve
2. Contains the uterine tubes
3. Overlies the origin of the internal iliac artery
4. Transmits the internal pudendal nerve
5. Lies within the deep perineal pouch

Answers

1 B; 2 A; 3 F; 4 BC; 5 D

APPLIED QUESTIONS

1. **Discuss the functions of the pelvic diaphragm.**

1. The pelvic diaphragm (levator ani and coccygeus) is the only striated muscle to possess resting tonus during sleep. It has an important role in the support of the pelvic viscera, greatly aided by its attachment to the fibrous focal point of the perineum, the perineal body. It supports the prostate and indirectly the bladder and, in females, the vagina and uterus. It resists the downward displacement of the pelvic organs that accompanies increases in intra-abdominal pressure, e.g. in lifting, coughing, micturition and defecation. The anorectal angle, maintained by the puborectalis part of levator ani, plays a very important role in faecal continence.

---

2. **What structures can one normally palpate during a bimanual pelvic examination in a female?**

2. During a bimanual pelvic examination the clinician can feel the cervix and its external os, the vaginal fornices, and can assess the size and shape of the uterus. A normal ovary is often felt, but the uterine tubes are palpable only if enlarged. Examination of the posterior fornix may reveal abnormalities in the rectouterine pouch (Douglas) and, sometimes, a normal ovary. The size of the bony pelvis can also be assessed.

The perineum

The perineum lies below the pelvic diaphragm (levator ani and coccygeus). It is a diamond-shaped space between the pubic symphysis and the coccyx, bounded anterolaterally by the ischiopubic rami, posterolaterally by the sacrotuberous ligaments, and laterally by the ischial tuberosities. A line joining the ischial tuberosities divides the space into a posterior anal triangle and an anterior urogenital triangle.

THE ANAL TRIANGLE

The anal triangle contains the anal canal in the midline and the two ischioanal fossae laterally.

The **ischioanal fossa** (Figs 9.13, p. 133, and 10.1) is wedge shaped, with its base lying inferiorly between the ischium and the anal canal. It is bounded superomedially by levator ani's attachment to the obturator fascia above and its junction with the external anal sphincter below; laterally by the fascia over obturator internus, and inferiorly by perineal skin. Posteriorly it extends deep to gluteus maximus between the sacrotuberous and sacrospinous ligaments, and anteriorly it extends below levator ani, deep to the urogenital diaphragm. Its contents are identical in both sexes. The two fossae are separated by the anococcygeal body, the anal canal and the perineal body, but communicate behind the anal canal. Each fossa contains lobulated fat; the pudendal nerve and vessels lie on its lateral wall in a sheath of the fascia covering obturator internus (**the pudendal canal**), which lies about 3 cm above the ischial tuberosity. The perianal skin is supplied by the inferior rectal nerve, the perineal nerve and branches from the coccygeal plexus (S3, 4 and 5).

Infection of the glands of the anal canal frequently spreads through the anal wall into the ischioanal fossa (which clinicians still refer to as the ischiorectal fossa) to produce large **abscesses.** Should these discharge through the skin, a chronic **fistula** may develop between the anal canal and skin (fistula in ano).

THE UROGENITAL TRIANGLE

The urogenital triangle is divided by the inferior layer of the urogenital diaphragm – the perineal membrane – into superior and inferior compartments (pouches). The **urogenital diaphragm** is a triangular double layer of fascia (stronger in the male than in the female) that stretches across the pubic arch between the ischiopubic rami. Its free posterior border is attached to a central subcutaneous fibrous mass, the **perineal body.** The diaphragm is pierced by the urethra and, in the female, the vagina. Its inferior fascial layer, the **perineal membrane,** gives attachment to the bulb and crura of the penis or clitoris. Its superior (deep) layer is continuous with the pelvic fascia where the viscera pass through between the two levatores ani. The deep layer fuses posteriorly with the posterior border of the perineal membrane to make a fascial bound envelope, the deep perineal pouch (Fig. 9.13, p. 133). The superficial and deep perineal pouches differ markedly in males and females.

THE MALE UROGENITAL TRIANGLE

The **superficial perineal pouch** lies between the membranous layer of the superficial fascia and the urogenital diaphragm. The superficial fascia is attached to the posterior border of the diaphragm, laterally to the ischiopubic rami, and anteriorly is continuous with the superficial fascia of the anterior abdominal wall over the pubic symphysis (Fig. 9.5a, p. 125, and Fig. 9.6, p. 126). It provides a fascial

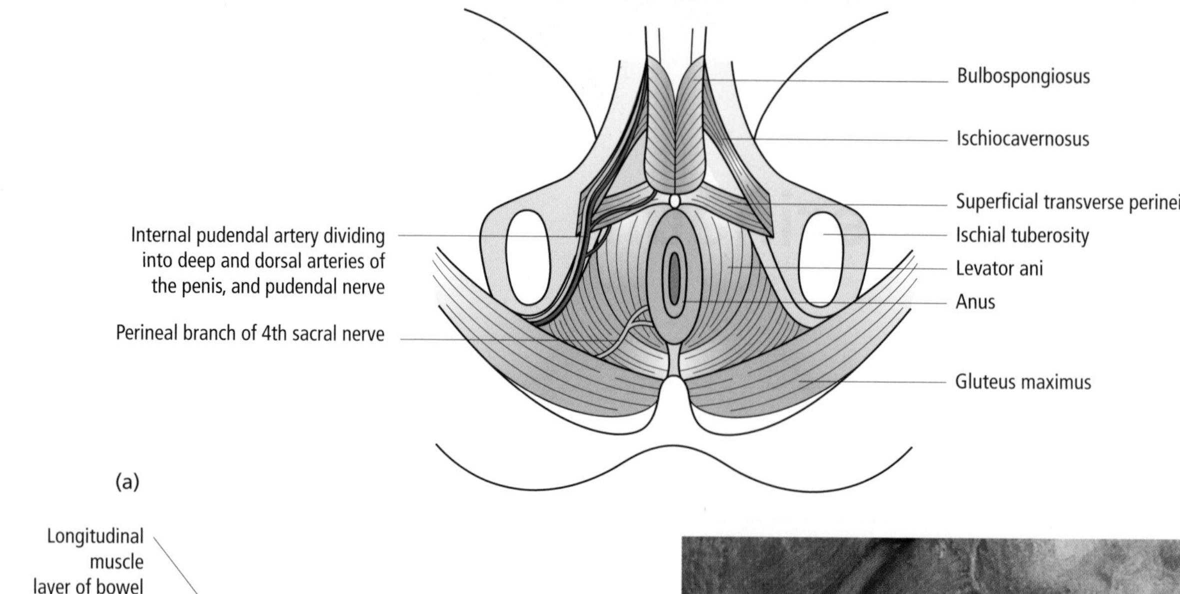

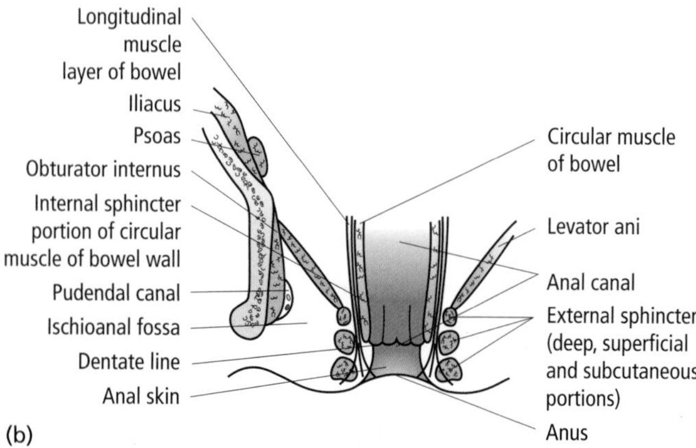

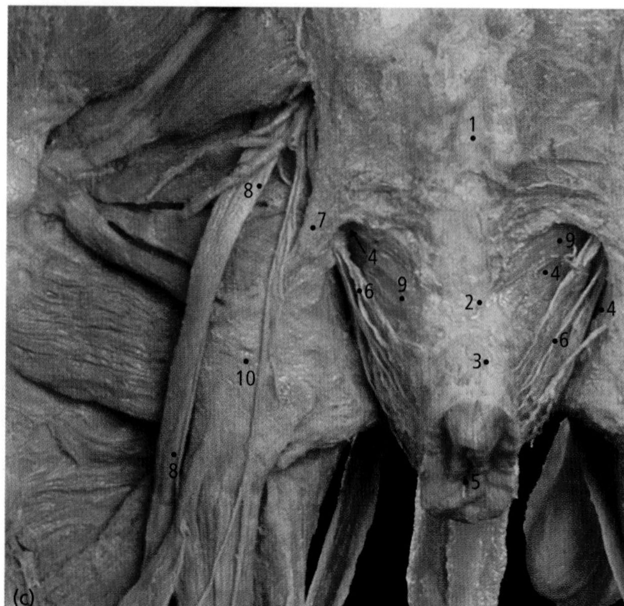

Figure 10.1 (a) Male perineum in the lithotomy position viewed from below. (b) Anal canal – coronal section, showing ischioanal fossa. (c) Dissection of posterior view of anal triangle and gluteal region with gluteus maximus removed: 1, sacrum; 2, coccyx; 3, anococcygeal body; 4, ischioanal fossa; 5, anus; 6, pudendal neurovascular bundle, 7, sacrotuberous ligament; 8, sciatic nerve; 9, levator ani muscle; 10, ischial tuberosity

sheath which contains the root and body of the penis and superficial perineal muscles (Fig. 10.1). The penis, testes and other scrotal contents lie in this fascial space, known as the superficial perineal pouch.

The penis

The **penis** comprises three longitudinal cylinders of erectile tissue: the central corpus spongiosum containing the urethra, and the two lateral corpora cavernosa covered by fascia and skin (Fig. 10.2a,b). It has a body and a root, and the root attaches it to the perineal membrane. The **corpus spongiosum** lies ventral and is expanded to form the bulb of the penis posteriorly and the glans penis anteriorly. The bulb, covered by the bulbospongiosus muscle, is attached to the perineal membrane. The urethra traverses the corpus and opens externally on the apex of the glans. The two **corpora cavernosa** unite dorsally and are embedded in the glans anteriorly. Posteriorly, beneath the symphysis, they diverge to form the two **crura** of the penis, which are covered by the ischiocavernosus muscles. The corpus spongiosum and the corpora cavernosa are enclosed in a tough fibrous sheath, the tunica albuginea, which is itself enclosed by the deep fascia of the penis. This is attached dorsally by the suspensory ligament of the penis to the symphysis pubis. The skin of the penis forms a fold over the glans, the **prepuce or foreskin,** which is attached to the glans by a small skinfold, the frenulum.

Blood supply

This is by branches of the internal pudendal; the artery to the bulb supplies the bulb, the corpus spongiosum and glans; the deep artery of the penis the corpora cavernosa; and the dorsal artery of the penis the skin.

Special attention must be paid to ligating the small frenular artery during circumcision, otherwise severe blood loss may occur.

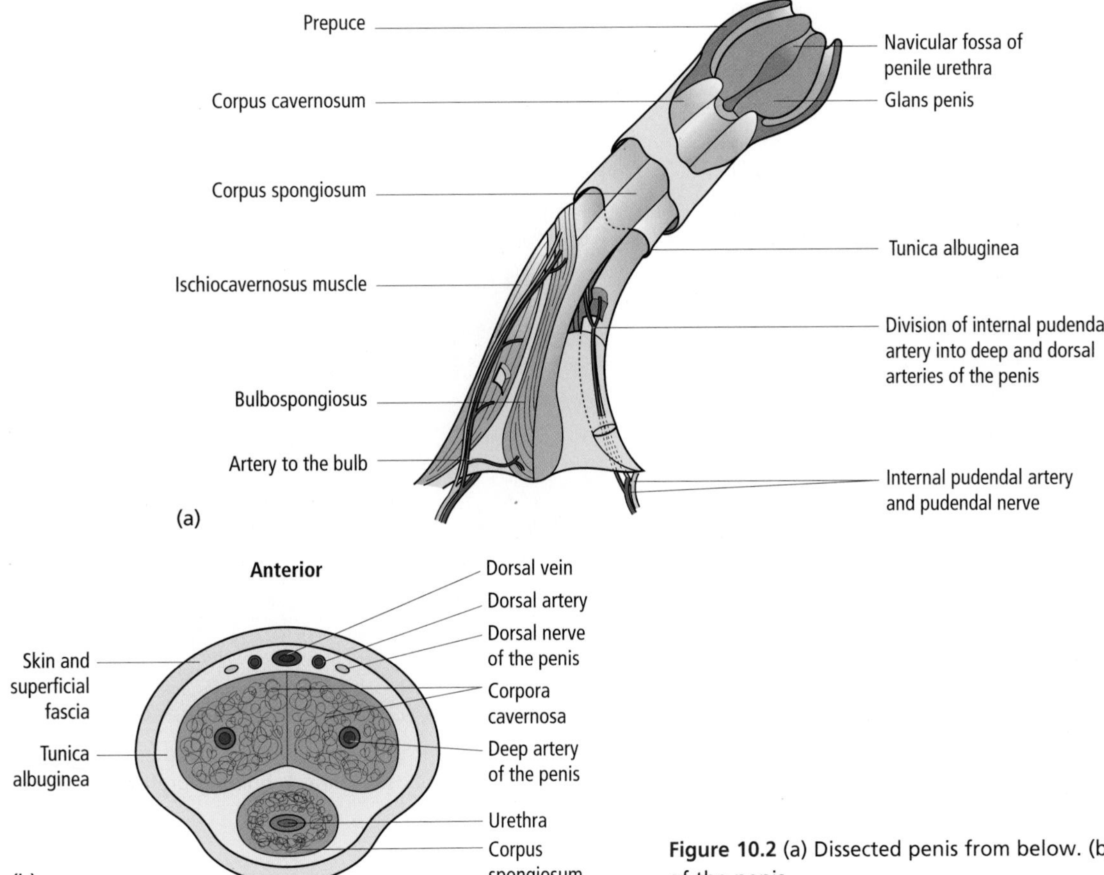

Figure 10.2 (a) Dissected penis from below. (b) Transverse section of the penis

Venous drainage is to the internal pudendal vein and, via the deep dorsal vein of the penis, to the prostatic plexus. Erection is achieved by engorgement of the cavernous spaces. The pelvic parasympathetic fibres cause dilation of the coiled penile arteries. Bulbospongiosus and ischiocavernosus muscles compress the venous drainage from the cavernous spaces. Ejaculation is mediated by the sympathetic fibres – there is closure of the bladder neck and the sphincter urethrae, together with somatic contractions of the bulbospongiosus muscles.

Lymphatic drainage

This is to the superficial inguinal and iliac nodes.

Nerve supply

Somatic supply is by the ilioinguinal nerve and the dorsal nerve of the penis. Parasympathetic vasodilator fibres from the pelvic splanchnics (S2, 3, 4) supply the erectile tissue.

The scrotum

The scrotum is a pouch of thin, rugose skin enclosing the two testes and spermatic cords, separated by a midline raphé and septum. Its walls contain smooth muscle fibres, the dartos muscle.

The superficial perineal pouch

The superficial perineal pouch contains the **superficial muscles of the perineum,** as well as the bulbospongiosus and ischiocavernosus muscles, both of which constrict the corpora and contribute to erection and ejaculation. There are also the paired **superficial transverse perineal muscles,** which lie in the posterior edge of the perineal membrane (Fig. 10.1a). All are supplied by branches of the perineal branch of the pudendal nerve. The penis and penile urethra lie within the pouch.

Leakage of urine from a ruptured penile urethra, an injury which usually follows direct trauma to the perineum or is the result of a fractured pelvis (Fig. 10.3), spreads into the superficial perineal pouch. Its spread is confined by the attachments of the perineal fascia; initially the spread is into the subfascial tissues of the scrotum and penis, and then the **extravasation** ascends the anterior abdominal wall deep to its superficial fascia. It cannot spread into the thigh because of the attachments of the perineal fascia to the fascia lata.

The deep perineal pouch

The **deep perineal pouch** is a closed space sandwiched between the two layers of the urogenital diaphragm. It contains the membranous urethra and the **sphincter urethrae muscle,** which surrounds the urethra. This voluntary muscle is attached on each side to the ischiopubic ramus and supplied by the pudendal nerves S2, 3, 4 (Fig. 9.13, p. 133).

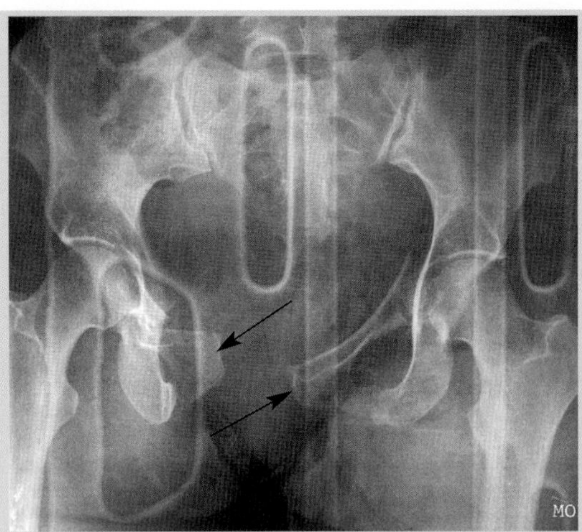

Figure 10.3 Fractured pelvis showing gross disruption of pubic symphysis and fracture of pubic bones (arrows), with associated injury to bladder

The urethra

The male urethra, about 20 cm long, runs from the internal urethral orifice in the bladder through the prostate, deep perineal pouch and corpus spongiosum to the external urethral orifice (Fig. 10.4). It is divided into prostatic, membranous and spongy parts:

- **The prostatic urethra,** about 3 cm long, is the widest part and descends through the gland. Its posterior wall possesses an elevation, the **urethral crest** (verumontanum), on whose summit is a small pit, the **prostatic utricle,** into which open the common ejaculatory ducts and numerous prostatic ducts.
- The **membranous urethra,** 1 cm long, is narrow. It descends through the deep perineal pouch surrounded by the sphincter urethrae muscle and the bulbourethral glands (Cowper's).
- The **spongy urethra,** about 16 cm long, traverses the whole of the corpus spongiosum. Its slit-like lumen is dilated posteriorly in the bulb of the urethra (Fig. 10.4) and is narrowest at the external urethral meatus.

Blood supply

This is by the inferior vesical and branches of the internal pudendal artery. The veins drain to the prostatic venous plexus and internal pudendal vein.

Nerve supply

The pudendal nerve.

Lymphatic drainage

The prostatic and membranous parts drain to the internal iliac nodes and the spongy part to the superficial inguinal nodes.

Urethral **catheterization** is often required in the male to relieve urinary obstruction. The narrow, thin-walled membranous urethra is most vulnerable to damage during this procedure. The male urethra is susceptible to infection and stricture. Dilatation is achieved by the passage of fine graduated urethral sounds.

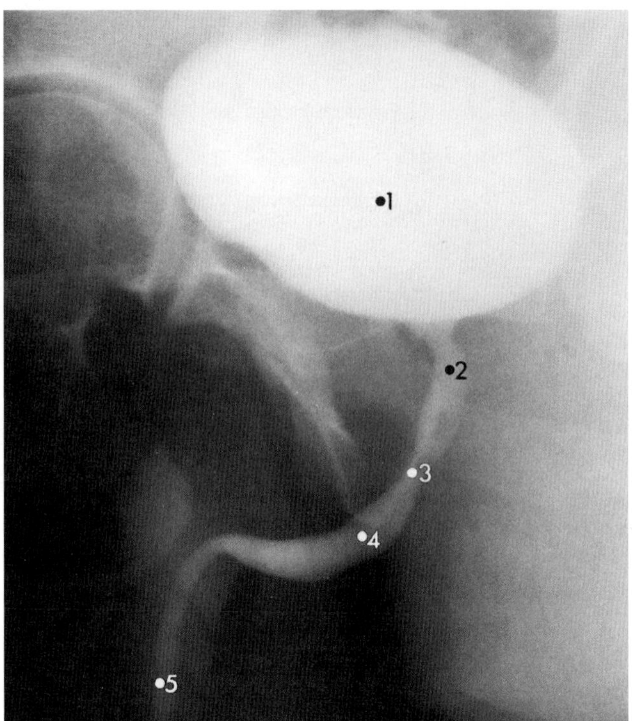

Figure 10.4 Male urethrogram: 1, urinary bladder; 2, prostatic urethra; 3, membranous urethra; 4, bulbous urethra; 5, spongy (penile) urethra

THE FEMALE UROGENITAL TRIANGLE

The superficial and deep pouches of the triangle are almost completely divided by the passage of the vagina through them. The **superficial pouch** contains the crura of the clitoris, the bulb of the vestibule, the greater vestibular glands, superficial perineal muscles and the terminal parts of the vagina and urethra (Fig. 10.5). The deep pouch is traversed by the vagina and membranous urethra and contains the sphincter urethrae and deep perineal muscles together with the pudendal nerve and internal pudendal vessels. The **female urethra** is about 3 cm long. From the bladder neck it descends through the deep perineal pouch, surrounded by its sphincter urethrae muscle, to open into the vestibule posterior to the clitoris. Also in the superficial pouch, alongside the vagina, are the bilateral **vestibular bulbs,** lying on the membrane covered by the bulbospongiosus muscles. Into this area drain the **greater vestibular glands** (Bartholin's).

Infection of the greater vestibular glands is not uncommon and produces a **Bartholin's abscess** at the side of the vaginal vestibule (Fig. 10.6). The perineum is examined most conveniently when the patient is lying in the 'lithotomy' position, i.e. supine with the hips flexed and abducted. If labour is prolonged and a perineal laceration looks likely, then an **episiotomy** may be performed, with the assistance of a pudendal nerve block, to prevent damage to the anal sphincter or rectal wall. A mediolateral incision 3 cm in length is made, cutting through skin, posterior vaginal wall and bulbospongiosus muscle. After delivery it is sutured in

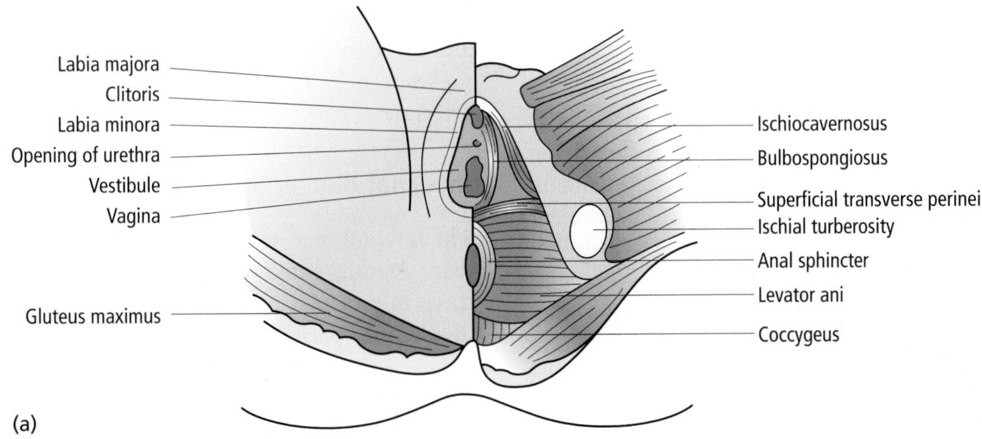

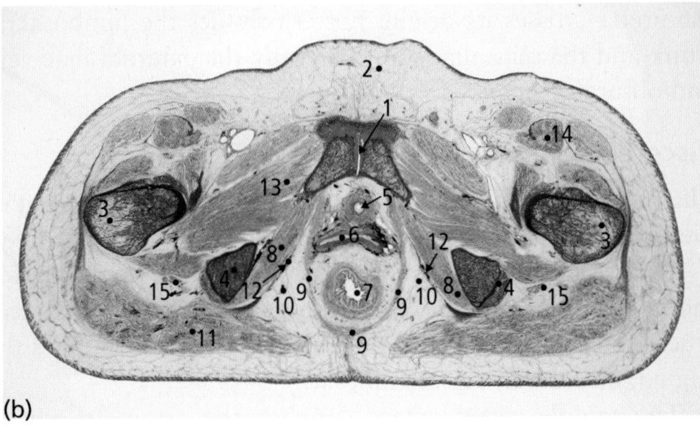

Figure 10.5 (a) Female pelvic floor as seen in the lithotomy position. (b) Axial plastination through female pelvis and perineum: 1, pubic symphysis; 2, mons pubis; 3, femur; 4, ischial tuberosity; 5, urethra with catheter *in situ*; 6, vagina; 7, anus; 8, obturator internus muscle; 9, levator ani muscle; 10, ischioanal fossa; 11, gluteus maximus muscle; 12, pudendal canal; 13, adductor muscles; 14, quadriceps muscle; 15 sciatic nerve

layers. A pudendal nerve block is achieved by infiltration of local anaesthetic into the pudendal nerve, which can be located 3 cm deep to the ischial tuberosity, with a needle inserted into the vaginal wall and directed towards the ischial spine (palpable per vaginum). A pudendal block will anaesthetize the posterior vulva. The lateral walls, supplied by the ilioinguinal nerve, will require local infiltration to achieve anaesthesia of the whole vulva.

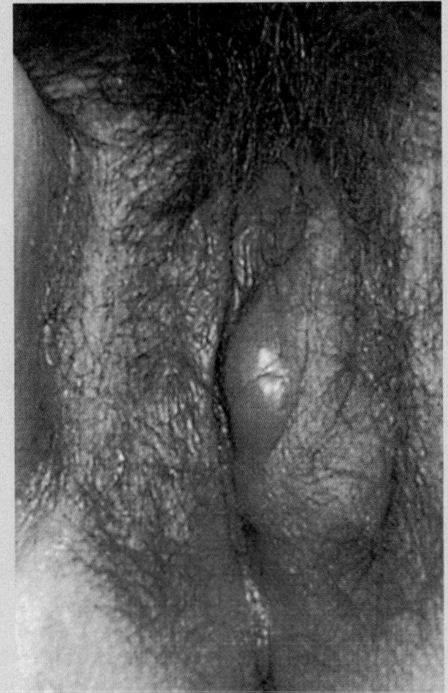

Figure 10.6 Bartholin's cyst on left vaginal wall (swollen greater vestibular gland)

The female external genitalia

The **female external genitalia** comprise the mons pubis, the two labia majora and two labia minora, clitoris and vestibule. The **mons pubis** is the mound of subcutaneous fat and hairy skin in front of the pubis. The **labia majora** are fatty folds of hairy skin forming the lateral boundaries of the vagina. The **labia minora** are thin cutaneous folds within the labia majora which unite anteriorly above the clitoris, a small, sensitive mass of erectile tissue, homologous with the penis, attached to the ischiopubic rami. It possesses two small corpora cavernosae and a diminutive glans. The **vestibule,** bounded by the labia minora, contains the external urethral meatus and the entrance of the vagina (Fig. 10.5).

The vagina

The vagina, a canal approximately 8 cm long, extends from the uterus to the pudendal cleft. It is supported by surrounding fascia and its supporting connections with the perineal body. It lies behind the bladder and urethra and in front of the rectum, its axis forming an angle of 90° with the uterus. Its anterior and posterior walls are normally in contact, except at its upper end, into which projects the cervix, surrounded by a sulcus, the fornix. The lower end is partially occluded at birth by a perforated membrane, the hymen.

Relations

Anterior – the uterus, bladder and urethra; posterior – above, the peritoneum of the rectouterine pouch (Douglas), separating the vagina and rectum; below, the anal canal and perineal body and levator ani. The lowest part of the vagina lies in the perineum (Fig. 9.9, p. 128).

Blood supply

This is by internal iliac and uterine arteries. Venous drainage is via lateral plexuses to the internal iliac veins.

Lymphatic drainage

The upper two-thirds drains to internal and external iliac nodes; the lower third to superficial inguinal nodes.

A bimanual digital vaginal examination is usually performed with the patient in the lithotomy position, lying on her back with hips flexed. When combined with a hand on the lower abdominal wall, this allows bimanual assessment of the cervix, uterus and ovaries. The uterus is usually felt to be in an anteverted and anteflexed position, although 20 per cent of healthy women have a retroflexed or retroverted uterus. The non-pregnant cervix is firm, the pregnant cervix soft. The ovaries may be felt in the lateral fornices of the vagina and the size of the uterus can be assessed.

BLOOD SUPPLY OF THE PELVIC FLOOR AND PERINEUM

Common iliac arteries

The common iliac arteries arise at the aortic bifurcation on the front of the 4th lumbar vertebra slightly to the left of the midline. Each descends laterally to the front of the corresponding sacroiliac joint and ends by dividing into internal and external iliac arteries (Figs 10.7 and 10.8).

Relations

Each artery is covered by peritoneum and surrounded by lymph nodes, sympathetic nerves and plexuses. It is crossed at its bifurcation by the ureter and, on the left, by the root of the sigmoid colon. Posteriorly it lies on the bodies of the 4th and 5th lumbar vertebrae and crosses over psoas muscle and the lumbosacral trunk. The common iliac veins lie behind the arteries.

Internal iliac artery

The internal iliac artery is a terminal branch of the common iliac. Arising anterior to the sacroiliac joint it descends on the posterior pelvic wall to the greater sciatic notch, where it divides into parietal and visceral branches.

Relations

It is covered by peritoneum, surrounded by lymph nodes, and the ureter crosses its origin; posteriorly lies the lumbosacral trunk and the sacroiliac joint; laterally the external iliac vein and obturator nerve.

Visceral branches

The **superior vesical artery** is a branch of the patent remnant of the largely obliterated umbilical artery and supplies the bladder.

The **uterine artery** passes medially over the ureter alongside the lateral fornix of the vagina to gain the broad ligament, where it anastomoses with the ovarian artery. It supplies the vagina, uterus and uterine tubes.

The **middle rectal artery** supplies the seminal vesicles, prostate and lower rectum.

The **vaginal artery** (**inferior vesical artery in males**) supplies the vagina (vas deferens and seminal vesicles), bladder and ureter.

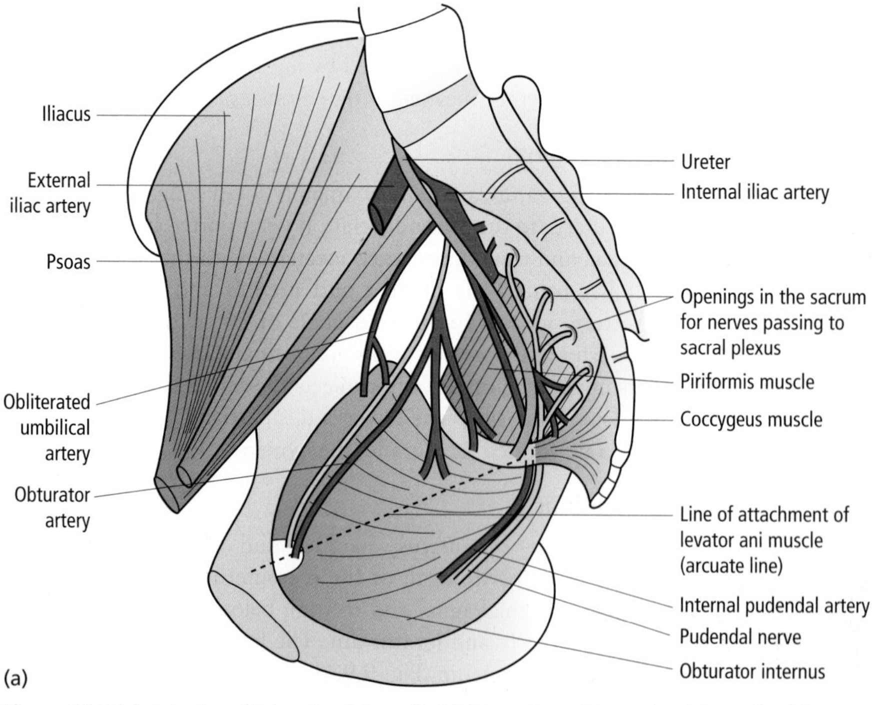

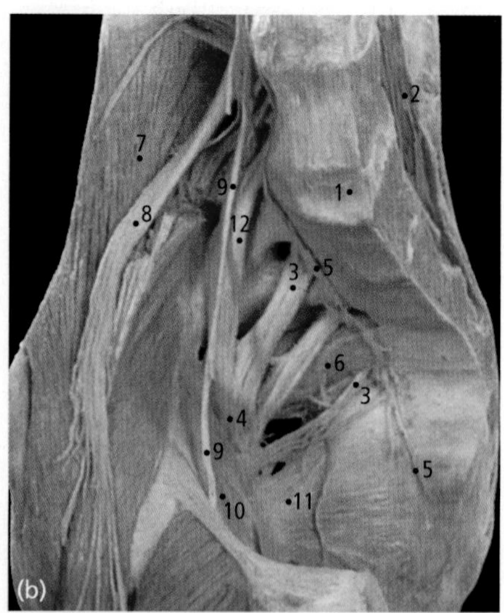

Figure 10.7 (a) Arteries of lateral pelvic wall. (b) Dissection of lateral pelvic wall with viscera removed to reveal neuronal components: 1, sacral promontory; 2, vertebral canal with cauda equina; 3, sacral spinal nerve roots; 4, formation of sacral plexus; 5, sympathetic chain terminating on coccyx; 6, piriformis muscle; 7, iliopsoas muscle; 8, femoral nerve; 9, obturator nerve, 10, obturator internus muscle; 11, levator ani muscle

Parietal branches

The **umbilical artery** is obliterated soon after birth, but it remains as a fibrous cord between the pelvic wall and umbilicus; forming the medial umbilical ligament.

The **obturator artery** runs forwards on obturator internus, leaving the pelvis by passing above the obturator membrane to supply local muscles, and, of importance in both children and adults, the hip joint.

The **internal pudendal artery** passes back to leave the pelvis through the greater sciatic foramen. It enters the pudendal canal on obturator internus (Fig. 10.1, p. 138) to give branches to the anal canal, scrotum (labia) and penis.

The **inferior gluteal artery** leaves the pelvis via the greater sciatic foramen below the piriformis to supply the gluteal muscles, the hip joint and the sciatic nerve.

The **superior gluteal artery** leaves the pelvis by the greater sciatic foramen above the piriformis and supplies gluteal muscles and the hip joint.

The **lateral sacral artery** supplies the contents of the sacral canal.

The **iliolumbar artery** ascends on the sacrum to supply the posterior abdominal wall muscles.

The external iliac artery

The external iliac artery, a terminal branch of the common iliac artery, begins over the sacroiliac joint and runs forwards around the pelvic brim. It enters the thigh below the mid-inguinal point to become the femoral artery.

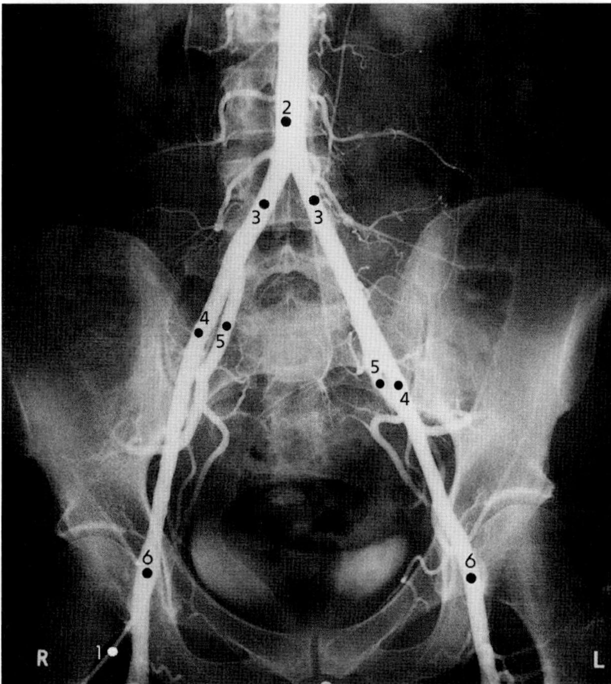

Figure 10.8 Angiogram showing iliac arteries: 1, fine plastic catheter which has been inserted percutaneously into the femoral artery and along which contrast media has been injected; 2, aorta; 3, common iliac arteries; 4, external iliac arteries; 5, internal iliac arteries; 6, femoral arteries

Relations

It lies extraperitoneally, surrounded by lymph nodes on psoas, lateral to the external iliac vein. Anteriorly, in the male it is crossed by the ductus deferens and the testicular vessels; in the female by ovarian vessels and the round ligament.

Branches (which both arise just above the inguinal ligament)

The **inferior epigastric artery** ascends medial to the deep inguinal ring behind the anterior abdominal wall to enter the posterior rectus sheath whose contents it supplies.

The **deep circumflex iliac artery** also supplies the abdominal wall.

Veins

These drain mainly to the internal iliac vein via tributaries corresponding to the branches of its artery. The viscera drain via the venous plexuses surrounding them; the intercommunicating prostatic, vesical, uterine, vaginal and rectal plexuses also communicate with the vertebral venous plexuses (Fig. 10.9).

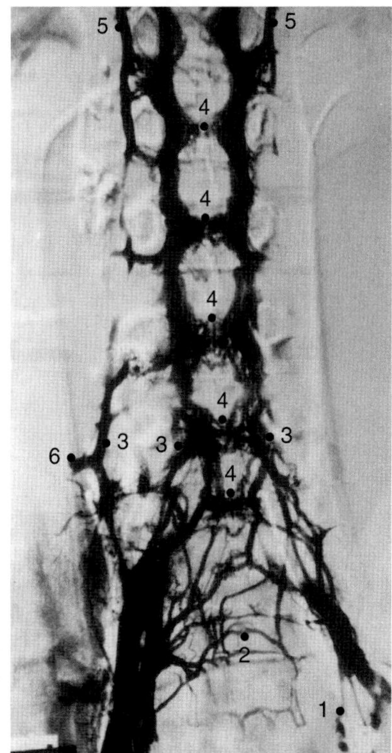

Figure 10.9 Subtracted lumbar venogram. Since the advent of CT and MR scanning these images are rarely performed, however they do illustrate the anatomy optimally. The drainage of the spinal cord, vertebrae and spinal musculature is via this complex internal and external venous plexus: 1, pelvic veins draining via the internal iliac veins to connections in the vertebral venous plexus; 2, pelvic bilateral venous drainage; 3, vertebral channels – up to six – along side the vertebral column: these are valveless and connect to 4; 4, basivertebral segmental veins draining each vertebral body – direct from the bone marrow; 5, venous channels passing up to the thoracic and cervical region; 6, segmental intervertebral veins connecting to the posterior lumbar and intercostal systems

This accounts for the frequency with which some of the cancers affecting the pelvic organs, especially the prostate, spread to the vertebrae and the bones of the skull.

The **internal and external iliac veins** unite to form the common iliac vein anterior to the sacroiliac joint, and lie posterior to the accompanying arteries. The **common iliac vein** ascends obliquely to meet its fellow to the right of the midline on the 5th lumbar vertebra to form the inferior vena cava (p. 118). The left vein is longer than the right and crossed by the right common iliac artery. The ovaries and testes drain via gonadal veins, which form pampiniform plexuses and drain into, on the right, the inferior vena cava, and on the left the left renal vein.

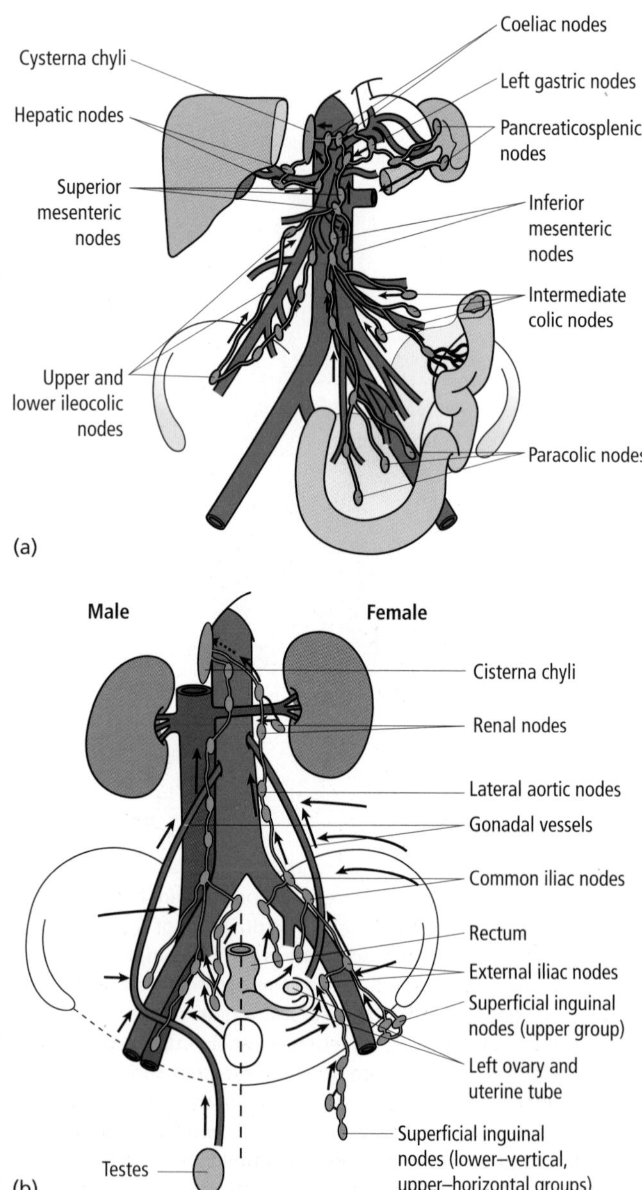

LYMPHATIC DRAINAGE OF THE PELVIS AND PERINEUM

Pelvis and perineum

The **internal iliac nodes** drain all of the pelvic viscera apart from the ovary and testis, together with all of the perineum and the gluteal region. Lymph drains from the gonads directly to the para-aortic nodes around the renal vessels. The **external iliac nodes** receive vessels from the lower limb, the lower abdominal wall, and also from the bladder, prostate, uterus and cervix. Lymph drains from the perineum, the lower anal canal, the vagina and the perineal skin to the **superficial inguinal nodes.** Efferent vessels from the iliac nodes pass to the common iliac and para-aortic nodes (Fig. 10.10a–c shows the general arrangement of the pelvic and abdominal lymph nodes).

Abdomen

The lymph vessels of the anterior abdominal wall pass to axillary, anterior mediastinal (p. 66) and superficial inguinal nodes (Fig. 10.10b). The abdominal viscera and posterior abdominal wall drain to para-aortic nodes. **Para-aortic nodes** lie alongside the aorta around the paired lateral arteries. They drain the posterior abdominal wall, the kidneys, suprarenals and gonads

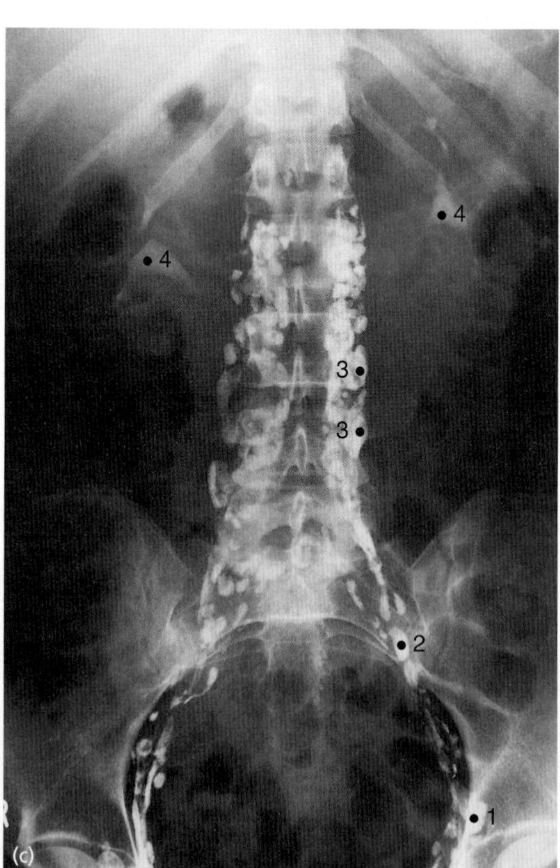

Figure 10.10 Lymph nodes of pelvis and posterior abdominal wall: (a) preaortic; (b) para-aortic; (c) lymphangiogram: 1, external iliac nodes; 2, common iliac nodes; 3, para-aortic nodes; 4, renal pelvis (outlined by excreted contrast material)

and, through the common iliac nodes, the pelvic viscera and lower limbs. Their efferents unite and form the right and left lumbar lymph trunks. **Preaortic nodes** are arranged around the origins of the three arteries supplying the alimentary tract, the coeliac, superior and inferior mesenteric arteries, and drain the intestinal tract supplied by the arteries. Their efferents unite to form the **intestinal lymph trunk,** which enters the cisterna chyli. The **cisterna chyli** is a thin-walled slender sac, 5–7 cm long, lying between the aorta and the right crus of the diaphragm in front of the upper two lumbar vertebrae. It receives the right and left lumbar lymph trunks and the intestinal lymph trunk, and leads directly to the thoracic duct (p. 67).

NERVES OF THE POSTERIOR ABDOMINAL WALL AND PELVIS

These comprise the lumbar and sacral plexuses, and the abdominal autonomic nervous system.

The **lumbar plexus** is formed from the ventral primary rami of L1–L4 on the surface of psoas (Fig. 8.13, p. 116). Its principal branches are the femoral nerve (p. 116 and p. 237) and the obturator nerve; these also give **muscular** branches to the thigh and leg (quadriceps, sartorius and pectineus) and cutaneous branches (**medial and intermediate cutaneous nerves of thigh, saphenous nerve**). The **obturator nerve** descends close to the medial border of psoas deep to the internal iliac vessels, and enters the thigh by passing through the obturator foramen. It supplies obturator internus, the adductor muscles of the thigh, and cutaneous branches to the medial thigh as well as the joints of the thigh.

The **sacral plexus** is formed from the ventral primary rami of L4/5 and S1–4 on the surface of piriformis in the pelvis. Note that L4 contributes to both plexuses (Figs 10.11 and 10.12), and that the contribution to the sacral plexus is by a branch that joins the L5 ramus to form the **lumbosacral trunk.** Branches from the plexus supply pelvic and hip muscles (p. 126), as well as cutaneous branches to the buttock and thigh, but its two major branches are the sciatic nerve (p. 231) and the **pudendal nerve.** The latter passes from the

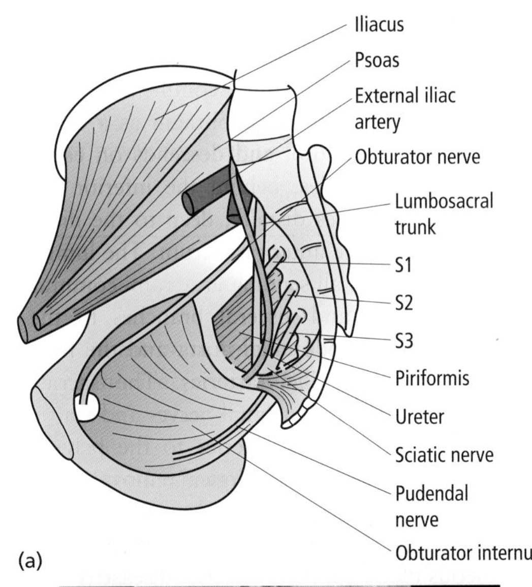

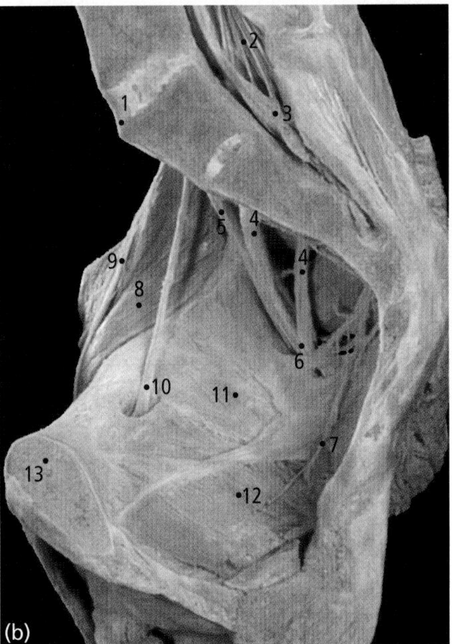

Figure 10.12 (a) Lateral pelvic wall demonstrating the position of the sacral plexus. (b) Dissection of lateral pelvis with viscera removed to reveal pelvic nerves and muscles: 1, sacral promontory; 2, vertebral canal with cauda equina; 3, terminal dural sac at S2; 4, sacral spinal nerve roots; 5, lumbosacral trunk; 6, formation of sacral plexus; 7, pudendal nerve; 8, iliacus muscle; 9, femoral nerve; 10, obturator nerve entering the obturator foramen; 11, obturator internus muscle; 12, levator ani muscle; 13, pubis

L4
L5
S1
S2
S3
S4
Lumbosacral trunk
Superior gluteal
Inferior gluteal
Posterior femoral cutaneous
Obturator internus
Quadratus femoris
Perforating cutaneous
Levator ani and sphincters
Pudendal
Anococcygeal
Sciatic — Common peroneal (fibular) / Tibial
Dorsal divisions
Ventral divisions

Figure 10.11 Sacral plexus

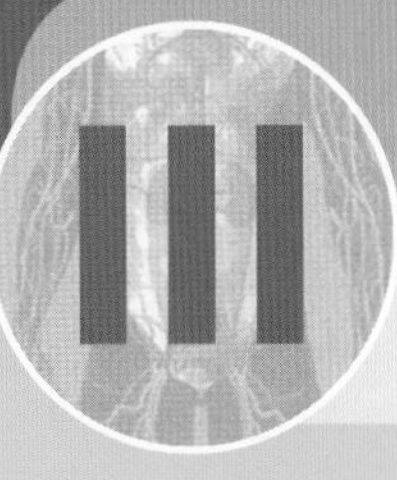

The back

11 The vertebral column and spinal cord

The curved, flexible column that forms the central axis of the skeleton, supports the weight of the head, trunk and upper limbs and transmits it through the pelvic girdle to the lower limbs. Its great strength derives from the size and articulation of its bones, the vertebrae, and the strength of the ligaments and muscles which are attached to them. There are 33 vertebrae, united by cartilaginous discs (which contribute about one-quarter of its length) and ligaments. The column is about 70 cm long and within its canal contains and protects the spinal cord. There are five groups of vertebrae, each with specific characteristics: cervical (7), thoracic (12), lumbar (5), sacral (5) and coccygeal (4).

A **typical vertebra** (Fig. 11.1a–c) has an anterior body with a vertebral arch behind enclosing the vertebral foramen. The arch consists of paired anterior pedicles and posterior flattened laminae; it bears two transverse processes arising near the junction of the pedicles and laminae, and a spinous process posteriorly. There are two superior and two inferior articular processes.

The **body** is short and cylindrical, with flat upper and lower articular surfaces. The **pedicles** are short and rounded, extending backwards from the posterolateral part of the body. Adjacent pedicles bound intervertebral foramina which are traversed by spinal nerves. The **laminae** are flat and fuse posteriorly to form a projecting **spinous process.** Adjacent laminae overlap each other like tiles on a roof. The tips of the spinous process may be palpable posteriorly in the midline.

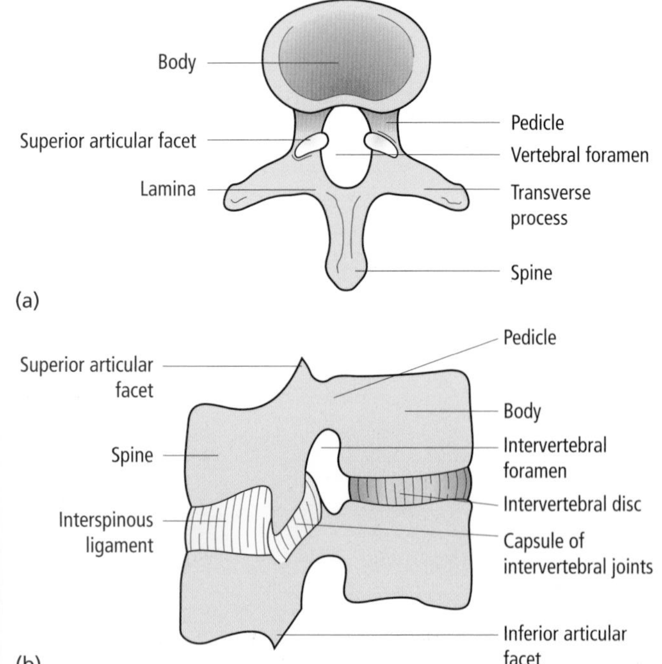

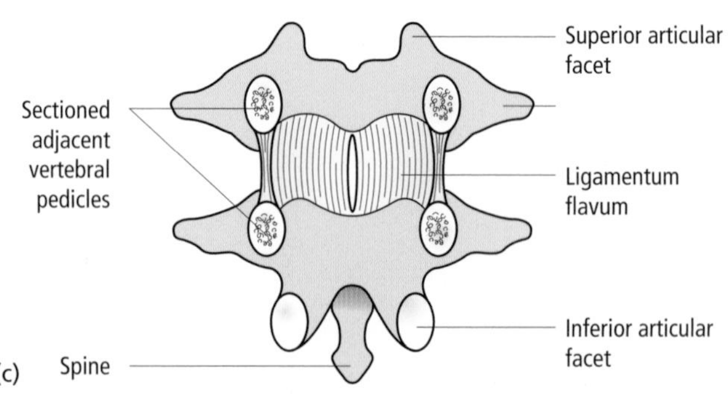

Figure 11.1 (a) Typical vertebra. (b) Intervertebral joints. (c) Ligamentum flavum viewed from within the vertebral canal – vertebral bodies removed

Superior and inferior pairs of **articular processes** lie near the junction of the pedicles and laminae and bear articular facets covered with hyaline cartilage, which articulate in synovial joints between adjacent vertebral arches. The stout **transverse processes** project laterally, giving attachment to muscles and, in the thorax, articulation with the ribs.

REGIONAL VARIATIONS

Cervical

The typical cervical vertebra (Fig. 11.2) has a small oval body and a relatively large vertebral foramen. Each short, but wide, transverse process encloses a **foramen transversarium** containing vertebral vessels, and bears anterior and posterior tubercles. The surface of the superior articular facet faces backwards and upwards, the inferior in the opposite direction. The spine is bifid. The first, second and seventh cervical vertebrae show variations from this pattern.

The **atlas** (first cervical) is modified to allow free movement of the head (Fig. 11.3). It is a ring of bone with neither body nor spine, but bearing two bulky articular **lateral masses.** The kidney-shaped upper articular facets articulate with the occipital condyles. The lower circular articular facets articulate with the second cervical vertebra. The transverse ligament of the atlas is attached to the medial aspect of the lateral masses. The **anterior arch** has a facet posteriorly for articulation with the dens of the axis. The **posterior arch** is grooved on each side superiorly by the vertebral artery. Its transverse processes are long and its tips, which are crossed by the spinal accessory nerve, are palpable behind the angle of the mandible.

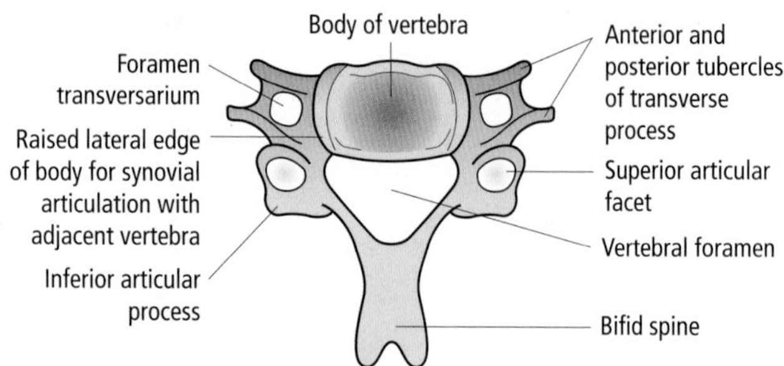

Figure 11.2 Typical cervical vertebra

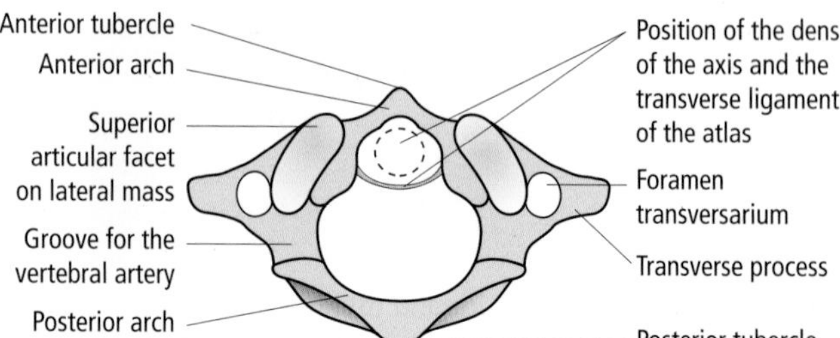

Figure 11.3 Superior surface of the atlas vertebra

The **axis** (second cervical) bears a conical projection, the dens, or odontoid peg, on the upper surface of its body (Figs 11.4a–e and 11.5). The dens articulates with the back of the anterior arch of the atlas, where it is held in position by the transverse ligament of the atlas. The alar ligaments connect its apex to the occiput. The superior articular facets are almost horizontal and face upwards.

The seventh cervical vertebra (**the vertebra prominens**) has a long non-bifid spine, easily palpable and often visible in the midline at the level of the shirt collar on the back of the neck (Fig. 11.6).

Thoracic

A thoracic vertebra (Fig. 11.7a,b) has a wedge-shaped body which is deeper posteriorly. The sides of each body articulate with paired ribs at **superior and inferior costal facets.** The transverse processes are directed backwards and laterally, and their ends bear a facet for articulation with the tubercle of the corresponding rib. The superior facets face backwards and laterally. The broad laminae and downward-projecting spines overlap with those below.

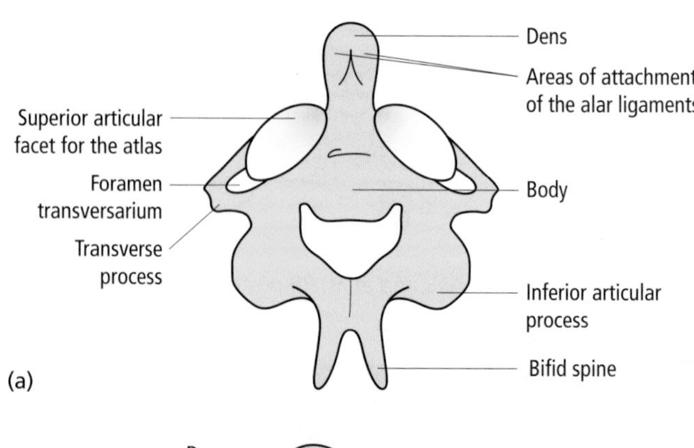

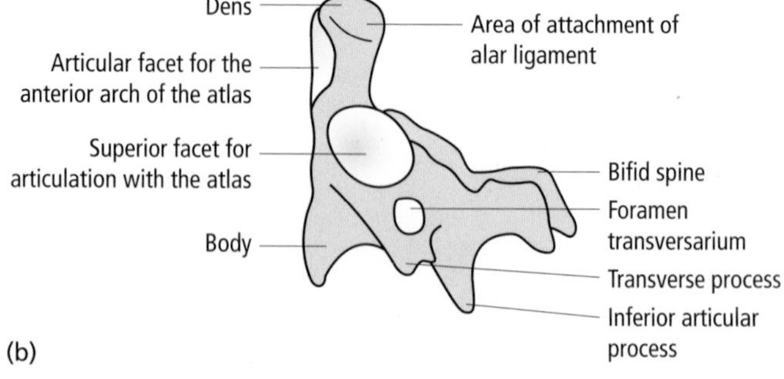

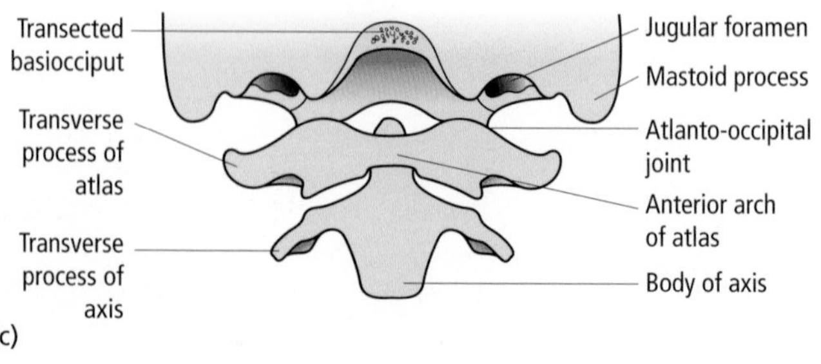

Figure 11.4 Axis and atlas: (a) posterosuperior view; (b) lateral view; (c) anterior view of atlantoaxial joint (*continued*)

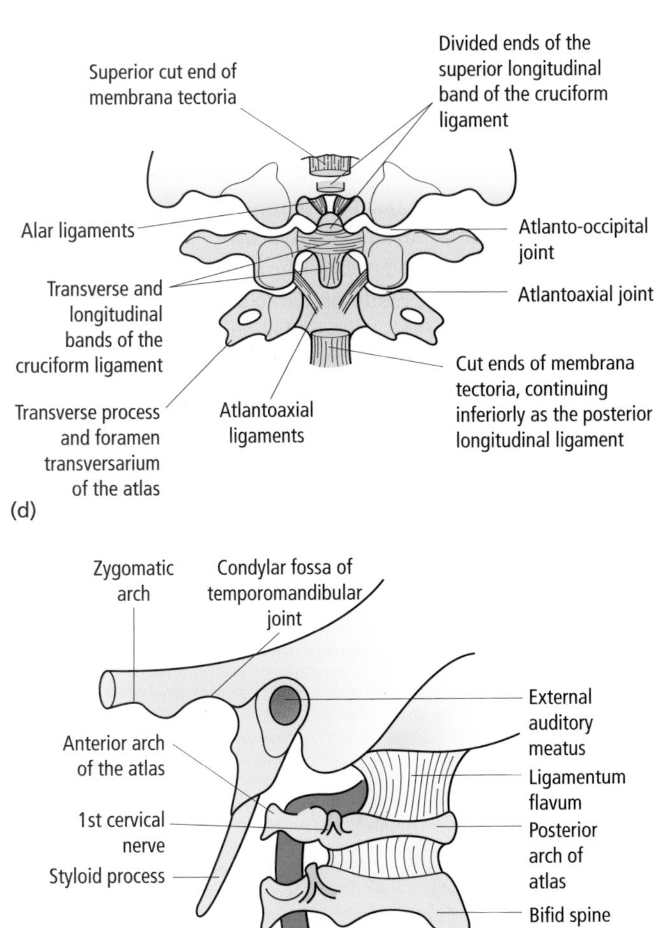

Figure 11.4 (*continued*) Axis and atlas: (d) posterior view; (e) lateral view

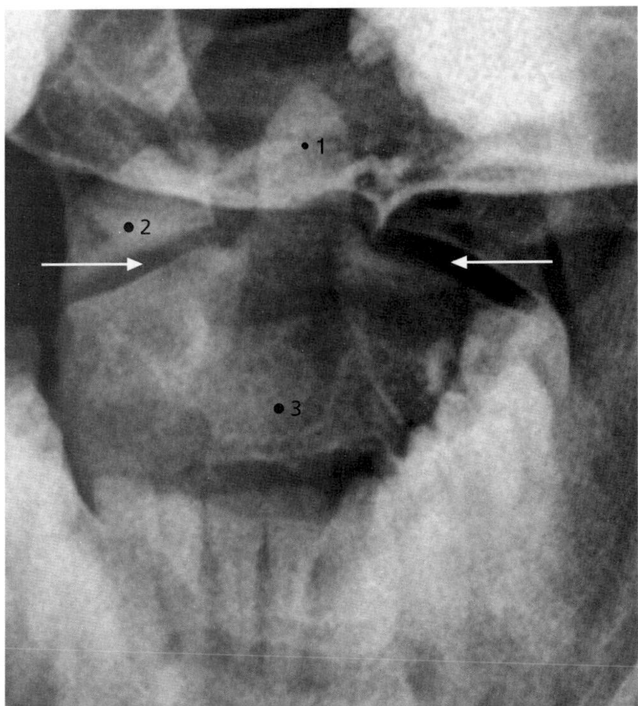

Figure 11.5 Transoral 'open mouth' view of atlantoaxial joints (arrows): 1, dens; 2, lateral mass of C1; 3, body of C2

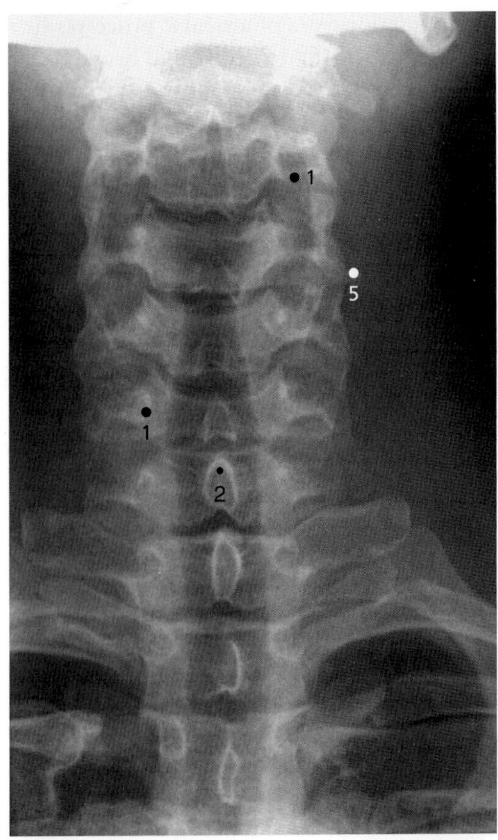

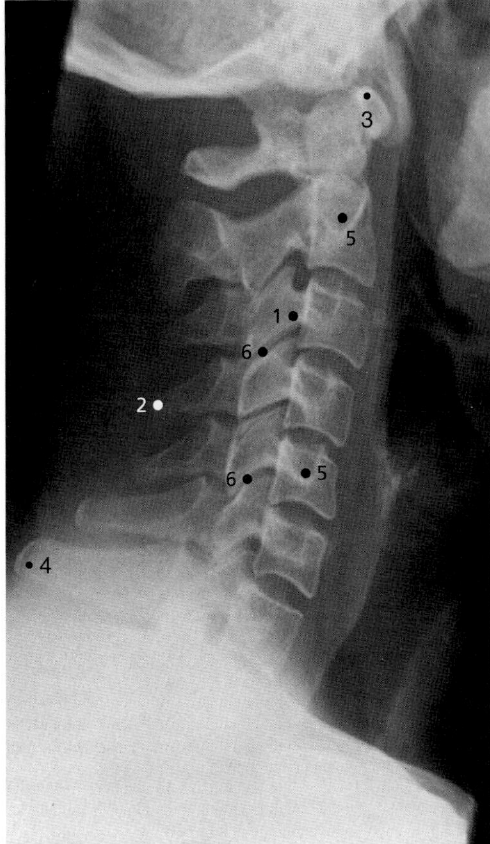

Figure 11.6 (a) Anteroposterior and (b) lateral views of cervical spine X-ray: 1, pedicle; 2, spinous process; 3, anterior arch atlas; 4, tip of spinous process of vertebra prominens; 5, transverse process; 6, facet joint

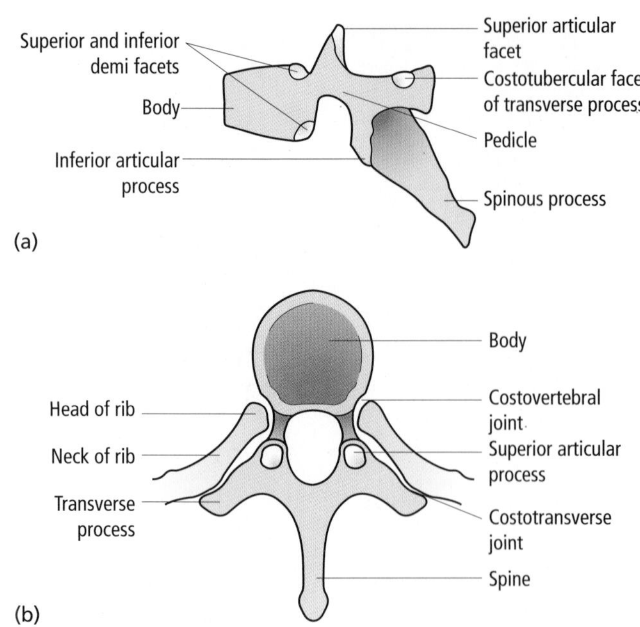

Figure 11.7 (a) Typical thoracic vertebra, lateral view. (b) Costovertebral articulation, superior view

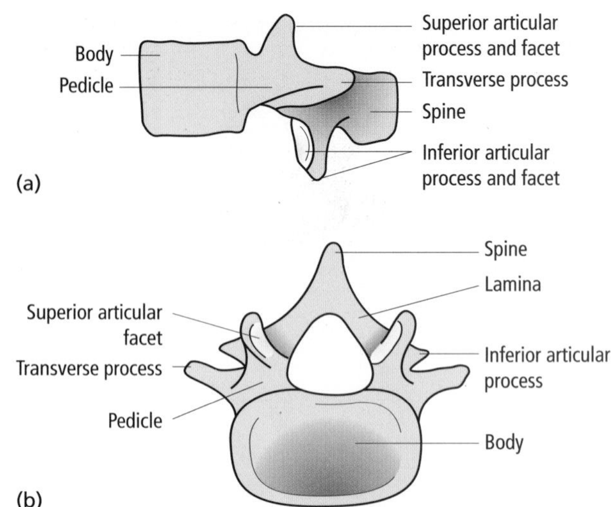

Figure 11.8 (a) Typical lumbar vertebra, lateral view. (b) 5th lumbar vertebra, superior view

The bodies of the upper vertebrae are small, whereas those of the lower are larger and their spines more horizontal. The costal facets on the bodies of the 10th, 11th and 12th vertebrae are usually single and complete.

Lumbar

A lumbar vertebra (Fig. 11.8a,b) has a large kidney-shaped body, wider from side to side. Its bulky transverse processes project laterally and its superior articular facets face backwards and medially. The broad rectangular spinous process projects horizontally backwards. The **fifth lumbar vertebra** is atypical – its body, being thicker anteriorly, is wedge-shaped and its transverse process is small and conical. Its forward-facing inferior articular facet prevents it sliding anteriorly over the top of the sacrum.

Spina bifida occulta is a common congenital abnormality in which the laminae of L5 or S1 fail to develop. The bony defect usually causes no problems but rarely the defect is larger and the meninges and sometimes the spinal cord herniate (spina bifida cystica), with associated neurological symptoms such as lower limb paralysis.

The cervical, thoracic and lumbar vertebrae can be readily distinguished from each other: all cervical vertebrae have a foramen in the transverse process, all thoracic vertebrae have costal facets on each side of the body, whereas lumbar vertebrae have neither a foramen in their transverse process nor costal facets.

Sacrum and coccyx

The sacrum and coccyx are described on p. 123.

JOINTS AND LIGAMENTS

The articular surfaces of the bodies of adjacent vertebrae are covered by hyaline cartilage and united by a thick fibrocartilaginous **intervertebral disc.** The centre of the disc (**nucleus pulposus**) is gelatinous, with the consistency of toothpaste, and surrounded by a fibrous part, **the annulus fibrosus.** The disc is a shock absorber (Fig. 11.16, p. 160).

Occasionally the semisolid nucleus protrudes through a defect in the annulus (**prolapsed disc**) and then may press on the spinal cord or a spinal nerve, to produce symptoms and signs of nerve compression (Fig. 11.9d). The majority of symptomatic disc protrusions occur at the L4/L5 or L5/S1 levels where the intervertebral foramina are small and the spinal nerve roots are relatively large.

The vertebral bodies are also united by **anterior and posterior longitudinal ligaments.** The anterior ligament extends from the occiput to the sacrum, and the posterior from the axis to the sacrum (Fig. 11.4d), and each is attached to each vertebral body and disc. Adjacent vertebrae articulate by two synovial joints between the paired articular processes. Additional support to the vertebral column is provided by:

- The **ligamenta flava** (Fig. 11.1c), which unite adjacent laminae. These ligaments contain a large amount of yellow elastic tissue and are strong. They maintain the curvatures of the spinal column and support it when it is flexed.
- The **supraspinous, interspinous** and **intertransverse ligaments,** which help unite adjacent vertebrae.

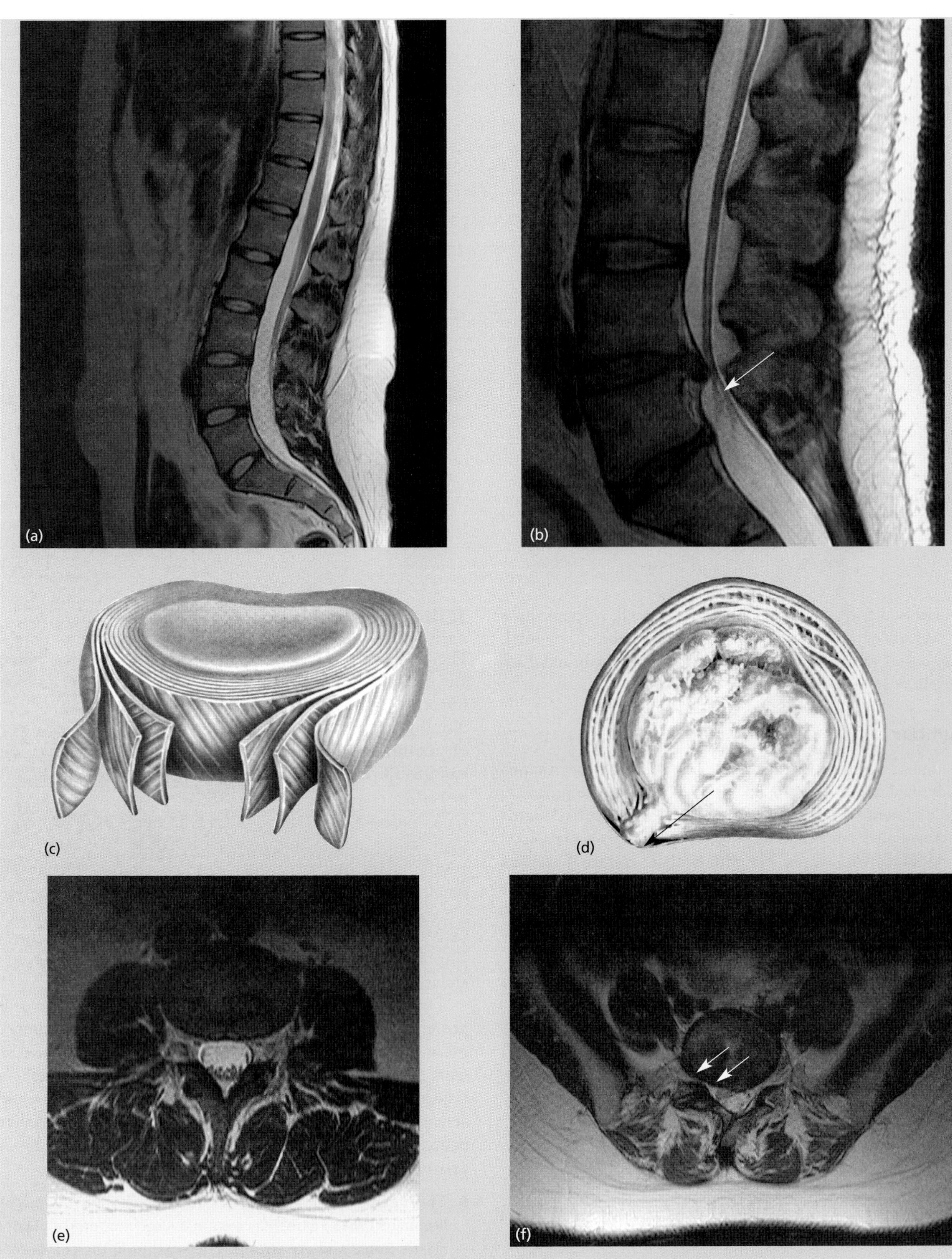

Figure 11.9 (a and c) Lateral MRI view showing normal spine and spinal cord, and diagram of normal intervertebral disc. (b and d) Lateral MRI view and diagram showing disc protrusion (arrow). (e and f) Axial MRI views showing normal vertebral body and disc protrusion (arrows)

Variations

The atlanto-occipital and atlantoaxial joints are modified to allow free movement of the head.

X-rays taken through the wide-open mouth are used to demonstrate these joints (Fig. 11.5).

The **atlanto-occipital joints** are condyloid synovial joints between the convex occipital condyles and the concave upper articular surfaces of the atlas. They are strengthened by anterior and posterior atlanto-occipital membranes. The atlantoaxial joints comprise two lateral synovial plane joints between the lateral mass of the atlas and the pedicle of the axis and a midline synovial pivot between the dens and a ring formed by the anterior arch and the transverse ligament of the atlas. The joint is strengthened by accessory ligaments, the **membrana tectoria,** which connect the back of the axis and the occiput and the adjacent **cruciate (cruciform) ligament** (Fig. 11.4d).

FUNCTIONAL ASPECTS

Curvatures and mobility

In fetal life the vertebral column is flexed – its primary curvature. After birth two secondary curvatures develop: extension of the cervical region by the muscles that raise the head, and extension of the lumbar region after adoption of the erect posture. The primary curvature is retained in the thoracic and sacral regions. These curves and the intervertebral discs give some resilience and spring to the column (Figs 11.10 and 11.11).

Abnormalities in the curvature of the vertebral column occur. **Lordosis** gives an excessive hollowness to the back and an exaggerated lumbar curvature may be caused by weakened trunk muscles and is often present temporarily in late pregnancy. **Scoliosis,** an excessive lateral curvature, is always associated with rotation of the vertebral bodies so that the spinous processes point toward the concavity of the curve. It is often the result of weak back muscles or associated with failed growth of a vertebra (hemivertebra). **Kyphosis,** an exaggeration of the thoracic curvature, is usually the result of osteoporosis, a generalized bone atrophy, which causes erosion and collapse of several neighbouring vertebrae. The collapse of a single vertebra from tuberculous infection or fracture produces a localized kyphosis (kyphus).

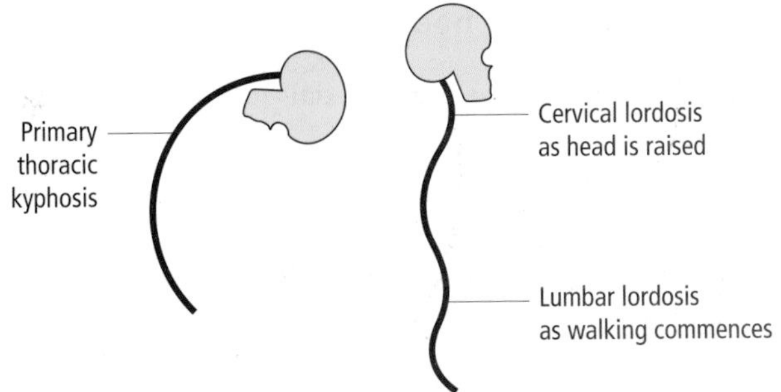

Figure 11.10 Primary and secondary vertebral curves

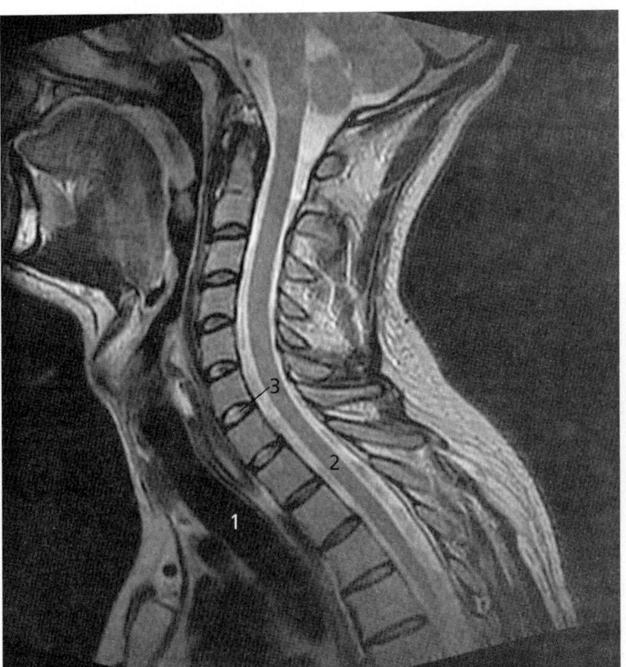

Figure 11.11 MRI mid-sagittal section of cervical spine showing normal cervical lordosis: 1, trachea; 2, spinal cord; 3, intervertebral disc

MUSCLES

The extensor muscles of the back and neck extend the head and vertebral column. They form a large composite mass lying deep to trapezius and girdle muscles, and extend from the sacrum to the occiput. The largest and most powerful are the erector spinae, but these are supported by shorter muscles attached to adjacent vertebrae and to nearby ribs (Fig. 11.12). These muscles play a large part in maintaining posture and are in constant action when standing at rest, as the centre of gravity lies anterior to the vertebral column. The muscles attached to the skull produce extension, lateral flexion and rotation of the head.

Movements

Only limited movements are possible between adjacent vertebrae, but because these can augment each other it is possible to produce extensive movement of the whole vertebral column. Flexion is most marked in the cervical region, rotation in the thoracic, and rotation and lateral flexion in the lumbar region:

- **Flexion** – rectus abdominis and prevertebral muscles.
- **Lateral flexion** – in the neck by sternocleidomastoid and trapezius; in the trunk by the oblique abdominal muscles and quadratus lumborum.
- **Rotation** – sternocleidomastoid and oblique abdominal muscles.
- **Extension** – erector spinae muscles of the back.

Movements of the head

Rotation occurs at the atlantoaxial joints and all other movements, flexion, extension and lateral flexion, at the atlanto-occipital joints:

- **Rotation** – sternocleidomastoid, trapezius.
- **Flexion** – longus capitis and the muscles depressing the fixed mandible.
- **Extension** – postvertebral muscles.
- **Lateral flexion** – sternocleidomastoid and trapezius aided and supported by stout muscles joining the atlas and axis to each other and to the base of the skull.

Stability

This depends almost entirely on the pre- and postvertebral muscles, helped by the ligamenta flava; neither the bones nor the ligaments alone could withstand the large forces that occasionally act on the vertebral column.

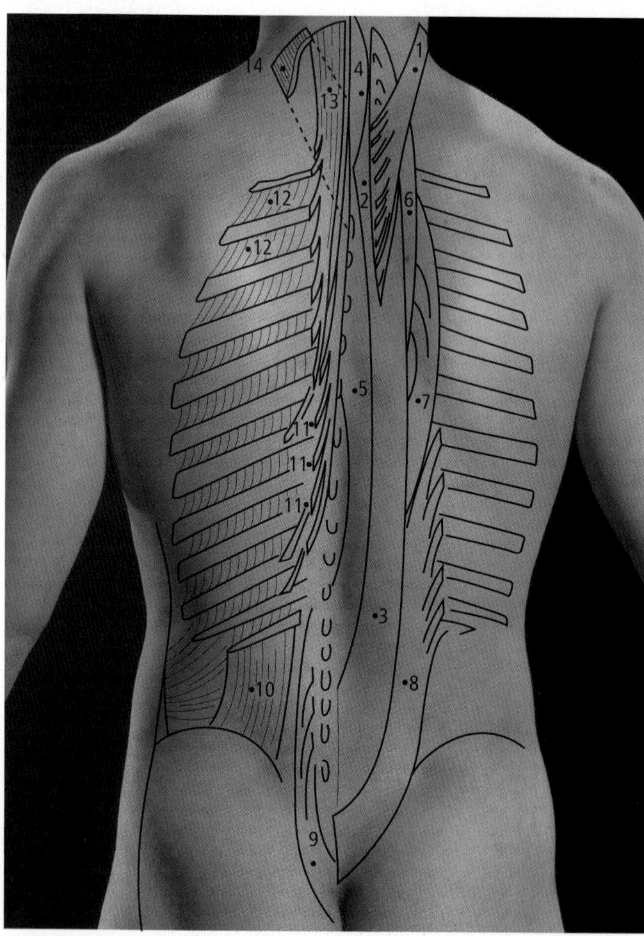

Figure 11.12 Surface anatomy of back muscles: **Longissimus**: 1, capitis; 2, cervicis cord; 3, thoracis; **Spinalis**: 4, cervicis; 5, thoracis; **Iliocostalis**; 6, cervicis; 7, thoracis; 8 lumborum; 9, multifidus; 10, quadratus lumborum; 11, levator costae; 12, intercostals; 13, semispinalis capitis; 14, splenius capitis

The commonest cause of vertebral fracture is a flexion-compression injury and this most commonly occurs at the thoracolumbar junction involving T12 and/or L1 and causes 'wedging' of the affected vertebrae. In the majority of such fractures the posterior longitudinal ligament remains intact and there is no instability of the vertebral column (Fig. 11.14a). If, however, severe flexion is accompanied by forcible rotation of the vertebral column, the ligamenta flava (Fig. 11.1c) and interspinous ligaments are ruptured, and the vertebral column becomes unstable. Subsequent displacement may produce compression of the spinal cord and irreversible nerve damage.

Fracture-dislocation of a cervical vertebrae may have serious consequences especially if the transverse ligament of the atlas ruptures to cause atlantoaxial subluxation (incomplete dislocation) or complete dislocation: there is a risk of the dens impacting onto the spinal cord and paralysis of all four limbs (quadriplegia) – the injury may be fatal. **Fractures of the vertebral bodies** (Fig. 11.14) are usually the result of forcible flexion of the vertebral column and may occur in any part of the column, but often occur at the thoracolumbar junction where the inflexible thoracic region meets the more mobile lumbar spine. A common genetic defect is a gap in the pars interarticularis of the pedicle of a lumbar vertebra (spondylolisthesis); it may give rise to slipping of the vertebrae. This is seen in an oblique X-ray of the lumbar spine. Disc prolapse posterolaterally (the most common type) often causes compression of a nerve root. The rarer posterocentral protrusion may produce pressure on the spinal cord. The diagnosis of disc prolapse has been made much easier by the use of MRI scans (Figs 11.11 and 11.13). Prolapse of the L4/5 disc presses on the 5th lumbar nerve, and that of the disc below on the 1st sacral nerve.

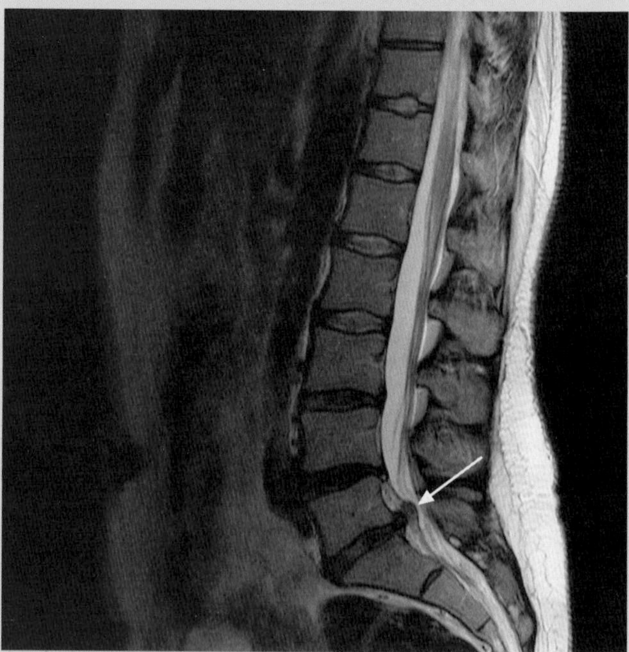

Figure 11.13 MRI, lumbar disc protrusion (arrow)

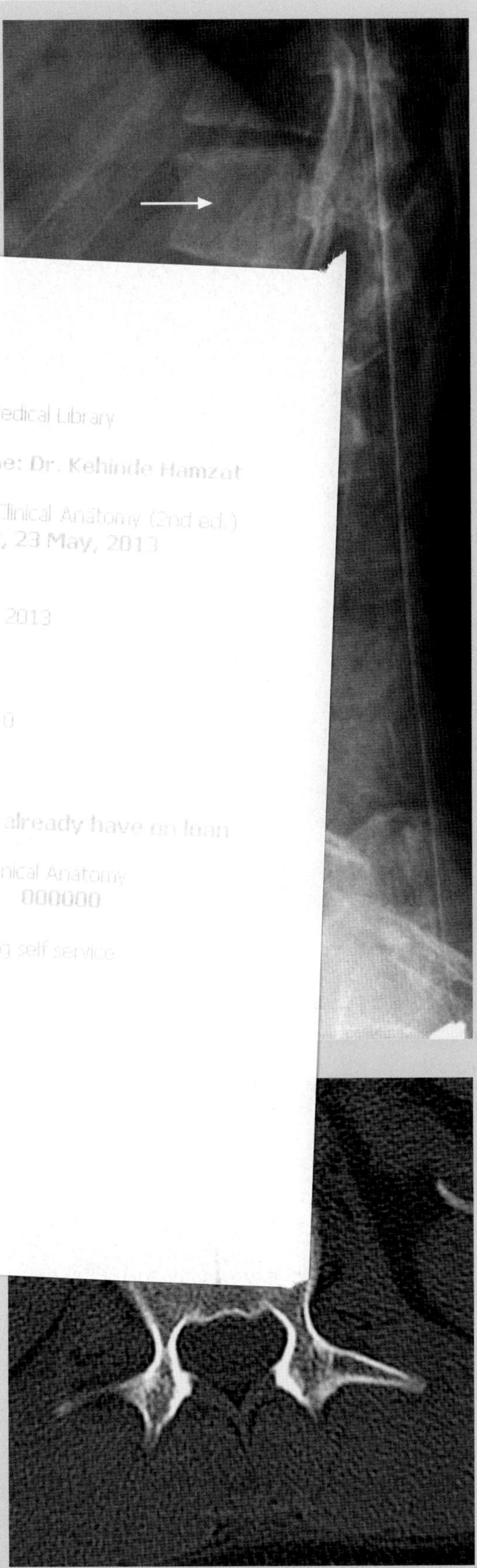

Either of these events produces pain along the posterior thigh and leg. The diagnosis may be confirmed clinically by the 'straight leg raising' test (Fig. 15.27, p. 232); this produces pain along the irritated nerve root.

Back pain is a common but poorly understood condition. Acute cases frequently follow extreme movements of the vertebral column or unaccustomed physical activity involving bending and/or lifting. It is likely that the cause in these cases is minor tearing of muscle fibres or ligaments. Longstanding cases of back pain are common: they are often caused by poor stance, the body weight is not well balanced on the vertebral column and unequal strain is placed on part of the erector spinae muscles. In both types of back pain there is associated protective muscle spasm in the extensor muscles of the spine.

(b)

Figure 11.14 Lumbar crush fracture: (a) lateral X-ray (fracture arrowed); and (b) axial CT showing fragmented rim of vertebral body

THE VERTEBRAL CANAL AND SPINAL CORD

The bony-ligamentous vertebral canal is formed by the series of vertebral foramina and the ligaments joining them. It extends from the foramen magnum to the sacral hiatus, becoming continuous below with the sacral canal. It contains the spinal meninges, the spinal cord and nerve roots. The bony wall of the canal is separated from the meninges by the epidural (extradural) space that contains the emerging spinal nerves, fat and the internal vertebral venous plexus (Fig. 11.15). The spinal cord ends at the 2nd lumbar vertebra, and the **dural sac** at the 2nd sacral. The latter is separated from the walls of the vertebral canal by extradural fat and the internal vertebral venous plexus (Fig. 11.15 and p. 143), but is pierced by the ventral and dorsal nerve roots of the spinal nerves. It ensheathes the nerves as far as the intervertebral foramina. The spinal subarachnoid space communicates above the foramen magnum with the subarachnoid space of the posterior cranial fossa. Below the termination of the spinal cord at the level of L2 the space contains only the cauda equina.

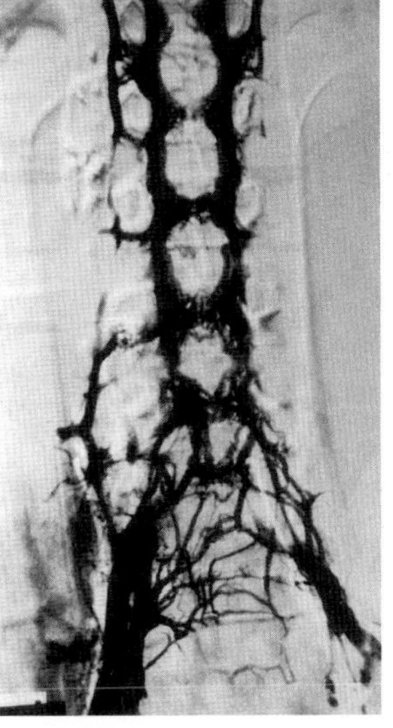

Figure 11.15 Vertebral venous plexus ascending from pelvis throughout the vertebral column

When performing **lumbar puncture** a needle is inserted just below the fourth lumbar spine in the midline (this level is found on the intercristal plane, which lies between the highest points of the iliac crests (Fig. 8.1, p. 110, and Fig. 24.2, p. 369). The needle is passed through the interspinous ligament to enter first the epidural space, and then pierces the dura to enter the spinal canal, from which cerebrospinal fluid can be drawn off for examination. This site is used also for the injection of local anaesthetic solution into the epidural (extradural) space (epidural anaesthesia) or into the spinal canal (spinal anaesthesia) (Figs 11.16 and 24.2, p. 369).

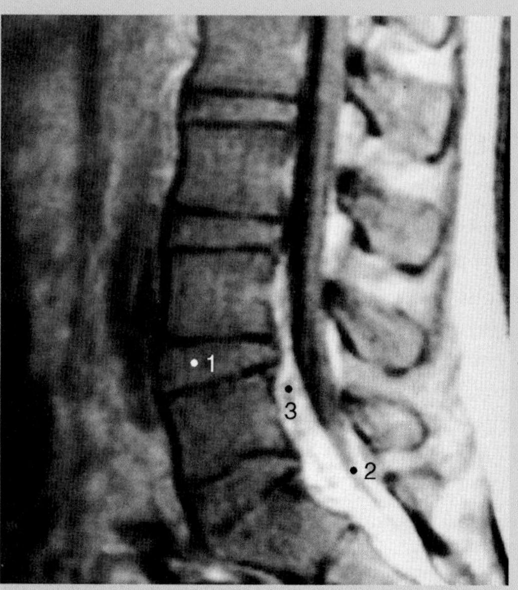

Figure 11.16 MRI, mid-sagittal view showing: 1, L4/5 intervertebral disc; 2, cauda equina; 3, epidural space

Blood supply

The **vertebral column** is supplied by small segmental spinal arteries. The veins drain into the external and internal vertebral venous plexuses, which in turn drain into the internal iliac, lumbar, azygos and basivertebral veins, which drain the vertebrae and communicate with both the pelvic plexuses and the intracranial sinuses.

The arterial supply is from a single **anterior spinal artery** (from both vertebral arteries) and two **posterior spinal arteries** (branches of the posterior inferior cerebellar or vertebral arteries). The anterior artery descends in the anterior median fissure of the cord, and each posterior artery descends posterior to the nerve rootlets. These three arteries receive reinforcement in the lower parts of the spinal cord by branches from the vertebral, deep cervical, posterior intercostal, lumbar and lateral sacral arteries. Venous drainage is by midline anterior and posterior spinal veins, which drain to the **vertebral venous plexus.**

The segmental additions to the longitudinal arteries are a most important contribution to the cord's blood supply. Thus spinal trauma, fractures and fracture-dislocations may each be attended by **spinal cord ischaemia.** Similarly, occlusive arterial disease in these small vessels, and especially in the particularly important segmental vessel, the **great radicular artery (of Adamkiewicz)**, which contributes to the blood supply of the lower half of the spinal cord, may contribute to spinal cord ischaemia, muscle weakness and paralysis. If the aorta is clamped during surgery there is a risk of spinal cord ischaemia. The **vertebral venous plexus** (Batson's valveless plexus) (Fig. 11.15) has up to six longitudinal channels and numerous connections to each vertebral body via the basivertebral veins, which drain the newly formed cells from the vertebral marrow. It interconnects both outside and inside the spinal canal from pelvis to skull, and serves as an easy transport system for metastases, especially those of the prostate, ovary and breast, to both the vertebral column and the cranial cavity.

MCQs

1. In the vertebral column: **T/F**

- **a** the individual vertebrae are all separately identifiable in the adult (___)
- **b** cervical vertebrae all have bifid spines (___)
- **c** all thoracic vertebrae have articular surfaces for articulation with ribs (___)
- **d** the vertebral bodies bear articular processes arising near the base of their pedicles (___)
- **e** in the adult the primary fetal curvatures are retained in the thoracic and sacral regions (___)

Answers

1.

- *a* ***F*** – *Five vertebrae fuse to form the sacrum and several to form the coccyx.*
- *b* ***F*** – *C1 has no spine, and that of C7 is not usually bifid.*
- *c* ***T*** – *This is an identifying feature of thoracic vertebrae.*
- *d* ***F*** – *The articular processes arise near the junction of the pedicles and laminae …*
- *e* ***T*** – *… and secondary curvatures develop after birth in the cervical and lumbar regions (these are the most mobile regions and most liable to injury).*

---

2. In the cervical region of the vertebral column: **T/F**

- **a** the atlas has no body (___)
- **b** the superior articular facets of the atlas face anterolaterally (___)
- **c** the sixth cervical spine is the most prominent and palpable (___)
- **d** atlantoaxial dislocation is prevented by the alar and apical ligaments (___)
- **e** the upper vertebrae are related to the oropharynx (___)

Answers

2.

- *a* ***T*** – *In early fetal life the body of the atlas is attached to the axis to form the dens.*
- *b* ***F*** – *The facets face upwards.*
- *c* ***F*** – *C7 is known as the vertebra prominens.*
- *d* ***F*** – *The cruciate (cruciform) ligament stabilizes the joint.*
- *e* ***T*** – *X-rays of the atlanto-occipital and atlantoaxial joints are best taken through the open mouth.*

---

3. In the vertebral canal: **T/F**

- **a** the dural covering of the spinal cord fuses with the periosteum of adjacent vertebrae (___)
- **b** the adult spinal cord ends at about the level of the second lumbar vertebrae (___)
- **c** internal vertebral veins have large branches (basivertebral veins) draining the vertebral bodies (___)
- **d** spinal nerve roots fuse in the intervertebral foramina (___)
- **e** the spinal cord cannot be damaged by a lumbar puncture performed between the first and second lumbar spines (___)

Answers

3.

- *a* ***F*** – *The bony–ligamentous wall of the canal is separated from the dura by a fat-filled epidural space containing emerging spinal nerves and the internal vertebral venous plexus …*
- *b* ***T*** – *… and in a child it ends somewhat lower.*
- *c* ***T*** – *The bone marrow of the vertebral bodies is haemopoietic throughout life.*
- *d* ***T*** – *The dorsal root ganglion is situated near the point of fusion.*
- *e* ***F*** – *The spinal cord is still present at this level. The site of election for a lumbar puncture is above or below the spine of the fourth lumbar vertebra (interspace).*

EMQs

Each question has an anatomical theme linked to the chapter, and a list of 10 related items (A–J) placed in alphabetical order: these are followed by five statements (1–5). Match **one or more** of the items A–J to each of the five statements.

Vertebrae

A. 1st lumbar
B. 1st thoracic
C. 3rd lumbar
D. 4th cervical
E. 5th lumbar
F. 7th cervical
G. 7th thoracic
H. 12th thoracic
I. Atlas
J. Axis

Match the following statements with the appropriate vertebra(e) in the above list.

1. Has a bifid spine
2. Has no vertebral body
3. Has the longest transverse process
4. Has a costovertebral joint
5. Gives attachment to psoas major muscle

Answers

1 DJ; 2 I; 3 C; 4 BGH; 5 ACEH

APPLIED QUESTIONS

1. Why should the cervical vertebrae be prone to dislocation in whiplash injuries?

1. Because of the almost horizontal alignment of their articular facets.

---

2. What might be an immediate consequence of a fracture dislocation of the dens?

2. Death, being caused by the fractured dens being driven into the cervical spinal cord. Judicial hanging produces this effect. One of the most essential ligaments in the body is the transverse part of the cruciate ligament, which stabilizes the dens against the anterior arch of the atlas and prevents it from compressing the spinal cord.

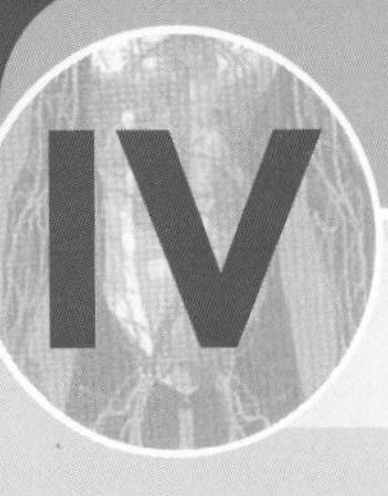

The upper limb

12 The shoulder region

The human upper limbs are specialized for prehension, sensation and grasping. They show little of their primitive functions of locomotion and support. Their ability to perform finely controlled movements is due to a well-developed sensory nerve supply, a large cerebral representation and a great mobility; pronation of the forearm and opposition of the thumb each contribute to this.

THE SHOULDER (PECTORAL) GIRDLE

This consists of the scapula (with which the humerus articulates), the clavicle and its articulation with the sternum, and the first costal cartilage. The shoulder girdle provides a very mobile connection of the upper limb with the axial skeleton, with two small joints, the sternoclavicular and the acromioclavicular, each with strong ligaments, and with a large muscular element.

The clavicle

The **clavicle** (Fig. 12.1) is a long bone but atypical in that it lacks a medullary cavity. Its expanded medial end articulates with the manubrium sterni and the first costal cartilage at the sternoclavicular joint (Fig. 12.2). It is subcutaneous throughout its length. The body is convex anteriorly in its medial two-thirds and concave in its lateral third. The flattened lateral end articulates with the acromion at the acromioclavicular joint. On the inferior surface of its medial end is attached the costoclavicular ligament, and on the inferior surface of its lateral end the strong coracoclavicular ligament. Four powerful muscles gain attachment: pectoralis major anteromedially, deltoid anterolaterally, sternocleidomastoid superomedially and trapezius posterolaterally.

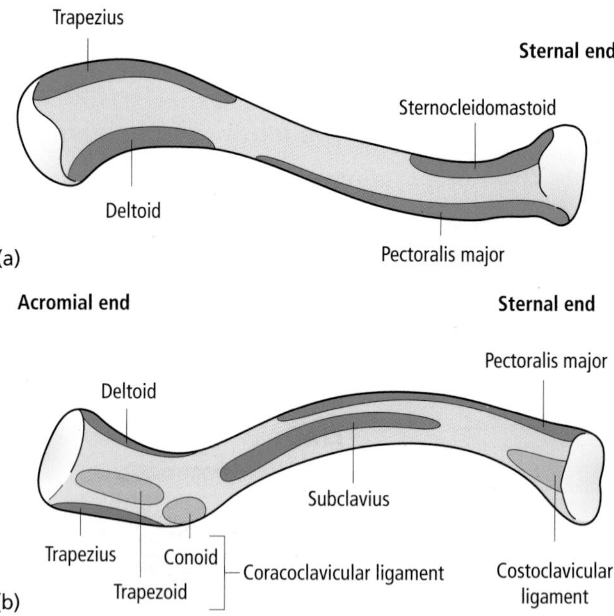

Figure 12.1 The clavicle. (a) Superior surface; (b) inferior surface

Functions

The clavicle transmits part of the weight of the limb to the trunk and also allows it to swing clear of the trunk. It transmits shocks – commonly sustained by falling on to the outstretched hand – from the upper limb to the trunk, and thus is one of the most commonly fractured bones.

The scapula

The **scapula** (Fig. 12.3) is a flat triangular bone situated on the posterolateral part of the chest wall over the second

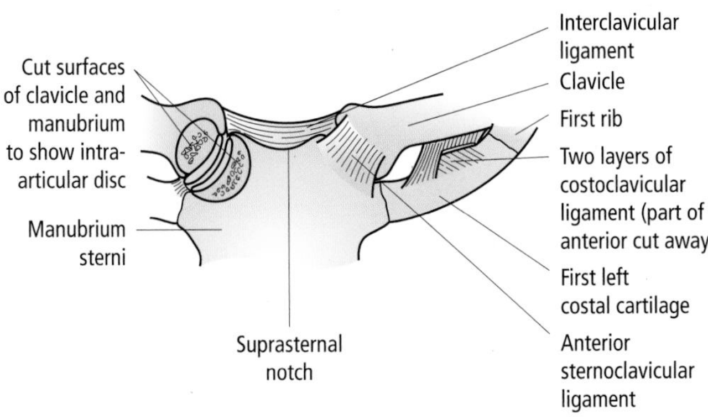

Figure 12.2 Sternoclavicular joint

to the seventh ribs. Its costal surface gives attachment to subscapularis; its dorsal surface, divided by the projecting spine, gives attachment to the supraspinatus and infraspinatus muscles. The spine is expanded laterally into a flattened acromion, which articulates with the clavicle. The acromion and spine give attachment to trapezius and deltoid muscles. Near the lateral end of the superior border the beak-like coracoid process projects upwards and then forwards; it gives attachment to coracobrachialis, the short head of biceps and pectoralis minor muscles, and the coracoclavicular ligament.

The lateral angle is expanded to form the glenoid fossa for articulation with the humerus. Tubercles above and below it give attachment to the long heads of biceps and triceps, respectively. Latissimus dorsi, teres major and serratus anterior are attached to the stout inferior angle. Strong thick muscles cover much of the bone. Only the spine, acromion, coracoid process and inferior angle are palpable. The inferior angle overlies the seventh rib in the resting position and is an important surface landmark.

The humerus

The **humerus** is a long bone possessing an upper end, a shaft and a lower end (Fig. 12.4). The upper end has a humeral head and greater and lesser tubercles (tuberosities). The head articulates with the glenoid cavity of the scapula; it is bounded by the anatomical neck. The greater tubercle lies laterally behind the lesser tuberosity, separated from it by the bicipital (intertubercular) groove. To the greater tubercle are attached some of the muscles of the rotator cuff: supraspinatus, infraspinatus and teres minor. Subscapularis is attached to the lesser tubercle; the long head of biceps lies in the bicipital groove. The narrow junction between the upper end and the shaft of the humerus, its weakest part because of its propensity for fracture, is known as the surgical neck. The axillary nerve is in close relation to the bone at this point. The deltoid muscle gains attachment to a tuberosity halfway down its lateral border. Posteriorly, the oblique radial (spiral) groove, along which runs the nerve of the same name, separates the attachments of the lateral head of triceps above from the medial head below. The lower end of the shaft bears

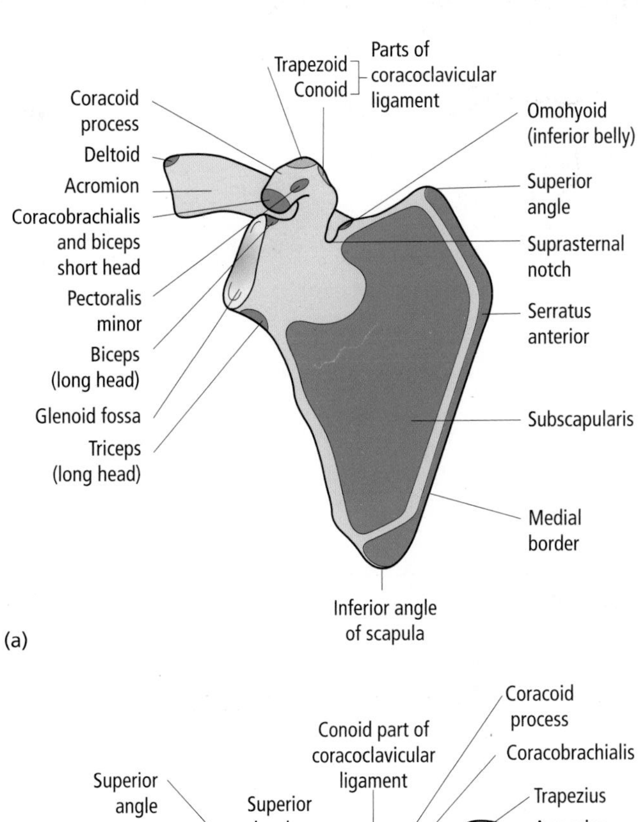

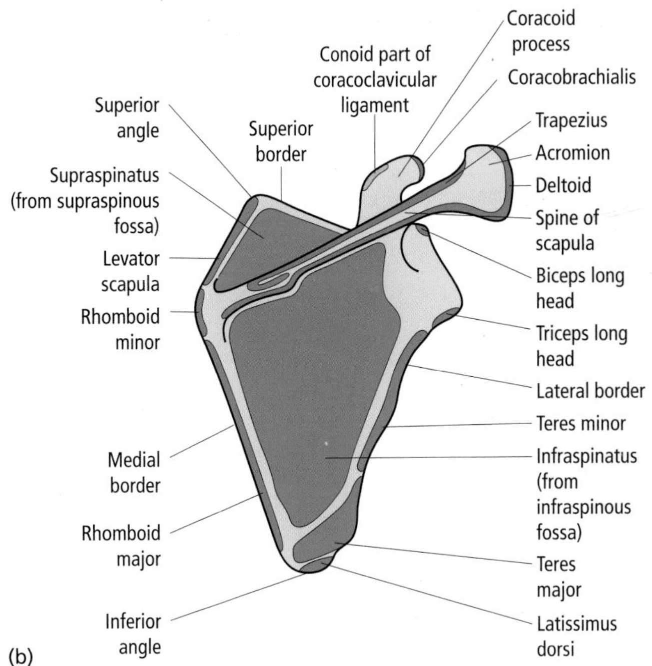

Figure 12.3 Scapula. (a) Anterior view; (b) posterior view

prominent lateral and medial supracondylar ridges; to the lateral ridge are attached brachioradialis and extensor carpi radialis longus. Brachialis is attached to the anterior surface of the body.

The supracondylar ridges lead into the lateral and medial epicondyles, from which the common extensor and flexor origins, respectively, gain attachment. On the distal articular surface are a rounded capitulum laterally and a pulley-shaped trochlea medially; these articulate with the radius and ulna, respectively. Fossae, or concavities, are present anteriorly to accommodate the head of the radius and the coronoid process of the ulna during flexion, and posteriorly to accommodate the olecranon during extension.

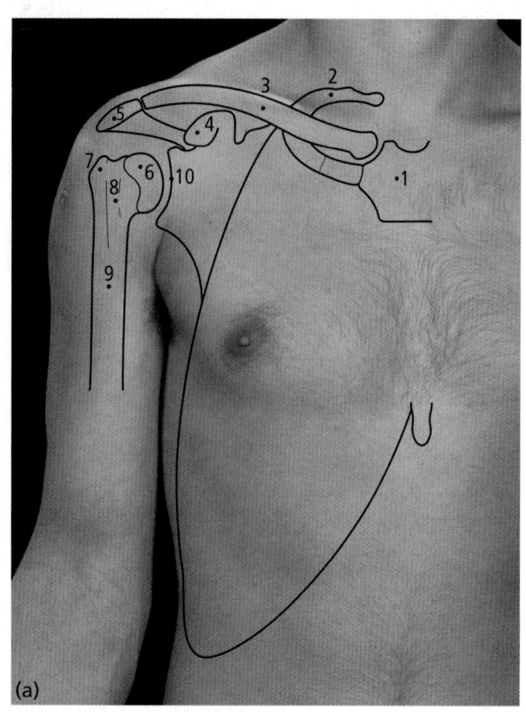

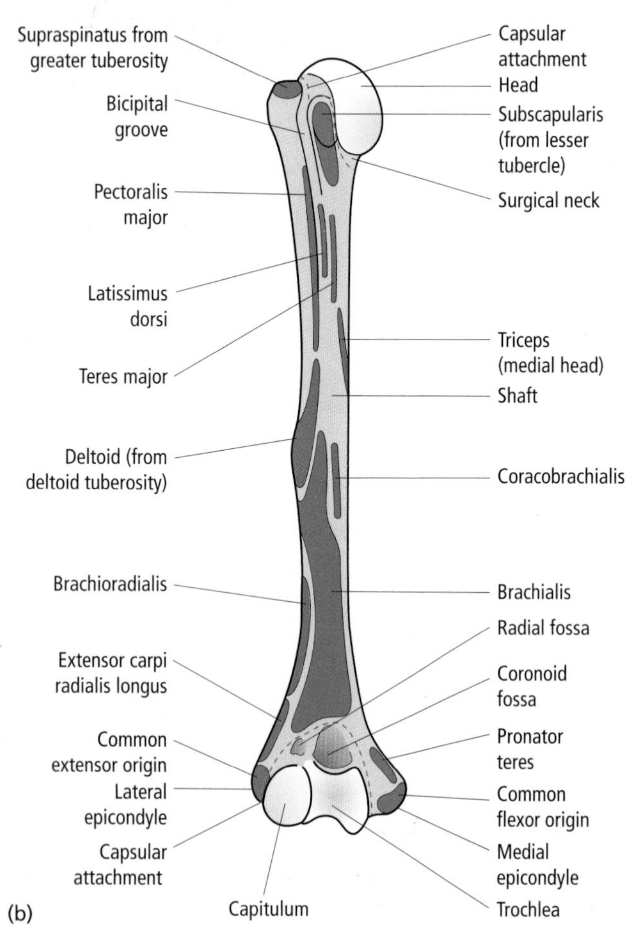

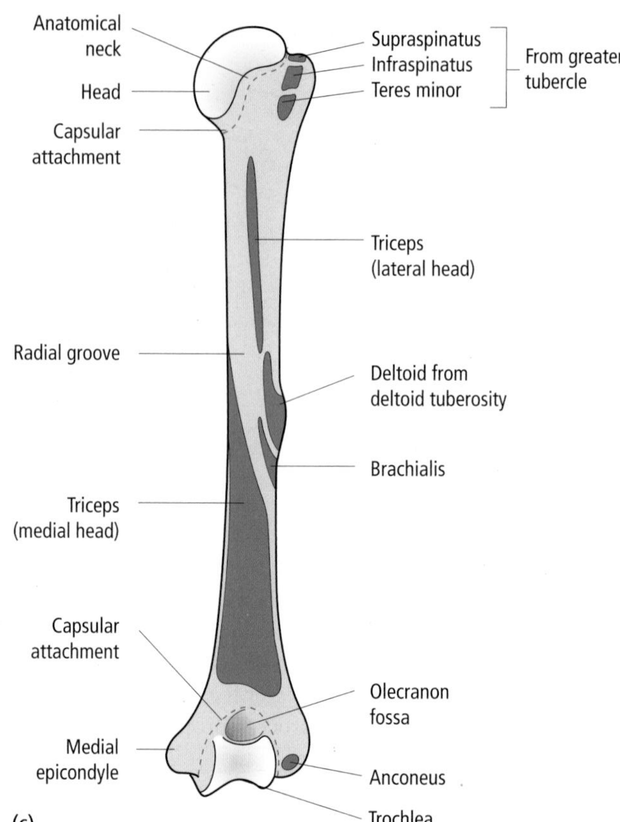

Figure 12.4 Bones of the shoulder joint. (a) Surface anatomy: 1, manubrium sterni; 2, first rib; 3, clavicle; 4, coracoid process; 5, acromion; 6, head of humerus; 7, greater tuberosity; 8, intertubercular groove; 9, shaft of humerus; 10, glenoid fossa. (b) Humerus anterior view and (c) humerus posterior view each showing features, muscle attachments and capsular attachments (dotted red lines)

Fractures of the neck of the humerus (Fig. 12.5a), which usually follow a fall on the outstretched arm, may be complicated by injury to closely related nerves and vessels. The axillary nerve, lying close to the surgical neck, may be injured by a fracture at this level as it may be following dislocation of the shoulder joint (Fig. 12.5b) and result in paralysis of the deltoid and inability to abduct the arm. There is associated sensory loss over the lateral upper arm. If the axillary nerve is severely injured then the normal rounded contour of the shoulder is lost because of the atrophy of the deltoid muscle. The radial nerve in the radial groove may be injured by fractures of the midshaft (Fig. 12.5d). A more common injury to the radial nerve is that of 'Saturday night palsy', wherein prolonged pressure to the radial nerve in the axilla after a drunken sleep resting with the arm thrown over a chairback results in prolonged paralysis of elbow and wrist extension. The ulnar nerve, lying subcutaneously behind the medial epicondyle, is often injured after trauma to the elbow region. The supracondylar region in children is a relatively weak spot and is often fractured (Fig. 13.4g, p. 188). In these cases the brachial artery may be occluded. Urgent attention is then required to prevent ischaemic contracture of the forearm muscles (Volkmann's contracture) (Fig. 12.6).

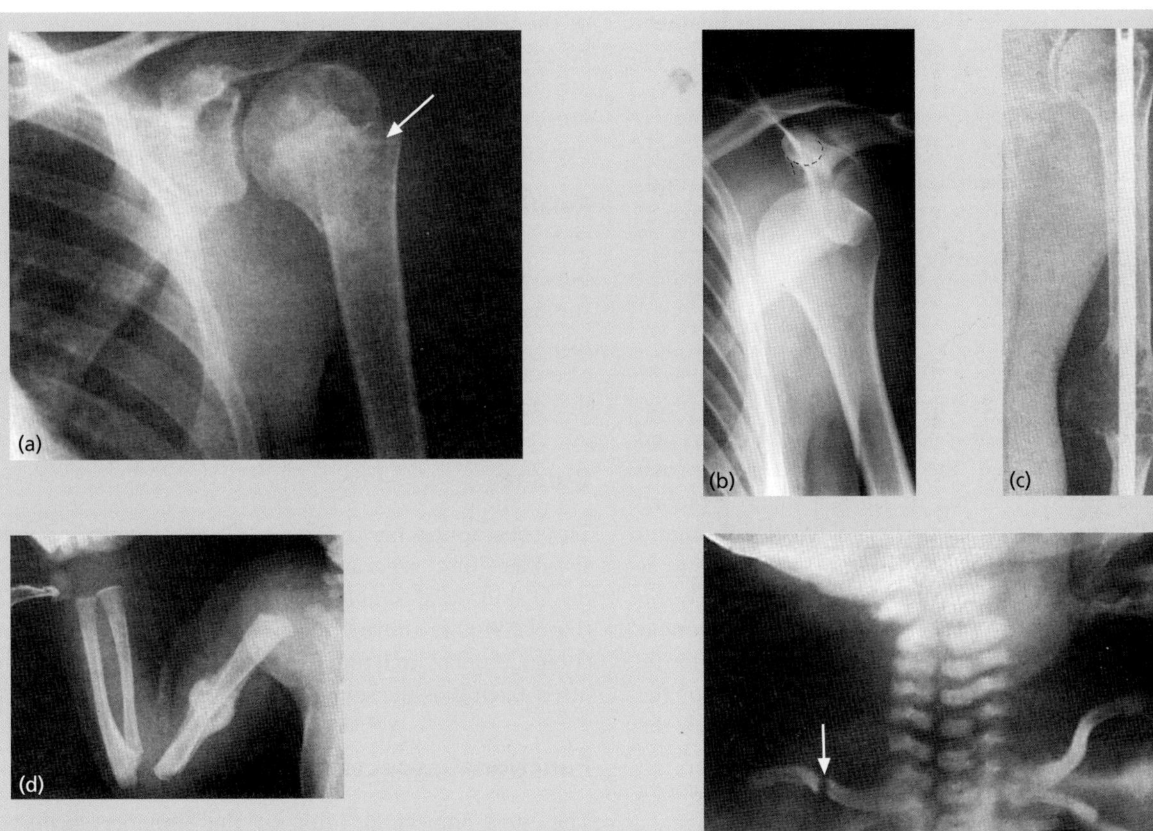

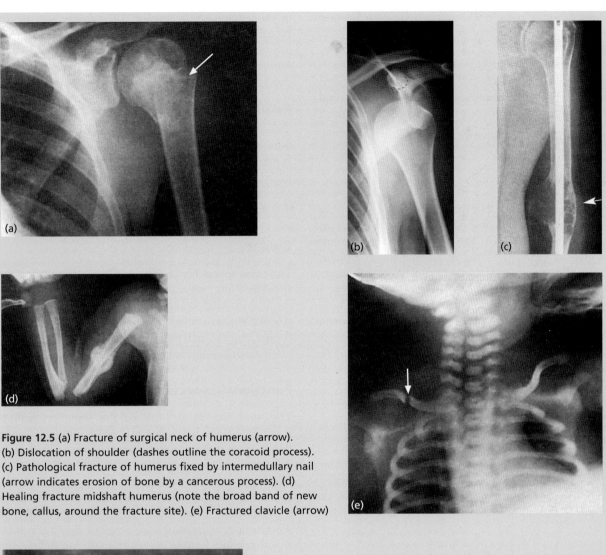

Figure 12.5 (a) Fracture of surgical neck of humerus (arrow). (b) Dislocation of shoulder (dashes outline the coracoid process). (c) Pathological fracture of humerus fixed by intermedullary nail (arrow indicates erosion of bone by a cancerous process). (d) Healing fracture midshaft humerus (note the broad band of new bone, callus, around the fracture site). (e) Fractured clavicle (arrow)

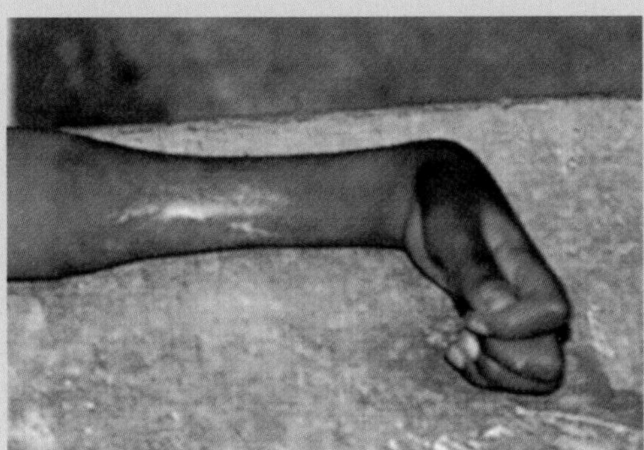

Figure 12.6 Volkmann's ischaemic contracture showing contracture of the wrist and finger flexors

The sternoclavicular joint

The **sternoclavicular joint** (Fig. 12.2) comprises the shallow concavity formed by the manubrium sterni and the first costal cartilage articulating with the medial end of the clavicle. It is lined by fibrocartilage and its capsule strengthened by anterior and posterior sternoclavicular ligaments. The joint's stability is due to the strong accessory ligament, the **costoclavicular ligament**, and its fibrocartilaginous articular disc, which prevent the clavicle overriding the sternum. The costoclavicular ligament acts as a fulcrum around which clavicular movements occur.

The acromioclavicular joint

The **acromioclavicular joint** lies subcutaneously. It permits a slight degree of gliding movement. It is a synovial joint with weak capsular ligaments and strong accessory ligaments. The **coracoclavicular ligament** provides a strong union between the scapula and the clavicle, and conveys much of the upper limb's weight to the clavicle. The **acromioclavicular ligament** covers the upper aspect of the joint and lends strength to it (Fig. 12.7a).

Acromioclavicular joint separation, a rather uncommon injury, can follow severe downward blows to the shoulder. Usually the coracoclavicular ligament remains intact and subluxation rather than complete dislocation occurs. Confirmation is easier to obtain if the X-ray is taken with a heavy weight in the hand (Fig. 12.7).

The shoulder joint

The **shoulder joint** (Fig. 12.8) is synovial of the ball and socket variety, between the hemispherical head of the humerus and the shallow glenoid fossa of the scapula. This is deepened by the glenoid labrum, a ring of fibrocartilage attached to its rim. The capsule is strengthened by glenohumeral ligaments but it is lax, a necessity for a joint as mobile as the shoulder; it extends onto the diaphysis inferiorly on the medial side of the neck. The **coracohumeral ligament** gives some support. This is a broad band passing from the base of the coracoid process to the greater tubercle of the humerus. The synovial membrane communicates with the subscapular bursa and encloses the tendon of the long head of biceps as it crosses the joint in the intertubercular groove (Fig. 12.8). .

Stability

The lax capsule and the shallow glenoid cavity would, alone, make the shoulder joint very unstable, but its potential for instability is reduced by strong contributions from the glenohumeral and coracohumeral ligaments and the fusion of the tendons of the rotator cuff muscles with the capsule. Nonetheless the shoulder joint is frequently dislocated, most commonly in a downwards direction because of the lack of muscles and tendons inferiorly. The coracoacromial arch prevents upward dislocation occurring very frequently.

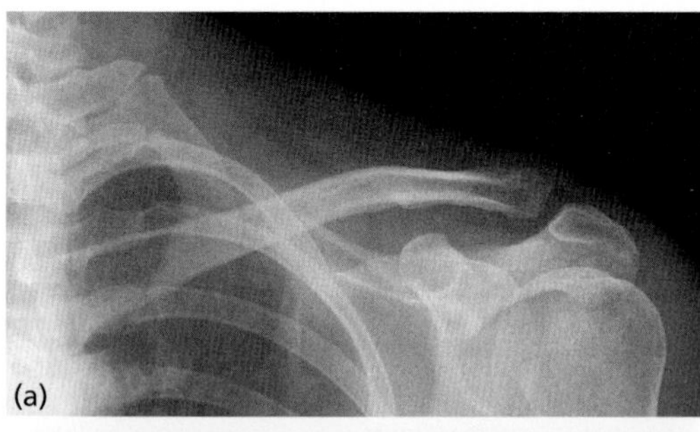

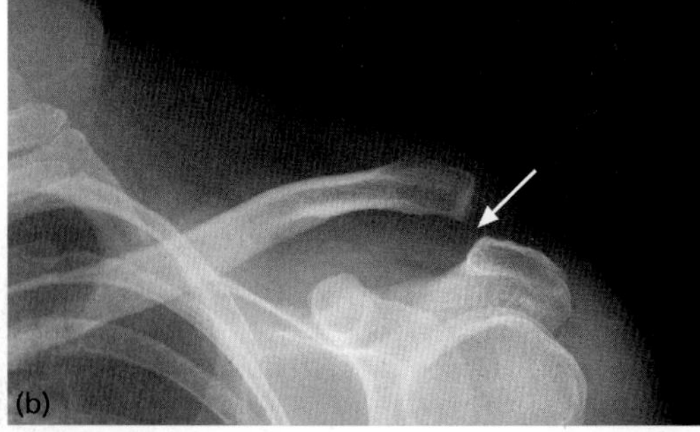

Figure 12.7 Acromioclavicular joint: (a) normal; (b) traumatic separation: weight distraction (arrow) – the scapula is dragged away from the acromion

Relations

These are seen in Figure 12.9; *anterior* – subscapularis and bursa; *posterior* – infraspinatus and teres minor; *superior* – supraspinatus, subacromial bursa and coracoacromial arch; inside the joint is the long head of biceps; *inferior* – long head of triceps and the axillary nerve. The deltoid muscle embraces the joint.

Bursae

The **subscapular bursa** (Fig. 12.9) communicating with the shoulder joint separates subscapularis from the neck of the scapula and shoulder joint; a large **subacromial bursa** (Fig. 12.9b) lies above supraspinatus and separates it from the coracoacromial arch and the deep surface of deltoid, where it often extends as the subdeltoid bursa.

Functional aspects of the shoulder girdle

The most important joint of the shoulder girdle is the muscular **scapulothoracic joint**, which allows movements of the scapula on the posterolateral thoracic wall: elevation and depression, as in shrugging of the shoulder, protraction, as in pushing or opening a door, and retraction, as in bracing the shoulders, are each usually combined with movements of the shoulder joint. Even when the shoulder joint has restricted movement or is fused, a wide range of upper arm movement is still possible by this scapulothoracic movement, in which the scapula pivots on the costoclavicular ligament and levers against the sternoclavicular joint (note that in forward movement and retraction of the scapula the medial end of the clavicle moves in the opposite direction).

Abduction of the arm is begun by supraspinatus and continued by deltoid (Fig. 12.10); **adduction** is by pectoralis major and latissimus dorsi; **flexion** is by pectoralis major, biceps brachii and the anterior fibres of deltoid, and **extension** is by the posterior fibres of deltoid, long head of triceps and latissimus dorsi. In most of these movements there are associated movements of the shoulder girdle. The scapula moves easily over the thoracic wall: elevated by trapezius, depressed by serratus anterior and lower fibres of trapezius, and it moves forward as in punching by the action of serratus anterior and pectoralis minor, with latissimus dorsi holding the inferior angle to the chest wall. Retraction, as in bracing the shoulders, is effected by trapezius. Fixation of the humerus and shoulder girdle, achieved by placing the elbows on a table, or hands on thighs, allows some of these muscles to act as accessory muscles of respiration during forced respiration. Their attachments to the ribs are then approximated to the now fixed humerus or scapula, and the chest wall is pulled up to increase the capacity of the thoracic cavity.

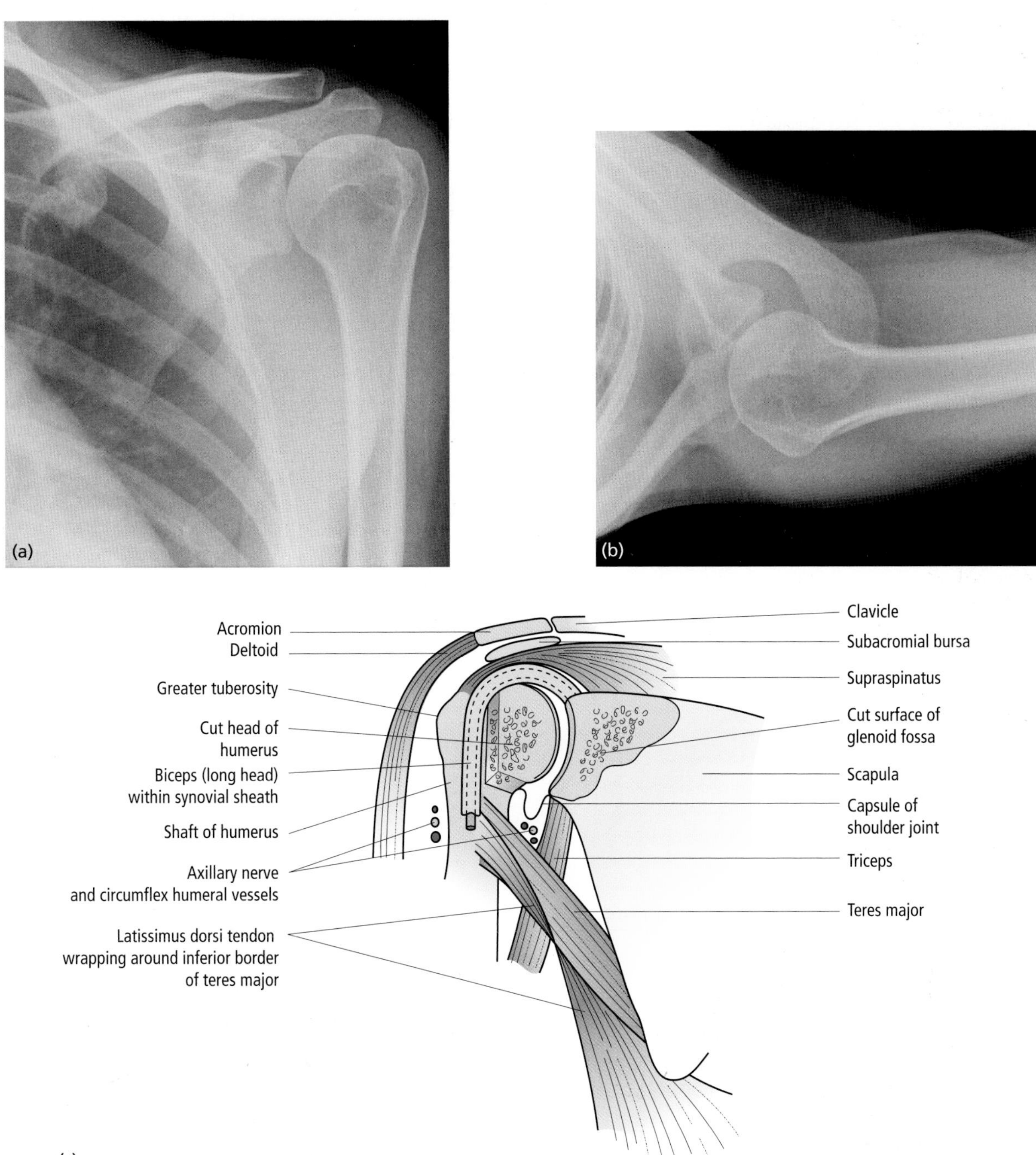

Figure 12.8 Shoulder: (a) X-ray, anteroposterior view; (b) X-ray, axial view; (c) shoulder joint anterior view, some bone removed

Dislocation of the shoulder (Fig. 12.5b) is a relatively common injury, usually caused by a blow on to the fully abducted arm – for example a backstroke swimmer colliding with the end of the pool. The dislocation is usually through the inferior capsule with the head of the humerus coming to lie anterior to the glenoid cavity. Such a dislocation frequently recurs due to tearing of the shoulder capsule and the rotator cuff muscles. The dislocation can be reduced by gentle traction on the hand, which is met by counterforce provided by a bare foot in the patient's axilla (Hippocratic method) or by Kocher's method, in which, while the operator grips and pulls on the epicondyles, the externally rotated arm is first adducted across the body and then internally rotated. Check for axillary nerve damage before and after reduction – it lies directly below the joint capsule and is thus subject to damage with this injury. The **rotator cuff syndrome** is painful and arises from impingement or injury of the tendons, particularly that of supraspinatus, under the coracoacromial arch (see below).

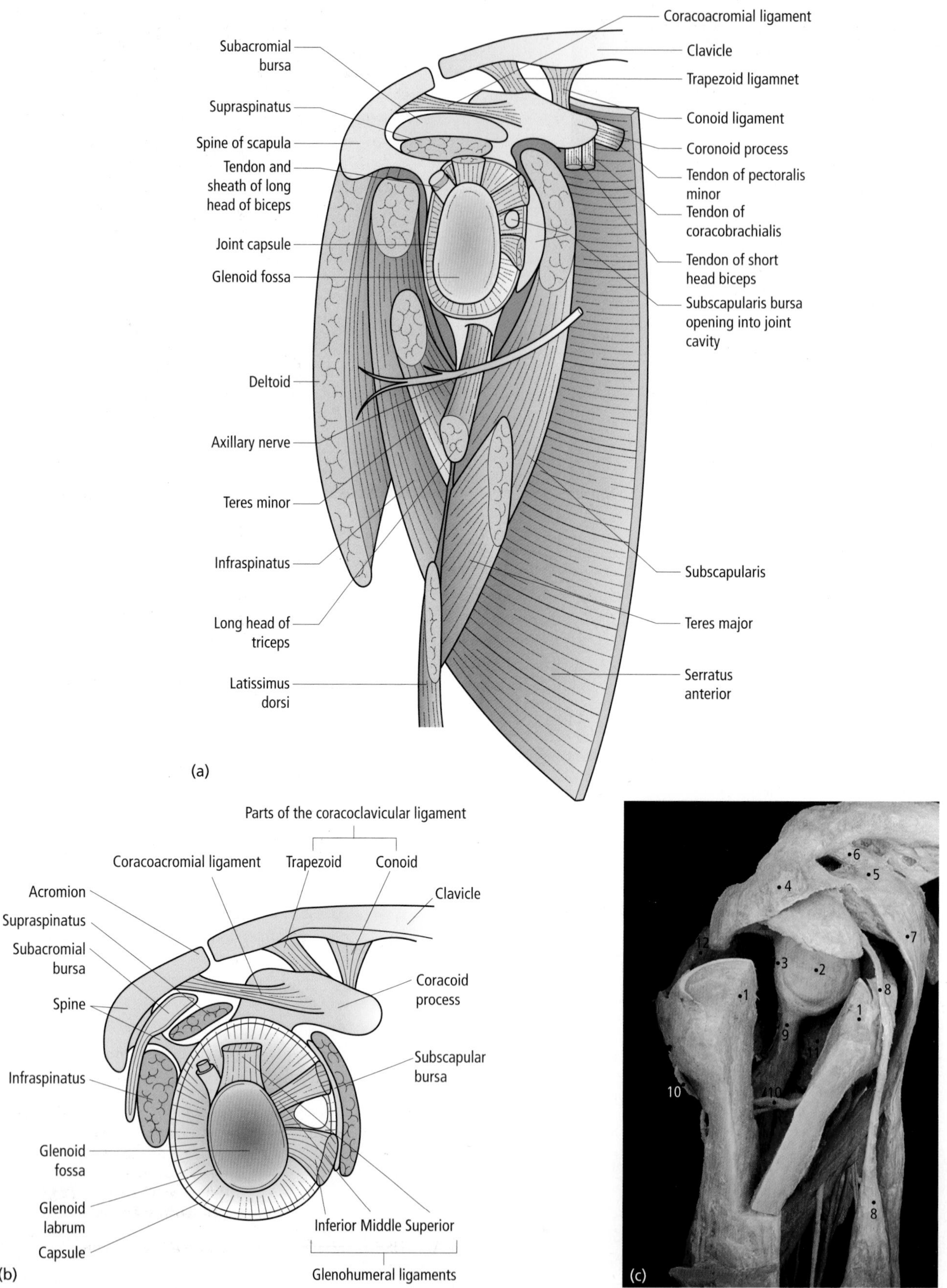

Figure 12.9(a) Lateral view of right shoulder joint (humerus removed) showing rotator cuff muscles. (b) Lateral view of right shoulder joint (humerus removed) showing bursae and ligaments. (c) Dissection of shoulder with division of humeral head to reveal glenoid fossa: 1, humeral head (split); 2, glenoid fossa; 3, glenoid labrum; 4, acromion; 5, coracoid process, 6, coracoclavicular ligament; 7, short head biceps muscle; 8, long head biceps tendon; 9, long head triceps muscle; 10, axillary nerve; 11, subscapularis muscle; 12, deltoid muscle

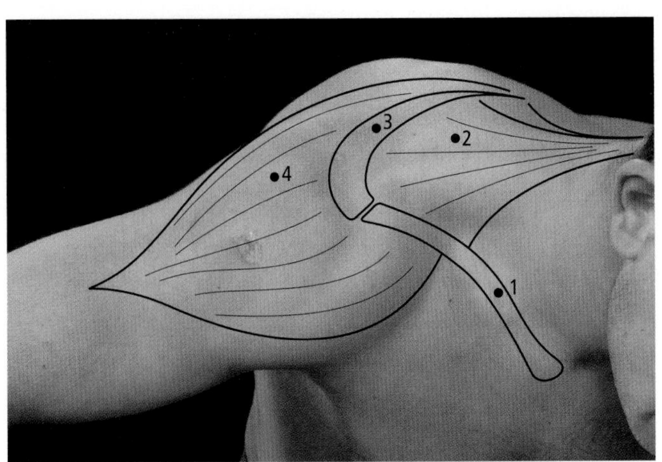

Figure 12.10 Deltoid muscle, superior view: 1, clavicle; 2, trapezius; 3, spine and acromion of scapula; 4, deltoid

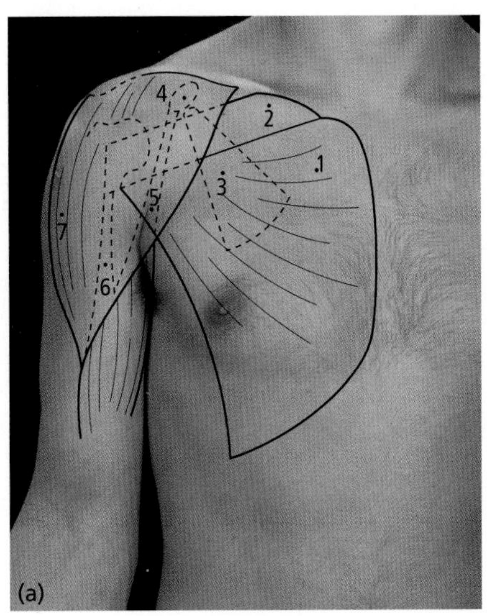

MUSCLES CONNECTING THE UPPER LIMB TO THE TRUNK

Anterior group

Four pectoral muscles move the shoulder girdle and attach it to the thoracic wall (Table 12.1 and Fig. 12.11). Pectoralis major covers the upper chest and its lower border forms the anterior wall of the axilla. Superiorly it is separated from deltoid muscle along the clavicle by the **deltopectoral triangle** (Fig. 12.11b). Pectoralis minor lies covered by pectoralis major in the anterior axillary wall. Serratus anterior lies on the lateral thoracic wall, forming the medial wall of the axilla. Subclavius lies below the clavicle and has no significant function.

Posterior group

These four muscles, trapezius, latissimus dorsi, levator scapulae and the rhomboids, attach the upper limb to the vertebral column (Table 12.2 and Fig. 12.12). Trapezius, levator scapulae and the rhomboids are attached to the shoulder girdle; only latissimus dorsi is attached to the humerus.

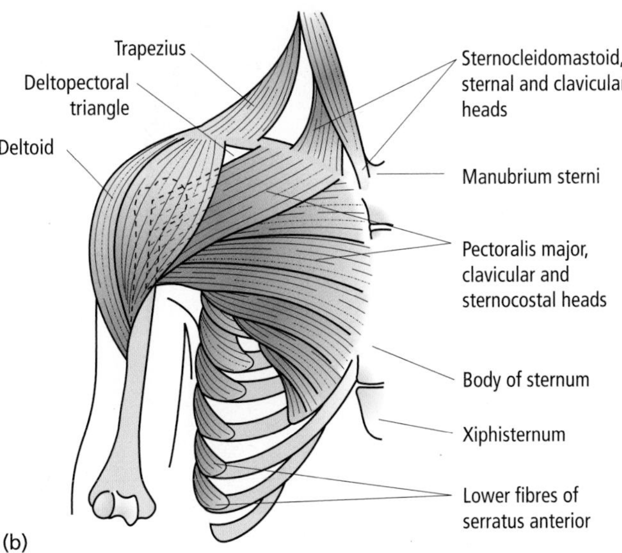

Figure 12.11 Shoulder. (a) Surface anatomy: 1 and 2, sternocostal and clavicular heads of pectoralis major; 3, underlying pectoralis minor; 4, coracoid process; 5 short and 6 long heads of biceps; 7 deltoid; (b) muscles, anterior view

Table 12.1 Shoulder girdle muscles

Muscle	Proximal attachment	Distal attachment	Nerve supply	Function
Pectoralis major	By two heads: Clavicular: medial half of clavicle. Sternocostal: anterior sternum, upper six costal cartilages and external oblique aponeurosis	Intertubercular groove of the humerus	Medial and lateral pectoral nerves (C5, 6, 7)	Adduction and medial rotation of humerus, pulls scapula anteriorly; anterior fibres flexion of shoulder, posterior fibres extend shoulder
Pectoralis minor	Anterior surfaces of 3rd–5th ribs	Coracoid process of scapula	Medial pectoral nerve (C8, T1)	Stabilization of scapula
Serratus anterior	External surface of lateral surface of 1st–8th ribs	Medial border of scapula	Long thoracic nerve (C5, 6, 7)	Protraction of scapula, holds scapula against chest wall

Table 12.2 Muscles of the shoulder girdle

Muscle	Proximal attachment	Distal attachment	Nerve supply	Function
Trapezius	Occipital bone, ligamentum nuchae, all the thoracic spines and supraspinous ligaments	Lateral third of clavicle, acromion, spine of scapula	Spinal accessory nerve, cervical nerves (C3, C4)	Elevates, retracts, and rotates the scapula; upper fibres elevate, middle retract and lower depress. Both act to extend the head and neck
Latissimus dorsi	Spinous processes of lower six thoracic vertebrae, thoracolumbar fascia, posterior iliac crest and lower four ribs	Intertubercular groove of humerus	Thoracodorsal nerve (C6, 7, 8)	Adduction, extension and medial rotation of humerus; in climbing it raises body on the arms
Levator scapulae	Transverse processes of 1st four cervical vertebrae	Medial border of scapula	Dorsal scapular nerve (C5)	Elevation of scapula
Rhomboids	Spinous processes of cervical and upper thoracic vertebrae	Medial border of scapula	Dorsal scapular nerve (C4, 5)	Retraction of scapula

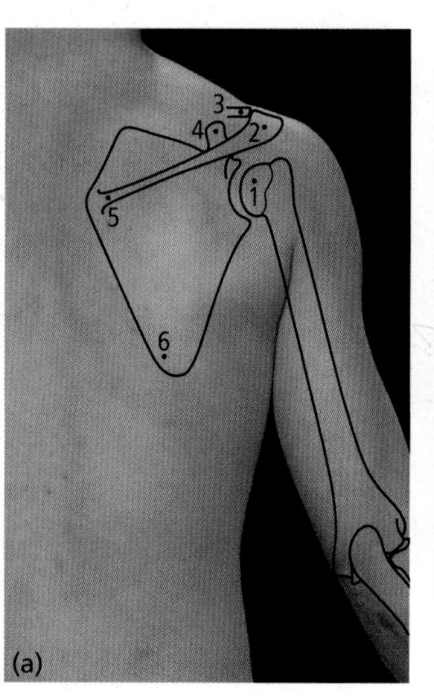

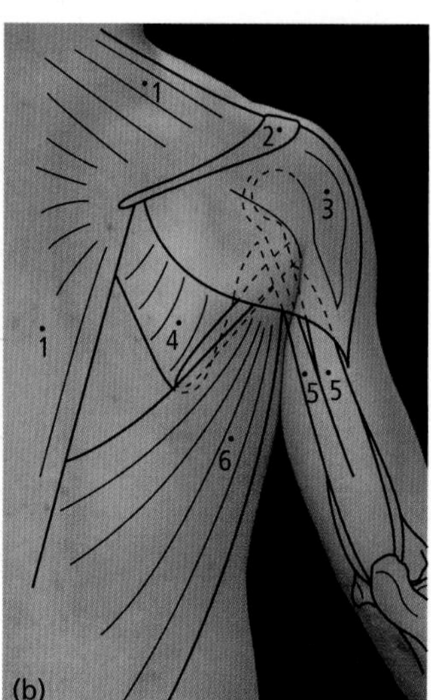

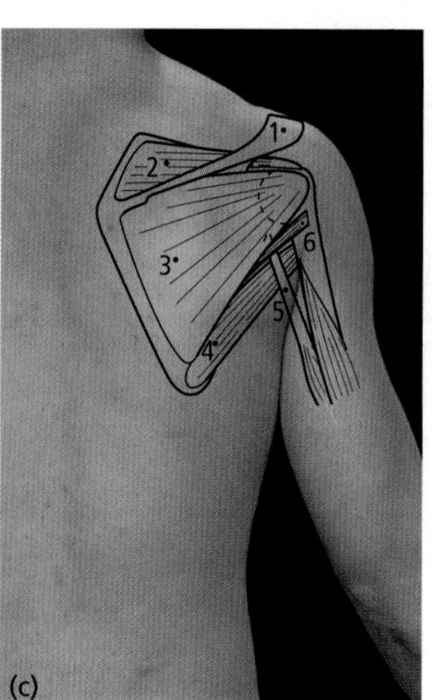

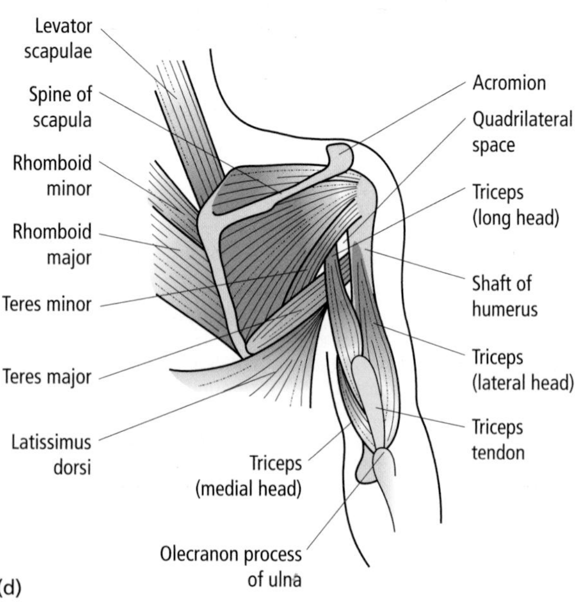

Figure 12.12 Shoulder, posterior view. (a) Bones, surface anatomy: 1, head of humerus; 2, acromion; 3, clavicle; 4, coracoid process; 5, spine of scapula; 6, inferior angle of scapula. (b) Superficial muscles, surface anatomy: 1, trapezius; 2, acromion; 3, deltoid; 4, infraspinatus; 5, long and lateral heads of triceps; 6, latissimus dorsi. (c) Deep muscles, surface anatomy: 1, acromion; 2, supraspinatus; 3, infraspinatus; 4, teres major; 5, long head of triceps; 6, teres minor. (d) Diagram of deep posterior muscles of shoulder joint

MUSCLES OF THE SHOULDER REGION

Deltoid (Fig. 12.10) forms the contour of the shoulder and is functionally divided into anterior, middle and posterior parts. Teres major, with the tendon of latissimus dorsi, forms the posterior axillary fold. Deep to deltoid are the four rotator cuff muscles: supraspinatus, teres minor, infraspinatus (all rotators of the humerus) and subscapularis (Table 12.3). Their tendons blend to form the **rotator cuff**, which gives stability to the shoulder joint.

Intramuscular injections, when necessary, can be made into deltoid's anterior fibres. Avoidance of the posterior part of the muscle prevents accidental injury to the axillary nerve.

If the **supraspinatus tendon** is torn after injury then initiation of abduction is difficult without the trick manoeuvre of dipping the shoulder towards the injured side so that gravity can assist abduction of the arm away from the trunk. Repetitive injury may occur in sportsmen using a strong throwing action, and can result in inflammation of the supraspinatus tendon and associated inflammation of the underlying subacromial bursa (**rotator cuff syndrome**). This causes abduction to be painful, particularly during the middle range of this movement. This 'painful arc' of abduction, usually from 45 to 100°, is diagnostic of this inflammatory condition. Rotator cuff tears are nowadays commonly diagnosed on MRI scans (Fig. 12.13).

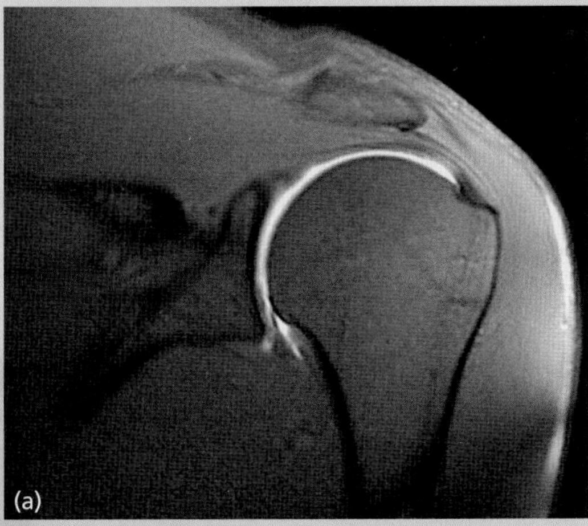

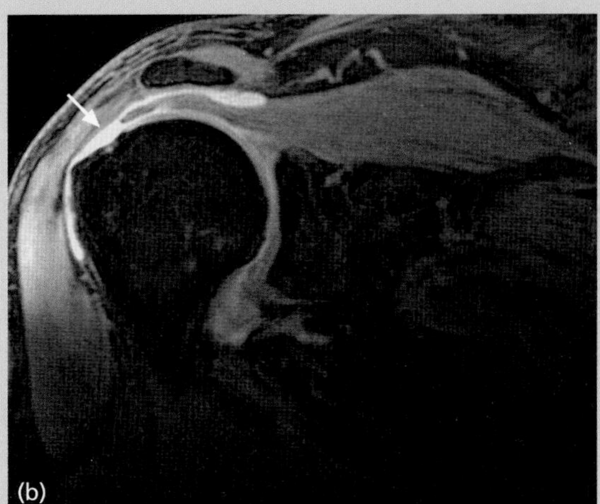

Figure 12.13 MR arthrogram of shoulder joint. (a) Normal; (b) tear in supraspinatus tendon – arrow shows gap in tendon

Table 12.3 Muscles of the shoulder joint

Muscle	Proximal attachment	Distal attachment	Nerve supply	Function
Deltoid	Lateral third of clavicle, acromion and scapular spine	Deltoid tuberosity of humerus	Axillary nerve (C5, 6)	Anterior – flexion, medial rotation of arm Middle – abduction of arm Posterior – extension and lateral rotation of arm
Supraspinatus	Supraspinous fossa of scapula	Greater tuberosity of humerus	Suprascapular nerve (C5)	Initiate abduction
Infraspinatus	Infraspinous fossa of scapula	Greater tuberosity of humerus	Suprascapular nerve (C5)	Adduction and lateral rotation of arm
Teres minor	Lateral border of scapula	Greater tuberosity of humerus	Axillary nerve (C5)	Adduction and lateral rotation of arm
Subscapularis	Subscapular fossa of scapula	Lesser tuberosity of humerus	Subscapular nerve (C6)	Adduction and lateral rotation of arm
Teres major	Inferior angle of scapula	Intertubercular groove of humerus	Subscapular nerve (C6)	Adduction, medial rotation of arm

THE AXILLA AND UPPER ARM

The **axilla** is a fat-filled pyramidal space between the lateral thoracic wall and the upper arm (Fig. 12.14). Its apex, which allows the axillary vessels, brachial plexus and lymphatics to pass from the neck to the axilla via the cervicoaxillary canal, is bounded by the first rib, scapula and the middle third of the clavicle. Its base is formed by hairy axillary skin. Its anterior wall comprises pectoralis major and minor (Fig. 12.11); its posterior wall, lower than the anterior, comprises subscapularis, latissimus dorsi and teres major, which cover the scapula (Fig. 12.12). The medial wall is formed by the upper four ribs, their intercostal muscles and the overlying serratus anterior, and the narrow lateral wall is the intertubercular groove of the humerus, whose lips give attachment to the muscles of the anterior and posterior axillary walls. It contains the axillary artery and vein, the cords and branches of the brachial plexus, coracobrachialis and biceps, axillary lymph vessels, lymph nodes and fat.

Deep fascia

Around the shoulder region the deep fascia invests all the muscles and is drawn out as a tubular prolongation over the arm. Proximally it encloses pectoralis minor and extends above the clavicle as the clavipectoral fascia. Around the elbow the fascia ensheathes the muscles and gives attachment to some of their fibres; in the cubital fossa it is reinforced by the bicipital aponeurosis. In the forearm the fascia is attached to the posterior border of the ulna along its subcutaneous border; at the wrist it forms the flexor and extensor retinacula, and in the hand the palmar aponeurosis and fibrous flexor sheaths. Both the arm and forearm are divided into fascial compartments by strong fascial sheaths, each of which contain a nerve and blood vessels.

Clinically their importance is that if during trauma bleeding occurs, this can then cause compression within a compartment.

Lymphatic drainage

There are two groups of vessels, superficial and deep. The **superficial group** drain the skin. The medial vessels lie with the basilic vein and drain to axillary nodes; the lateral vessels lie with the cephalic vein and drain into infraclavicular nodes, and thence to the apical group of axillary nodes. The **deep group** drain bone and muscle and run with the deep veins to drain into the lateral group of axillary nodes.

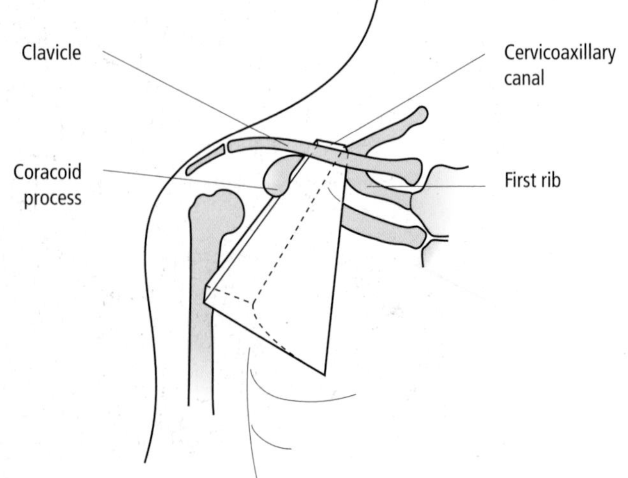

Figure 12.14 Pyramidal shape of axilla

The axillary nodes are arranged in five groups (Fig. 1.17, p. 30):

- **Pectoral** – deep to pectoralis major; drain the lateral and anterior chest wall, the breast and upper anterior abdominal wall
- **Lateral** – on the lateral axillary wall; drain the efferents of the upper limb
- **Posterior** (subscapular) – on the posterior axillary wall; drain the back of the upper trunk
- **Central** – lie around the axillary vessels
- **Apical** – at the axillary apex; drain from all the preceding groups. They are continuous with the inferior deep cervical nodes.

Infection in the superficial tissues of the upper limb results in tender enlargement of the axillary nodes. Skin malignancies arising in the upper limb or anterolateral chest wall may spread lymphatically to produce enlarged axillary nodes. Blockage of the axillary nodes after, for example, radiotherapy treatment, may lead to lymphatic swelling of the limb (lymphoedema) (Fig. 1.20b, p. 31).

The **infraclavicular group** are grouped around the termination of the cephalic vein and drain to the apical nodes. Efferent vessels from the apical nodes form the **subclavian lymph trunk**, which, on the left, joins the thoracic duct and, on the right, opens into the right lymphatic duct, or the internal jugular or subclavian vein.

Blood supply

The **axillary artery** (Figs 12.15 and 12.16) commences at the lateral border of the 1st rib as the continuation of the third part of the subclavian artery and ends at the lower border of teres major, where it becomes the **brachial artery.** Pectoralis minor divides it into three parts, the first above, the second behind and the third below the muscle. It is enclosed in the axilla by the axillary sheath, a continuation of the prevertebral fascia and surrounded by the cords and branches of the brachial plexus (p. 177). The **axillary vein** (Fig. 12.16) lies medial to this neurovascular bundle; coracobrachialis and the short head of biceps are lateral. The brachial plexus lies above and behind the first part of the artery, but below this its cords surround it closely in relationships according to their names, i.e. posterior, medial and lateral.

Branches

The first part has one branch, the superior thoracic artery. The second part has two branches, the thoracoacromical artery and the lateral thoracic artery, which supply the anterolateral aspects of the upper thoracic wall. The third part has three branches, the subscapular artery which follows the lower border of subscapularis and gives a circumflex scapular branch to supply the infraspinous fossa; and the anterior and posterior circumflex humeral arteries which supply the shoulder region and anastomose around the surgical neck of the humerus. The **scapular anastomosis** acquires importance if the upper parts of the axillary artery are occluded. It comprises anastomoses between the **subclavian artery** via its thyrocervical trunk and the **third part of the axillary artery** via its subscapular and circumflex scapular branches.

Venous drainage

The veins are divided into superficial and deep groups that communicate via perforating veins, which under normal circumstances drain from superficial to deep systems.

Superficial group

The digital veins drain into a **dorsal venous arch** on the back of the hand. From its lateral side arises the cephalic vein; from its medial the basilic vein. The **cephalic vein** ascends the radial side of the forearm, crossing the cubital fossa to lie lateral to biceps in the upper arm. In the deltopectoral groove it pierces the clavipectoral fascia to join the axillary vein. The **basilic vein** ascends the ulnar side of the forearm, crosses the cubital fossa and lies medial to biceps. In the upper arm it pierces the deep fascia to join the brachial veins. The **median cubital vein**, frequently chosen for venepuncture, unites the cephalic and basilic veins superficial to the bicipital aponeurosis in the roof of the cubital fossa (Fig. 12.16).

The veins of the forearm and hand are most frequently chosen for intravenous infusions; patient comfort is more easily obtained when the puncture site is not too close to the wrist or elbow joint. The cephalic vein just proximal to the wrist is a popular site.

Deep group

The radial and ulnar veins accompany the arteries and join in the floor of the cubital fossa to form the brachial vein, which forms the axillary vein at the lower border of teres major.

The **axillary vein** is the continuation of the **basilic** and **brachial veins** above the lower border of teres major; it ascends medial to the axillary artery to the outer border of the first rib, where it becomes the subclavian vein. It gains tributaries that correspond to the branches of the axillary artery and the **cephalic vein**, which enters through the fascia in the deltopectoral groove.

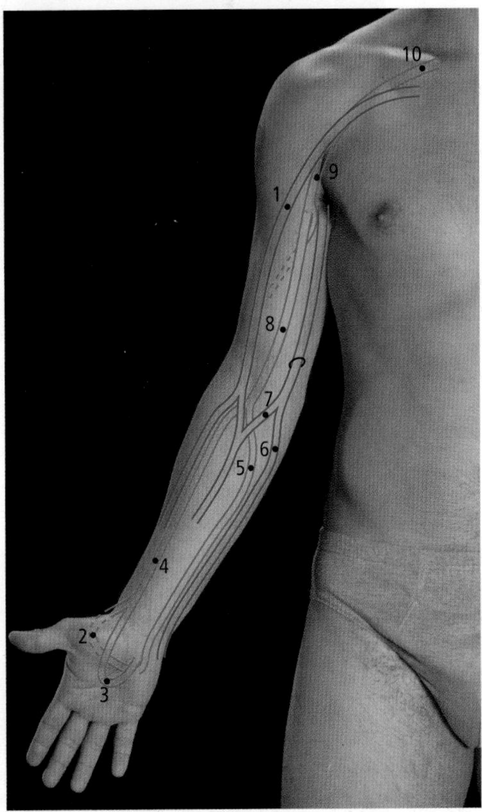

Figure 12.16 Upper limb arteries and veins: 1, cephalic vein; 2, deep palmar arch; 3, superficial palmar arch; 4, radial artery; 5, ulnar artery; 6, basilic vein; 7, medial cubital vein; 8, brachial artery; 9, axillary artery; 10, subclavian artery

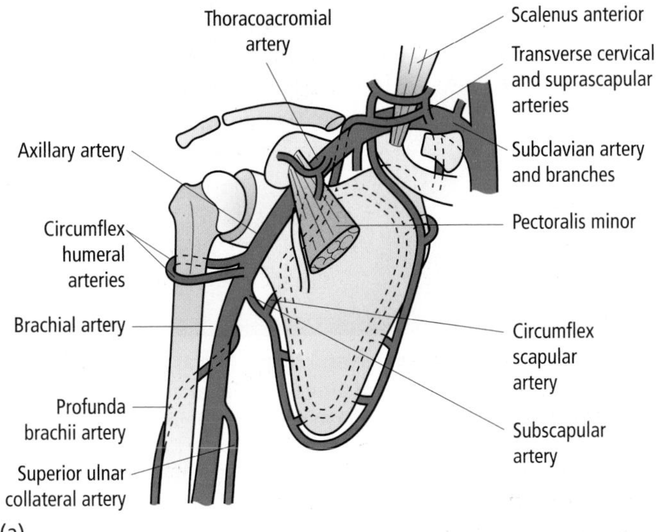

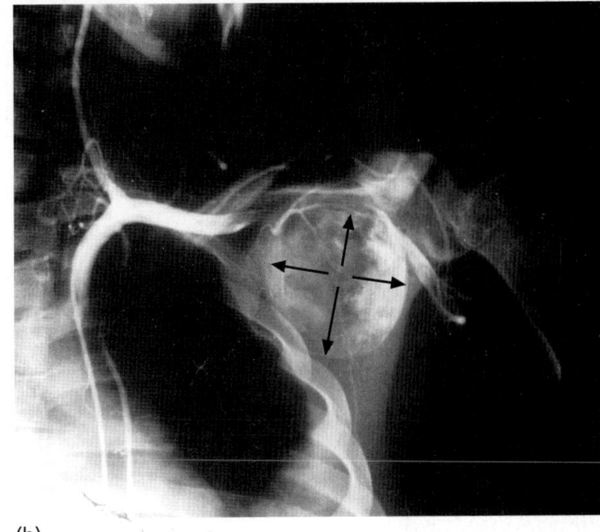

Figure 12.15 (a) Axillary artery and shoulder girdle anastomoses. (b) Angiogram showing aneurysm of axillary artery (arrows)

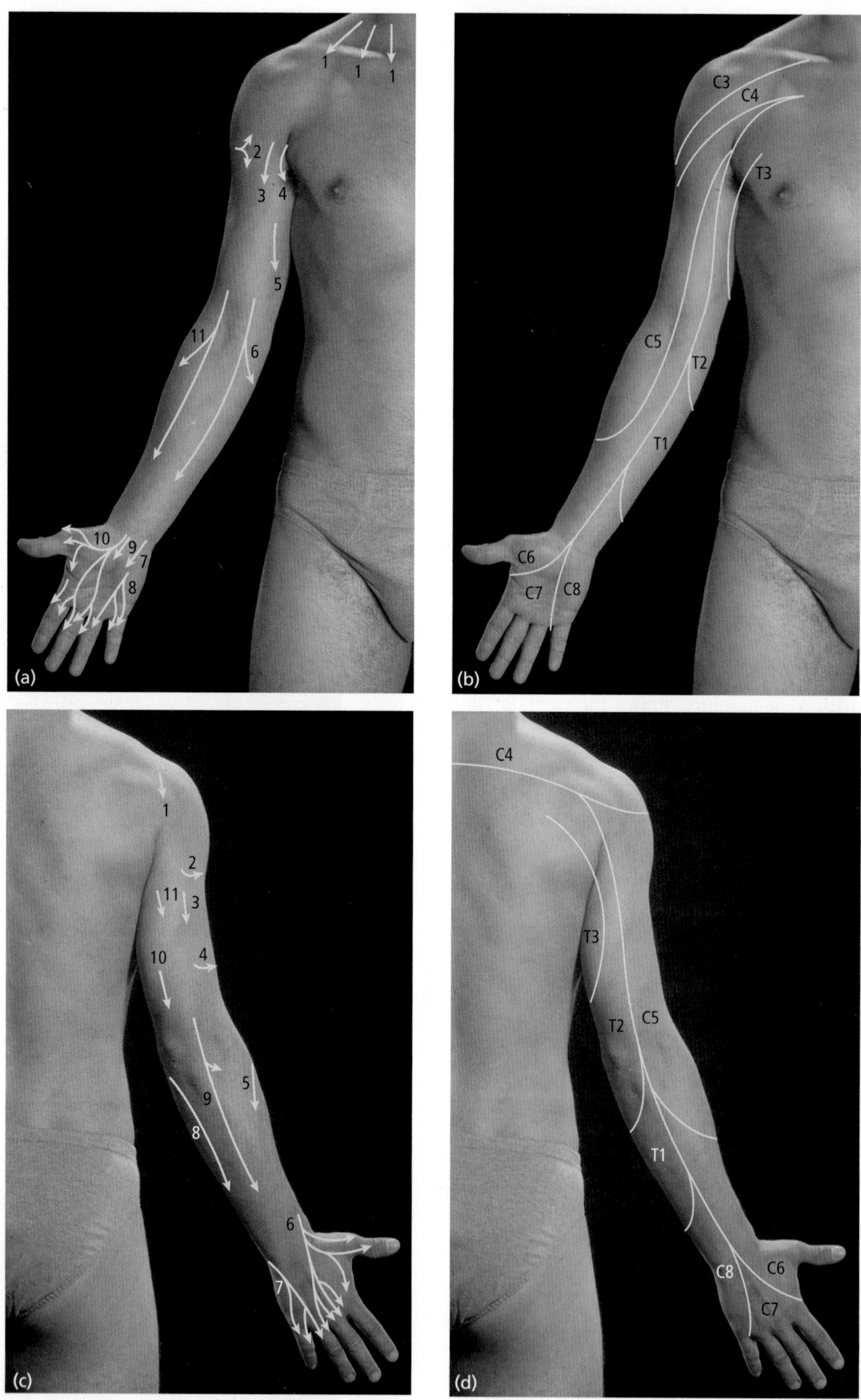

Figure 12.17 (a) Surface anatomy of anterior cutaneous branches of brachial plexus: 1, supraclavicular nerves; 2, upper lateral cutaneous nerve of arm; 3, intermediate cutaneous nerve of arm; 4, intercostobrachial nerve; 5, medial cutaneous nerve of arm; 6, medial cutaneous nerve of forearm; 7, palmar branch of ulnar nerve; 8, ulnar nerve; 9, palmar branch of median nerve; 10, median nerve and its cutaneous branches to the lateral three and a half digits; 11, lateral cutaneous nerve of forearm. (b) Dermatomes of upper limb, anterior view: the numbers denote the dermatomes of the brachial plexus and their distribution. (c) Posterior view, cutaneous nerves: 1, supraclavicular nerve; 2, axillary nerve; 3, posterior cutaneous nerve of arm; 4, lower lateral cutaneous nerve of arm; 5, lateral cutaneous nerve of forearm; 6, superficial radial nerve; 7, dorsal branch of ulnar nerve; 8, medial cutaneous nerve of forearm; 9, posterior cutaneous nerve of forearm; 10, posterior cutaneous nerve of arm; 11, intercostobrachial nerve. (d) Posterior view: dermatomes. C = cervical, T = thoracic

NERVES

The brachial plexus

The **brachial plexus** (Fig. 12.17) supplies the upper limb. It is formed from the anterior primary rami of the lower four cervical and the first thoracic nerves. These **five roots** of the plexus appear between the middle and anterior scalene muscles and unite to form three **trunks** in the posterior triangle of the neck. The upper two roots (C5, 6) form at the apex of the axilla. Each trunk divides into **anterior** and **posterior divisions.** The three posterior divisions join to form the posterior cord, the anterior divisions of the upper and middle trunks form the lateral cord, and the anterior division of the lower trunk continues as the medial cord.

The cords lie close to the axillary artery, disposed around it according to their names. The posterior cord and its branches supply structures on the dorsal surface of the limb and end by dividing into axillary and radial nerves. The medial and lateral cords and their branches supply structures on the flexor surface of the limb; the lateral cord ends by dividing into the musculocutaneous nerve and the lateral head of the median nerve, the medial cord ends as the ulnar nerve and the medial head of the median nerve.

The plexus and its branches can be best understood by study of Fig. 12.18b.

From the **roots**: small branches to the back muscles; C5 contributes to the phrenic nerve, the long thoracic nerve passes behind the vessels to the medial wall of the axilla to supply serratus anterior.

Segmental nerve supply

Although the course of the nerve roots in the brachial plexus is complex the skin of the upper limb has perfectly regular dermatomes (Fig. 12.17b,d). They originate from segments C4 to T2 (Fig 12.8).

It is worth noting that the segmental innervation of the skin over the deltoid muscle, C4, is identical to that segment supplying the diaphragm, which explains the referral of pain originating in the diaphragm to the shoulder region.

C5 supplies the upper outer arm, C6 the radial side of forearm and thumb, C7 the palm of hand and first three fingers, C8 the ulnar forearm, T1 the ulnar upper arm and T2 the axillary skin (dermatomal patterns are subject to variation and overlap). Autonomic sympathetic nerves are carried in the branches of the brachial plexus and supply blood vessels, sweat glands and arrector pili muscles throughout the upper limb.

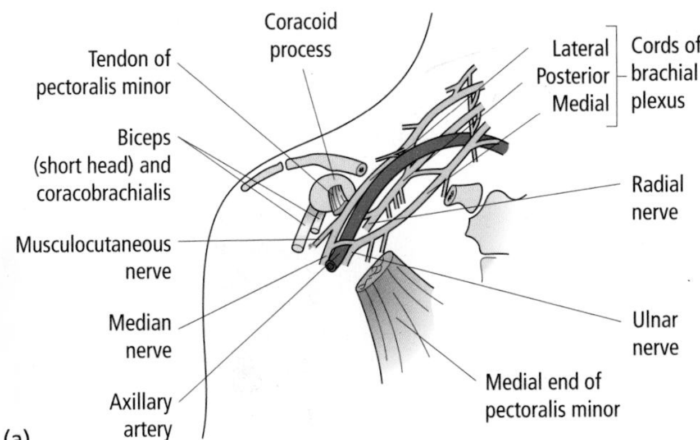

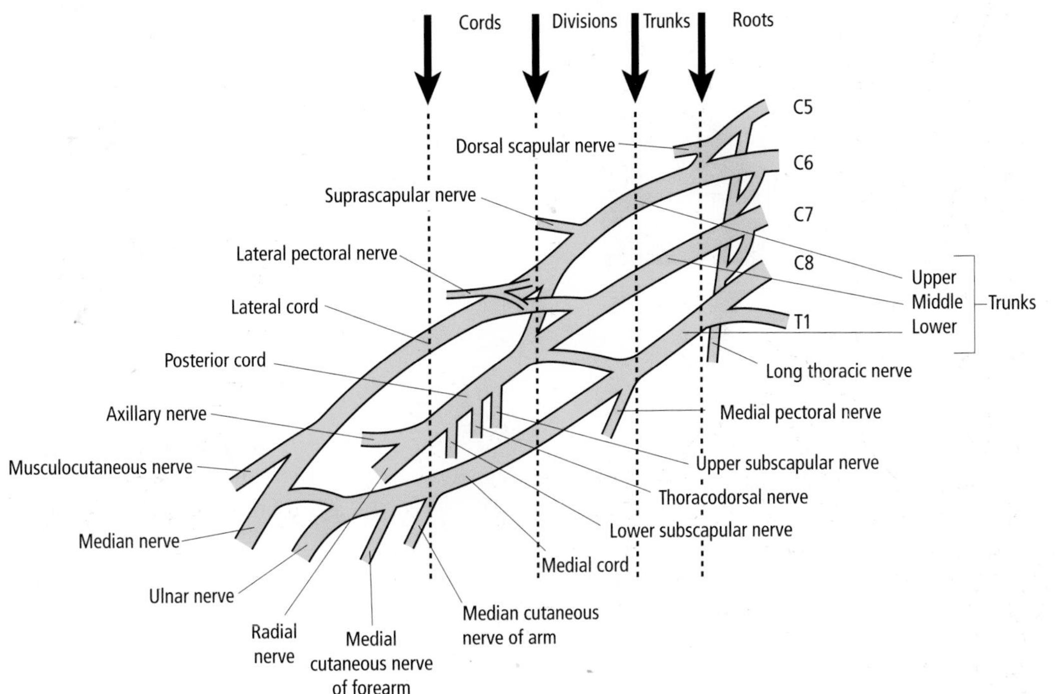

Figure 12.18 (a) Diagram of brachial plexus showing relationship of cords to axillary artery with segment of clavicle and pectoralis minor removed. (b) Brachial plexus – diagram showing its roots, trunks, cords and branches

THE UPPER ARM MUSCLES

In the anterior compartment of the arm there are three flexor muscles: biceps, brachialis and coracobrachialis (Table 12.4 and Fig. 12.20). The tendon of the long head of biceps lies in the shoulder joint, retained in the intertubercular groove by the transverse humeral ligament, surrounded by a synovial sheath. It unites with the short head in the lower arm. One extensor, triceps, occupies the posterior compartment. Anconeus lies close to triceps, but the bulk of it lies in the forearm.

Injuries to the brachial plexus

Brachial plexus injuries, which are usually the result of forceful stretching or direct wounding, will produce signs of a segmental nature. **Upper trunk injury** is usually the result of forceful and excessive separation of the neck and shoulder, such as may happen when a motorcyclist is thrown forwards at high speed on to his shoulder, or following a difficult birth delivery which has been associated with excessive traction on the baby's head. Upper trunk damage produces sensory loss on the radial side of the arm and forearm (C5, 6) and paralysis of deltoid, biceps and brachialis. The limb hangs limply, medially rotated and fully pronated (the 'waiter's tip' position) (Erb's palsy; Fig. 12.19a). **Lower trunk injuries** are uncommon but may occur when the upper limb is pulled forcibly upwards. This may result from pulling too hard on an infant's arm during a difficult delivery. Injury to C8 and T1 results in paralysis of the small muscles of the hand, and the unopposed action of the long flexors (flexing the interphalangeal joints) and the long extensors (extension of the metacarpophalangeal joints) produces the typical 'claw-hand' deformity (Klumpke's paralysis; Fig. 12.19d).

Non-traumatic causes of brachial plexus pathology occur: a cervical rib (Fig. 12.19c) may put undue pressure on the lower cord, as may direct invasion of an apical lung cancer to result in similar paralysis.

When viewed pushing against a wall, the patient in Fig 12.19e is seen to have an obvious 'winging' of his scapula due to damage to the long thoracic nerve (C5, 6, 7) which arises from the roots of the brachial plexus and supplies serratus anterior muscle. This muscle, which normally holds the scapula against the chest wall when pushing, is here paralysed.

Peripheral nerve injuries are described on pp. 211–12.

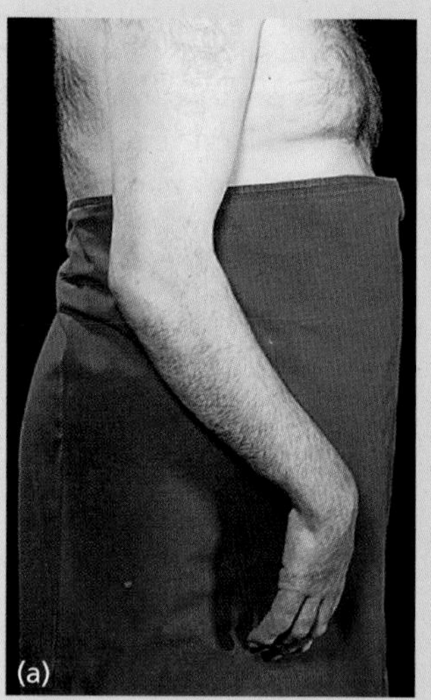

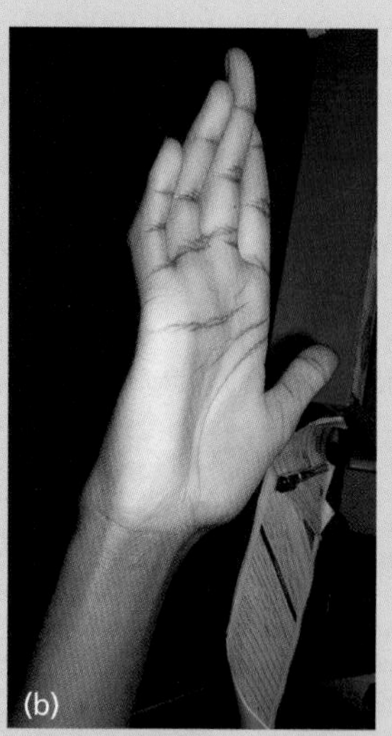

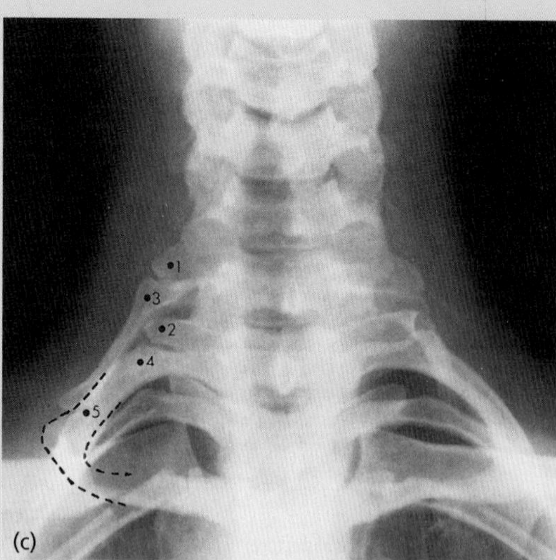

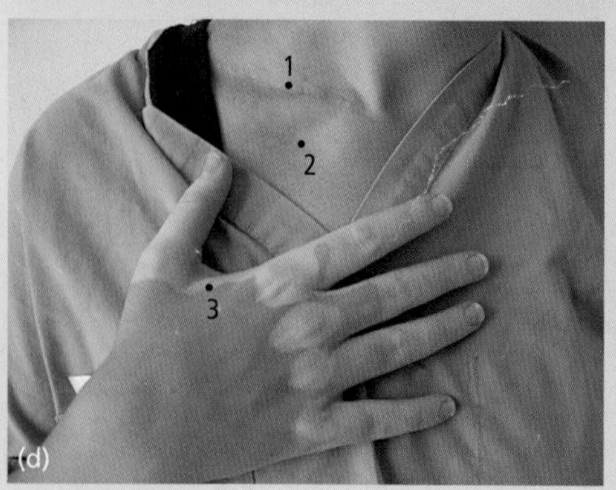

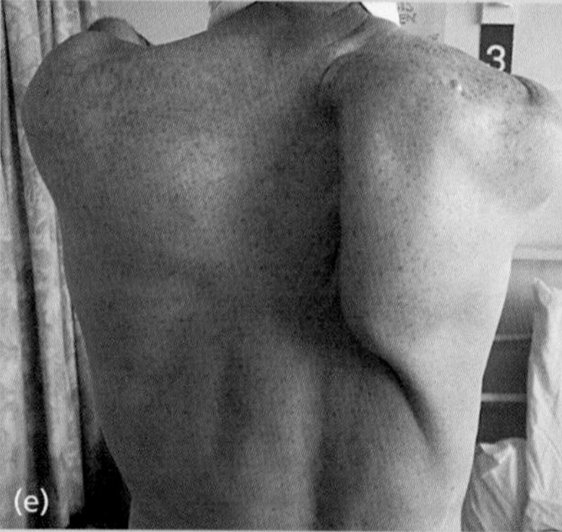

Figure 12.19 (a) Erb's palsy. (b) Injury to T1 producing claw hand. (c) Cervical rib X-ray: 1, transverse process of 7th cervical vertebra; 2, transverse process of 1st thoracic vertebra; 3, abnormal cervical rib; 4, 1st rib; 5, prominent articulation between cervical and 1st rib. (d) This patient has: 1, a cervical rib scar; 2, a hollow where 1st rib has been removed; 3, wasting of 1st dorsal interosseous muscle due to cervical rib pressure on T1 nerve root, 'Klumpke's palsy'. (e) 'Winging' of the scapula

Table 12.4 Muscles of the arm

Muscle	Proximal attachment	Distal attachment	Nerve supply	Function
Biceps brachii	By two heads: Short head: coracoid process of scapula Long head: supraglenoid tubercle of scapula	Radial tuberosity and by bicipital aponeurosis to the deep fascia of forearm	Musculocutaneous nerve (C6)	Flexion of forearm, supinator
Brachialis	Distal half of anterior humerus	Coronoid process of ulna	Musculocutaneous nerve (C6)	Flexion of forearm
Coracobrachialis	Coracoid process of scapula	Medial side of mid-humerus	Musculocutaneous nerve (C6)	Adduction and flexion of humerus (the newspaper under the arm when running for a bus)
Triceps	By three heads: Long head: infraglenoid tubercle of scapula Lateral head: posterior upper humerus Medial head: posterior humerus below radial groove	Olecranon of the ulna	Radial nerve (C7, 8)	Chief extensor of forearm
Anconeus	Lateral epicondyle of humerus	Olecranon and upper part of posterior surface of ulna	Radial nerve (C8, T1)	Weak extensor of forearm; abducts the ulna during pronation

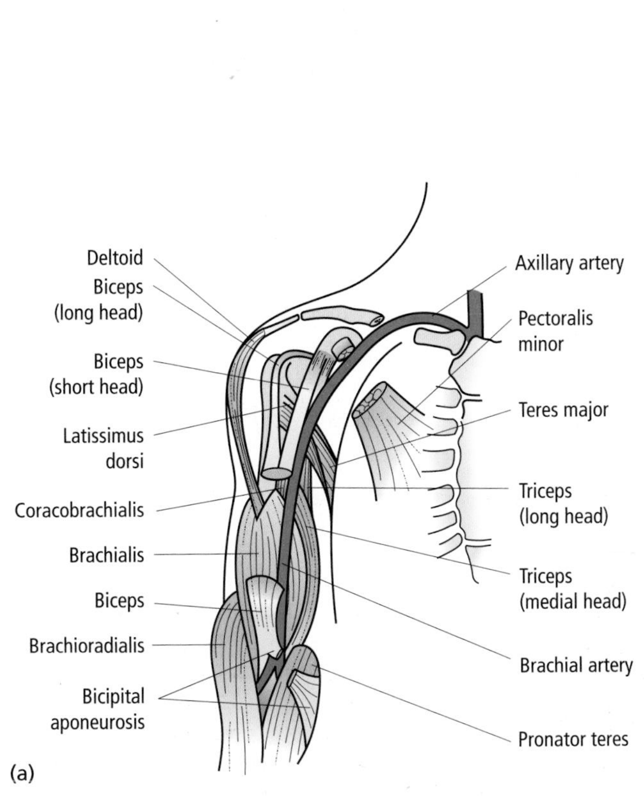

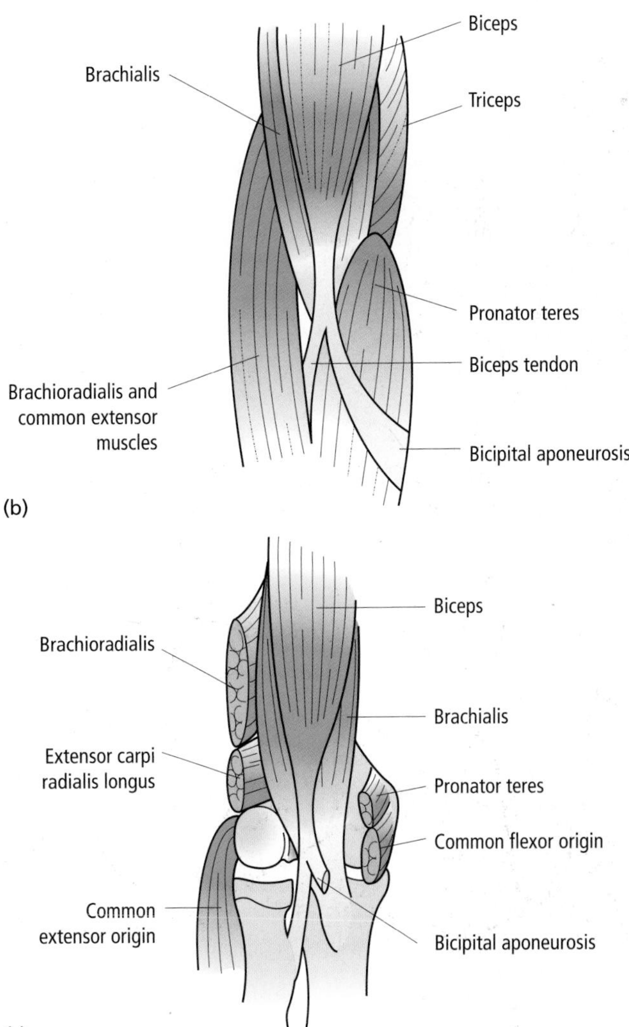

Figure 12.20 Upper arm. (a) Anterior muscles – pectoralis minor and biceps divided to reveal artery. (b) Anterior elbow – bicipital aponeurosis. (c) Deep dissection of the elbow – attachment of biceps in cubital fossa

Biceps

Biceps arises proximally by two heads: the **short head** from the coracoid process and the **long head** from the supraglenoid tubercle of the humerus.

Degenerative disease around the shoulder joint may cause the long head of biceps to fray and weaken, resulting sometimes in rupture. A noticeable bulge appears low on the anterior surface of the arm (Fig. 12.21) when the elbow is flexed, and supination against resistance is painful. Peripheral reflexes can be tested around the elbow joint: the biceps reflex (C5, 6) by tapping the thumb held against the biceps tendon in front of the elbow, and the triceps reflex by tapping the triceps tendon just above the olecranon (C6, 7).

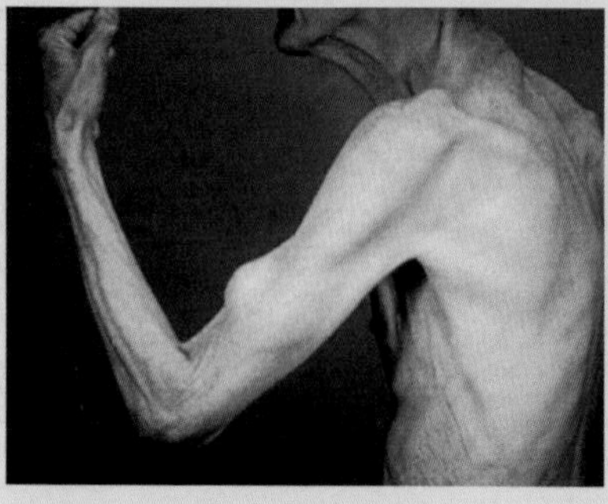

Figure 12.21 Rupture of long head of biceps.

The brachial artery

The **brachial artery** (Figs 12.15, 12.20 and 12.22), the continuation of the axillary artery, begins at the lower border of teres major and descends subcutaneously on the medial side of the upper arm within the anterior compartment. Throughout its course it lies medial to biceps and its tendon. It is accompanied by veins and is crossed by the **median nerve** from lateral to medial halfway down the arm. It ends in the cubital fossa by dividing into radial and ulnar arteries, and is here crossed by the **medial cubital vein** and separated from it by only the bicipital aponeurosis (Fig. 12.23).•

Because the vein is frequently here used for venepuncture this close relationship should be noted.

The artery provides branches to the muscles, the elbow joint and humerus and the **profunda brachii artery**, which runs with the radial nerve in the radial groove.

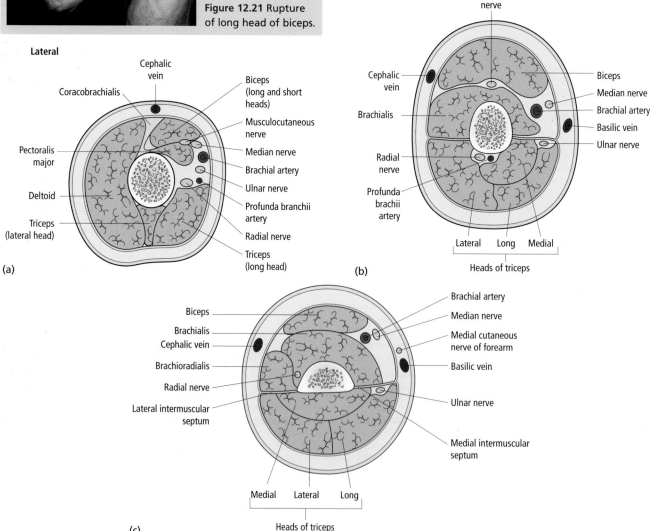

Figure 12.22 Transverse sections of upper limb: (a) upper third; (b) middle third; (c) lower third

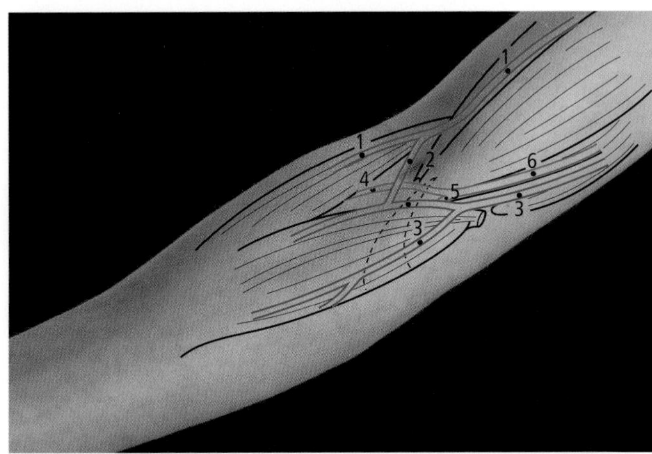

Figure 12.23 Surface marking of vessels and nerves in the cubital fossa (dotted lines show the bicipital aponeurosis separating the median cubital vein from the median nerve below): 1, cephalic vein; 2, median cubital vein; 3, basilic vein; 4, radial artery; 5, ulnar artery; 6, brachial artery.

The brachial artery is palpable through most of its course on the medial side of the arm and in the cubital fossa medial to the bicipital tendon under the aponeurosis. In the latter situation it is usually palpated and auscultated when taking the blood pressure. The sphygmomanometer cuff is inflated until the arterial pulse can no longer be palpated, the stethoscope placed over the artery and the cuff slowly deflated. The pressure at which the arterial pressure waves are first heard is the systolic and the pressure at which they disappear is the diastolic. Laceration of the brachial artery or occlusion due to, for instance, displacement of an elbow fracture, is a surgical emergency because ischaemia and paralysis of the forearm muscles follows within a few hours. Subsequent fibrosis of the muscles results in contracture of the long forearm extensor and flexor muscles (Fig. 12.6).

The musculocutaneous nerve

The **musculocutaneous nerve** is a terminal branch of the lateral cord of the brachial plexus. Initially it lies lateral to the axillary artery and then pierces coracobrachialis to descend between biceps and brachialis. It finally emerges lateral to these muscles to end, after piercing the deep fascia, as the **lateral cutaneous nerve of the forearm.** It supplies muscular branches to coracobrachialis, biceps and brachialis, and articular branches to the elbow joint. The lateral cutaneous nerve of the forearm supplies flexor and extensor surfaces of the radial side of the forearm.

The nerve is rarely injured, but this occasionally occurs after a dislocation of the shoulder, producing paralysis of coracobrachialis, biceps and brachialis and a resultant weakness in elbow flexion and supination, together with loss of sensation on the lateral side of the forearm.

The radial nerve

The **radial nerve** (Fig. 12.22a–c), a terminal branch of the posterior cord of the brachial plexus, arises on the posterior wall of the axilla and descends between the long head of triceps and the shaft of the humerus to reach the posterior compartment of the arm. Here it descends with the profunda brachii artery between the medial and lateral heads of triceps in the radial groove of the humerus.

At this site it is susceptible to injury in midshaft fractures of the humerus.

It divides anterior to the elbow joint between brachioradialis and brachialis.

In the axilla it gives branches to triceps and the posterior cutaneous nerve of the arm, which supplies the skin of the posteromedial aspect of the upper arm.

In the posterior compartment of the arm it supplies triceps, brachioradialis and extensor carpi radialis longus, and gives off two sensory branches, the lower lateral cutaneous nerve of the arm, supplying the skin of the lower lateral aspect of the arm, and the posterior cutaneous nerve of the forearm, before piercing the lateral intermuscular septum.

The median nerve

The **median nerve** (Figs 12.22a–c) in the upper arm arises by the union of its medial and lateral heads, both terminal branches of the brachial plexus. It descends through the upper arm, at first lateral to the axillary and brachial arteries and then, halfway down the limb, crosses the latter to the medial side. It has no branches above the elbow.

The ulnar nerve

The **ulnar nerve** (Fig. 12.22a–c) in the upper arm arises as the continuation of the medial cord of the brachial plexus. It descends medial to the axillary and brachial arteries and, halfway down the arm, pierces the medial intermuscular septum to continue its descent on the medial head of triceps to enter the forearm by passing behind the medial epicondyle. It has no branches in the upper arm above the elbow.

MCQs

1. The shoulder joint: **T/F**

a has a scapular articular surface less than one-third that of the diameter of the humeral head (____)
b is surrounded by a tight capsular ligament (____)
c usually communicates with the subacromial bursa (____)
d depends for most of its stability on the capsular and accessory ligaments (____)
e is closely related inferiorly to the axillary nerve (____)

Answers

1.

a ***T*** – *Even though the scapular articular surface includes the ring of fibrocartilage, the glenoid labrum, around its margin.*
b ***F*** – *The capsule is lax, particularly inferiorly, and allows for a wide range of movement in this joint.*
c ***F*** – *The subscapular bursa communicates with the joint, not the subacromial.*
d ***F*** – *The lax capsule is of little support and the shallow glenoid cavity affords almost none. The tendons of the short articular (rotator cuff) muscles, subscapularis, supraspinatus, infraspinatus and teres minor, by their close fusion with the capsule, are the major stabilizing factors.*
e ***T*** – *Which is thus easily damaged in downward dislocations of the joint.*

---

2. Branches of the posterior cord of the brachial plexus include the: **T/F**

a axillary nerve (____)
b lateral pectoral nerve (____)
c long thoracic nerve (____)
d nerve to rhomboids (____)
e nerve to teres major (____)

Answers

2.

a ***T*** – *The branches of the posterior cord are the axillary, radial, thoracodorsal, upper and lower subscapular nerves.*
b ***F*** – *The lateral pectoral nerve is a branch of the lateral cord.*
c ***F*** – *The long thoracic nerve to serratus anterior is a branch from the roots C5, 6 and 7.*
d ***F*** – *The nerve to rhomboids is a branch from the root of C5.*
e ***T*** – *The nerve to teres major is a branch of the subscapular nerves, which are branches of the posterior cord.*

---

3. The axilla contains: **T/F**

a the trunks of the brachial plexus (____)
b the superior thoracic artery (____)
c latissimus dorsi muscle (____)
d the dorsal scapular nerve (____)
e the long thoracic nerve (____)

Answers

3.

a ***F*** – *The axilla contains the cords of the brachial plexus; the trunks lie in the posterior triangle of the neck.*
b ***T*** – *It arises in the upper axilla and supplies the upper thoracic wall.*
c ***F*** – *It is the tendon of latissimus dorsi, rather than the muscle that is in the axilla.*
d ***F*** – *The dorsal scapular nerve (nerve to rhomboids) lies posterior to the axilla.*
e ***T*** – *The long thoracic nerve (nerve to serratus anterior) lies on serratus anterior on the medial wall of the axilla.*

EMQs

Each question has an anatomical theme linked to the chapter, and a list of 10 related items (A–J) placed in alphabetical order: these are followed by five statements (1–5). Match **one or more** of the items A–J to each of the five statements.

Muscles of the shoulder and upper arm

A. Biceps
B. Brachialis
C. Deltoid
D. Latissimus dorsi
E. Pectoralis major
F. Serratus anterior
G. Subscapularis
H. Supraspinatus
I. Trapezius
J. Triceps

Match the following attachments to the appropriate muscle(s) in the above list.

1. Coronoid process of the ulna
2. Olecranon process of the ulna
3. Clavicle
4. Superior nuchal line of the skull
5. Infraglenoid tubercle of the scapula

Answers

1 B; 2 J; 3 CEI; 4 I; 5 J

Nerves of the shoulder and upper arm

A. Biceps
B. Brachialis
C. Deltoid
D. Latissimus dorsi
E. Pectoralis major
F. Serratus anterior
G. Subscapularis
H. Supraspinatus
I. Trapezius
J. Triceps

Match the following nerves to the appropriate muscle(s) in the above list.

1. Posterior cord of the brachial plexus
2. Axillary
3. Long thoracic
4. Thoracodorsal
5. Musculocutaneous

Answers

1 CDGJ; 2 C; 3 F; 4 D; 5 AB

APPLIED QUESTIONS

1. Where can the axillary artery be surgically ligated without compromise to the blood supply of the upper limb?

1. The scapular anastomosis, connecting the first part of the subclavian (via the thyrocervical trunk) with the third part of the axillary (via the subscapular artery), enables the blood supply to the upper limb to be uncompromised in all positions of the shoulder joint. Accurate identification of the subscapular artery is therefore needed, as the axillary artery must be ligated above it to ensure a continued blood supply to the upper limb.

---

2. A patient complained that after she had had a radical mastectomy her scapula stuck out like a wing when she pushed open a door. She also now found difficulty reaching the top shelves in her kitchen. Can you explain why?

2. A 'winged' scapula is seen in some thin women, but following a radical mastectomy one must immediately think of a weak serratus anterior muscle. The most likely cause is trauma to the long thoracic nerve (Bell), which lies along the medial axillary wall, sending twigs to each of the eight slips of the muscle. It is here that breast surgeons may traumatize it while clearing lymph nodes from the axillary fat. The resulting paralysis makes the patient unable to abduct the arm further than the horizontal, as the scapula cannot be rotated to raise the glenoid cavity.

---

3. Why is an intramuscular injection into the posterior part of the deltoid potentially dangerous?

3. The axillary nerve arises from the posterior cord of the brachial plexus. The anterior branch, accompanied by the posterior circumflex humeral vessels, winds posteriorly through the quadrangular (quadrilateral) space and round the surgical neck of the humerus to supply deltoid from its deep surface. This is usually some 6–8 cm inferior to the bony prominence of the acromion. Any injections below and posterior to the midpoint of the acromion endangers the axillary nerve. Muscular (and financial!) incapacity may result.

The elbow and forearm

THE RADIUS AND ULNA

The radius

The radius, the lateral bone of the forearm, has a head, a body and a lower end (Fig. 13.1). The **head** is a cupped circular disc which articulates with the capitulum of the humerus and the radial notch of the ulna (Fig. 13.2). It can be palpated in the depression behind the lateral side of the elbow in extension. Just below the head is the radial tuberosity, which gives attachment to the biceps tendon. The **body** has a slight lateral convexity and expands in its lower part for muscle attachments (see Fig. 13.1). Its medial side bears a ridge for the attachments of the interosseous membrane. The **lower end** extends into a palpable styloid process laterally; posteriorly lies a dorsal tubercle, which guides the tendon of extensor pollicis longus, and ridges to which septa from the extensor retinaculum are attached. Its medial surface articulates with the head of the ulna and its inferior surface has facets for the carpal bones, and it gives attachment to a fibrocartilaginous articular disc.

A fall on the outstretched hand causes the body weight to be transmitted via the thenar eminence onto the lower end of the radius and occasionally causes a Colles' fracture; the distal fragment being impacted and characteristically displaced laterally and posteriorly (see Fig. 14.4b, p. 206).

The ulna

The ulna (Fig. 13.1), the medial forearm bone, has an upper end, a body and a lower end. The **upper end** has a deep trochlear notch bounded by two projections, the olecranon giving attachment to the triceps, and the coronoid process to which brachialis is attached. The notch articulates with the trochlear notch of the humerus. On the lateral side of the coronoid process is an articular radial notch for the head of the radius; its borders give attachment to the annular ligament. Below the notch the anterior surface gives attachment to the supinator muscle. To the medial side of the body and upper end flexor digitorum profundus is attached. The **body** has anterior, medial and posterior surfaces, but towards the lower end it becomes cylindrical. The middle of the lateral border is prominently marked by the attachment of the interosseous membrane. The **lower end** possesses a rounded head and a prominent styloid process, between which lies the tendon of extensor carpi ulnaris; the head articulates with the lower end of the radius and with the articular disc attached to the base of the styloid process. The olecranon, the posterior border of the shaft, the lower medial surface and the styloid process are subcutaneous and palpable.

The cubital fossa

The cubital fossa (Fig. 12.23, p. 181) lies anterior to the elbow joint (Fig. 13.2). It is triangular, bounded by a line joining the humeral epicondyles, medially by pronator teres, and laterally by brachioradialis. It is roofed by deep fascia, here strengthened by the bicipital aponeurosis, across which the often-visible median cubital vein runs. The fossa contains, from medial to lateral, the median nerve, the brachial artery and its terminal branches, the radial and ulnar arteries and the biceps tendon. The radial and posterior interosseous nerves, lateral to the tendon, usually lie deep to brachioradialis. The brachial artery is palpable here lying medial to the tendon of biceps; a point taken advantage of when taking the blood pressure.

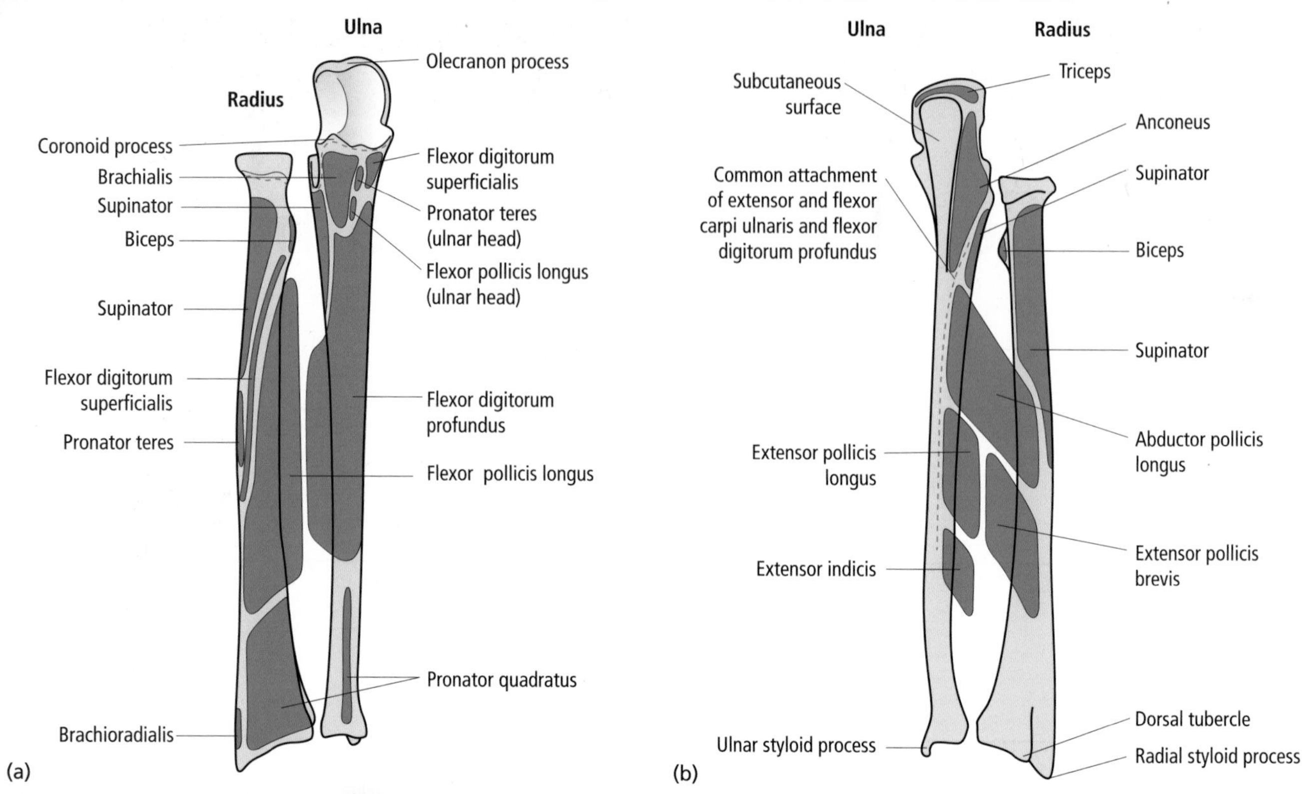

Figure 13.1 Radius and ulna with muscle attachments: (a) anterior view (dotted red lines show capsular attachments); (b) posterior view

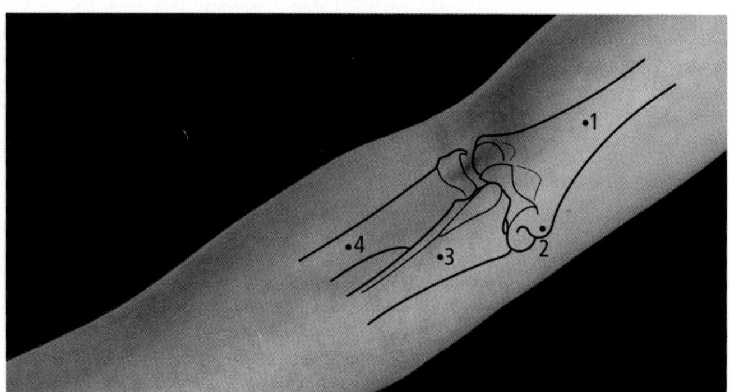

Figure 13.2 Bones of the elbow: 1, humerus; 2, medial epicondyle; 3, ulnar; 4, radius

THE ELBOW JOINT

The elbow joint (Fig. 13.3) is a synovial hinge joint between the lower end of the humerus and the upper ends of the radius and ulna. The humerus presents a rounded capitulum and a saddle-shaped trochlea for articulation with the cupped head of the radius and the trochlear notch of the ulna, respectively. In the anatomical position the forearm deviates laterally from the arm (carrying angle). The **capsular ligament** is attached to the humerus around the upper margins of its olecranon, coronoid and radial fossae, and inferiorly to the medial border of the trochlear notch and the annular ligament of the proximal radioulnar joint (Fig. 13.1). The capsule is thickened by strong **radial** and **ulnar collateral ligaments** (Fig. 13.4).

Functional aspects

The only movement permitted at the elbow is flexion and extension, but, in addition, the humeroradial articulation permits pronation and supination (Fig. 13.7).

- **Flexion** – brachialis and biceps are assisted by brachioradialis and the common flexor muscles.
- **Extension** – triceps.

The shapes of the bones, the strong capsule and the close envelope of brachialis and triceps contribute to the joint's sound stability.

The interosseous membrane

The radius and ulna are joined by the **interosseous membrane** (Figs 13.4 and 13.5) and the radioulnar joints. The interosseous membrane is a strong fibrous sheet joining the adjacent interosseous borders of the two bones and giving attachment to deep flexor and deep extensor muscles. The membrane's fibres are directed downwards and medially, hence a force passing from the hand to the radius, such as would occur in punching, is transmitted to the elbow by the ulna as well as through the head of the radius.

THE RADIOULNAR JOINTS

There are two radioulnar joints. The **proximal radioulnar joint** is a synovial joint of the pivot variety; the side of the disc-shaped radial head articulates within the osseoligamentous ring formed by the radial notch of the ulna and annular

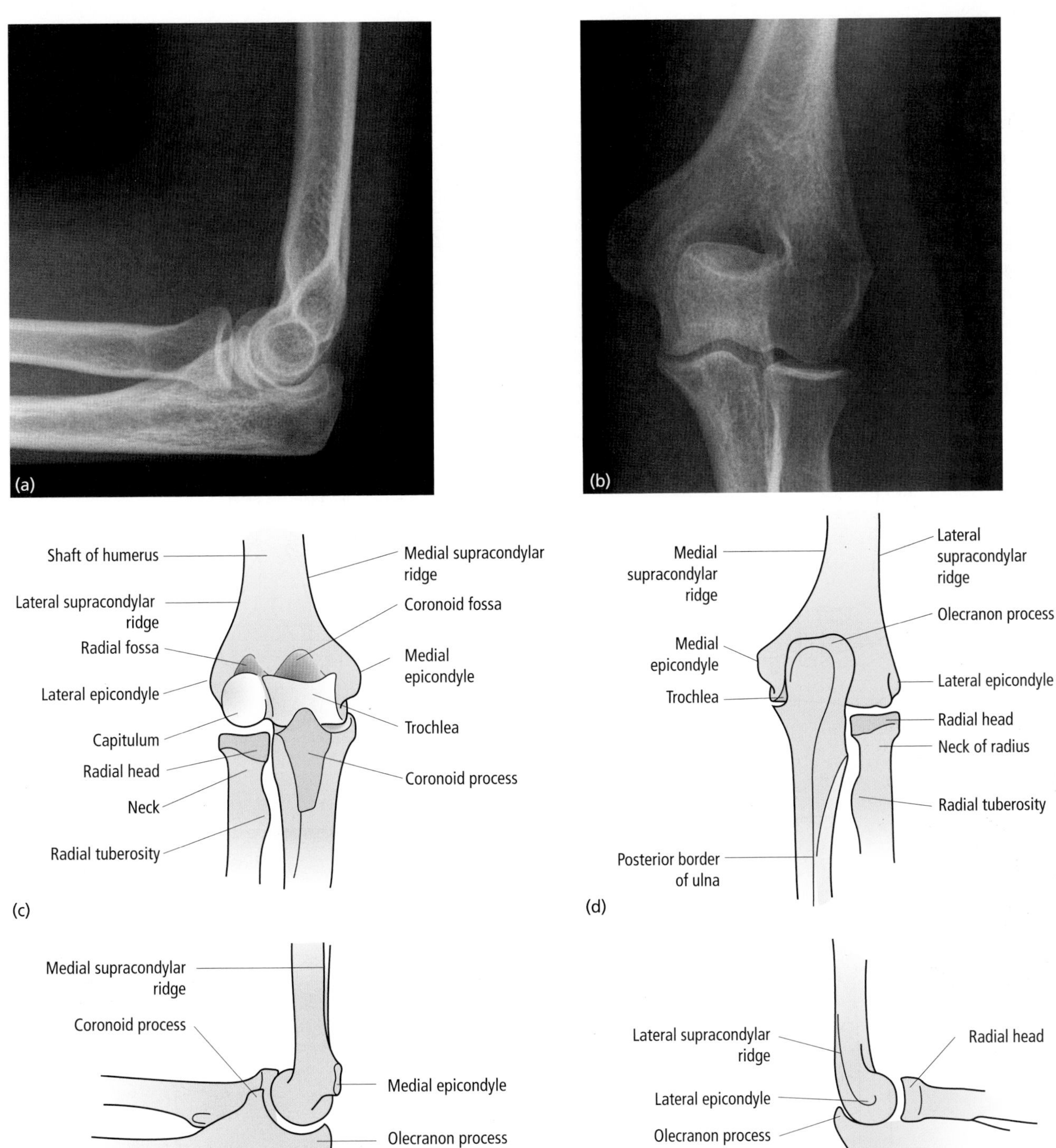

Figure 13.3 Elbow joint: (a) X-ray, lateral view; (b) X-ray, anteroposterior view; (c–f) diagrams showing bony features

ligament which encircles the radial head and is attached to the margins of the ulna's radial notch. Its synovial membrane is continuous with that of the elbow joint. It is a stable joint; the annular ligament, narrower below than above, firmly holds the adult radial head.

In the child, the radial head is less conical and therefore less firmly held by the annular ligament. A sharp tug on a child's arm can cause a dislocation (pulled elbow).

The **distal radioulnar joint** is also a synovial joint of the pivot variety; the head of the ulna articulating with the ulnar notch on the radius. A triangular fibrocartilaginous **articular disc** lies distal to the ulna and contributes to the articular surface of the wrist joint (Fig. 13.6). The weak capsular ligament is attached to the articular margin and the articular disc. The synovial membrane is not usually continuous with that of the wrist joint. Joint stability is dependent on the strength of the articular disc's attachments.

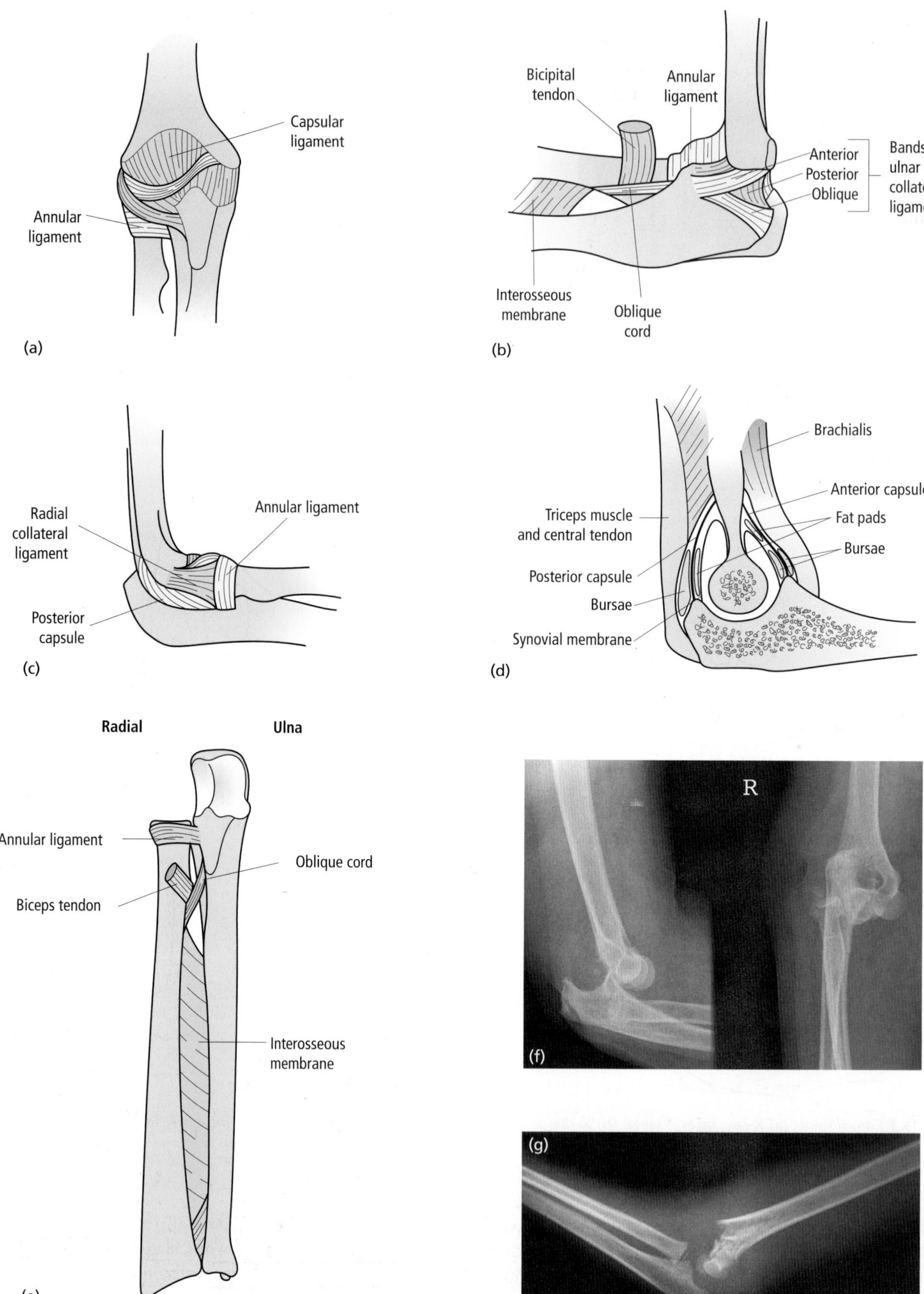

Figure 13.4 (a–c) Elbow joint ligaments. (d) Sagittal section showing relations of tendons and bursae to the joint. (e) Forearm bones and ligaments of superior radioulnar joint. (f) X-ray showing dislocation of the elbow – lateral and anteroposterior views. (g) Supracondylar fracture of humerus in a child

Functional aspects

Supination and pronation (Fig. 13.7) occur about an axis joining the centre of the radial head to the styloid process of the ulna. In the anatomical position the forearm is fully supinated. Pronation is produced by the radial head rotating within the annular ligament so that the lower end of the radius, tethered by the articular disc, moves ventrally around the head of the ulna. The palm of the hand then faces dorsally. The range of these movements is high – more than 180° – but can be increased further by simultaneous rotation of the humerus (provided the elbow joint is fully extended). Both supination and pronation are stronger when the elbow is flexed. Supination, produced by biceps and supinator, is

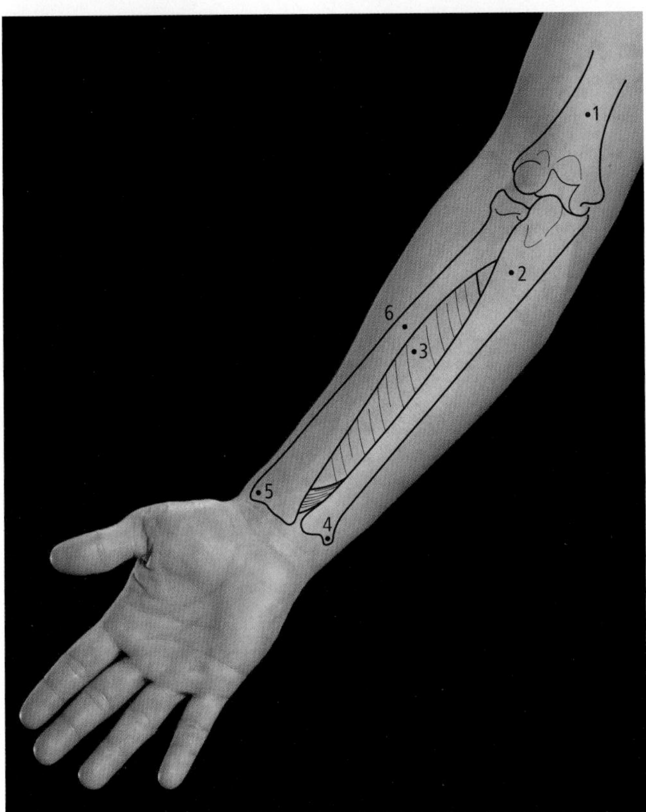

Figure 13.5 Surface anatomy of interosseous membrane: 1, humerus; 2, ulna; 3, interosseous membrane; 4, ulnar styloid process; 5, radial styloid process; 6, radius

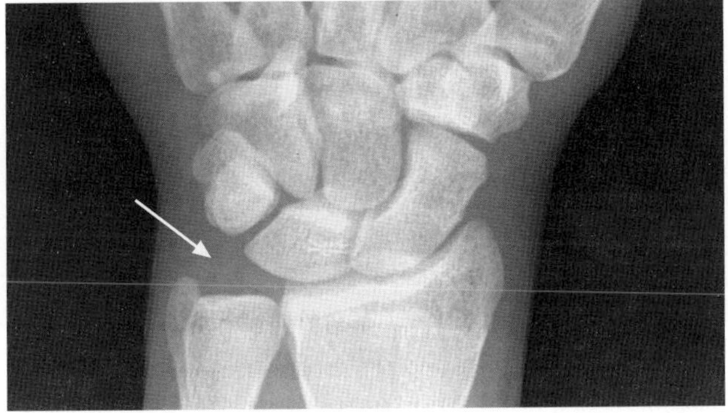

Figure 13.6 Wrist joint showing gap occupied by articular disc (arrow)

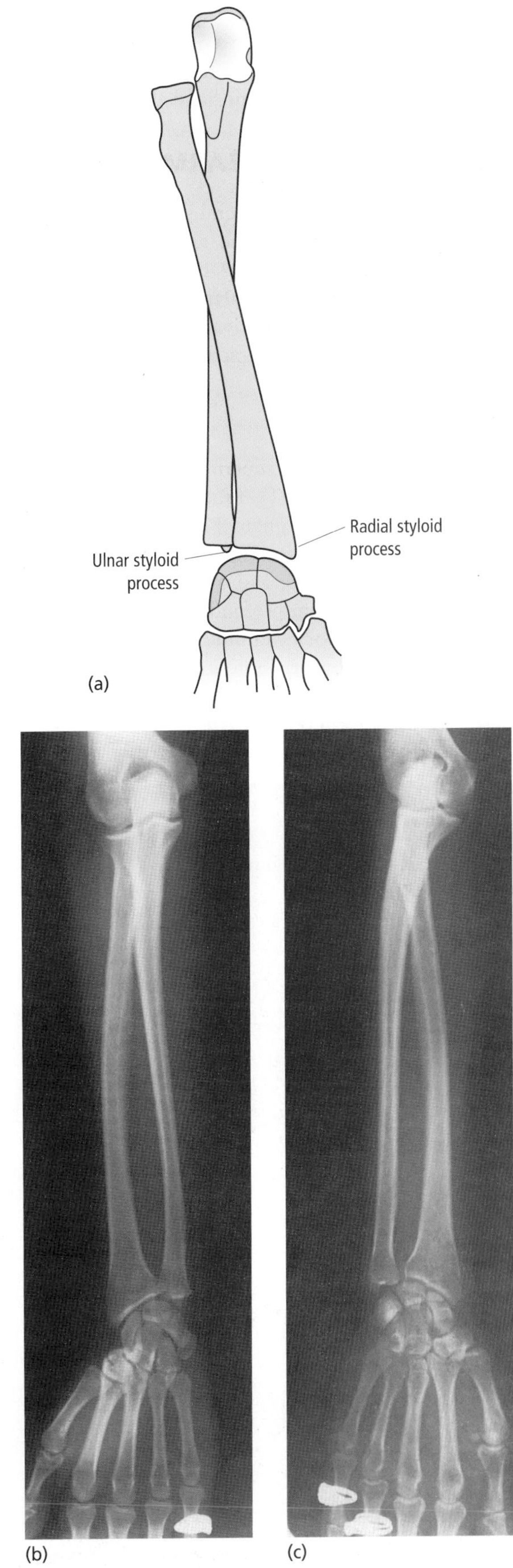

Figure 13.7 (a) Position of radius and ulna in pronation. (b) X-ray in supination. (c) X-ray in pronation

stronger than pronation, which is produced by pronator teres and pronator quadratus. The power of supination is taken advantage of in the design of most screws, which are tightened by the action of supination in right-handed individuals.

MUSCLES OF THE FOREARM

These muscles act variously on several joints: the elbow, wrist and the joints of the fingers. The anterior (flexor) group, which includes pronator teres, arises from the common flexor attachment, the medial epicondyle of the humerus. The extensor group, which includes supinator, arises from the common extensor attachment, the lateral epicondyle of the humerus.

Flexor muscles

These are divided into the **superficial group** (Fig. 13.8a) comprising pronator teres (PT), brachioradialis (BR), flexor carpi radialis (FCR), palmaris longus (PL) and flexor carpi ulnaris (FCU); an **intermediate group** (Fig. 13.8b) comprising flexor digitorum superficialis (FDS); and a **deep group** (Fig. 13.8c) comprising flexor digitorum profundus (FDP), flexor pollicis longus (FPL) and pronator quadratus. The tendons of all but the two pronators pass over the anterior aspect of the wrist and are there retained by the flexor retinaculum, a thickening of the deep fascia of the forearm (Fig. 13.10).

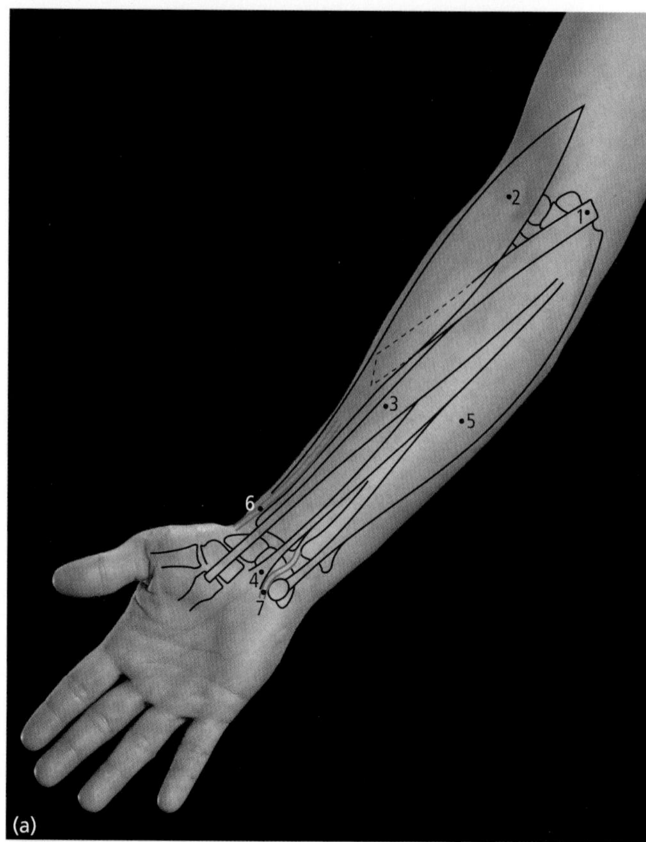

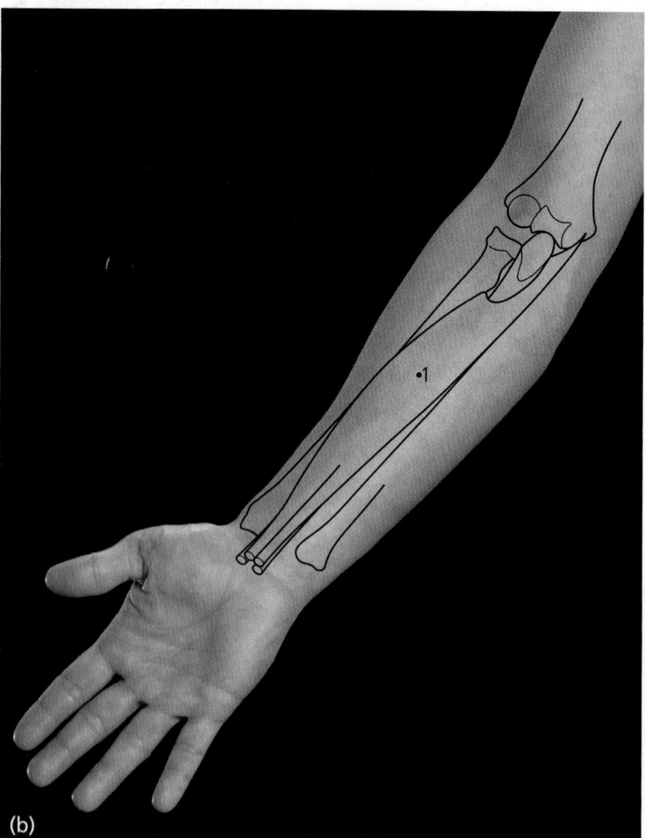

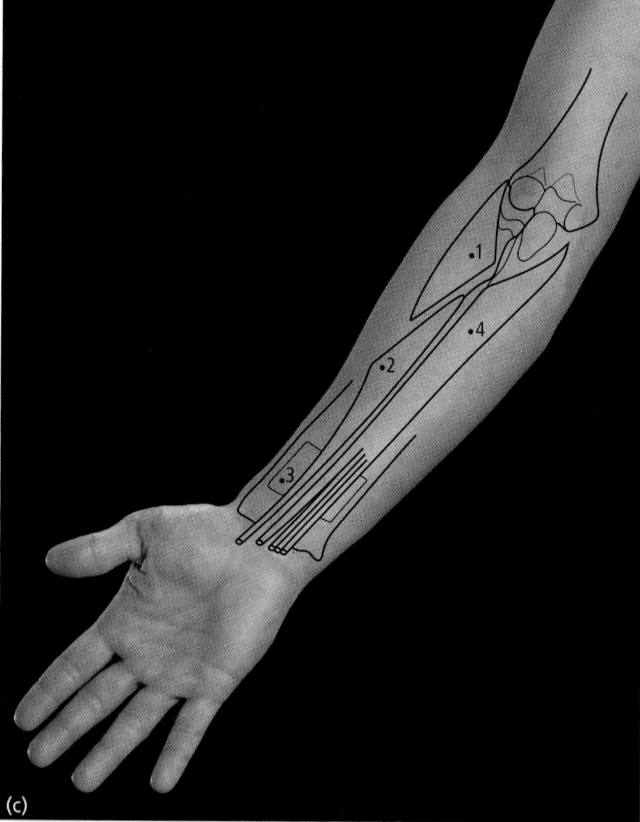

Figure 13.8 Surface anatomy of forearm. (a) Superficial muscles: 1, pronator teres; 2, brachioradialis; 3, flexor carpi radialis; 4, palmaris longus; 5, flexor carpi ulnaris; 6, radial artery; 7, ulnar artery. (b) Intermediate muscle: 1, flexor digitorum superficialis. (c) Deep muscles: 1, supinator; 2, flexor pollicis longus; 3, pronator quadratus; 4, flexor digitorum profundus

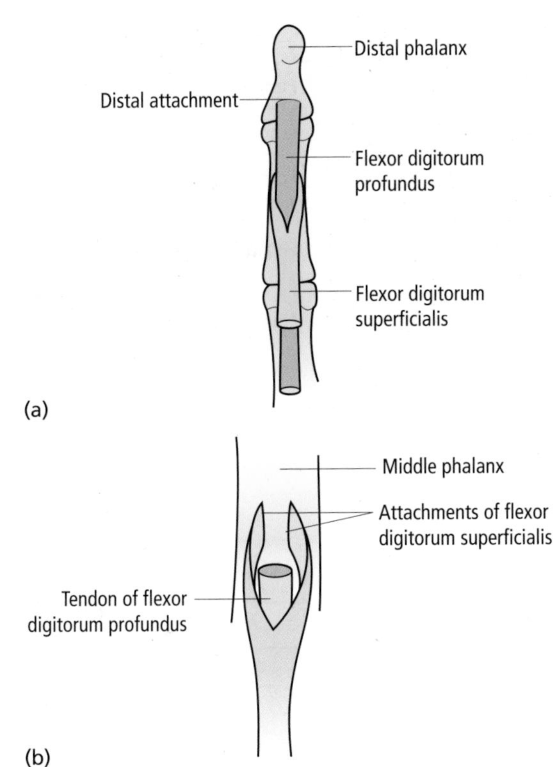

Figure 13.9 (a, b) Arrangement of long flexor tendons in the finger

The four tendons of FDS diverge in the palm, one passing to each finger. The tendon splits over the proximal phalanx to encircle the tendon of FDP and is attached to the sides of the middle phalanx (Fig. 13.10a,b).

All these forearm flexor muscles are supplied by the median or ulnar nerves. The long flexors of the fingers (FDS and FDP) flex the wrist, metacarpal and interphalangeal joints. Their attachments, nerve supply and functions are summarized below.

Brachioradialis is attached proximally to the lateral supracondylar ridge of the humerus and distally to the lower radius. It is a powerful flexor of the elbow, particularly when the forearm is in the midprone position, and it contributes to both pronation and supination, depending on the position of the forearm. It is supplied by the radial nerve.

Superficial group

All arise from the common flexor origin and all are supplied by the median nerve, apart from flexor carpi ulnaris, which is supplied by the ulnar nerve, and brachioradialis, which is supplied by the radial nerve (Table 13.1).

Deep group

All are supplied by the median nerve, but the ulnar half of FDP is also supplied by the ulnar nerve (Table 13.2).

Flexor synovial sheaths

The long flexor tendons are invested with synovial sheaths at points of maximum friction beneath the flexor retinaculum (Fig. 13.10 and p. 107) and within the digital fibrous flexor

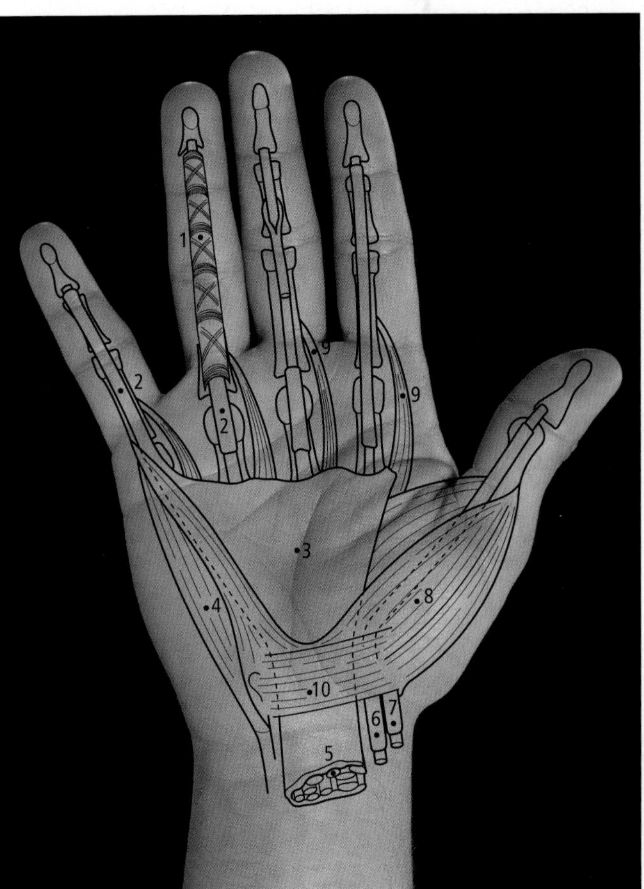

Figure 13.10 Surface anatomy of flexor synovial sheaths and flexor retinaculum: 1, fibrous flexor digital sheath; 2, synovial digital sheath, sheath of the little finger being continuous with the ulnar bursa; 3, ulnar bursa; 4, hypothenar muscles; 5, tendons of flexor digitorum superficialis and profundus within ulnar bursa; 6, synovial sheath round flexor pollicis longus; 7, sheath of flexor carpi radialis; 8, thenar muscles; 9, lateral two lumbricals; 10, flexor retinaculum

sheaths (Fig. 13.9 and p. 209). Deep to the retinaculum the tendons of FDS and FDP have a common sheath, the **ulnar bursa.** The tendon of flexor pollicis longus has its own sheath, the **radial bursa.** Each begins 2–3 cm above the wrist joint and they occasionally communicate with each other. The ulnar bursa ends in the palm, apart from a prolongation around the tendons of the little finger that extends to the distal phalanx. The radial bursa also continues to the distal phalanx of the thumb. There are separate digital synovial sheaths around the tendons to the index, middle and ring fingers. The tendons are nourished via membranous attachments called vincula (Fig. 14.7b, p. 208).

Penetrating wounds of the palm may cause infection of the digital synovial sheaths, **tenosynovitis.** Localized swelling of the fingers and painful limitation of finger movement soon follow. Infections of the sheaths of the index, middle and ring fingers are confined to those fingers but infection of the little finger's sheath, which is in continuity with the common synovial sheath in the palm, may spread through the palm and through the carpal tunnel to the forearm. Tenosynovitis of the thumb may similarly spread to infect the whole of the radial bursa.

Table 13.1 Superficial muscles of the forearm

Muscle	Proximal attachment	Distal attachment	Nerve supply	Function
Brachioradialis	Flexor origin of humerus	Styloid process of radius	Radial nerve (C5, 6)	Elbow flexion
Pronator teres	Flexor origin of humerus, coronoid process of ulna	Distal surface of radius	Median nerve (C6, 7)	Pronation
Flexor carpi ulnaris	Flexor origin of humerus, anterior surface of ulna	Pisiform, hamate and base of 5th metacarpal	Ulnar nerve (C8, T1)	Flexion and adduction of wrist
Flexor carpi radialis	Flexor origin of humerus	Bases of 2nd and 3rd metacarpals	Median nerve (C6, 7)	Flexion and abduction of wrist
Palmaris longus	Flexor origin of humerus	Palmar aponeurosis and flexor retinaculum	Median nerve (C6, 7)	Flexion of wrist
Flexor digitorum superficialis (intermediate group)	Flexor origin of humerus, neighbouring anterior surfaces of radius and ulna	Lateral surfaces of middle phalanges of fingers 2–5	Median nerve (C7, T1)	Flexion of proximal interphalangeal, metacarpophalangeal and wrist joints

Table 13.2 Deep muscles of the forearm

Muscle	Proximal attachment	Distal attachment	Nerve supply	Function
Flexor pollicis longus	Anterior shaft of radius, interosseous membrane	Base of distal phalanx of thumb	Median nerve (C8, T1)	Flexion of joints of thumb
Flexor digitorum profundus	Posterior surface of ulna, coronoid process and interosseous membrane	Bases of distal phalanges 2–5	Anterior interosseous branch of median nerve and ulnar nerve (C8, T1)	Flexion of distal interphalangeal joints and, to a lesser extent, the wrist
Pronator quadratus	Medial surface of distal ulna	Lateral surface of distal radius	Median nerve (C8, T1)	Pronation

Extensor muscles

The extensor (posterior) muscles of the forearm (Figs 13.11 and 13.12, Table 13.3) can be functionally described as of three groups:

- Muscles that act on the wrist joint – extensor carpi radialis longus (ECRL), extensor carpi radialis brevis (ECRB) and extensor carpi ulnaris (ECU)
- Extensor muscles of the fingers – extensor digitorum (ED), extensor indicis (EI) and extensor digiti minimi (EDM)
- Muscles extending/abducting the thumb (Fig. 13.13) – abductor pollicis longus (APL), extensor pollicis brevis (EPB) and extensor pollicis longus (EPL).

In addition to these muscles the posterior compartment of the forearm contains the supinator muscle. All are supplied by the radial nerve or its posterior interosseous branch.

The extensor muscle tendons pass under the **extensor retinaculum** (Figs 13.14 and 13.15) as they pass over the wrist joint, and are retained so that 'bowstringing' does not occur during wrist extension. Here, closely contained between bones of the wrist joint and the retinaculum, they are covered by synovial sheaths, reducing the effects of friction. Extensor indicis lies deeper. On the heads of the metacarpals and over the proximal phalanges the extensor tendons expand to form flat extensor expansions (Figs 13.15 and 13.16), which wrap around the dorsum and sides of these bones. They help to retain the tendon in line with the finger and give attachment to the interossei and lumbrical muscles (Fig. 13.16 and p. 208). The tendon divides over the proximal interphalangeal joint, into three slips; the middle is attached to the base of the middle phalanx and the outer two to the base of the terminal phalanx. The extensor muscles of the forearm may also be divided into superficial and deep groups. The superficial extensors (ECRB, ECU, ED, EDM) are all attached to the common extensor origin of the humerus, the lateral epicondyle, and are supplied by the posterior interosseous nerve. The deep extensors of the forearm, APL, EPL and EPB, act on the thumb and EI acts as a strong extensor on the forefinger. They lie deep to the superficial extensors and are all supplied by the posterior interosseous branch of the radial nerve (Fig. 13.17).

Tennis elbow – a common painful condition – is the result of repetitive flexion and extension of the wrist which, by putting strain on the common extensor origin, causes inflammation in the muscles' attachment to the lateral epicondyle. 'Mallet finger' is the name given to the deformity resulting from an unguarded forceful flexion of a finger's terminal interphalangeal joint, which avulses the attachment of the long extensor to the base of the terminal phalanx. It most commonly follows a failed attempt to catch a cricket- or baseball.

Extensor pollicis longus is attached proximally to the posterior surface of the ulna distal to abductor pollicis; distally the tendon descends under the extensor retinaculum on the medial side of the dorsal tubercle of the radius in its own synovial sheath. Here it forms the posterior margin of

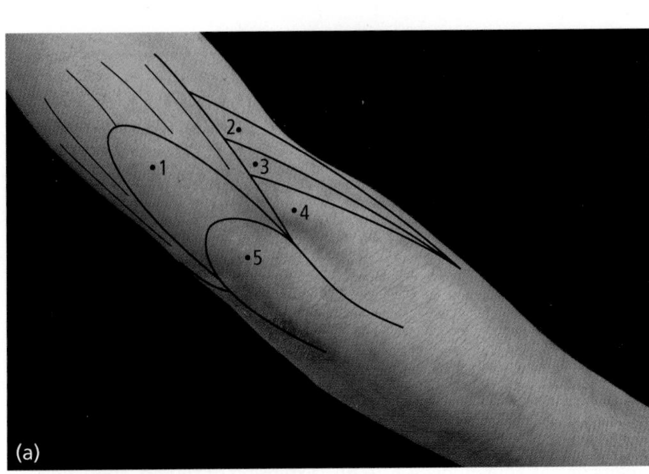

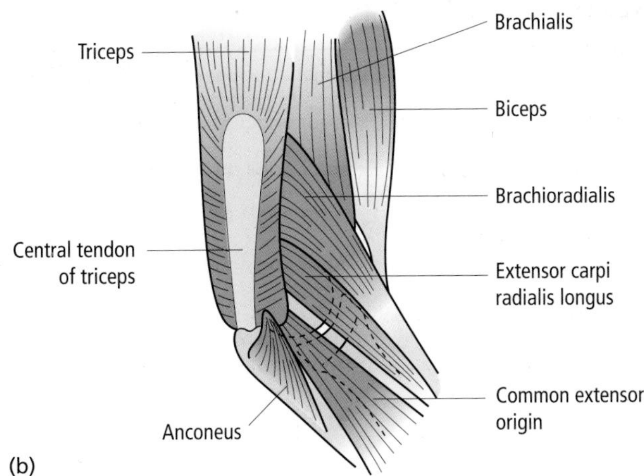

Figure 13.11 Extensor muscles of the forearm – (a) surface anatomy at elbow: 1, common extensor tendon of triceps muscle; 2, brachioradialis; 3, extensor carpi radialis longus; 4, common extensor origin; 5, olecranon process. (b) Diagram of posterior aspect of the elbow showing brachioradialis, and extensor carpi radialis longus

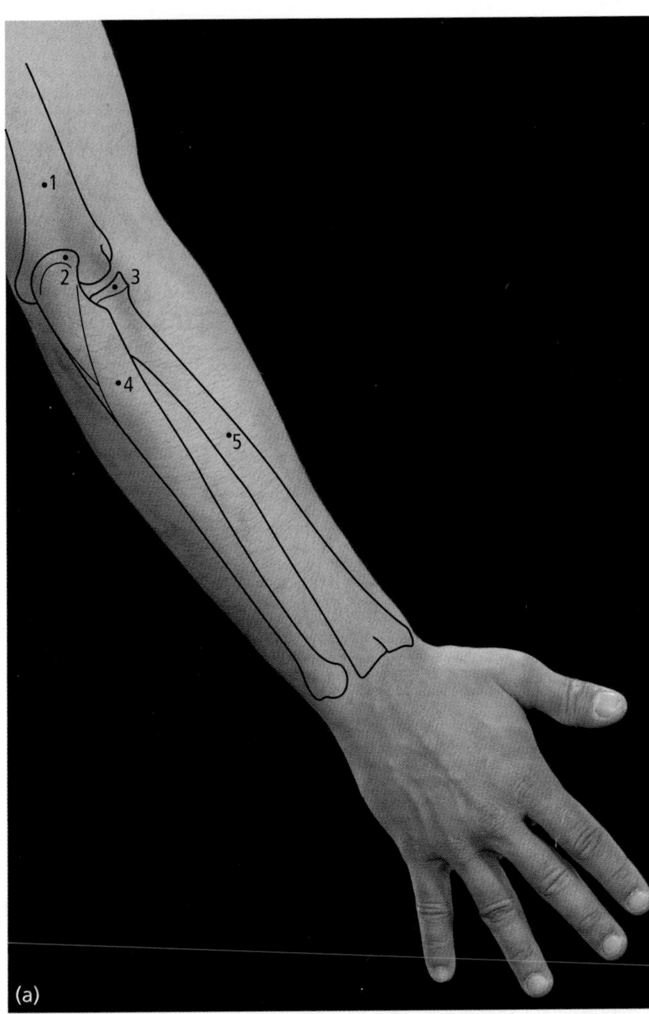

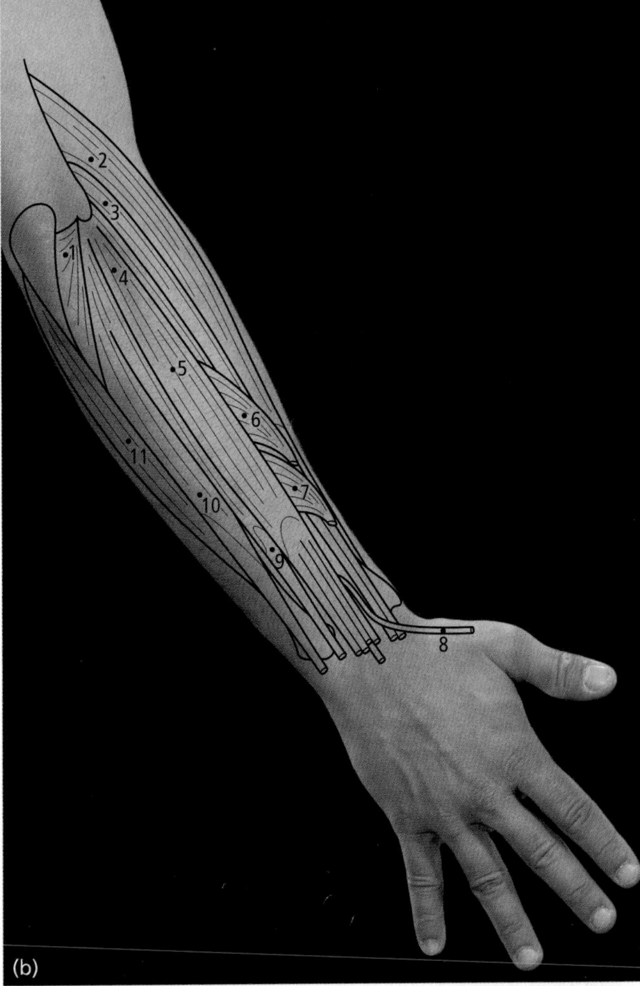

Figure 13.12 Surface anatomy. (a) Bones: 1, humerus; 2, olecranon process; 3, head of radius; 4, ulnar; 5, radius. (b) Superficial muscles: 1, anconeus; 2, brachioradialis; 3, extensor carpi radialis longus; 4, common extensor origin; 5, extensor digitorum; 6, abductor pollicis longus; 7, extensor pollicis brevis; 8, tendon of extensor pollicis longus; 9, extensor digiti minimi; 10, extensor carpi ulnaris; 11, flexor carpi ulnaris

Table 13.3 Extensor muscles of the forearm

Muscle	Proximal attachment	Distal attachment	Nerve supply	Function
Extensor carpi radialis longus	Extensor origin of humerus	Base of 2nd metacarpal	Radial nerve (C6, 7)	Extension and abduction of wrist
Extensor carpi radialis brevis	Extensor origin of humerus	Base of 3rd metacarpal	Radial nerve (C6, 7)	Extension and abduction of wrist
Extensor carpi ulnaris	Extensor origin of humerus	Base of 5th metacarpal	Radial nerve (C6, 7, 8)	Extension and adduction of wrist
Extensor digitorum	Extensor origin of humerus	Posterior surfaces of phalanges, fingers 2–5	Radial nerve (C6, 7, 8)	Extension of finger joints and wrist
Abductor pollicis	Proximal extensor surfaces of radius and ulna	Lateral aspect of 1st metacarpal	Radial nerve (C6, 7)	Abduction of thumb and wrist
Extensor pollicis brevis	Distal shaft of radius	Base of proximal phalanx of thumb	Radial nerve (C6, 7)	Extension of thumb, abduction of wrist
Extensor pollicis longus	Posterior shaft of ulna and interosseous membrane	Base of distal phalanx of thumb	Radial nerve (C6, 7, 8)	Extension of thumb, abduction of wrist
Extensor indicis	Posterior surface of ulna and interosseous membrane	With tendon of ED into posterior surface of phalanges of index finger	Radial nerve (C6, 7, 8)	Extension of joints of index finger
Extensor digiti minimi	Extensor origin of humerus	Posterior surface of prox. phalanx of little finger	Radial nerve (C6, 7, 8)	Extension of joints of little finger
Supinator	Extensor origin of humerus and proximal ulna	Anterolateral surface of radius	Radial nerve (C6, 7, 8)	Supination (Fig. 13.17)

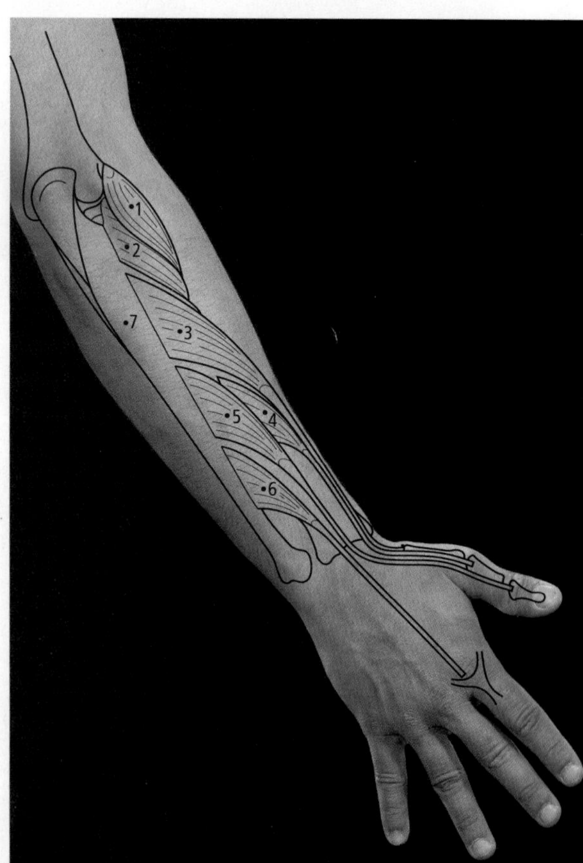

Figure 13.13 Surface anatomy of deep extensor muscles of the forearm: 1, supinator (humeral head); 2 supinator (ulnar head); 3, abductor pollicis longus; 4, extensor pollicis brevis; 5, extensor pollicis longus; 6, extensor indicis; 7, ulna

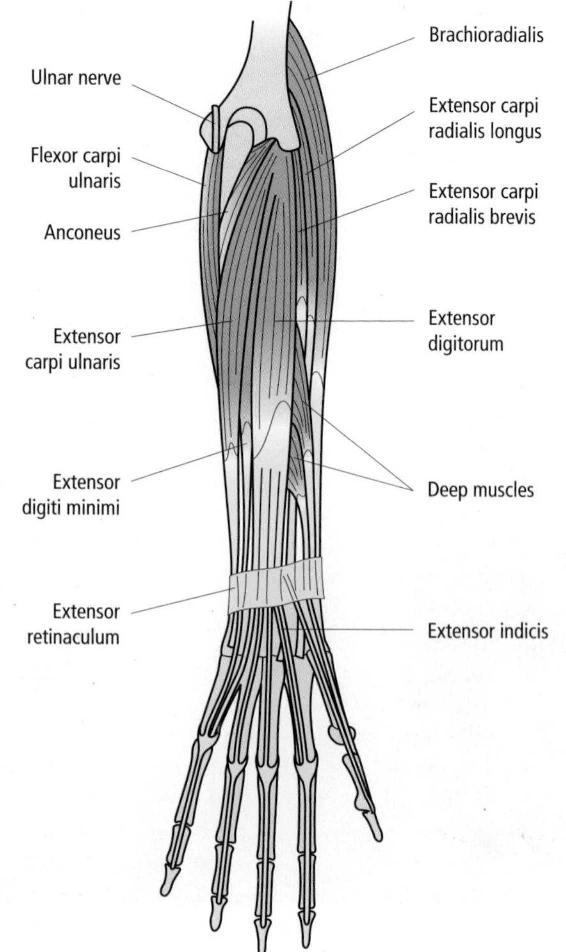

Figure 13.14 Extensor muscles, extensor retinaculum and tendons

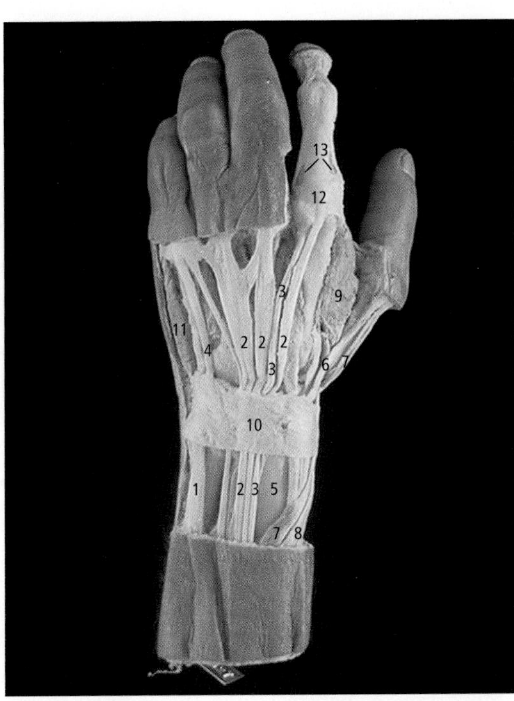

Figure 13.15 Dissection of extensor tendons and retinaculum: 1, extensor carpi ulnaris; 2, extensor digitorum tendons; 3, extensor indicis; 4, extensor digiti minimi; 5, radius; 6, extensor pollicis longus; 7, extensor pollicis brevis; 8, abductor pollicis longus; 9, first dorsal interosseous muscle; 10, extensor retinaculum; 11, abductor digiti minimi; 12, dorsal digital extensor expansion, 13, lateral 'wing' of extensor tendon expansion

the 'snuffbox' as it crosses over the two radial extensors and the radial artery, before becoming attached to the base of the thumb's distal phalanx. It extends all the joints of the thumb.

Tenosynovitis, an inflammatory thickening of the common sheath surrounding these two tendons, occurs sometimes after prolonged repetitive movements of the thumb. There is pain and swelling on movement of the thumb. It is given the name de Quervain's disease and usually responds to rest.

The **anatomical snuffbox** is the term applied to the depression formed on the lateral side of the wrist when the thumb is extended (Figs 13.18 and 13.19). Its boundaries are: *anterior* – tendons of abductor pollicis longus and extensor pollicis brevis; *posterior* – tendon of extensor pollicis longus. In its base are the wrist joint, the radial styloid process, the scaphoid bone and the base of the first metacarpal; crossing its floor are the tendons of the two radial extensors of the wrist and the radial artery. Superficially are the cephalic vein and cutaneous branches of the radial nerve; the latter can be palpated crossing over the tendons – they feel like threads of cotton over the tendon of brachioradialis.

The **extensor retinaculum** is a band of deep fascia 2–3 cm wide passing obliquely over the back of the wrist from the distal end of the radius to the medial side of the carpus. It is attached by fibrous septae to the radius and ulna, forming fibro-osseous tunnels for the passage of the tendons (Fig. 13.20). The tendons' synovial sheaths commence at the retinaculum's proximal border. Those of abductor pollicis and both radial extensors reach the tendons' distal attachments, but all others end in the middle of the dorsum of the hand.

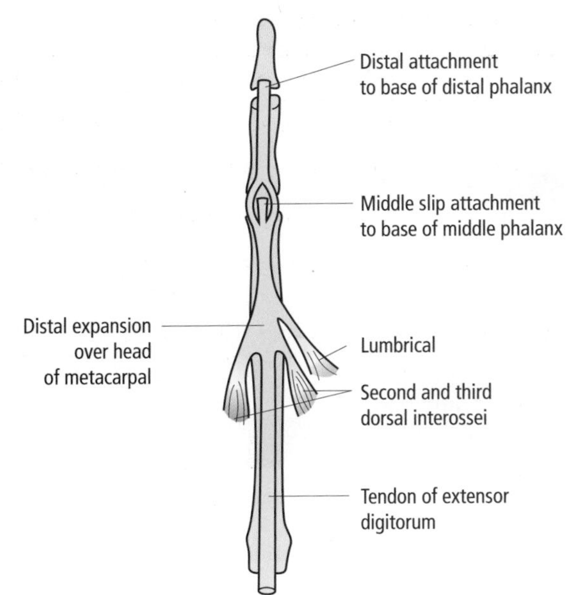

Figure 13.16 Extensor tendon of middle finger, its expansion and attachments of lumbricals and interossei

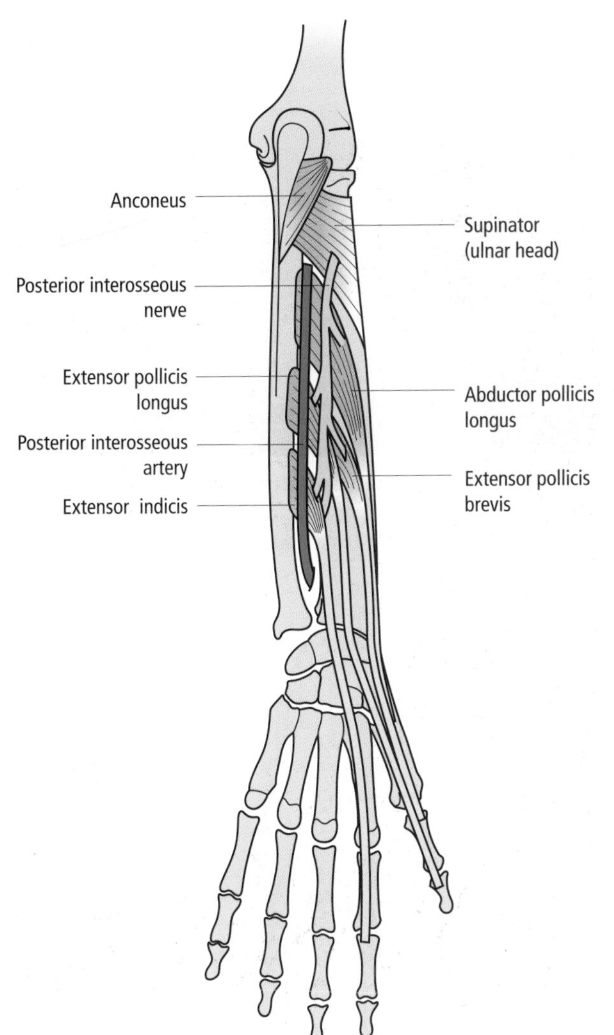

Figure 13.17 Deep extensors demonstrating supinator muscle and course of the posterior interosseous nerve and artery

The upper limb

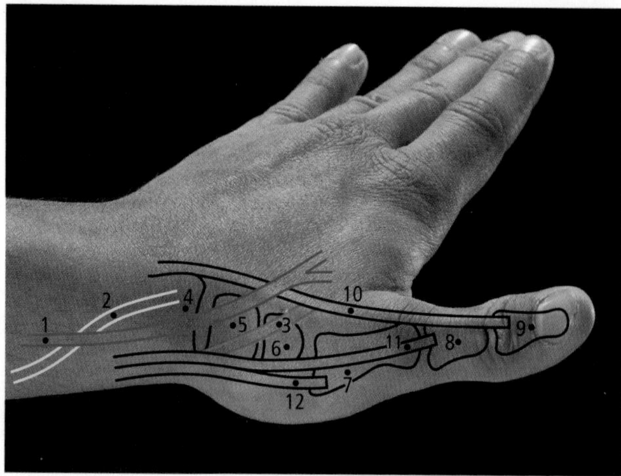

Figure 13.18 Surface anatomy of anatomical snuffbox: 1, cephalic vein (blue); 2, radial nerve (yellow); 3, radial artery (red); 4, lower end of radius; 5, scaphoid; 6, trapezium; 7, first metacarpal; 8, proximal phalanx; 9, distal phalanx; 10, extensor pollicis longus; 11, extensor pollicis brevis; 12, abductor pollicis longus

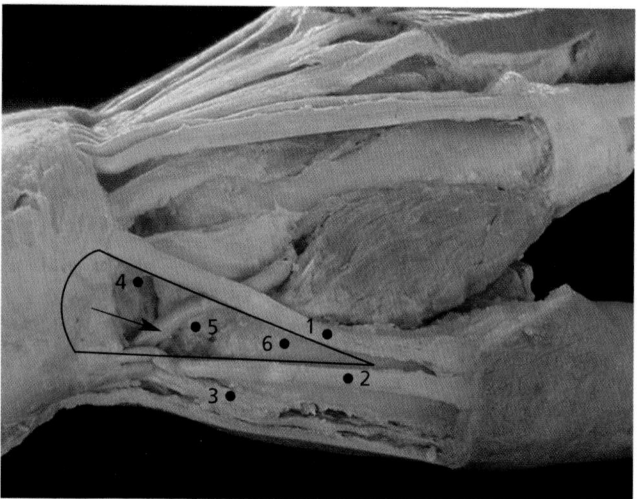

Figure 13.19 Snuffbox dissection, left hand: 1, extensor pollicis longus; 2, extensor pollicis brevis; 3, abductor pollicis longus; 4, scaphoid; 5, trapezium; 6, first metacarpal; arrow = radial artery

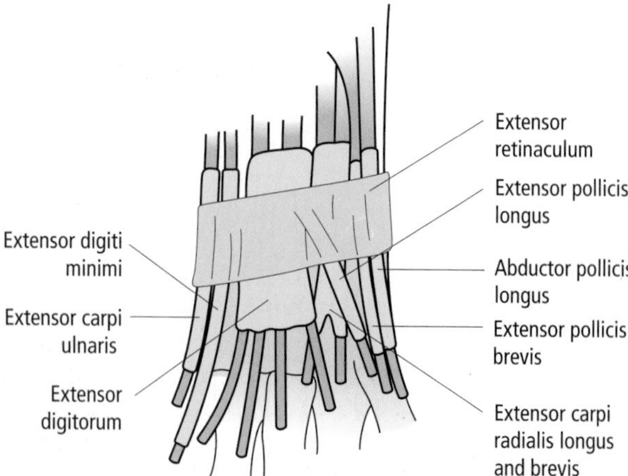

Figure 13.20 Extensor retinaculum and tendon sheaths across the dorsum of the wrist

BLOOD SUPPLY

The radial artery

The radial artery (Fig. 13.21), a terminal branch of the brachial, arises in the cubital fossa. It descends the anterior forearm, passes over the lateral side of the wrist to the dorsum of the hand and ends in the palm.

Relations

Leaving the cubital fossa deep to brachioradialis it descends close to the radius, with the radial nerve on its lateral side. At the wrist it is palpable on the front of the radius, but then it crosses lateral to the wrist joint deep to the tendons bounding the 'snuffbox', to reach the dorsum of the hand by passing through the first dorsal interosseous and adductor pollicis muscles.

The radial pulsation can be felt against the lower radius and against the scaphoid in the floor of the snuffbox (Fig. 13.19). Arterial blood samples can be obtained at the wrist because here the artery is easily palpable. It is very important, though, before taking the sample, to establish that there is a pulse in the ulnar artery, which would provide anastomotic blood should any damage or spasm follow the radial puncture (Allen's test: occude both arteries, make a fist and then, opening hand, release arteries individually to see return of blood flow).

The radial artery supplies the forearm muscles, contributes to anastomoses around the elbow and wrist joints (Fig. 13.21b) and supplies the elbow and wrist joints; it also contributes to the deep palmar arch and has a minor contribution to the superficial palmar arch (Fig. 13.22). It may be palpated in the floor of the anatomical snuffbox.

The ulnar artery

The ulnar artery (Fig. 13.21), also a terminal branch of the brachial, arises in the cubital fossa, descends in the anterior forearm, passes anterior to the flexor retinaculum near the wrist, and ends mainly in the superficial palmar arch; a minor branch contributes to the deep palmar arch.

Relations

Leaving the cubital fossa it lies on flexor digitorum profundus, deep to the muscles arising from the common flexor origin. In the lower forearm, under flexor carpi ulnaris, the ulnar nerve is medial to it. It crosses the wrist superficial to the flexor retinaculum and ends by continuing as the superficial palmar arch lateral to the pisiform bone. It supplies forearm muscles and the elbow and wrist joints. Its largest branch, the common interosseous artery, arises in the cubital fossa and then descends close to the interosseous membrane. It contributes to both the superficial and deep palmar arches.

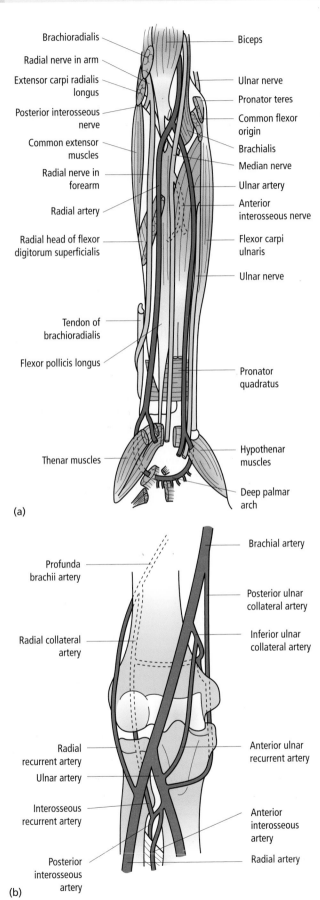

Figure 13.21 (a) Vessels and nerves of the forearm. (b) Arterial anastomoses around the right elbow joint

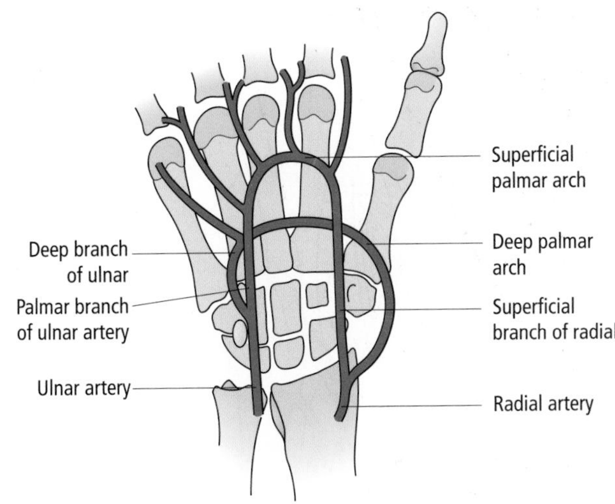

Figure 13.22 Palmar arterial arches of the right hand

NERVES

The radial nerve

The radial nerve lies on the anterolateral aspect of the forearm under brachioradialis (Fig. 13.23), lateral to the radial artery. Its largest branch, the **posterior interosseous nerve**, arises in the cubital fossa and passes posteriorly through the supinator muscle to gain the posterior compartment of the forearm, where it descends on the interosseous membrane supplying adjacent extensor muscles. Proximal to the wrist the superficial radial nerve turns posteriorly under the tendon of brachioradialis and superficial to the tendons bounding the 'snuffbox', to end on the dorsum of the hand as digital branches. It and its posterior interosseous branch supply brachioradialis, all extensor muscles, elbow, wrist and intercarpal joints and, by cutaneous branches, the lateral side of the dorsum of the hand and posterior aspects of the lateral 2½ digits, usually as far as the distal interphalangeal joints.

The median nerve

The median nerve descends in the anterior compartment of the forearm. In the cubital fossa it is medial to the brachial artery (Fig. 13.24a). Its largest branch, the **anterior interosseous nerve**, descends deep and close to the interosseous membrane, supplying most of the deep flexors and pronator quadratus. The median nerve then descends between the superficial and deep flexors to emerge, at the wrist, between the tendons of the FDS and the FCR, deep to palmaris longus. It enters the hand deep to the flexor retinaculum (Fig. 13.24b). It and its anterior interosseous branch supply all the forearm flexor muscles except the ulnar half of FDP and the FCU; in the hand it supplies abductor pollicis brevis, flexor pollicis brevis and opponens pollicis. Its palmar cutaneous branch supplies the radial side of the palm and, by digital branches, the palmar surface of the lateral 3½ digits, their fingertips and their nail beds. These digital branches lie anterior to the digital arteries, and the two lateral branches also supply the lateral two lumbrical muscles.

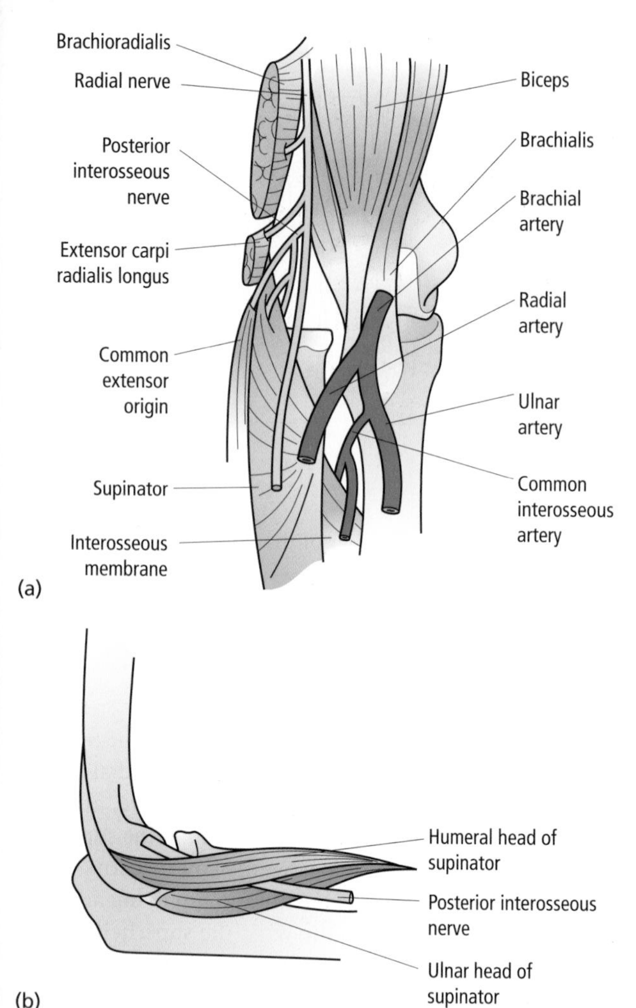

Figure 13.23 (a) Right cubital fossa, anterior aspect. (b) Passage of posterior interosseous nerve through the fibres of supinator muscle

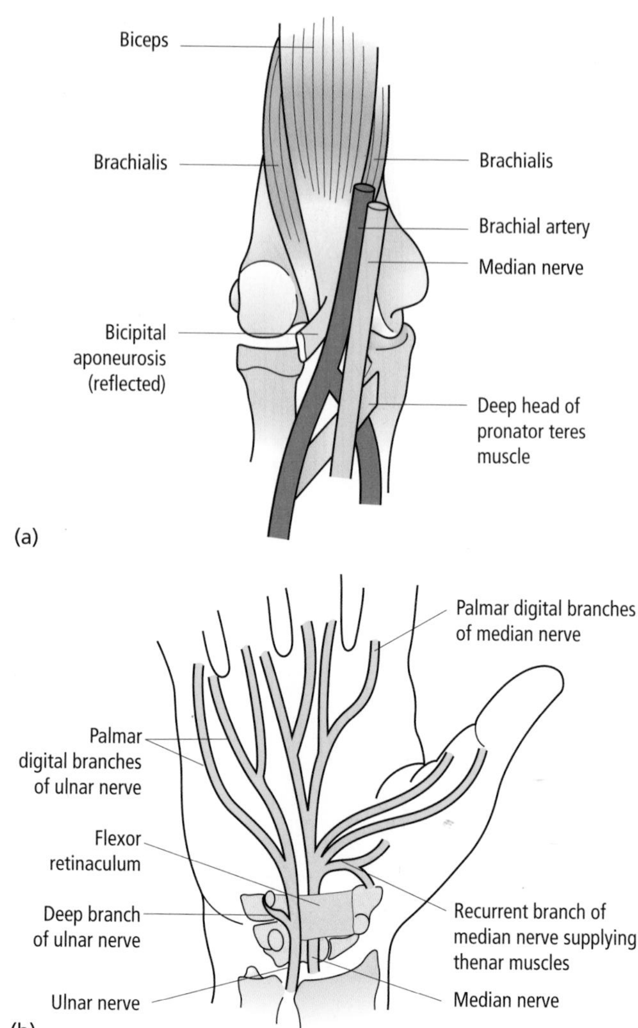

Figure 13.24 (a) Deep structures in the right cubital fossa. (b) Median and ulnar nerves in the hand

The ulnar nerve

From behind the medial epicondyle (Figs 13.21a, 13.24, 13.25) the **ulnar nerve** descends deep to flexor carpi ulnaris on the medial side of the forearm (Fig. 13.26a–c). At the wrist it lies superficially, lateral to the tendon, and passes into the hand superficial to the flexor retinaculum, lateral to the pisiform, to end by dividing into superficial and deep branches (Fig. 13.24). In the forearm it supplies FCU and the ulnar half of FDP. Its dorsal cutaneous branch arises above the wrist and supplies the ulnar half of the dorsum of the hand and the medial 2½ fingers as far as the distal interphalangeal joints. In the hand digital branches supply the palmar surface of the medial 1½ fingers, their fingertips and their nail beds, and a deep branch supplies all the hypothenar muscles (p. 212), all the interossei, the third and fourth lumbricals and adductor pollicis.

Nerve injuries

Nerve injuries and clinical testing for the functional integrity of these nerves are described on p. 212.

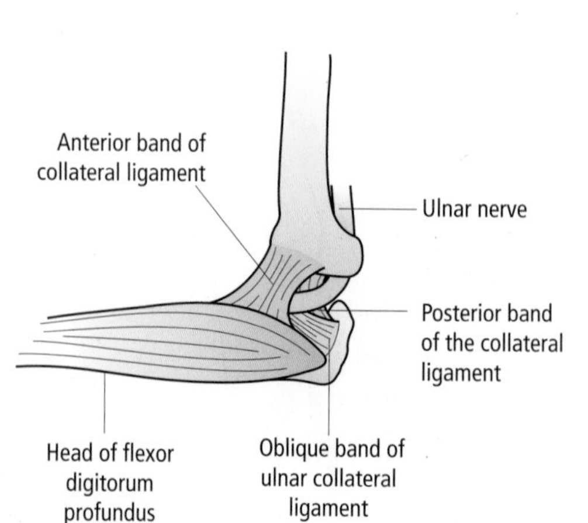

Figure 13.25 Medial view of elbow joint – ulnar nerve passing behind the medial epicondyle of the right humerus and into the cubital tunnel

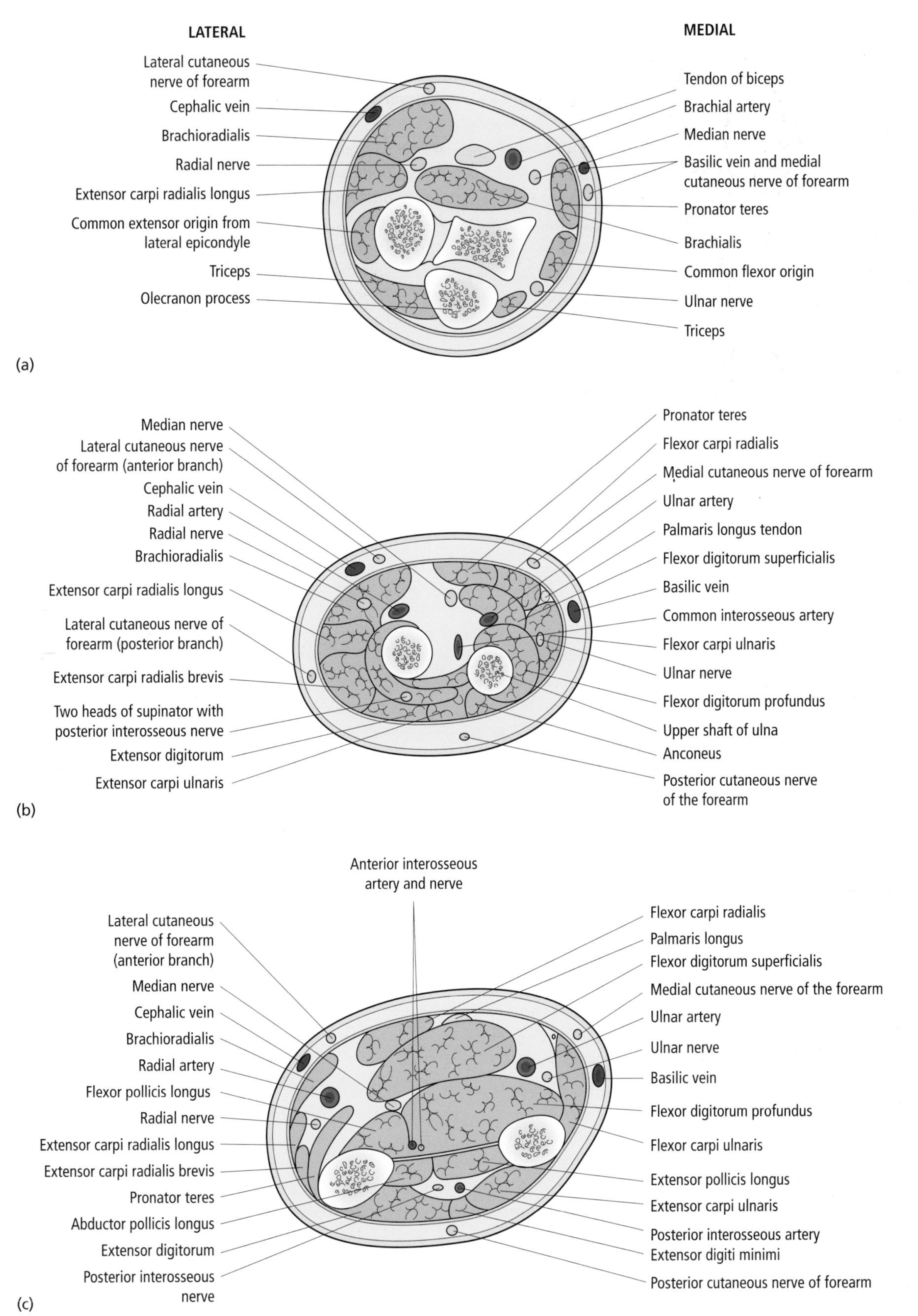

Figure 13.26 Transverse sections, viewed from below, through: (a) the right elbow; (b) the right upper forearm; (c) the right mid-forearm

MCQs

1. The anatomical snuffbox: **T/F**

- **a** is bounded anteriorly by the tendons of extensor pollicis longus and brevis (___)
- **b** is bounded posteriorly by the tendon of abductor pollicis brevis (___)
- **c** overlies the scaphoid and the trapezium (___)
- **d** contains the tendons of extensors carpi radialis longus and brevis in its floor (___)
- **e** contains the basilic vein in its roof (___)

Answers

1.

- *a* **F** – *Its boundaries are, anteriorly, the tendons of abductor pollicis longus and extensor pollicis brevis, and posteriorly, the tendon of extensor pollicis longus.*
- *b* **F**
- *c* **T** – *Together with the radial styloid process, the wrist joint and the base of the first metacarpal bone.*
- *d* **T** – *Together with the radial artery.*
- *e* **F** – *The cephalic vein overlies the snuffbox.*

---

2. The radial nerve: **T/F**

- **a** is the main branch of the posterior cord of the brachial plexus (___)
- **b** is derived from the posterior primary rami of C5, 6, 7, 8 and T1 nerve roots (___)
- **c** is the main nerve supply to the extensor muscles of arm and forearm (___)
- **d** gives rise to the anterior interosseous nerve (___)
- **e** supplies the skin of the extensor aspect of the radial 3½ digits (___)

Answers

2.

- *a* **T** – *The other branches of the posterior cord are the axillary, thoracodorsal, and upper and lower subscapular nerves.*
- *b* **F** – *It arises from the anterior primary rami of these nerves.*
- *c* **T**
- *d* **F** – *In the supinator muscle the radial nerve gives rise to the posterior interosseous nerve. The median nerve gives rise to the anterior interosseous nerve.*
- *e* **T**

EMQs

Each question has an anatomical theme linked to the chapter, and a list of 10 related items (A–J) placed in alphabetical order: these are followed by five statements (1–5). Match **one or more** of the items A–J to each of the five statements.

Muscles of the elbow and forearm

A. Brachioradialis
B. Extensor carpi radialis brevis
C. Extensor carpi ulnaris
D. Extensor digitorum
E. Flexor carpi radialis
F. Flexor carpi ulnaris
G. Flexor digitorum profundus
H. Flexor digitorum superficialis
I. Flexor pollicis longus
J. Pronator teres

Match the following attachments to the appropriate muscle(s) in the above list.

1. Flexor origin of the humerus
2. Extensor origin of the humerus
3. Distal phalanx
4. Mid lateral border of the radius
5. Styloid process of the radius

Answers

1 EFHJ; 2 BCD; 3 DGI; 4 J; 5 A

Nerves of the elbow and forearm

A. Brachioradialis
B. Extensor carpi radialis brevis
C. Extensor carpi ulnaris
D. Extensor digitorum
E. Flexor carpi radialis
F. Flexor carpi ulnaris
G. Flexor digitorum profundus
H. Flexor digitorum superficialis
I. Flexor pollicis longus
J. Pronator teres

Match the following nerves to the appropriate muscle(s) in the above list.

1. Median
2. Ulnar
3. Radial
4. Ulnar nerve passes between its two heads
5. Crosses anterior to the median nerve at the level of the cubital fossa

Answers

1 EGHIJ; 2 FG; 3 ABCD; 4 F; 5 J

APPLIED QUESTIONS

1. What surface anatomical clues aid clinical diagnosis of a fractured distal radius?

1. A fall onto the outstretched hand may fracture the distal radius. In the common Colles' fracture the distal radial fragment is displaced posteriorly and impacted, shortening the bone. Normally the radial styloid is palpated approximately 1 cm distal to the ulnar styloid, but their palpation at the same horizontal level indicates bony displacement.

---

2. You notice in 'cops and robbers' films that, to make a person drop a knife, the defender often forces the attacker's hand into acute flexion. Why is this a very sensible move?

2. Try this yourself and you will find that the power grip is very weak in acute wrist flexion. Normally, the wrist extensors work synergistically with the flexors of the fingers. Flexion of the wrist deprives the long flexor tendons of the ability to contract further and make a strong grip. Flexing the wrist will therefore make someone relax the grip and drop whatever is in the hand.

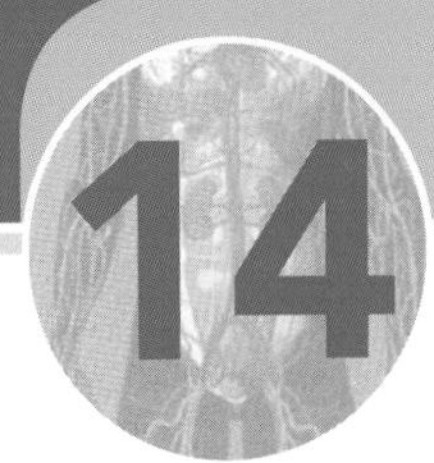

14 The wrist and hand

THE BONES OF THE HAND

The carpus (Figs 14.1 and 14.2) has eight carpal bones arranged as a proximal row of three, from lateral to medial the scaphoid, lunate and triquetral; a distal row of four, from lateral to medial the trapezium, trapezoid, capitate and hamate; and an anteromedially placed sesamoid bone – the pisiform. The square flexor retinaculum is attached to the scaphoid, trapezium, pisiform and hamate. All its points of attachment are palpable, as is the scaphoid in the anatomical snuffbox.

The **metacarpals** have expanded bases which articulate with the distal row of carpal bones (Figs 14.1 and 14.2) and the medial four also articulate with each other. Their slender bodies give attachment to the interossei, opponens pollicis

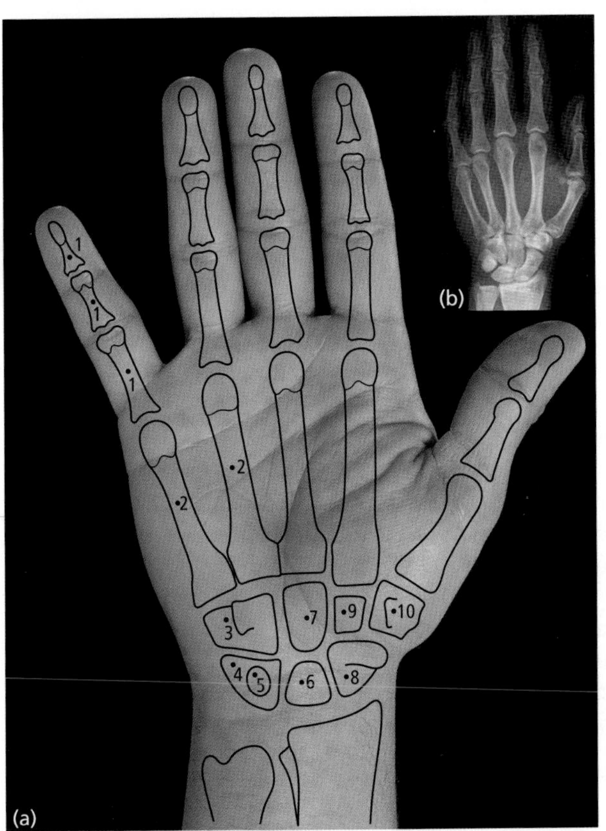

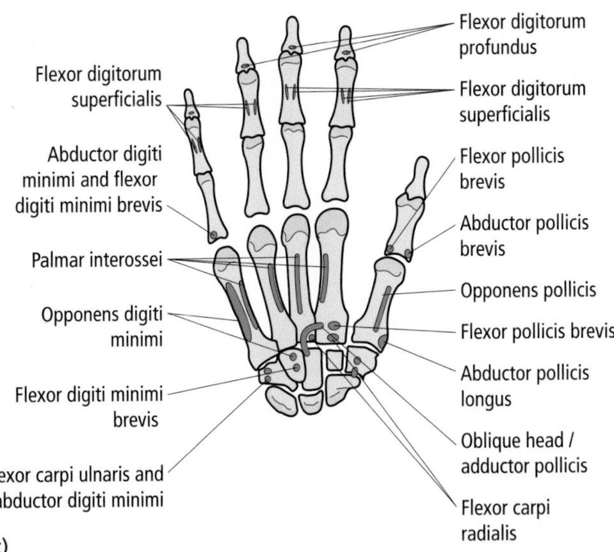

Figure 14.1 Hand. (a) Palmar surface surface anatomy: 1, proximal, middle and distal phalanges; 2, metacarpals; 3, hamate; 4, triquetral; 5, pisiform; 6, lunate; 7, capitate; 8, scaphoid; 9, trapezoid; 10, trapezium. (b) X-ray, dorsopalmar view. (c) Bones and muscle attachments, palmar aspect

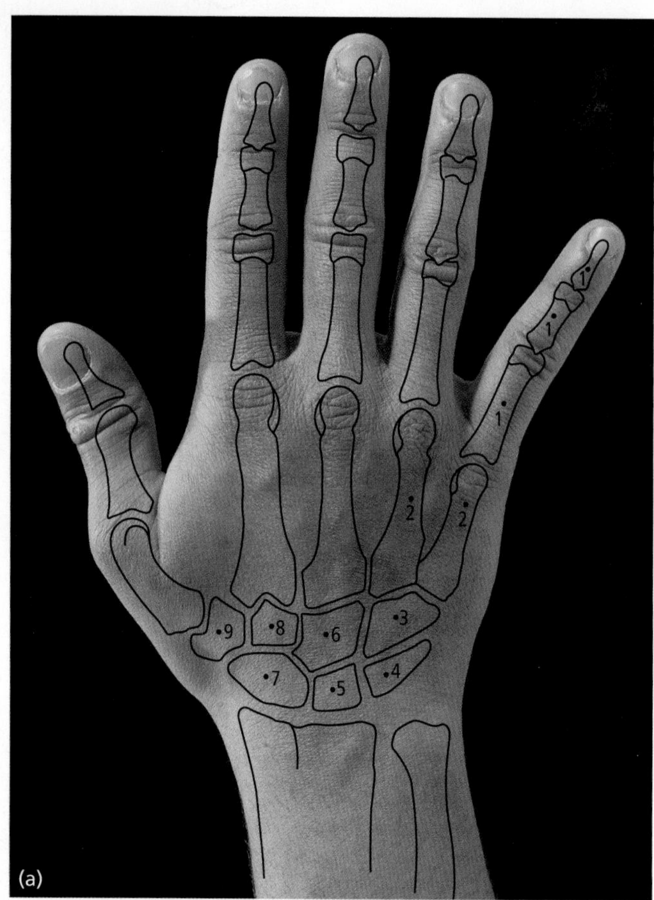

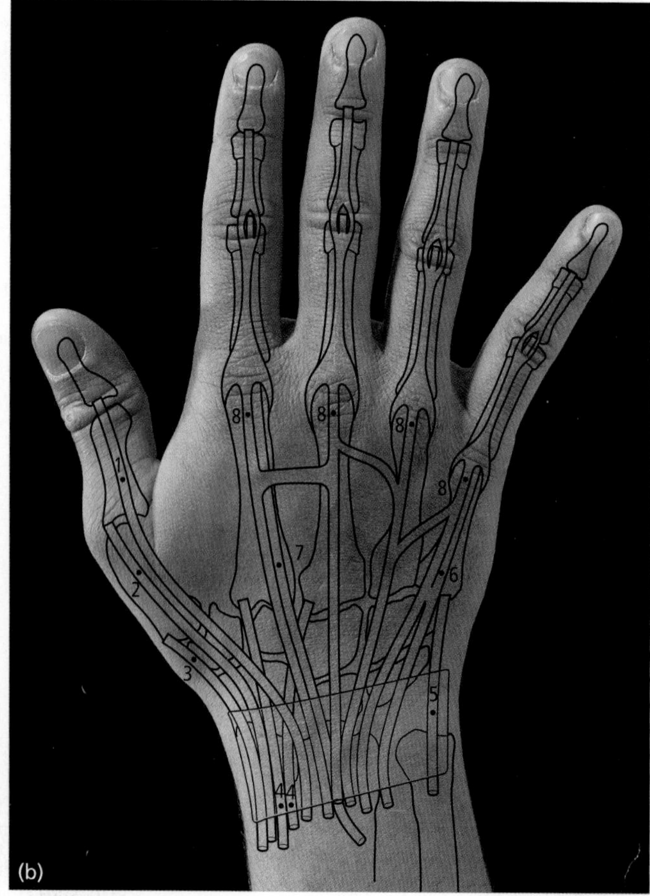

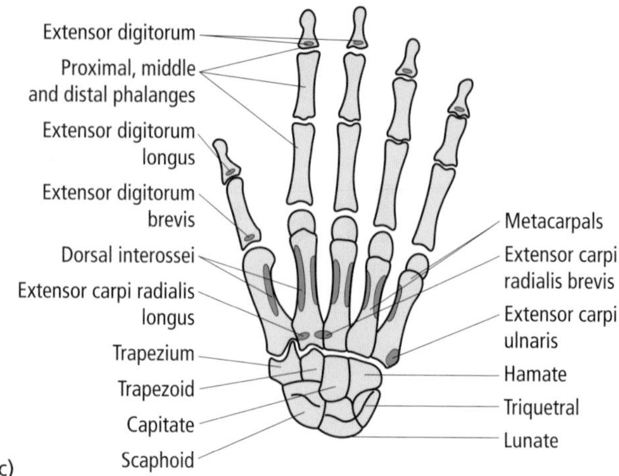

Figure 14.2 Dorsum of hand. (a) Surface anatomy – bones, posterior view: 1, proximal, middle and distal phalanges; 2, metacarpals; 3, hamate; 4, triquetral; 5, lunate; 6, capitate; 7, scaphoid; 8, trapezoid; 9, trapezium. (b) Surface anatomy – extensor tendons: 1, extensor pollicis longus; 2, extensor pollicis brevis; 3, abductor pollicis longus; 4, extensor carpi radialis longus and brevis; 5, extensor carpi ulnaris; 6, extensor digiti minimi; 7, extensor indicis; 8, tendons of extensor digitorum. (c) Bones and muscle attachments

and adductor pollicis muscles, and their heads articulate with the proximal phalanges. The first metacarpal is the shortest, strongest and most mobile; its axis is rotated to lie almost at a right-angle to that of the other metacarpals. It articulates proximally with the trapezium.

The **phalanges** are long bones, three in each finger and two in the thumb. The proximal phalanges have cupped surfaces for proximal articulation with the metacarpals; the heads of the proximal and middle phalanges have paired articular condyles, and the distal phalanges taper distally. The phalanges give attachment to the long flexors and extensors of the fingers and thumb, and to all the small muscles of the hand, apart from the opponens muscles.

The wrist joint

The **wrist (radiocarpal) joint** is a biaxial synovial joint – the lower end of the radius and the fibrocartilaginous disc over the head of the ulna articulate with the proximal row of carpal bones (scaphoid, lunate and triquetral). The **capsule,** attached to the articular margins, is thickened by medial and lateral collateral ligaments. The triangular articular disc is intracapsular, its apex being attached to the base of the ulnar styloid and its base to the lower end of the radius. Only if the disc is perforated does the wrist joint communicate with the distal radioulnar joint.

The **intercarpal joints** are synovial joints; the extensive composite joint between the proximal and distal row of carpal bones is known as the **midcarpal joint,** and it is here that most of the flexion and abduction of the wrist occurs. The stability of the joints is dependent on ligaments: palmar, dorsal and interosseous.

Functional aspects

Flexion, extension, abduction, adduction and circumduction are possible and both the wrist and midcarpal joints contribute to each movement. **Flexion** (flexor carpi radialis and ulnaris aided by the long digital flexors) is greater than **extension** (extensor carpi ulnaris and radialis longus and brevis assisted by the long digital extensors). **Adduction** (extensor and flexor carpi ulnaris) is greater than **abduction** (flexor carpi radialis and extensor carpi radialis longus and brevis).

The stability of the wrist depends on capsular ligaments assisted by the many long tendons crossing it (Fig. 14.3). Very few dislocations occur.

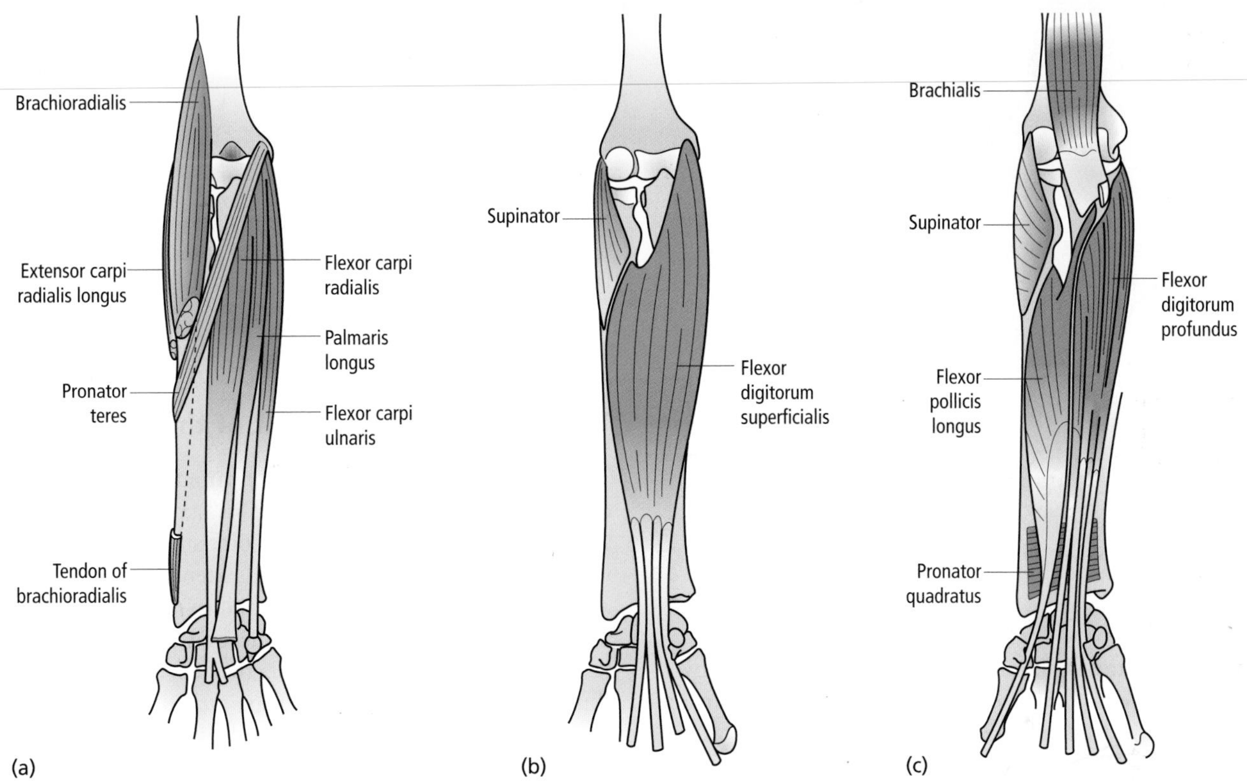

Figure 14.3 Anterior aspect of right forearm showing (a) superficial muscles; (b) intermediate muscle layer; (c) deep muscles. The tendons of these muscles cross the wrist joint to flex both wrist and fingers (Fig. 13.10, p. 191 and Tables 13.1 and 13.2)

A fall on the outstretched hand results in force being transmitted through the thenar eminence to the lateral bones of the carpus, the trapezoid and trapezium and scaphoid. In young adults the scaphoid may fracture across its waist (Fig. 14.4), and non-union of the fracture is not uncommon because of associated damage to the scaphoid's blood supply. In older people a similar fall may result in fracture of the lower end of the radius (Colles' fracture), producing a typical 'dinner-fork' deformity in which the distal fragment is displaced dorsally. In a child, this injury may result in separation of the distal radial epiphysis.

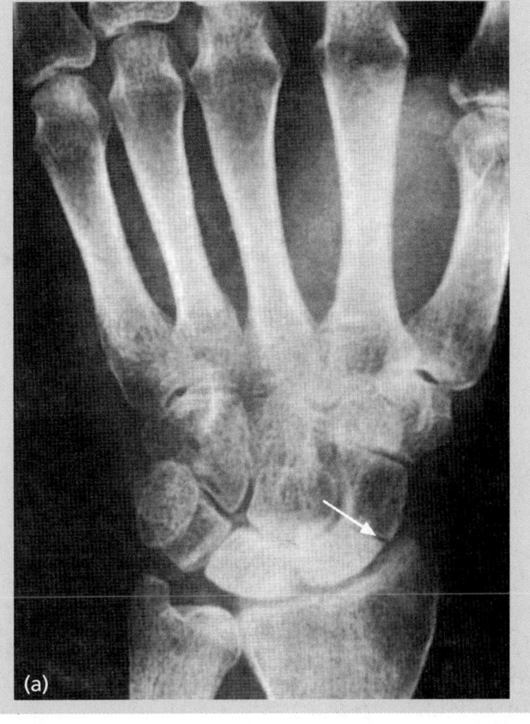

Figure 14.4 (a) Scaphoid fracture (arrow) (*continued*)

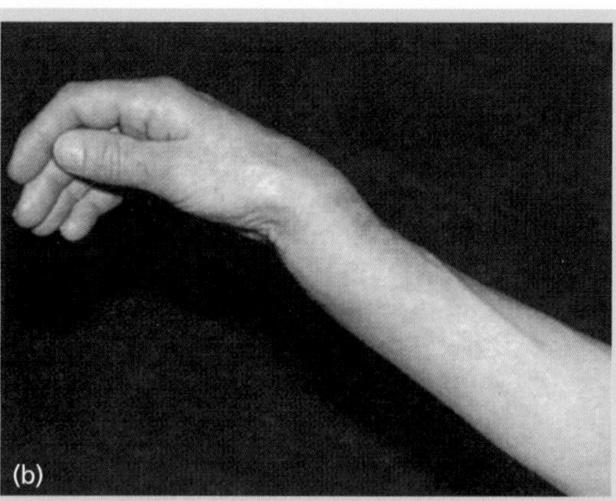

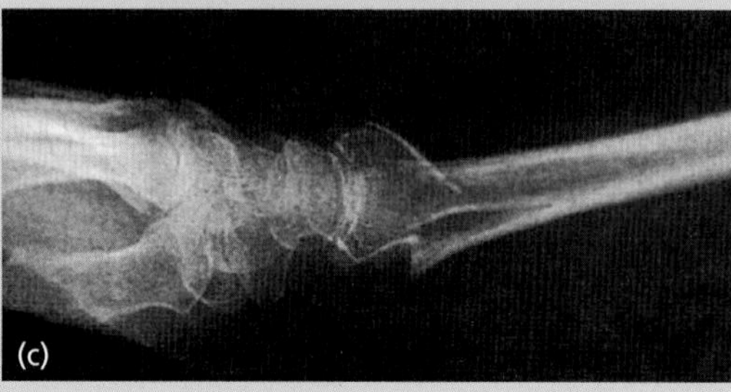

Figure 14.4 (*continued*) (b) Colles' fracture showing 'dinner fork' deformity. (c) Colles' fracture, X-ray

The **carpometacarpal joints of the fingers** are synovial plane joints. The second and third are less mobile than the fourth and fifth, and all are less mobile than that of the thumb; the metacarpal heads articulate with the cupped bases of the proximal phalanges. The joint capsules have strong palmar thickenings which are joined to each other by the deep transverse ligaments of the palm (Fig. 14.5). Flexion, extension, abduction, adduction and circumduction are all possible.

Relations of the wrist joint

These are complex but important (Fig. 14.6). Superficial veins and cutaneous nerves lie in the superficial fascia, the terminal branches of the radial nerve crossing the tendon of abductor pollicis longus. Dorsally the deep fascia thickens above the wrist joint to form the extensor retinaculum (Fig. 13.20, p. 197), which is attached to the lower ulna and radius. Beneath it pass the long extensor tendons and their synovial sheaths, each being retained by fibrous septae within fibro-osseous tunnels. The tendons bounding the anatomical snuffbox are visible when the thumb is extended (Figs 13.18 and 13.19, pp 197 and 210). The fascia over the ventral surface of the wrist thickens to form the flexor retinaculum (Fig. 14.6b). Proximal to this the radial artery can be readily palpated as it lies on the radius. Medial to this are the tendons of flexor carpi radialis and palmaris longus, and under the latter the median nerve crosses the joint deep to the retinaculum. Medially the tendon of flexor carpi ulnaris lies over the ulnar artery and nerve. Lying centrally on a deeper plane are the tendons of flexor digitorum superficialis and profundus and flexor pollicis longus.

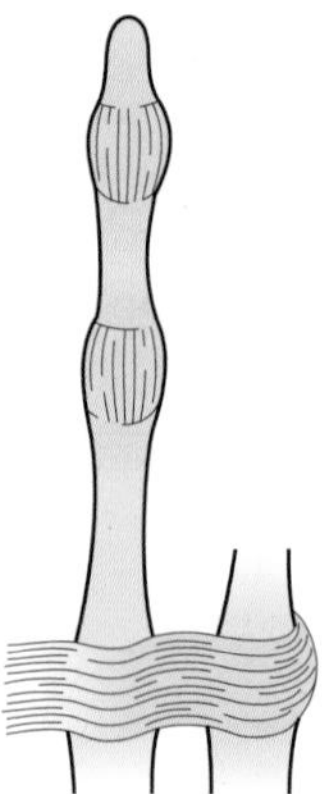

Figure 14.5 Deep transverse metacarpal ligament passing anterior to the metacarpophalangeal joints and anterior capsules of the interphalangeal joints

The carpometacarpal joint of the thumb

The carpometacarpal joint of the thumb is a synovial joint of considerable mobility owing to its lax capsule and saddle-shaped articulation. Because this joint's axis is at right-angles to those of the fingers, flexion and extension occur in a plane at right-angles to the thumbnail (and to the palm); abduction and adduction occur in the plane of the thumbnail. When these four movements combine then circumduction of the thumb can occur. The shape of the articular surfaces ensures that flexion is always accompanied by medial rotation, and extension by lateral rotation. One of the most specific thumb movements is that of **opposition**, in which the tip of the thumb is brought into contact with the tips of the fingers. It requires a combination of flexion, medial rotation and adduction of the thumb, and is very much a human attribute:

- **Flexion/medial rotation** – flexor pollicis longus and brevis and opponens pollicis
- **Extension/lateral rotation** – abductor pollicis longus and extensor pollicis longus and brevis
- **Abduction** – abductor pollicis longus and brevis
- **Adduction** – adductor pollicis
- **Opposition** – opponens pollicis.

The metacarpophalangeal joints

The metacarpophalangeal joints are synovial joints, the metacarpal heads articulating with the cupped bases of the proximal phalanges. The joint capsules have palmar thickenings which join with each other to form the deep transverse ligaments of the palm.

Flexion, extension, abduction and adduction and circumduction are possible, except for the thumb, whose metacarpophalangeal joint is limited to flexion and extension:

- **Flexion** – long digital flexors and flexor pollicis longus, assisted by the interossei, lumbricals, flexor pollicis brevis and flexor digiti minimi

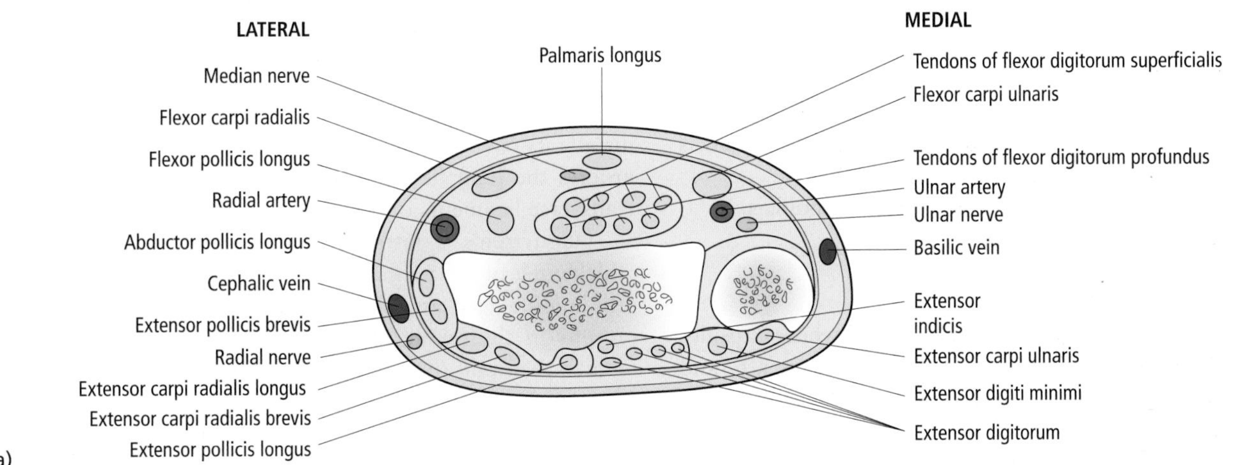

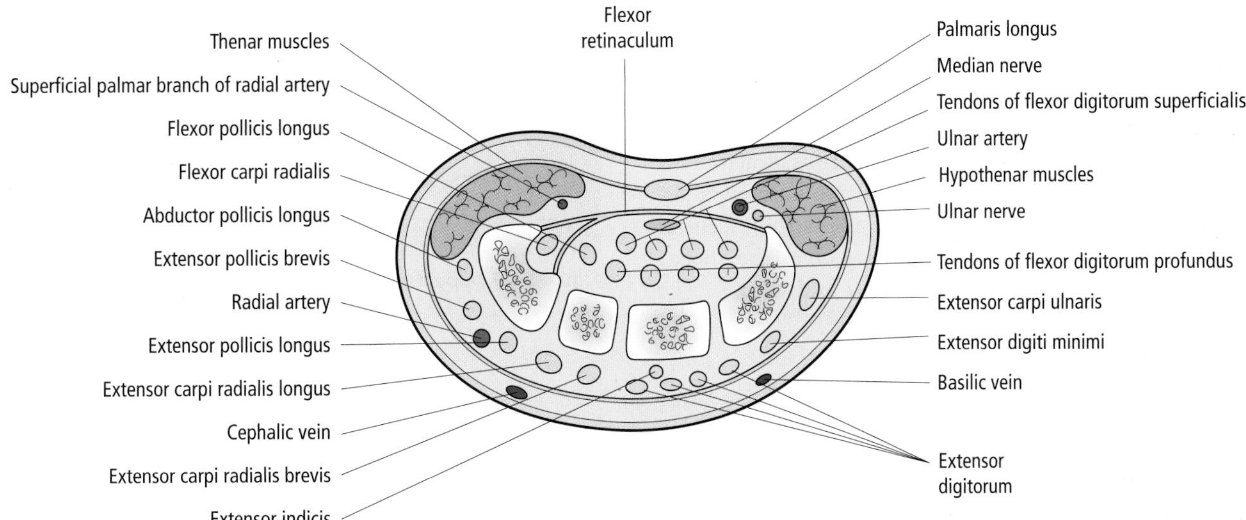

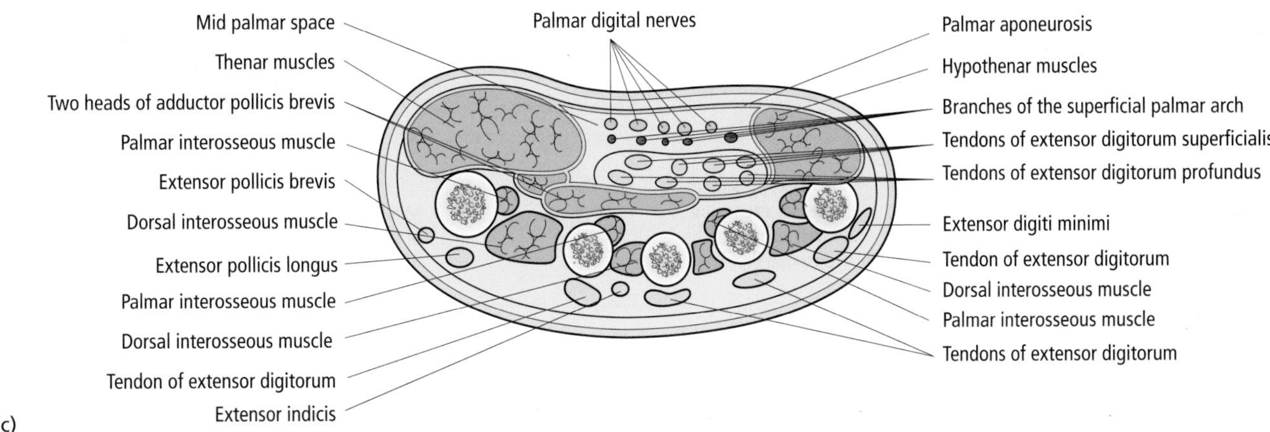

Figure 14.6 Transverse sections, viewed from below, through: (a) the right wrist; (b) the proximal carpus at the level of the flexor retinaculum; (c) the right palm at the mid-metacarpal level

- **Extension** – in the fingers, extensor digitorum, extensor indicis and extensor digiti minimi; in the thumb, extensor pollicis longus and brevis
- **Abduction** – in the fingers, the dorsal interossei and abductor digiti minimi; in the thumb, abductor pollicis longus and brevis
- **Adduction** – palmar interossei and adductor pollicis.

The interphalangeal joints

The interphalangeal joints are synovial joints whose capsules are thickened by palmar and collateral ligaments and strengthened posteriorly by the extensor tendons and their expansions (Fig. 13.16, p. 195). Flexion is by the long digital flexors, and extension mainly by the lumbrical and interosseous muscles with the long extensor tendons (Fig. 14.7a–d).

THE PALM

To facilitate grasping, the skin of the palm is thick, ridged, without hairs or sebaceous glands, and bound to the underlying palmar aponeurosis by strong fibrous attachments which give the palm its creases, and the grip to unscrew a jar.

The **palmar aponeurosis** comprises the strong central triangular part of the palm's deep fascia. Over the thenar and hypothenar muscles it is rather thinner and weaker. The aponeurosis, firmly attached to the palmar skin, overlies the superficial palmar arch and long flexor tendons (Fig. 14.3a–c). Its proximal apex is continuous with the flexor retinaculum and receives the attachment of the tendon of palmaris longus; distally its base divides into four digital slips, which bifurcate around the long flexor tendons to be attached to the deep transverse ligaments of the palm.

Dupuytren's contracture (Fig. 14.8), an abnormal thickening of the palmar aponeurosis, is not uncommon in the middle-aged and elderly. Its cause is unknown, but it results in shortening and thickening of the digital bands, which then pull the fingers into flexion, especially the ring and little fingers. Eventually the metacarpophalangeal and proximal interphalangeal joints become permanently flexed. Surgical excision of the contracture is often effective.

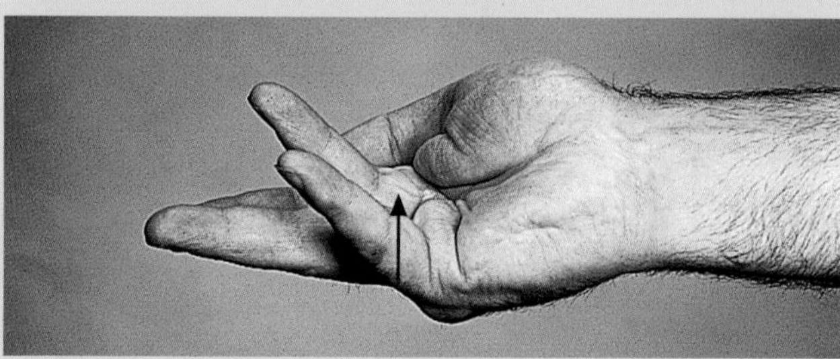

Figure 14.8 Dupuytren's contracture (arrow)

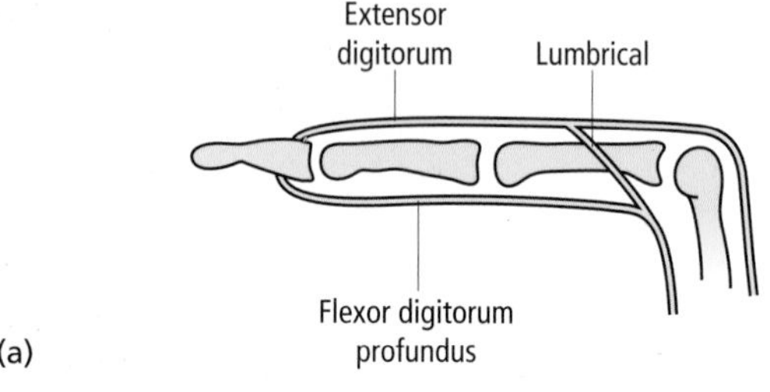

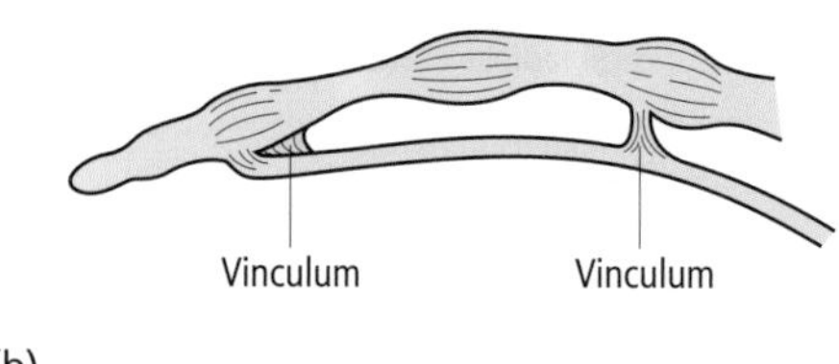

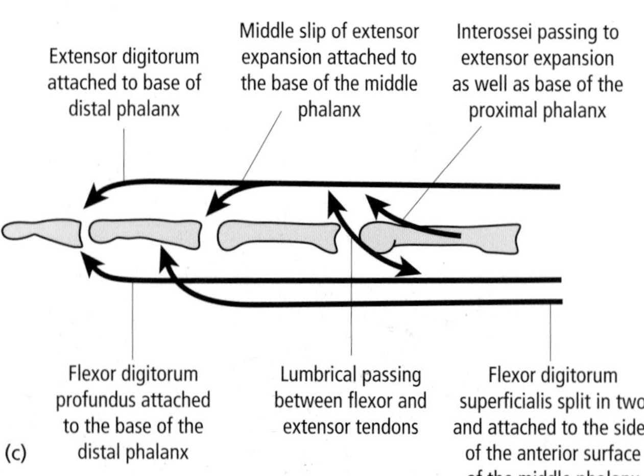

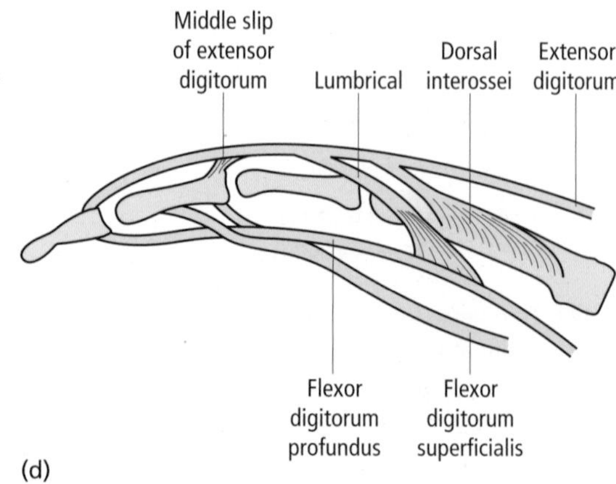

Figure 14.7 Diagram showing: (a) a lumbrical passing between tendons of extensor digitorum and flexor digitorum profundus; (b) the vincula carrying fine vessels to the adjacent tendons; (c) the digital tendon attachments; (d) the long tendons and small digital muscles

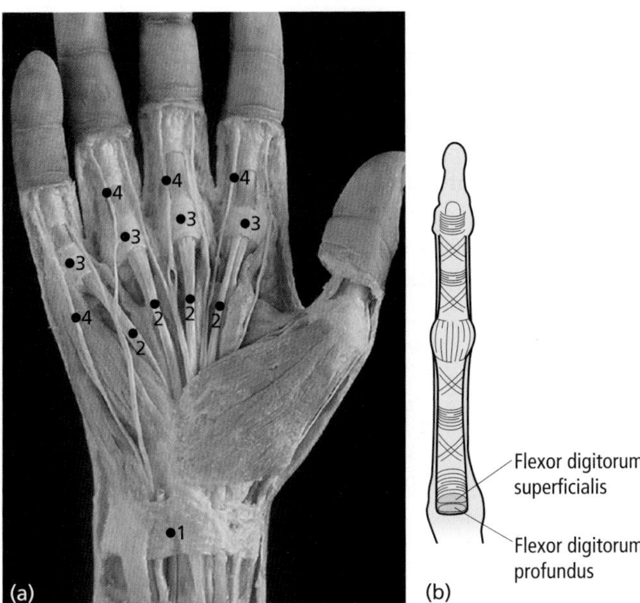

Figure 14.9 (a) Flexor surface of the hand, dissection: 1, flexor retinaculum; 2, long flexor tendons passing into, 3, fibrous sheaths; note the digital nerves, 4, lying superficially. (b) Fibrous digital sheaths of long flexor tendons

The **flexor retinaculum** (Figs 14.9 and 14.10) is a thickening of deep fascia, 2–3 cm square, which crosses the concavity of the carpus to form an osseofascial **carpal tunnel** to convey the long flexor tendons. Medially it is attached to the pisiform and hamate; laterally to the scaphoid and trapezium. Thenar and hypothenar muscles arise from its superficial surface, and the ulnar artery and nerve and its palmar branches cross it. Beneath it the carpal tunnel conveys the long flexor tendons, the radial and ulnar bursae, and the median nerve and its digital branches.

Whenever the size of the tunnel is reduced, as it may be following the tissue swelling of rheumatoid arthritis or pregnancy, symptoms are produced by compression of the median nerve deep to the retinaculum (carpal tunnel syndrome). Compression of its cutaneous digital branches produces pain, tingling (paraesthesia) and anaesthesia over the lateral 3½ digits. If the motor branches are affected then weakness, eventual paralysis and wasting of those small muscles of the hand supplied by the median nerve results. There will be progressive loss of coordination and strength in the thumb, and a loss of muscle bulk in the thenar eminence may be noted. Relief of symptoms is obtained by dividing the flexor retinaculum surgically.

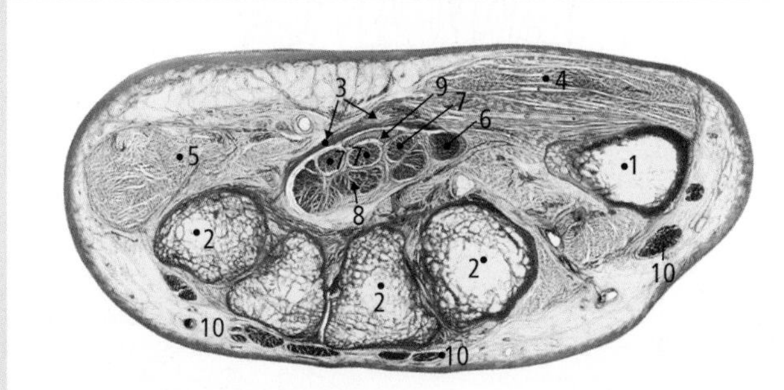

Figure 14.10 Axial plastination through the wrist to show contents of the carpal tunnel: 1, base of first metacarpal; 2, row of carpal bones; 3, flexor retinaculum; 4, thenar eminence – ball of thumb; 5, hypothenar eminence; 6, flexor pollicis longus; 7, flexor digitorum superficialis; 8, flexor digitorum profundus; 9, median nerve; 10, extensor tendons

The deep fasciae of the fingers and thumb form **fibrous flexor sheaths** (Fig. 14.9b) in continuity with the digital slips of the palmar aponeurosis. The tendons are confined within osseofascial tunnels that arch over the tendons and which are attached to the sides of the phalanges. Each extends to the base of the distal phalanx. These sheaths, together with the palmar aponeurosis and the flexor retinaculum, prevent the long flexor tendons 'bowstringing' across the palm during contraction.

Septa pass from the lateral and medial margins of the palmar aponeurosis to the shafts of the first and fifth metacarpals to create three **palmar spaces** (Fig. 14.6c): the thenar, containing the thenar muscles, the hypothenar, containing the hypothenar muscles, and the central, containing the superficial palmar arch, median nerve, long flexor tendons and lumbricals, and the deep palmar arch.

These potential fascial spaces may become infected, either by direct trauma from a puncture wound or by spread from a tendon sheath infection, and in these circumstances the infection can spread proximally deep to the flexor retinaculum to reach the lower forearm. The thick palmar fascia usually prevents the signs of infection appearing in the palm. The painful swelling is generally most evident on the dorsum where the fascia is thinner.

The fingertips are particularly liable to minor trauma and, should that cause infection, then the onset of pain soon follows because the soft tissue of the fingertip is tightly packed between firm fascial septa. Pus may spread from the fingertip proximally alongside the neurovascular bundle. Surgical drainage by an incision along the side of the finger may be required (Fig. 14.11).

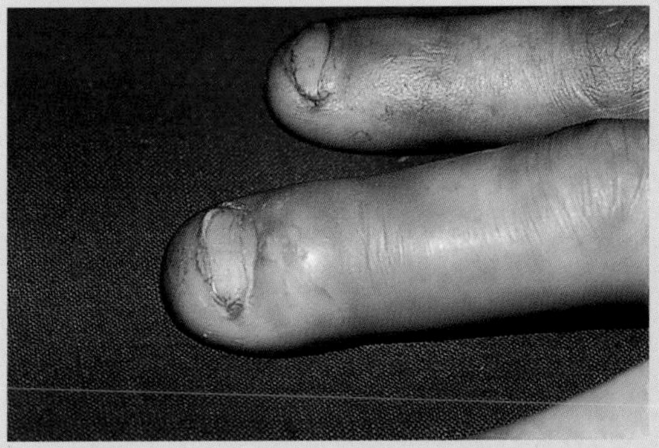

Figure 14.11 Acute paronychia (infection often starts under the edge of a nail)

Muscles of the palm

The **thenar muscles** (Fig. 14.12) are all supplied by the recurrent branch of the median nerve.

Abductor pollicis brevis lies superficial, immediately deep to the fascia. It is attached to the scaphoid and adjacent flexor retinaculum, and its tendon passes to the radial side of the base of the proximal phalanx of the thumb. It abducts the thumb.

Opponens pollicis is attached proximally to the trapezium and adjacent flexor retinaculum, and distally to the radial side of the first metacarpal. It flexes, adducts and medially rotates the thumb (otherwise known as opposing the thumb) to bring the pulp of the thumb tip into contact with the tips of the flexed fingers.

Flexor pollicis brevis, attached proximally to the trapezium and adjacent flexor retinaculum, is attached distally to the base of the thumb's proximal phalanx. It flexes the carpometacarpal and metacarpophalangeal joints of the thumb.

The **hypothenar muscles** are small mirror images of the thenar muscles and are supplied by the deep branch of the ulnar nerve. They each arise from the medial side of the flexor retinaculum and pisiform or hamate bones. **Abductor digiti minimi** and **flexor digiti minimi** gain distal attachment to the base of the proximal phalanx of the little finger; **opponens digiti minimi** is attached distally to the ulnar margin of the fifth metacarpal shaft. Their action is indicated by their names.

The deep muscles of the hand

Adductor pollicis is attached laterally to the base of the thumb's proximal phalanx and, by a tendon, into the radial side of the same bone; medially it is attached by two heads into (a) the palmar surface of the base of the second and third metacarpals, and (b) the palmar surface of the body of the third metacarpal. It adducts and assists in opposition of the thumb. Its nerve supply is the deep branch of the ulnar nerve.

The **interossei** (Fig. 14.13) lie deep between the metacarpals: four dorsal and four palmar muscles. Proximally these are attached to the shafts of the metacarpals: the palmar to the palmar surfaces of the first, second, fourth and fifth bones; the larger, more powerful dorsal muscles are attached by two heads to adjacent metacarpals. Distally both palmar and dorsal muscles are attached to the base of the corresponding

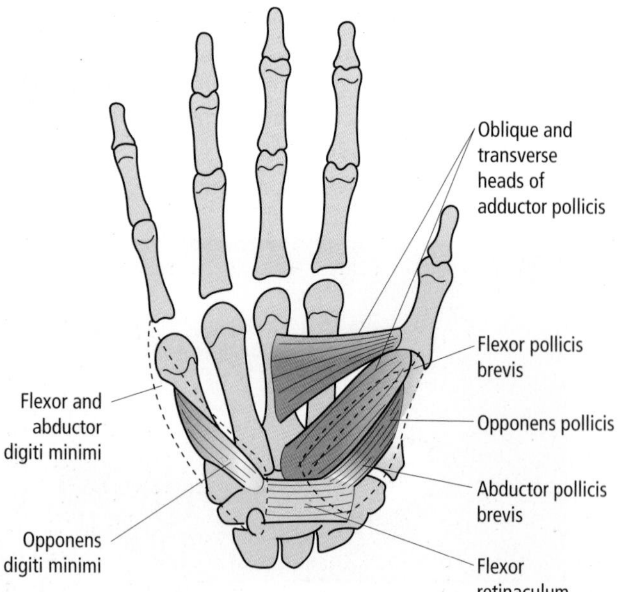

Figure 14.12 Thenar and hypothenar muscles; superficial muscles outlined (dashed)

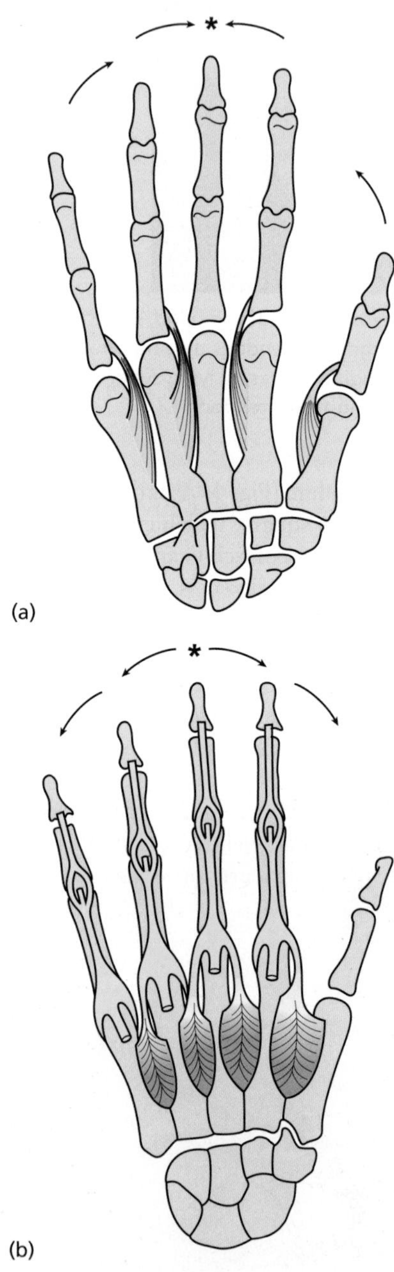

Figure 14.13 (a) Palmar interossei muscles pass from the sides of the metarcarpals to the adjacent base of the proximal phalanx, the arrangement producing adduction of the thumb and fingers towards the central axis that passes through the middle finger*. (b) The dorsal interossei pass from adjacent sides of the metacarpals to be attached distally to the bases of the proximal phalanges and the dorsal digital expansions; their action serves to abduct the digits away from the central axis that passes through the middle finger*

proximal phalanx and the extensor expansion. The **p**almar **ad**duct (**Pad**) and the **d**orsal **ab**duct (**Dab**) the fingers about the axis of the middle finger (Fig. 14.13). Both groups, acting with the lumbricals, flex the proximal phalanx and, by their attachment to the extensor expansion, help to extend the middle and distal phalanges. The nerve supply is the deep branch of the ulnar nerve.

The **lumbricals** (Fig. 14.14) are slender, worm-like muscles arising in the palm from the radial side of the four tendons of flexor digitorum profundus. Each is attached distally to the radial side of the extensor expansion of its tendon. Their action is similar to that of the interossei, but it is in the finer control of the upstroke in writing that they are most important. The two lateral are supplied by the median nerve, the two medial by the ulnar nerve. The power grip involves the long finger flexors and intrinsic flexors of the four fingers, locked down and reinforced by thumb flexion and adduction. A precision grip is much more a combination of mainly the interossei and lumbricals with assistance from the thenar and hypothenar opponens. In all hand movements it is a combination of ulnar median and radial nerves as there is normally synergism between the wrist extensors and finger flexor groups.

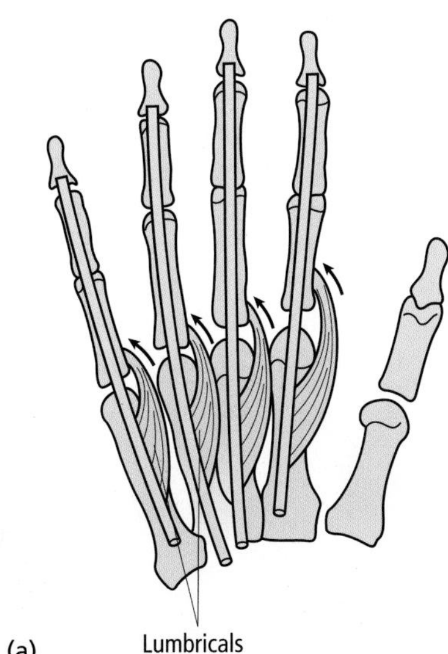

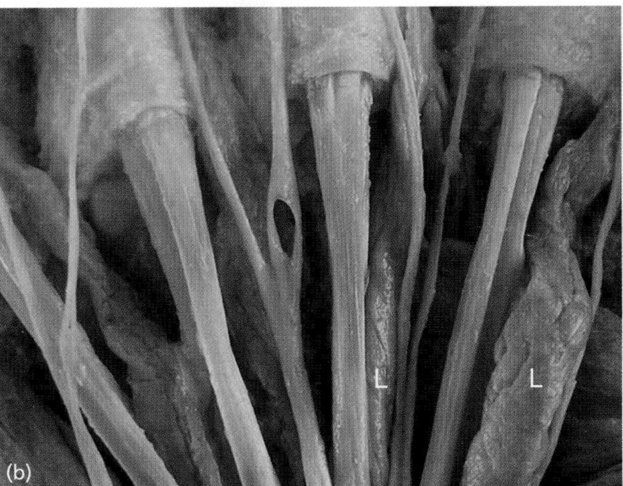

Figure 14.14 (a) Lumbrical muscles seen from the anterior aspect of the right hand, passing from the flexor digitorum profundus tendons around the lateral aspect of the four fingers to be attached to the dorsal digital expansion. They extend the interphalangeal joints by traction on the extensor tendons and flex the metacarpophalangeal joints by releasing tension in the digital aspect of the long flexor tendons. (b) Dissected right hand showing lumbricals (L)

BLOOD SUPPLY

The **superficial palmar arch** (Fig. 13.22, p. 197) provides an anastomosis between the radial and ulnar arteries in the hand. The superficial palmar branch of the ulnar artery passes laterally deep to the palmar aponeurosis to join the terminal branch of the radial artery superficial to the long flexor tendons. It provides four palmar digital branches which, by bifurcating, supply adjacent sides of the fingers and also join with the **deep palmar arch**, another anastomosis, formed largely by the radial artery and a smaller branch from the ulnar artery. It lies deep to the long flexor tendons and provides palmar metacarpal arteries and perforating arteries to the dorsum of the hand.

NERVES

The course of the nerves in the hand is described on pp 197, 198.

Upper limb sensory testing (with eyes closed) of dermatomes and individual nerves:

Touch (cotton wool); Pain (sterile needle); Temperature (side of finger v cold side of tuning fork); Vibration (base of tuning fork on head of ulna); Graphasthesia (writing numbers on forearm with a blunt instrument); Stereognosis (recognizing coin by touch); Position sense (recognising direction of movement – hold sides of index finger).

Motor testing:

Power (grip); Tone (passive flexion and extension of relaxed elbow joint); Coordination (finger to tip of nose – eyes open and then closed); Reflexes (biceps C5,6; supinator, triceps C 6,7); note wasting and abnormal movements; individual muscles – active and passive movements, and against resistance.

Peripheral nerve injuries

Radial nerve

In the arm, radial nerve injuries proximal to the attachment of triceps (most commonly in association with a fractured humerus) results in paralysis of triceps, brachioradialis, supinator, wrist and digital extensors. The characteristic deformity of wrist-drop occurs and there is loss of sensation over the radial side of the dorsum of the hand and lateral 3½ fingers and a variable part of the posterior surface of the forearm.

In the axilla, the nerve may be injured by the pressure of a crutch, or by the pressure on the nerve when the patient falls asleep with their arm thrown over the back of a chair (such as commonly happens to drunken people). Wrist-drop and sensory loss over the radial side of the palm and lateral fingers result.

In the forearm, superficial injuries cause no more than a small area of diminished sensation over the radial side of the dorsum of the hand because the radial nerve contains no muscular branches. Deeper forearm injuries or fractures of the radial neck may damage the posterior interosseous nerve and result in inability to extend the thumb and the metacarpophalangeal joints of the fingers, because of the paralysis of the long extensors. Extension of the wrist is maintained because extensor carpi radialis is supplied by a branch of the radial nerve that arises above the elbow. In this case there is no sensory loss because the posterior interosseous nerve is entirely motor. •

Median nerve

At the wrist (Fig. 14.15a), injuries are usually caused by lacerations over the wrist and result in paralysis of the thenar muscles and the first and second lumbricals and a loss of sensation over the radial two-thirds of the palm, the palmar surface of the thumb and lateral 2½ fingers. No opposition of the thumb is possible and the index and middle fingers are flexed and partly 'clawed'.

At the elbow, a median nerve injury produces a serious disability; pronation of the forearm is lost and wrist flexion is weakened (being retained only by flexor carpi ulnaris and the ulnar half of flexor digitorum profundus; Fig. 12.19d).

Ulnar nerve

At the wrist, lacerations may cause division of the nerve and produce paralysis of many of the intrinsic hand muscles: the interossei, adductor pollicis, the hypothenar muscles and the third and fourth lumbricals, resulting in a clawed hand (similar to Fig. 12.19b, p. 178), with diminished sensation over the ulnar side of the palm. The 'clawed hand' is the result of the long digital flexors, now unopposed by the paralysed lumbricals and interossei, flexing the middle and distal phalanges. The consequent pull of the long digital extensors produces hyperextension of the metacarpophalangeal joints. Adduction of the thumb is lost. A damaged ulnar nerve may result in paralysis of adductor pollicis with a resultant positive Froment's sign – the long flexors compensating for adductor loss (Fig. 14.15c).

At the elbow, the ulnar nerve is vulnerable to trauma, as it lies close to the subcutaneous medial epicondyle of the humerus, and injury results in paralysis of the ulnar half of flexor digitorum profundus and of flexor carpi ulnaris being added to the effects described above (Fig. 14.15d). This results in clawing of the hand and some radial deviation at the wrist (see Fig. 12.19b, p. 178, and Fig. 14.15d).

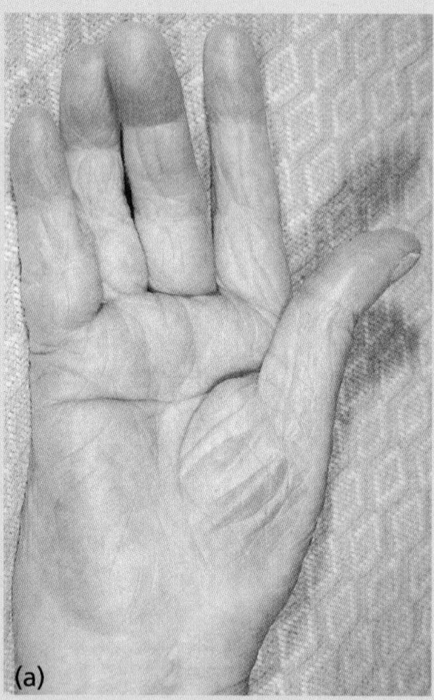

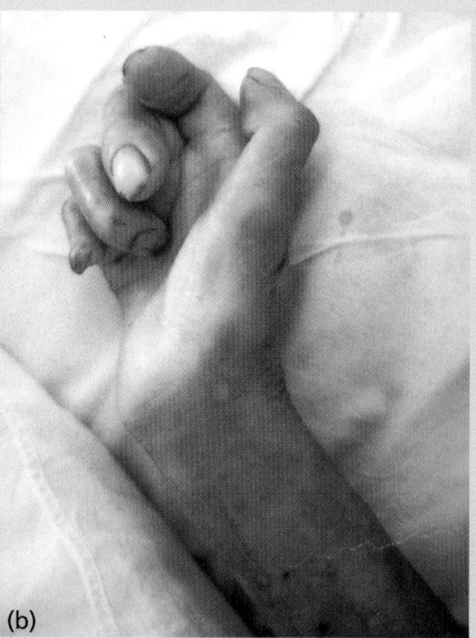

(c)

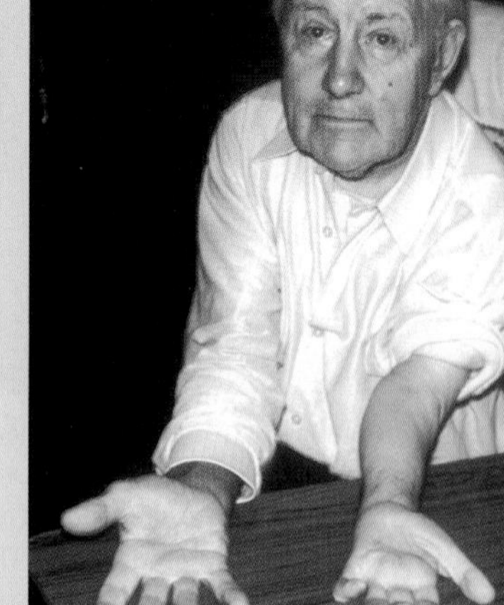

Figure 14.15 (a) Median nerve injury. (b) Median and ulnar nerve damage due to leprosy. (c) Ulnar nerve injury and inability to adduct right thumb, which is replaced by flexing (Froment's sign). (d) Chronic ulnar nerve injury resulting in left clawed hand and growth retardation

MCQs

1. The following muscles contribute to the extensor expansions of the fingers: **T/F**

- **a** extensor digitorum longus (___)
- **b** extensor indicis (___)
- **c** palmar interossei (___)
- **d** extensor pollicis longus (___)
- **e** the two medial lumbricals (___)

Answers

1.

a ***T*** – *The dorsal extensor expansion of the fingers has contributions from the ...*

b ***T*** – *... extensor digitorum longus, extensor indicis, both the dorsal and palmar ...*

c ***T*** – *... interossei and the four lumbrical muscles which pass from the flexor digitorum longus into the dorsal hood and expansion.*

d ***F*** – *There is no extensor expansion in the thumb.*

e ***T***

---

2. The following structures pass superficial to the flexor retinaculum: **T/F**

- **a** palmar branch of the ulnar nerve (___)
- **b** palmar branch of the median nerve (___)
- **c** anterior interosseous nerve (___)
- **d** the tendon of palmaris longus (___)
- **e** the tendon of flexor pollicis longus (___)

Answers

2.

a ***T*** – *The ulnar nerve and its palmar branch lie superficial to the flexor retinaculum.*

b ***T*** – *Although the median nerve passes deep to the retinaculum, its palmar branch lies superficial to it.*

c ***F*** – *The anterior interosseous nerve ends proximal to the retinaculum in pronator quadratus.*

d ***T*** – *The tendon of palmaris longus passes superficial to the retinaculum to end in the palmar aponeurosis.*

e ***F*** – *The tendon of flexor pollicis longus lies in its own compartment deep to the retinaculum.*

---

3. Palpation of the wrist reveals that: **T/F**

- **a** the palmaris longus tendon is present only in a minority of people (___)
- **b** the median nerve can usually be rolled under the fingers over the tendons of flexor digitorum superficialis (___)
- **c** the superficial branches of the radial nerve can be rolled over the flexor pollicis longus (___)
- **d** the radial pulse is usually medial to the tendon of flexor carpi radialis (___)
- **e** the scaphoid bone lies in the floor of the anatomical snuffbox (___)

Answers

3.

a ***F*** – *Palmaris longus is present in the great majority of people.*

b ***F*** – *The median nerve lies deep to palmaris longus tendon [in the minority, in whom the muscle is absent, the nerve can be rolled over the tendons of flexor digitorum].*

c ***F*** – *Branches of the radial nerve can be palpated over the tendon of extensor pollicis longus as it crosses the roof of the anatomical snuffbox.*

d ***F*** – *It is lateral to the tendon.*

e ***T*** – *Tenderness in the floor of the snuffbox may indicate a fracture of the scaphoid.*

---

4. The median nerve: **T/F**

- **a** arises from medial and lateral divisions of the brachial plexus (___)
- **b** passes between the two heads of pronator teres (___)
- **c** is situated at the wrist between palmaris longus and flexor carpi radialis longus (___)
- **d** lies on the centre of the flexor retinaculum (___)
- **e** may, when subject to pressure in the carpal tunnel, produce anaesthesia over the thenar eminence (___)

Answers

4.

a ***F*** – *The median nerve arises from the medial and lateral cords of the plexus.*

b ***T*** – *To lie deep to the muscle.*

c ***T*** – *In this position it passes deep to the flexor retinaculum centrally.*

d ***F*** – *It lies deep to the retinaculum.*

e ***F*** – *Compression within the carpal tunnel does not affect the palmar branch of the median nerve, which passes into the hand superficial to the retinaculum. Its innervation of the skin of the thenar eminence is not affected.*

EMQs

Each question has an anatomical theme linked to the chapter, and a list of 10 related items (A–J) placed in alphabetical order: these are followed by five statements (1–5). Match **one or more** of the items A–J to each of the five statements.

Relationships at the wrist

A. Flexor retinaculum
B. Median nerve
C. Pisiform bone
D. Radial artery
E. Radial nerve
F. Scaphoid bone
G. Styloid process of the radius
H. Styloid process of the ulna
I. Ulnar artery
J. Ulnar nerve

Match the following statements with the item(s) in the above list.

1. Lies in the floor of the anatomical snuff box
2. Lies superficial to the median nerve
3. Passes medial to the pisiform bone
4. Overlain by the palmaris longus tendon
5. Gives attachment to the flexor retinaculum

Answers

1 DFG; 2 A; 3 IJ; 4 AB; 5 CF

Bones of the upper limb

A. Clavicle
B. Distal phalanx of the little finger
C. First metacarpal
D. Humerus
E. Pisiform
F. Proximal phalanx of the middle finger
G. Radius
H. Scaphoid
I. Scapula
J. Ulna

Match the following statements with the bone(s) of the above list

1. Has a styloid process
2. Gives attachment to the abductor pollicis longus
3. Gives attachment to flexor carpi ulnaris
4. Gives attachment to the short head of biceps
5. Gives attachment to the flexor digitorum profundus

Answers

1 CGJ; 2 C; 3 EJ; 4 I; 5 JB

APPLIED QUESTIONS

1. An old woman falls downstairs and sustains a midshaft fracture of the humerus, damaging the radial nerve in the spiral groove. What are the effects, both motor and sensory, on the hand and wrist?

1. Wrist-drop is the most noticeable injury, owing to loss of all finger and wrist extensors. This also considerably weakens the power grip. The sensory loss, however, is often limited, owing to overlap of the nerves' sensory distribution, but may include a strip down the posterior aspect of arm and forearm as well as a small area of anaesthesia over the first dorsal interosseous muscle, in the posterior web between thumb and index finger.

---

2. In the hand, which nerve lesion is the most serious, and why?

2. The median nerve lesion is the most disabling because thumb opposition is lost, as well as the sensation over the thumb, index and middle fingers. Consequently, all fine pincer movements, such as writing, are almost impossible.

---

3. How might a swelling proximal to the wrist joint be connected with infection in the tip of the thumb (tenosynovitis)?

3. The long flexor tendons of the thumb are surrounded by synovial sheaths. An infection in the pulp might readily spread proximally where, in some people, it joins the ulnar bursa, both of them passing deep to the retinaculum and extending for 2–3 cm to the level of the wrist.

---

4. An attempted suicide cuts his wrists fairly deeply. After repair of the arteries, which other important structures would you also wish to test and how would you do this?

4. The two major nerves of the hand are both vulnerable. The median nerve lies just deep to palmaris longus and the ulnar nerve lies between the ulnar artery and the pisiform bone. To test the median nerve, the patient is asked to abduct his thumb against resistance (note that thumb opposition can be mimicked by the long flexor tendons). True thumb opposition is impossible in long-standing median nerve lesions, as the thumb is laterally rotated and adducted and consequently looks like a monkey's or ape's hand. To test the ulnar nerve, the hand is placed palm downwards and the fingers straightened, then abducted and adducted against resistance. Or try the paper-holding test between adducted fingers. When pulling on a sheet of paper held between thumb and side of index finger of both hands, adductor pollicis maintains the downward pressure; if the ulnar nerve is damaged additional pressure is applied by flexor pollicis with flexion of the interphalangeal joint (Froment's sign).

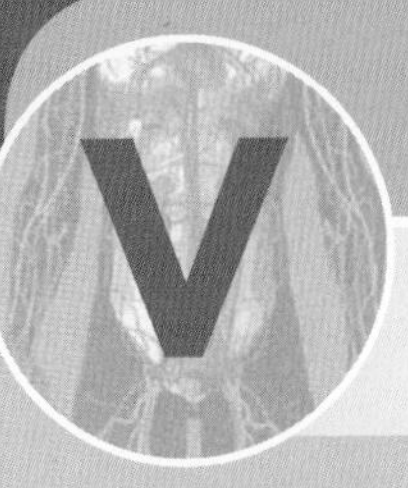

The lower limb

15 The hip and thigh

The lower limb, similar in structure to the upper, is modified by its functions of support and propulsion of the body. During its development there is rotation medially on its long axis, so that the flexor surface lies posteriorly and the sole of the foot faces backwards and then downwards. The pelvic girdle (Fig. 9.1a, p. 122), unlike the pectoral girdle, is firmly attached to the vertebral column, which allows the transmission of the body's weight through it to the lower limb. In the standing position the centre of gravity passes behind the hip and in front of the knee and ankle joints. The weight is distributed between the heel and the balls of the toes, most of it being carried by bones and ligaments, with only a minimal amount of muscle activity being required to maintain balance.

THE FASCIA

The membranous layer of the superficial fascia of the abdomen extends into the thigh, fusing with the deep fascia at the level of the skin crease in front of the hip joint. The deep fascia of the gluteal region and thigh forms a firm investing layer, the **fascia lata.** Proximally it is attached in a continuous line to the inguinal ligament, iliac crest, posterior sacrum, sacrotuberous ligament, ischiopubic ramus and the body of the pubis. Medial and lateral intermuscular septa spread from it to divide the thigh muscles into distinct compartments (Fig. 15.1a,b).

Three centimetres below and 1 cm lateral to the pubic tubercle an oval deficiency in the fascia, the **saphenous opening** (Fig. 15.2a), transmits the great saphenous vein. The

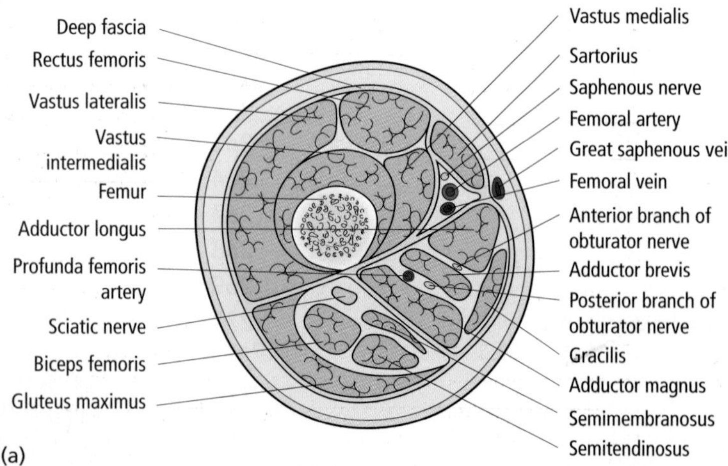

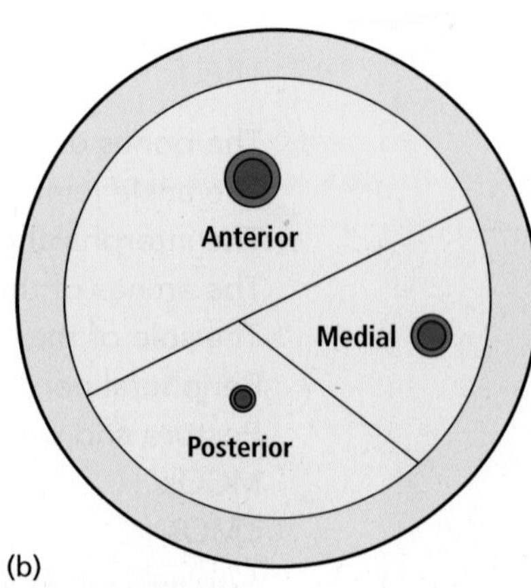

Figure 15.1 (a) Transverse section of the right thigh through the upper thigh, viewed from below (see dotted line in 15.2a for level): the deep fascia (fascia lata) divides the thigh into anterior, medial and posterior compartments as shown in schematic (b)

fascia lata is thickened on the lateral side of the thigh, forming the **iliotibial tract**, which is attached distally to the lateral tibial condyle. Gluteus maximus and tensor fasciae latae gain attachment to the tract and because of this attachment assist in extension and stabilization of the knee. Over the popliteal fossa the fascia is pierced by the small saphenous vein (Fig. 15.3).

The deep fascia of the lower leg is continuous with the fascia lata. It is attached to bone around the margins of the patella, the medial surface of the tibia and, inferiorly, to both malleoli. It ensheathes the muscles and contributes to intermuscular septa which separate the anterior, lateral and posterior muscle compartments. The posterior muscles are further divided by a fascial envelope into superficial and deep compartments, the former enclosing gastrocnemius and soleus. Around the ankle the fascia thickens to form the retinacula, restraining the tendons as they enter the foot. On the dorsum of the foot the fascia is thin, but on the sole it is thickened to form the **plantar aponeurosis**. Throughout the leg and thigh, the fascia is pierced by perforating (communicating) veins joining the superficial to the deep veins, and by cutaneous nerves, arteries and lymph vessels.

The fascial compartments of the leg are rather rigid envelopes for the soft tissues contained within them; trauma and bleeding, such as may follow a leg fracture, may cause compartmental swelling and rise in pressure of sufficient severity to compromise the arterial supply to the contents of the compartment. It is essential in these circumstances that close observation is maintained on the pulses in the leg, and if the circulation is found to be threatened then a fasciotomy (incision along the length of the fascial sheath) must be undertaken urgently to relieve the pressure in that compartment.

Venous drainage

There are three types of vein in the lower limb: superficial, deep and communicating (perforating) (Figs 15.2a–d and 15.3). Valves are present in the larger veins and all the communicating veins: they direct blood flow towards the heart, or from the superficial to the deep veins. The **superficial**

(a)

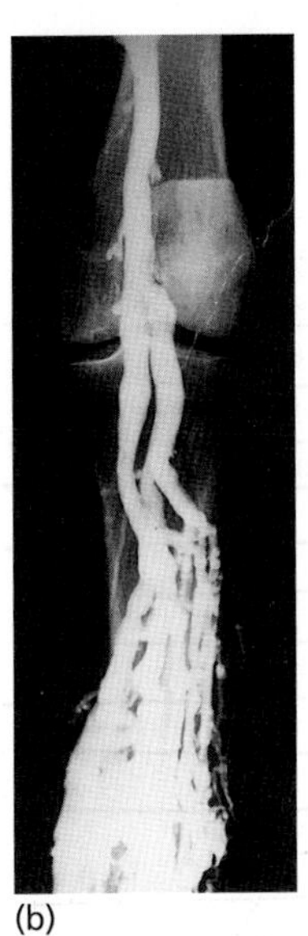

(b)

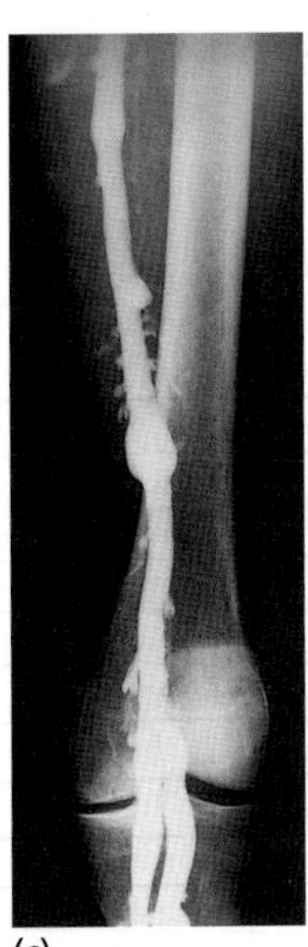

(c)

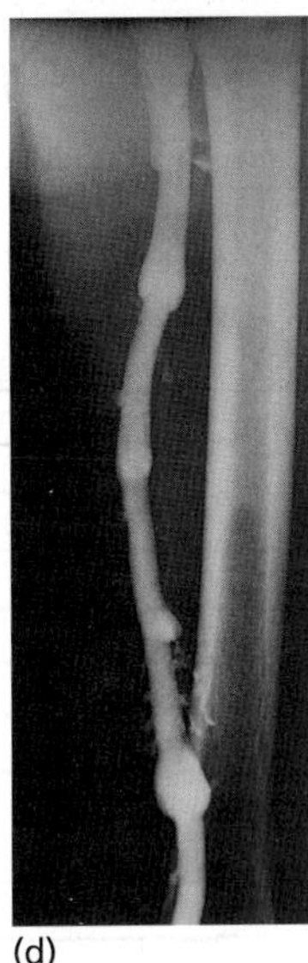

(d)

Figure 15.2 (a) Surface anatomy of lower limb vessels: 1, femoral artery; 2, profunda femoris; 3, adductor hiatus; 4, popliteal artery; 5, anterior tibial artery; 6, posterior tibial artery; 7, peroneal (fibular) artery; 8, dorsalis pedis artery; 9, saphenous opening; 10, great saphenous vein; 11, dorsal venous arch. N.B. the dotted line indicates the level of the transverse section in Fig. 15.1a. (b–d) Lower limb venograms: (b) Numerous deep veins within soleus and gastrocnemius draining into popliteal vein. (c) Popliteal vein becoming the femoral vein at adductor hiatus. (d) Femoral vein on medial side of thigh – note the bulges above the valves

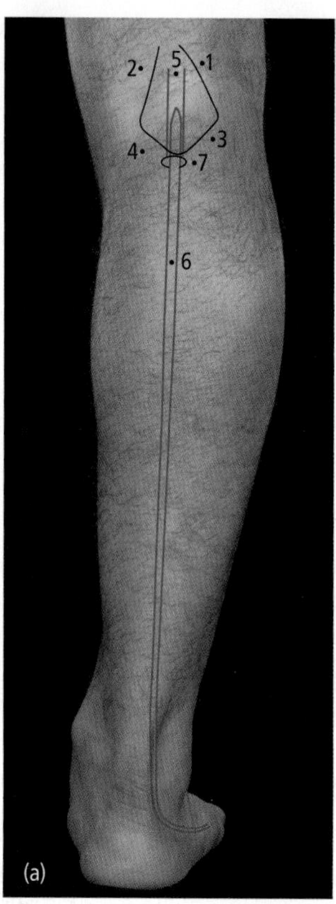

Figure 15.3 Surface anatomy of the small saphenous vein: 1, biceps femoris; 2, semitendinosus and semimembranosus; 3, lateral head of gastrocnemius; 4, medial head of gastrocnemius; 5, popliteal vein; 6, small saphenous vein; 7, opening for small saphenous vein in deep fascia

veins drain skin and superficial fascia into two main channels, the great and small saphenous veins. These originate in the **dorsal** and **plantar venous arches** of the forefoot.

The **great saphenous vein** (Fig. 15.2a), from the medial end of the dorsal arch, ascends anterior to the medial malleolus, lying subcutaneously along the medial calf and thigh, accompanied in the calf by the saphenous nerve. It enters the deep venous system by passing through the saphenous opening into the femoral vein (Fig. 15.6a below). It receives tributaries from the small saphenous vein, and connects by communicating branches to the deep veins of the thigh and calf just behind the medial border of the tibia.

Just anterior and superior to the medial malleolus the great saphenous vein can readily be located and is frequently used for an emergency venous 'cutdown'. The great saphenous vein is also commonly used to bypass blocked coronary arteries in a coronary artery bypass graft (CABG) operation – known as a 'cabbage' procedure. It is reversed so that its valves do not obstruct the arterial blood flow.

The **small saphenous vein** (Fig. 15.3) originates at the lateral end of the dorsal venous arch, ascends behind the lateral malleolus up the posterior calf, and ends by passing through the fascia over the popliteal fossa into the popliteal vein. It receives cutaneous tributaries and communicates with the deep veins of the calf by perforating veins.

The **deep veins** comprise those of the foot and the soleal plexuses of veins, the popliteal and the femoral vein (p. 237). The superficial veins drain to them by communicating veins that perforate the deep fascia.

All the veins of the lower limb possess valves which only permit blood flow up the limb, or from superficial veins to deep veins. Flow in the deep veins towards the heart is aided by the contraction of the calf muscles, the 'muscle pump'.

If the valves of the communicating veins become incompetent the blood flow within them becomes reversed and the 'muscle pump' is less effective at helping the venous return to the deep veins. The result is that the superficial veins become distended (**varicose veins**) (Fig. 15.4) with the increased amount of venous return that they are carrying, and their valves become incompetent veins. The deep plexuses of veins are emptied by foot and calf muscle contraction, and in prolonged recumbency, when leg activity is minimal, stagnation of blood occurs within them, often followed by thrombosis (Fig. 15.5). This is one of the factors that accounts for the high frequency of

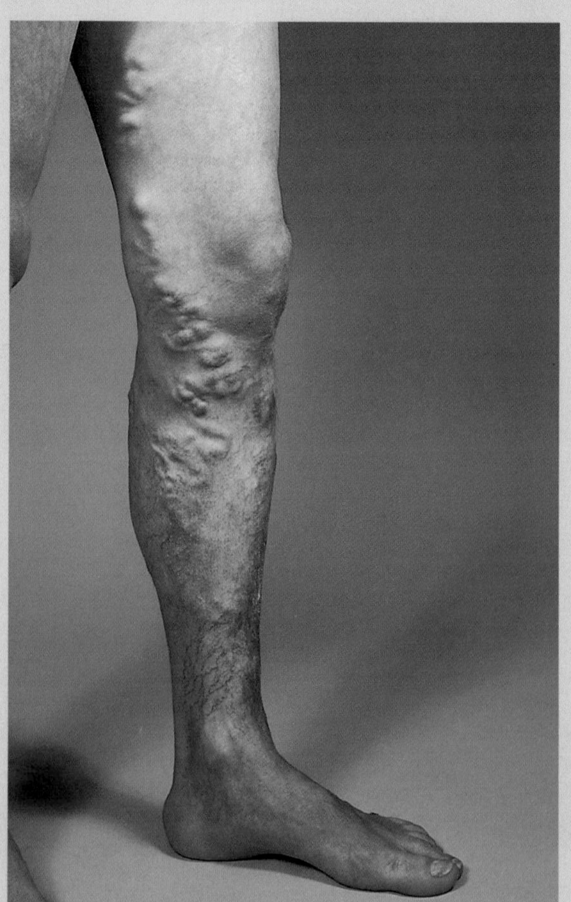

Figure 15.4 A varicose great saphenous vein distended with blood because the valves of the communicating veins are incompetent

deep vein thrombosis postoperatively. When deep venous thrombosis occurs there is always a risk that part of the thrombus can break off and cause a pulmonary embolus. More usually the thrombus resolves but damages the vein's valves, with the result that defective venous return from the lower limb may result in varicose veins, chronic leg swelling, skin changes and ulceration of the skin over the ankle – the postphlebitic limb.

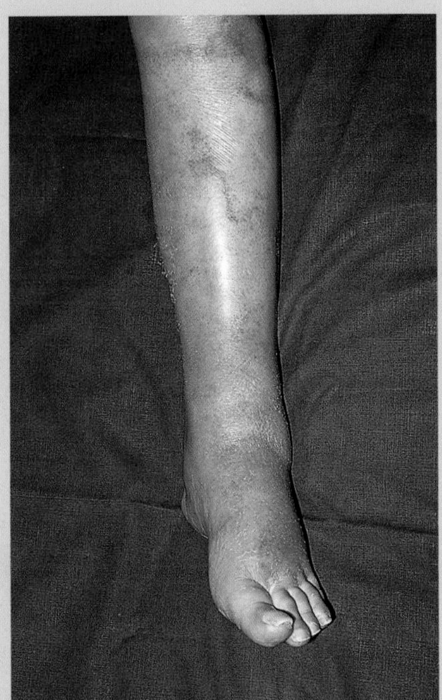

Figure 15.5 Deep venous thrombosis of left leg. Note swelling and skin changes

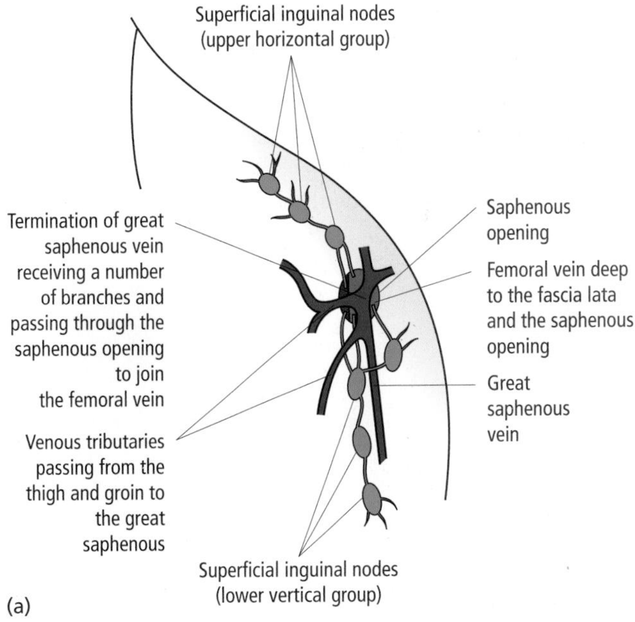

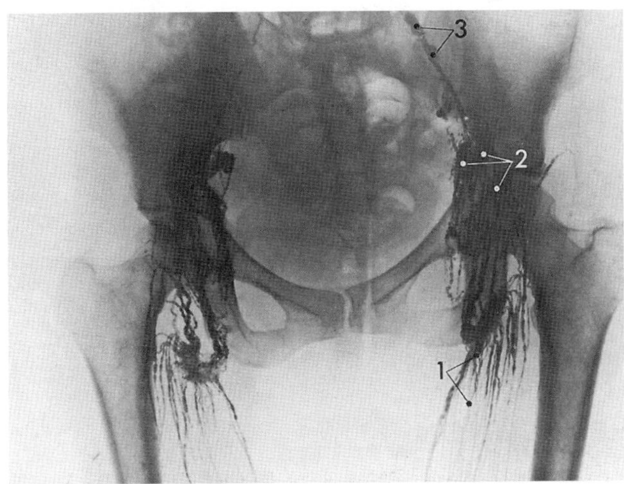

(b)

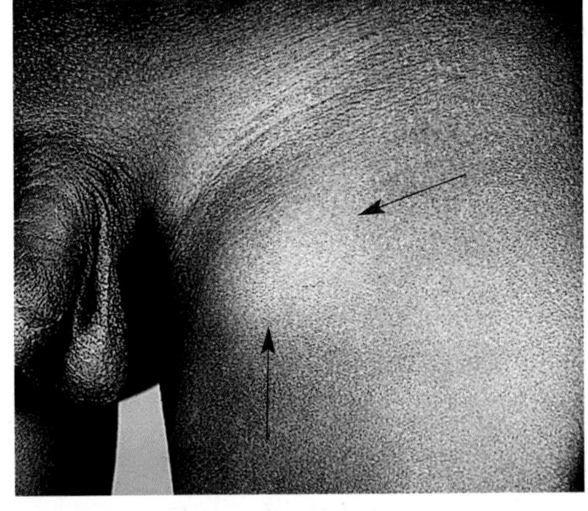
(c)

Figure 15.6 (a) Inguinal lymph nodes, the saphenous opening and the great saphenous vein. (b) Lower limb lymphangiogram: 1, lymphatic vessels of upper thigh; 2, inguinal lymph vessels; 3, external iliac lymph vessels. (c) Enlarged inguinal lymph nodes from a foot infection (arrows)

Lymphatic drainage

There are two groups of lymph nodes in the lower limb, superficial and deep.

The **superficial groups** lie in the inguinal region (Fig. 15.6a–c): the **upper superficial (horizontal) inguinal group** is in the femoral triangle, just below the inguinal ligament. It receives lymph from the lower abdominal wall, the perineum, external genitalia, anal canal and the gluteal region, and drains to the lower superficial inguinal group and the deep nodes. The **lower superficial inguinal (vertical) group** lies around the saphenous opening and receives lymph from the upper group and the skin of the thigh and the medial leg and foot. Its efferent vessels drain through the saphenous opening to the deep inguinal or external iliac group.

The **deep groups** lie under the deep fascia in the popliteal and inguinal regions. The **popliteal group**, a small group, lies in the popliteal fossa around the small saphenous vein and drains the skin of the lateral foot and calf and the deep tissues of the leg. Its efferents drain to the deep inguinal group. The **deep inguinal group** is around the femoral canal and receives the lymph of all the superficial nodes and deep lymphatic vessels of the lower limb. Its efferents drain to the external iliac nodes.

Enlargement of the inguinal nodes (Fig. 15.6c) follows soft tissue infection anywhere in the lower limb and perineum. Cancers arising in the external genitalia or in the anal canal may spread to and enlarge these inguinal nodes. Maldevelopment of the lymph vessels, or blockage of the vessels or nodes by disease, produces soft tissue swelling because of the interference with lymph flow. This is termed **lymphoedema** (Fig. 15.7).

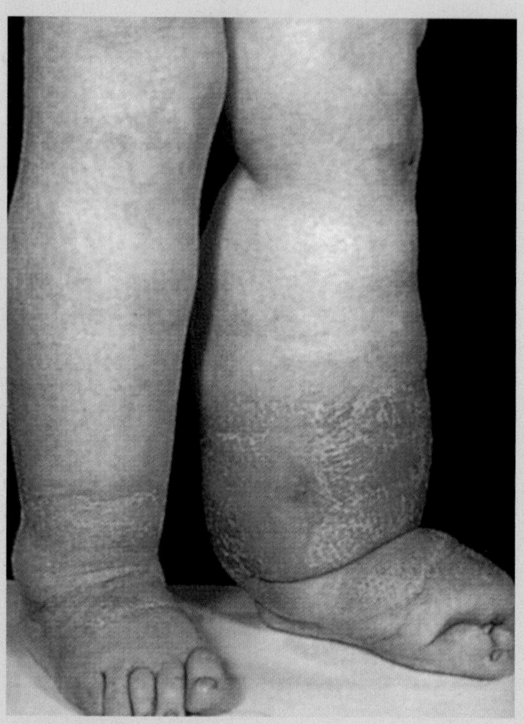

Figure 15.7 Lymphoedema

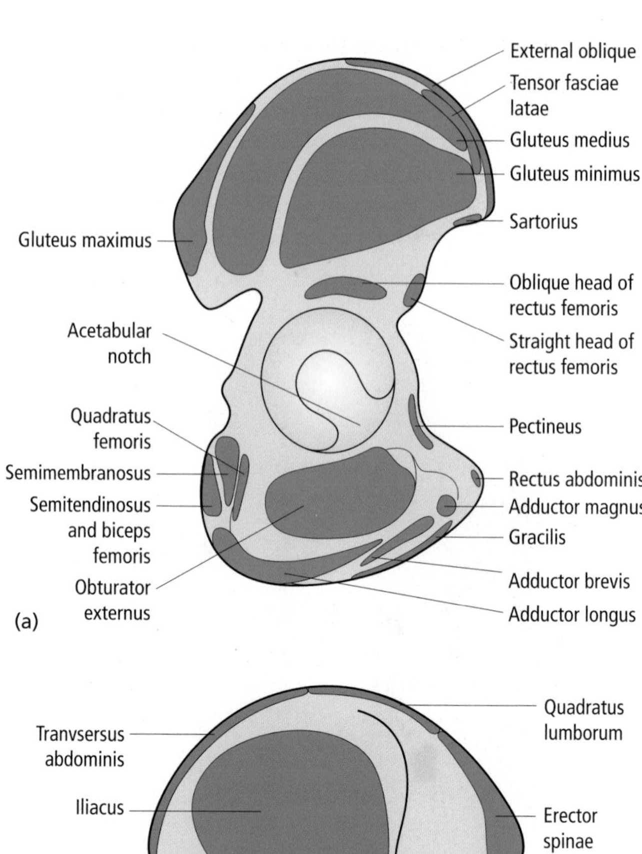

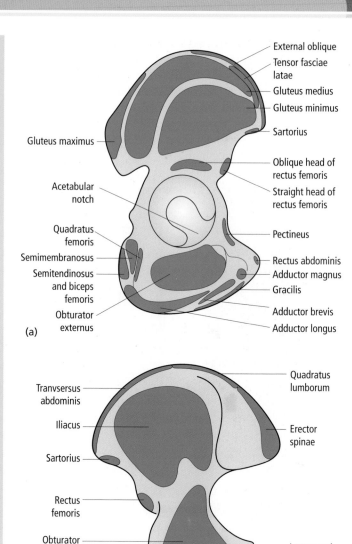

Figure 15.8 Right innominate bone showing muscle attachments: (a) lateral aspect (b) medial aspect

THE SKELETON

For the **hip bone** (**os innominatum**) (Figs 15.8, 15.9 and 15.10), see also p. 121.

The lateral surface of the hip bone

The gluteal surface of the **ala of the ilium** is smooth and faces laterally; it is bounded by the iliac crest above and by the greater sciatic notch and the acetabulum below. It gives attachment to gluteus medius and minimus centrally and to gluteus maximus posteriorly. Rectus femoris gains attachment to its anterolateral border. The **ischial spine** separates the greater and lesser sciatic notches; below the lesser notch is the **ischial tuberosity**. The anterior border of the ilium has prominent **superior** and **inferior iliac spines**. The **obturator foramen** is bounded by the inferior and superior pubic rami (Fig. 15.10).

Fractures of the pelvis are the result of violent blows such as may result from road traffic accidents. Fractures of the acetabulum result from severe lateral forces; compression in an anteroposterior direction may cause fractures of the pubic rami and if the fragments are displaced then injuries to the adjacent bladder may occur.

The femur

The femur (Fig. 15.11) possesses a proximal end, a shaft and a distal end. The **proximal end** consists of a head, a neck, and greater and lesser trochanters. The **head** articulates with the **acetabulum** of the hip bone; in the centre of the head is a small pit (fovea) for the ligament of the head of the femur.

The narrow **neck** forms an angle of about 125° with the shaft. Much of it lies within the hip joint capsule. The **greater trochanter**, a projection from the lateral part of the bone, gives attachment to the short rotators of the hip joint, gluteus medius and minimus, the obturator muscles and piriformis. The **lesser trochanter**, at the junction of the body and the neck, gives attachment to psoas major and

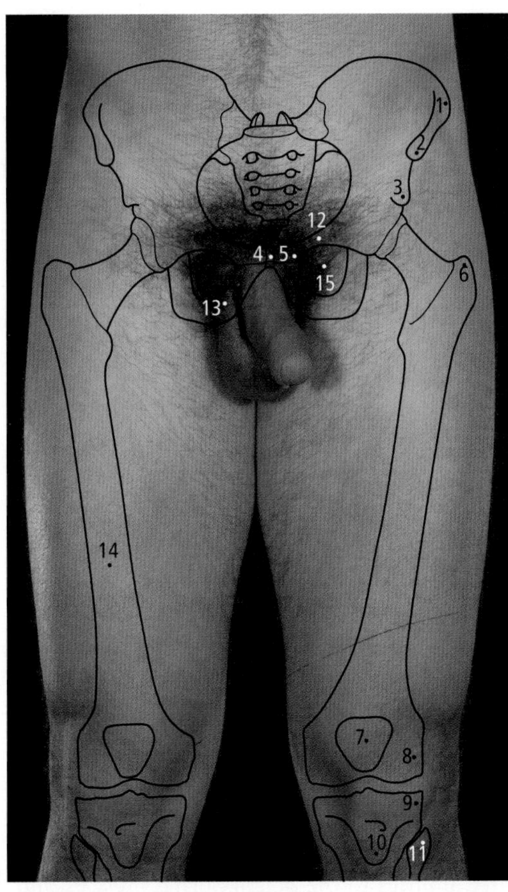

(a)

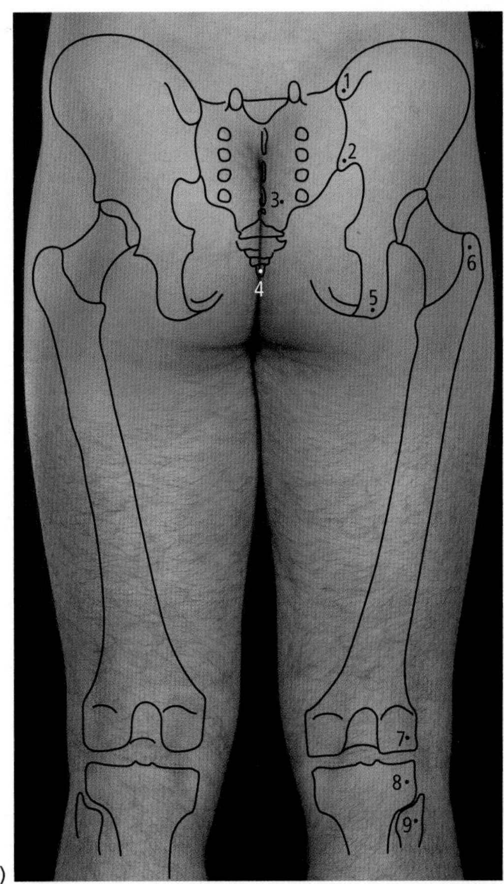

(b)

Figure 15.9 Surface anatomy of the pelvis and thigh. (a) Anterior view: 1, iliac crest; 2, anterior superior iliac spine; 3, anterior inferior iliac spine; 4, symphysis pubis; 5, pubic tubercle; 6, greater trochanter; 7, patella; 8, lateral condyle of femur; 9, lateral condyle of tibia; 10, tibial tuberosity; 11, head of fibula; 12, superior pubic ramus; 13, inferior pubic ramus; 14, shaft of femur; 15, obturator foramen. (b) Posterior view: 1, posterior superior iliac spine; 2, posterior inferior iliac spine; 3, posterior aspect of sacrum; 4, tip of coccyx; 5, ischial tuberosity; 6, greater trochanter; 7, lateral femoral condyle; 8, lateral condyle of the tibia; 9, head of fibula

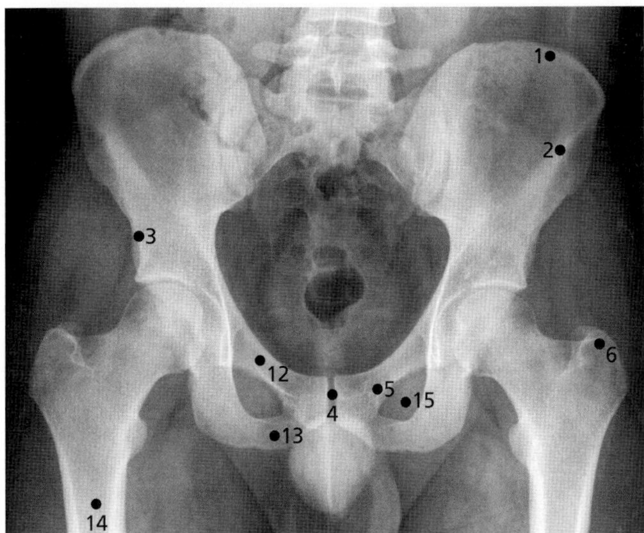

Figure 15.10 X-ray of hip joint and pelvis (labels as in Fig. 15.9a)

iliacus; the **intertrochanteric line** joins it and the greater trochanter anteriorly, and the **intertrochanteric crest** joins them posteriorly (Fig. 15.11).

The **shaft** of the femur inclines medially at an angle of about 10°. It is more oblique in the female because of the greater width of the female pelvis. It bears posteriorly, in its middle third, a longitudinal ridge, the **linea aspera**, which gives attachment to the adductors, short head of biceps and part of the quadriceps. In the lower third the linea aspera splays out into the **medial** and **lateral supracondylar lines;** the medial line ends at the **adductor tubercle** above the medial condyle.

The **distal end** is expanded into two masses, the **medial** and **lateral condyles**, for articulation with the tibial condyles and patella. The articular surfaces of the condyles are separated posteriorly by the intercondylar notch and united anteriorly by the concave articulation for the patella. The tibial articular surface of each condyle is markedly convex anteroposteriorly and slightly convex from side to side; the medial tibial surface is longer than the lateral. The side of each condyle bears a small elevation, the **epicondyle,** which gives attachment to the medial and lateral ligaments of the knee. Much of the lower end of the femur is subcutaneous and palpable (Fig. 16.2a, p. 242).

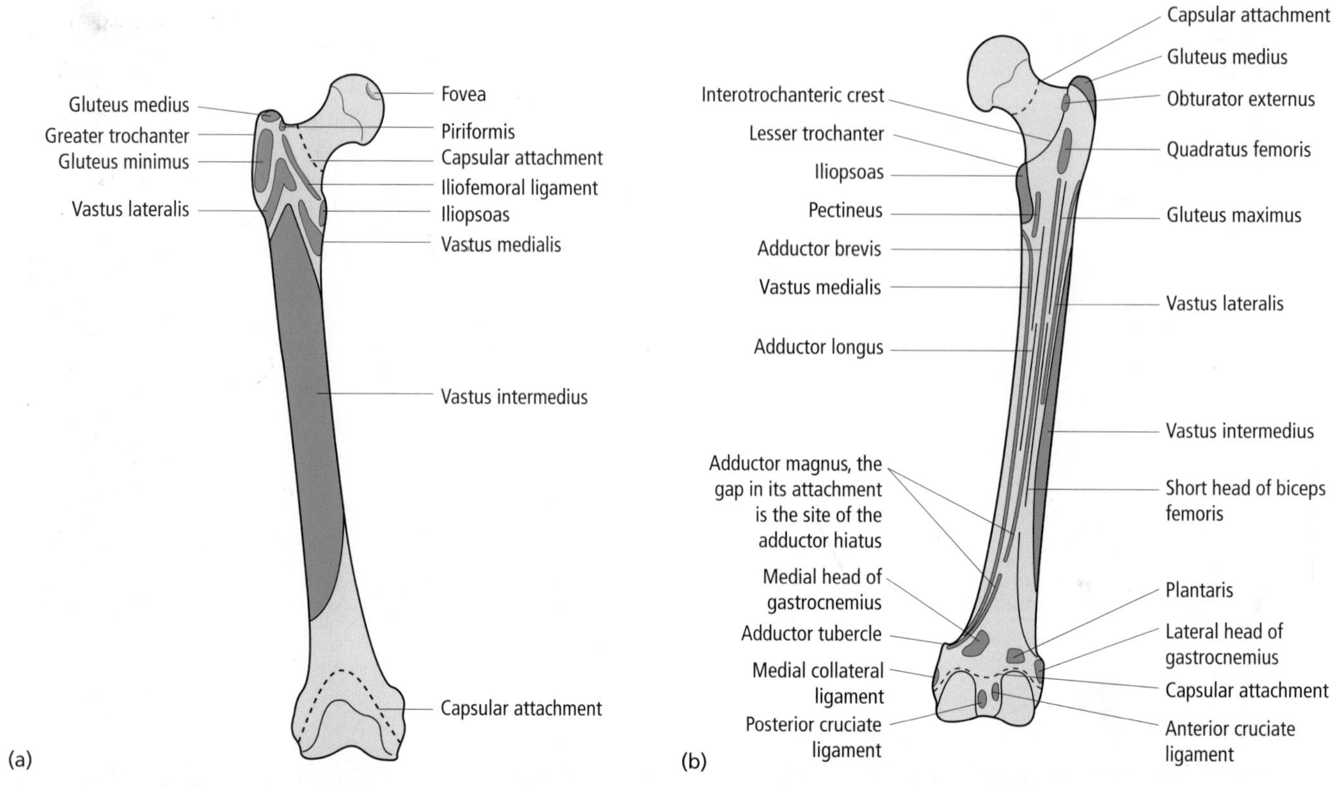

Figure 15.11 Right femur: (a) anterior view; (b) posterior view showing muscle and some ligament attachments

Fractures of the femoral neck are common in the elderly because of thinning of the bone structure (osteoporosis). It may fracture near to the trochanters, near the midpoint of the neck or below the head (subcapital, Fig. 15.12a–c). The subcapital fracture may be complicated by necrosis of the femoral head because of damage to the small arteries within the capsule supplying the femoral head. Pertrochanteric or midcervical fractures generally leave the retinacular vessels within the capsule undisturbed, and thus avascular necrosis does not occur and non-union is less frequent (Figs 15.13).

Fractures of the shaft of the femur (Fig. 15.14) are accompanied by considerable blood loss because of associated injuries to the neighbouring muscles and blood vessels. There is a characteristic deformity produced by fractures of the midshaft of the femur: namely a considerable shortening because of the now-unresisted contraction of the strong thigh muscles and the proximal fragment is flexed by the unopposed action of iliopsoas and abducted by the glutei, whereas the distal fragment is pulled medially by the adductors. Satisfactory reduction of the fracture must take account of these factors – strong traction to overcome the shortening, with the limb abducted to bring the distal fragment into line with the proximal fragment.

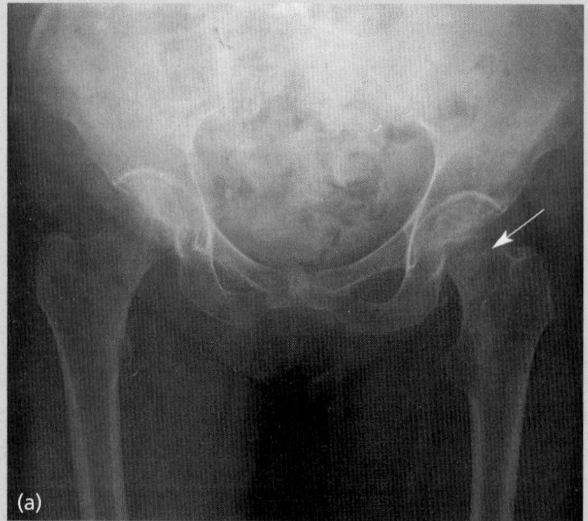

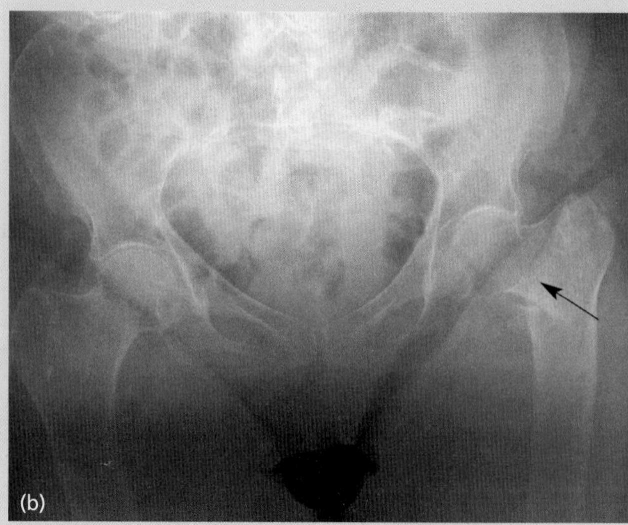

Figure 15.12 (a–b) Intra- and extracapsular fracture of neck of femur (arrows indicate site of fracture)

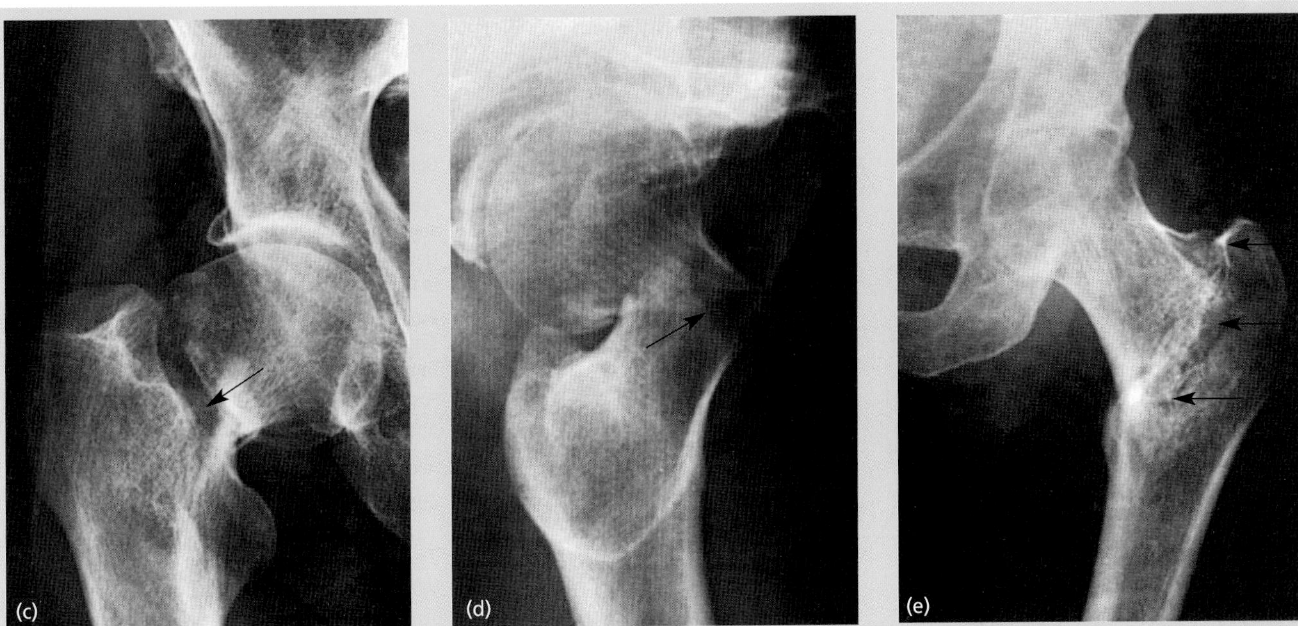

Figure 15.12 (*continued*) (c–e) Intra- and extracapsular fracture of neck of femur (arrows indicate site of fracture)

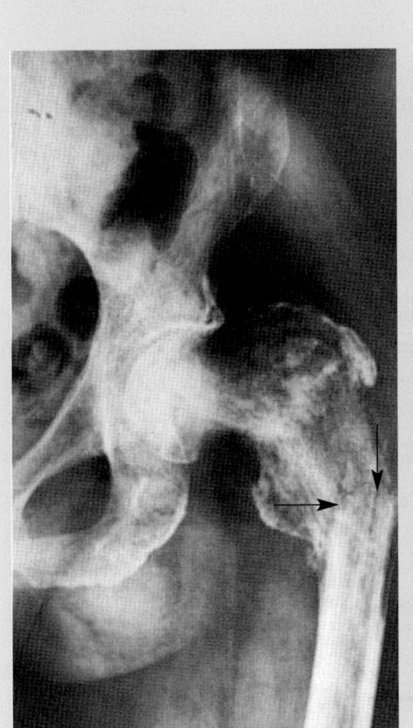

Figure 15.13 Subtrochanteric fracture of femur (arrows)

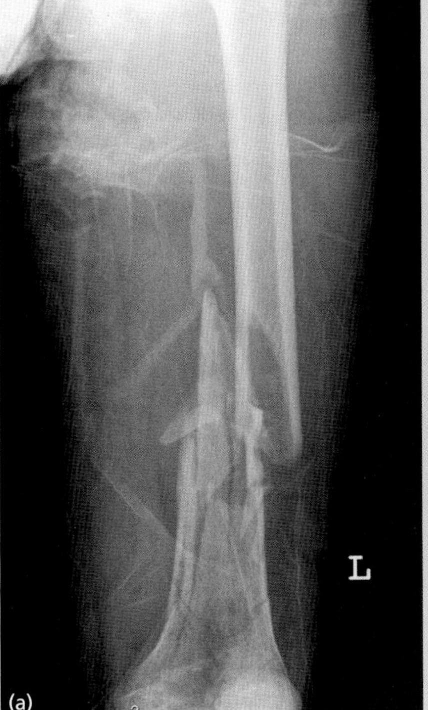

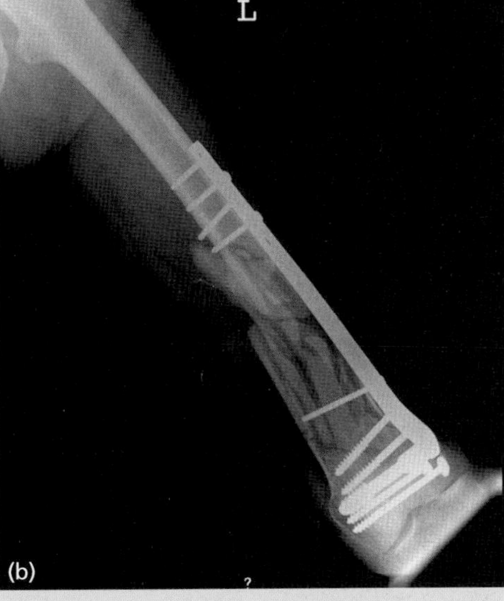

Figure 15.14 (a) and (b) Mid-shaft and lower-third fractures of femur – these often need internal nail fixation or external plates as in (b)

THE HIP JOINT

The **hip joint** is a synovial joint of the ball and socket variety between the head of the femur and the acetabulum. The acetabular articular surface is horseshoe-shaped, being deficient below at the acetabular notch. It is deepened by the fibrocartilaginous **acetabular labrum** (Fig. 15.15), and bridging the acetabular notch is the transverse acetabular ligament. Figure 15.16 shows the surface anatomy of the lateral side of the hip joint.

Ligaments

The **capsule** is strong and dense, attached proximally to the acetabular labrum and rim, distally to the femur along the intertrochanteric line anteriorly and, posteriorly, above the

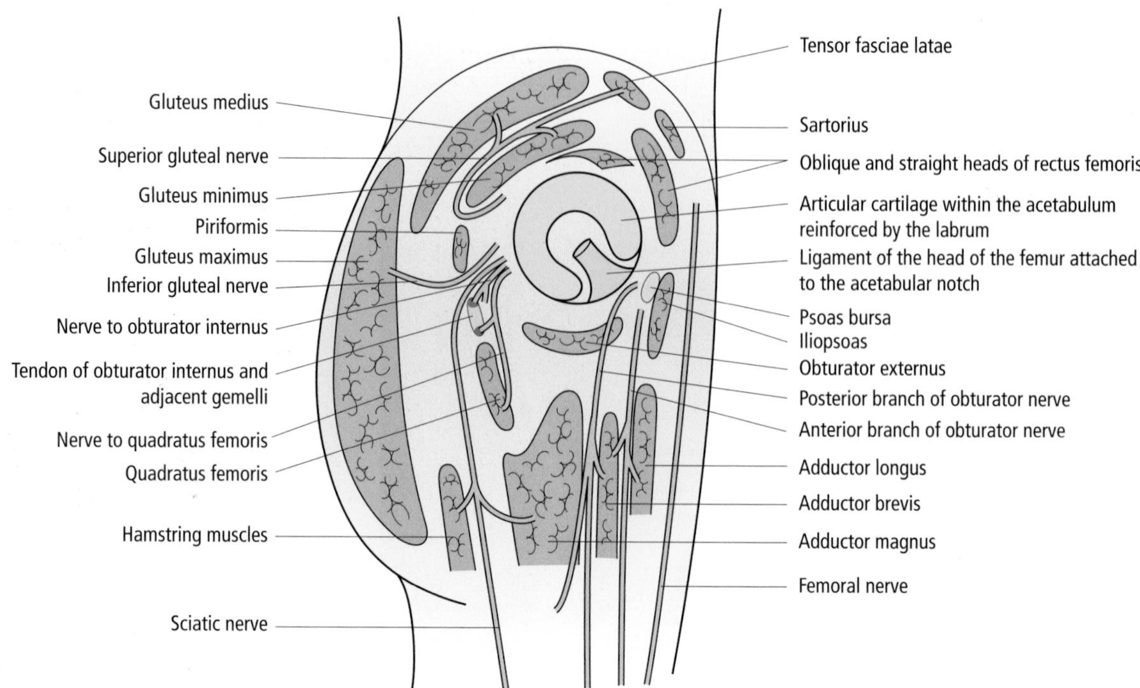

Figure 15.15 Diagram of lateral aspect of the right hip following removal of the femur

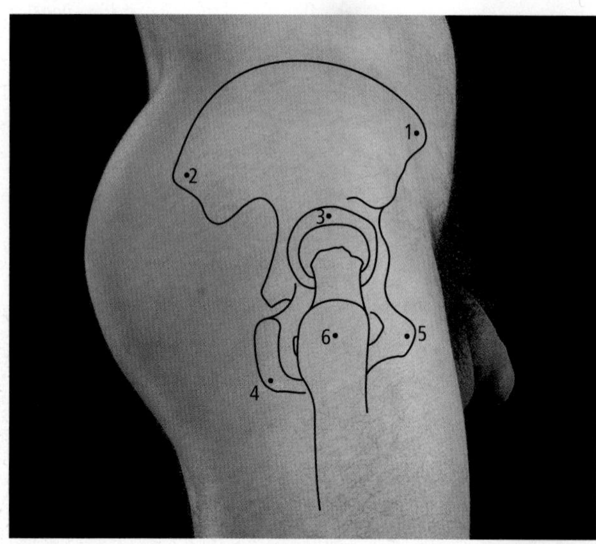

Figure 15.16 Surface anatomy of the pelvis and hip joint: 1, anterior superior iliac spine; 2, posterior superior iliac spine; 3, acetabulum; 4, ischial tuberosity; 5, symphysis pubis; 6, greater trochanter

intertrochanteric crest (Fig. 15.17a–c). In the reflection of the capsule on to the femoral neck are small blood vessels on which depends the nutrition of the femoral head.

The capsule is thickened by strong bands, namely the **iliofemoral ligament**, the **pubofemoral ligament** and the weaker **ischiofemoral ligament**. These three ligaments spiral around the capsule in such a way as to limit extension of the joint.

- The ligament of the head of the femur – this passes from the fovea on the head of the femur to the acetabular notch.
- The acetabular labrum and transverse acetabular ligament.
- The hip joint's synovial cavity may communicate with the psoas bursa.

Functional aspects

Movement

Flexion, extension, abduction, adduction, circumduction and medial and lateral rotation are possible. In the anatomical position the centre of gravity passes behind the axis of the joint, and thus gravity encourages extension of the joint, which is resisted by the capsular thickenings:

- **Flexion** – iliopsoas, helped by tensor fascia lata, rectus femoris and sartorius. Flexion is limited to about 110° by contact with the abdominal wall when the knee is flexed. Flexion is less when the knee is extended because of the tension in the hamstrings.
- **Extension** – limited to about 15–20°, and is by gluteus maximus and hamstrings, assisted by gravity.
- **Abduction** – gluteus medius and minimus, assisted by tensor fascia lata. Abduction occurs during every step in walking thus tilting the pelvis on the femur of the grounded leg to allow the opposite foot to clear the ground as it swings forward (pelvic tilt).

Damage to the abductors or their nerve supply results in a positive Trendelenburg sign, i.e. a patient standing on the affected leg, in the absence of satisfactory abductors, tilts the contralateral hip downwards. Such a disability makes the swing-through phase of walking very difficult and the patient walks with what is referred to as a waddling gait.

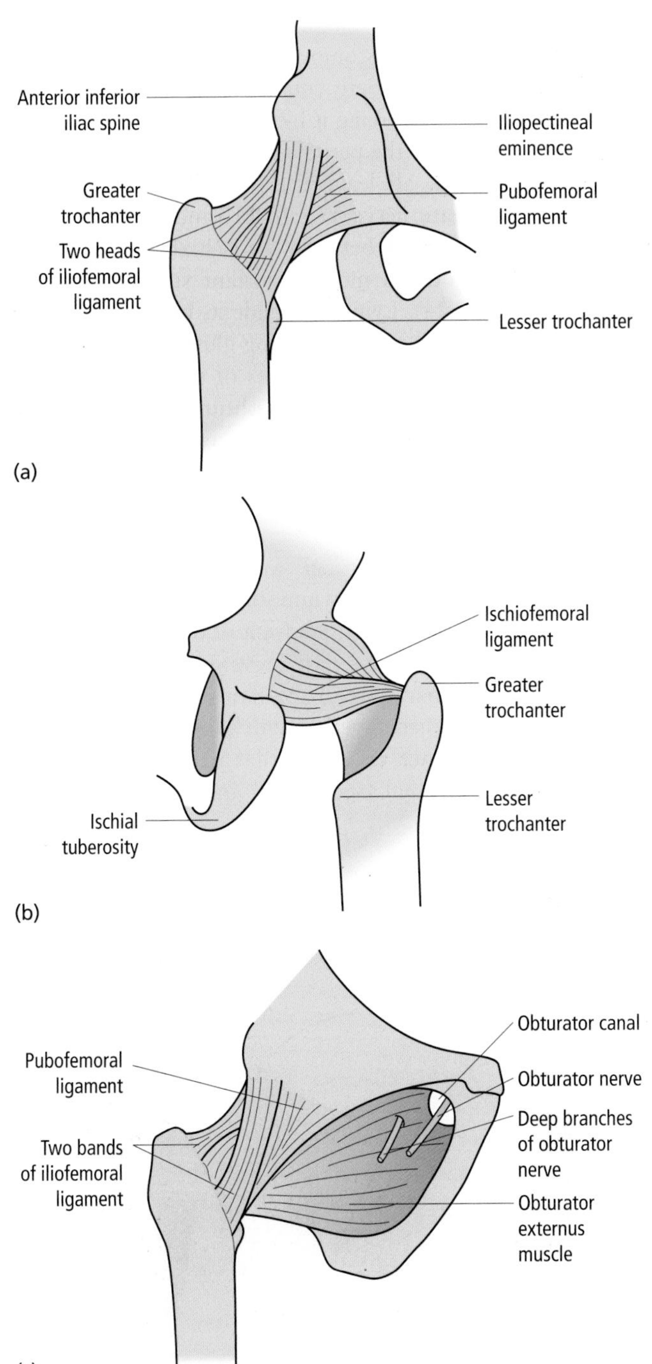

Figure 15.17 Ligaments of right hip joint. (a) Anterior aspect. (b) Posterior aspect of hip joint. (c) Anterior aspect of right hip joint showing obturator externus muscle

- **Adduction** – the thigh adductors and gracilis.
- **Medial rotation** – the adductor magnus, longus and brevis, assisted by iliopsoas.
- **Lateral rotation** – the short posterior muscles: piriformis, the obturator muscles, gemelli, quadratus femoris and gluteus maximus.

Stability

In spite of its great mobility the hip is a stable joint, its stability helped by the deep acetabulum, which clasps the femoral head, the strong capsule and its spiral thickenings, and the closely applied short lateral rotator muscles.

Congenital dislocation of the hip (Fig. 15.18) is associated with a shallow acetabulum. Its incidence is less in babies who are carried astride the back with the hips strongly abducted. A **slipped upper femoral epiphysis** (Fig. 15.19) tends to occur in overweight boys of 10–15 years of age. It presents as a 'coxa vara' deformity, in which the angle of the femoral neck on the shaft is reduced. **Traumatic dislocation** is rare and almost always the result of a posterior force acting on the flexed hip (the joint is least stable when flexed and adducted), such as when the flexed knee hits the dashboard in a car accident. It is usually associated with a fracture of the posterior acetabular rim, and sometimes with injury to the related sciatic nerve. .

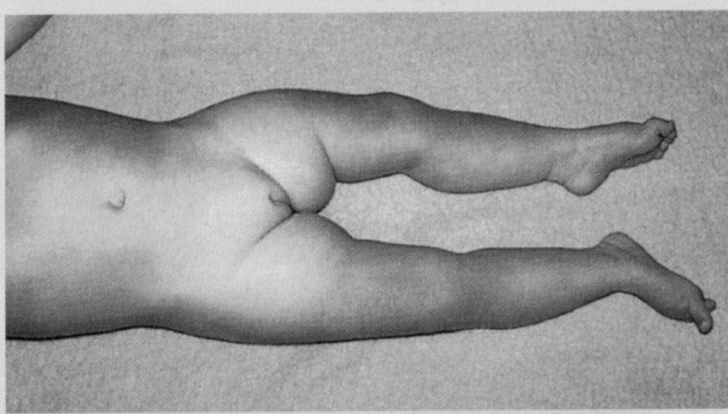

Figure 15.18 Congenital dislocation of left hip – note the extra skin creases in the upper thigh

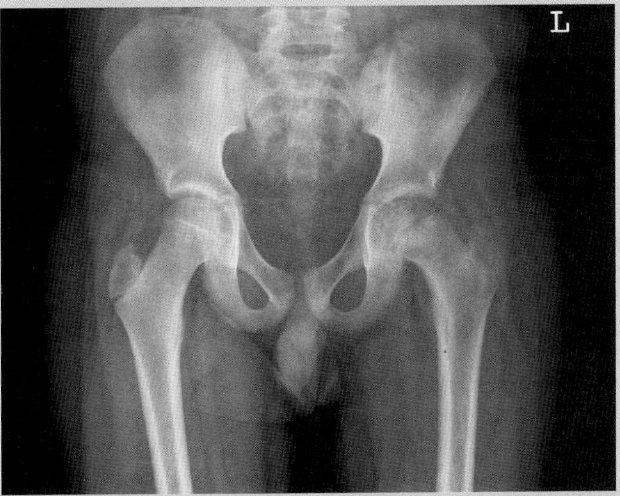

Figure 15.19 Slipped upper femoral epiphysis (left) showing that a line drawn along the upper border of the femoral neck remains superior to the femoral head (left) instead of passing normally through it (right)

Blood supply

This is via anastomoses between the gluteal arteries and branches of the femoral artery. The vessels are conveyed to the joint in reflections of the capsule of the joint (retinacula).

Nerve supply

This is by branches of the femoral, obturator and sciatic nerves.

Relations

Anteriorly, iliopsoas and pectineus muscles separate the joint from the femoral vessels and nerve; posteriorly the short lateral rotators, piriformis, obturator internus, gemelli and quadratus femoris separate the joint from the sciatic nerve. Rectus femoris is superior and obturator externus inferior (Fig. 15.15).

The psoas bursa lies between the iliopsoas tendon and the superior pubic ramus. It may communicate with the hip joint.

THE GLUTEAL REGION

The bulk of the buttock is composed of the three gluteal muscles (Table 15.1 and Fig. 15.20a,b), which overlie smaller rotator muscles of the hip and the nerves and vessels leaving the pelvis for the lower limb. They are supplied by branches of the internal iliac artery; the superior and inferior gluteal arteries traverse gluteus minimus to supply the muscles and contribute to the anastomosis around the hip joint; the internal pudendal artery briefly enters the region by the greater sciatic foramen before leaving it by the lesser sciatic foramen (Fig. 15.21a) to supply the perineum. The nerves, apart from the superior gluteal, all leave the pelvis below piriformis (Fig. 15.15); the **sciatic nerve** (Figs 15.21b and 15.22) emerges below piriformis midway between the ischial tuberosity and the greater trochanter (a most important surface marking; Figs 15.23 and 15.24). Lying alongside it, below piriformis, are the **inferior gluteal nerve** supplying gluteus maximus, the **pudendal nerve** supplying the muscles of the perineum, and the **nerves to quadratus femoris and obturator internus**. The **posterior femoral cutaneous nerve** emerges below piriformis superficial to the sciatic nerve and descends the midline of the thigh. It supplies the skin of the buttock, the perineum, the posterior thigh and the popliteal region.

The muscles of the buttock are frequently used for intramuscular injections. It is important that the needle is inserted into the upper outer quadrant of the buttock as far away as possible from the sciatic nerve. If the sciatic nerve is injured there is paralysis of the hamstrings and all the muscles below the knee, together with a loss of sensation to the skin below the knee, except for that area supplied by the saphenous nerve (medial aspect of leg and foot).

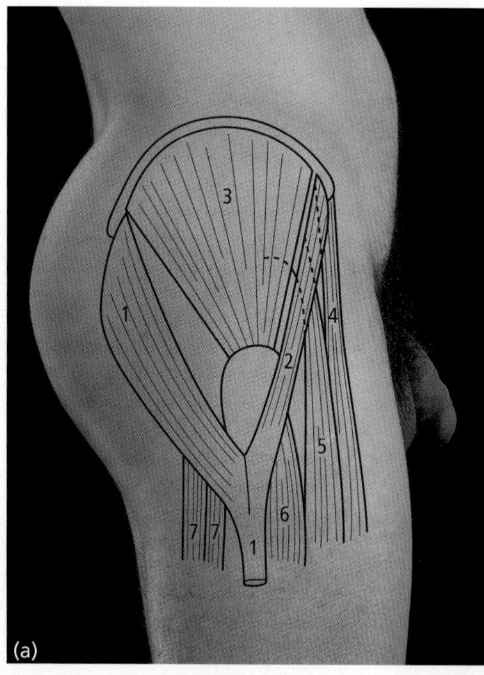

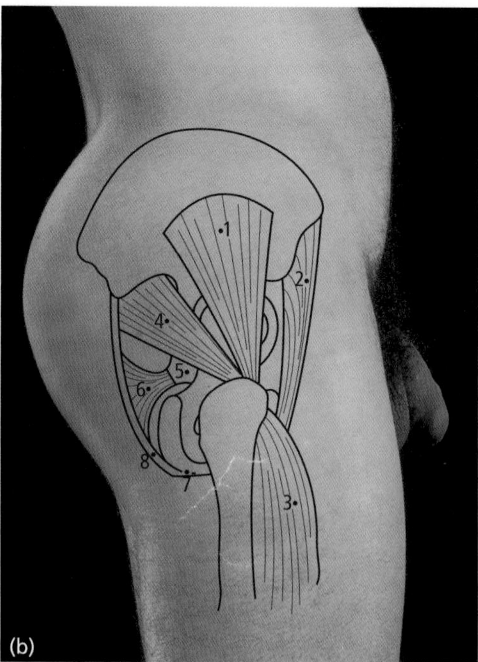

Figure 15.20 Surface anatomy of the gluteal region. (a) Most superficial muscles: 1, gluteus maximus has an extensive origin from pelvis and sacrum, the tendon to femur and iliotibial tract of fasciae latae; 2, tensor fasciae latae; 3, gluteus medius; 4, sartorius; 5, rectus femoris with straight and oblique heads; 6, vastus lateralis; 7, attachments of hamstring muscles to the ischium. (b) Gluteus maximus and medius removed: 1, gluteus minimus; 2, iliacus arising from superior aspect of the ilium; 3, vastus lateralis; 4, piriformis; 5, spine of the ischium; 6, sacrospinous ligament; 7, ischial tuberosity; 8, sacrotuberous ligament

Table 15.1 Muscles of the gluteal region (buttock)

Muscle	Proximal attachments	Distal attachments	Nerve supply	Actions
Gluteus maximus	Postero-external surface ilium and sacrum	Majority of fibres attach to iliotibial tract and some into posterior upper femur	Inferior gluteal nerve (L5, S1, 2)	Extends and assists in lateral rotation of the hip
Tensor fasciae latae	Anterior part of iliac crest	Iliotibial tract, a broad thickening of fasciae latae passing between iliac crest and upper end of tibia	Superior gluteal nerve (L4, 5, S1)	Flexes, abducts hip joint; extends and stabilizes knee joint (by iliotibial tract)
Gluteus medius	Gluteal surface of ilium, deep to gluteus maximus	Greater trochanter of femur	Superior gluteal nerve	Strong abductor and weak medial rotator of hip joint
Gluteus minimus	Gluteal surface of ilium deep to gluteus medius	Greater trochanter of femur	Superior gluteal nerve	Strong abductor and weak medial rotator of hip joint
Piriformis	Anterior surface of sacrum	Greater trochanter of femur	Branches of sacral plexus (S1, 2)	Lateral rotator of the hip joint
Quadratus femoris	Medially attached to the ischial tuberosity	Laterally to the intertrochanteric crest and posterior femur	Branch of sacral plexus (L5, S1)	Stabilization of hip joint; weak lateral rotator
Obturator externus	Outer surface of obturator membrane and adjacent bone	Greater trochanter of femur	Obturator nerve (L2, 3, 4)	Stabilization of hip joint; weak lateral rotator

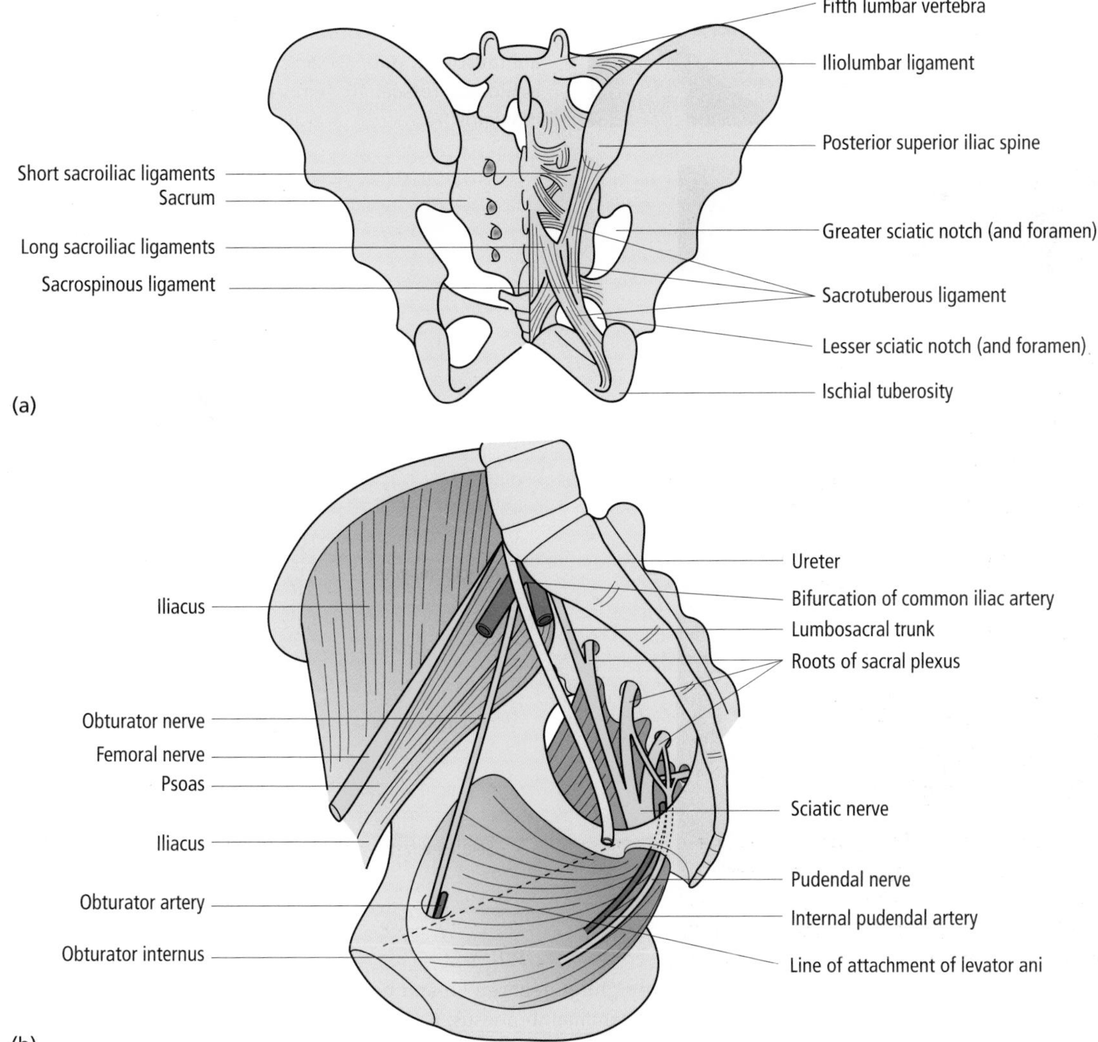

Figure 15.21 (a) Articulated pelvis – posterior aspect showing ligaments. (b) Muscles and nerves of lateral pelvic wall

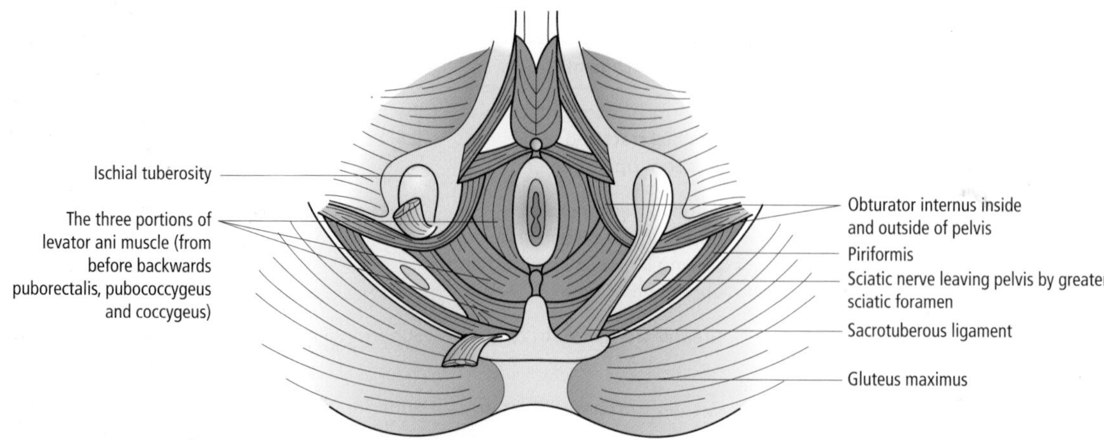

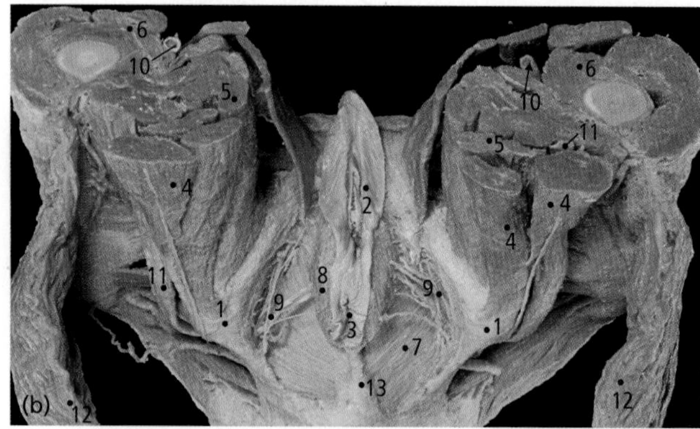

Figure 15.22 (a) Sciatic nerve passing through the male gluteal region from a perineal perspective. (b) Dissection of female perineum, seen in the lithotomy position: 1, ischial tuberosity; 2, labia and vestibule; 3, anus; 4, hamstring muscle group; 5,adductor muscle group; 6, quadriceps muscle group; 7, levator ani muscle; 8, puborectalis; 9, pudendal vessels and nerves in ischioanal fossae; 10, femoral artery; 11, sciatic nerve; 12, gluteus maximus (retracted laterally); 13, anococcygeal ligament

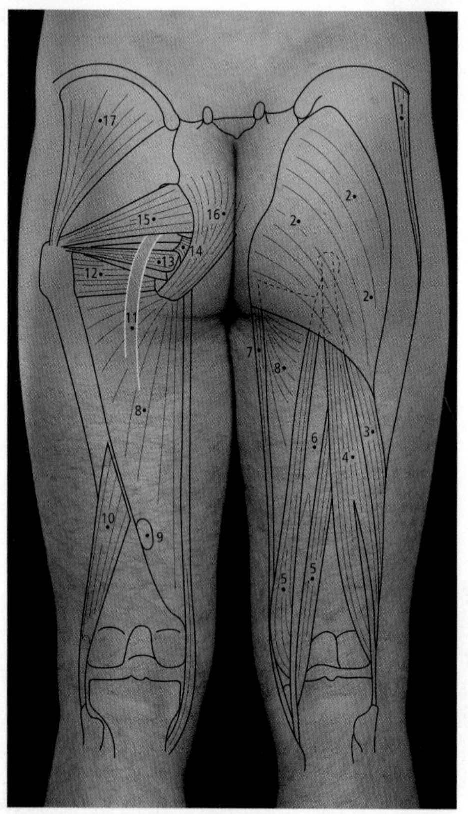

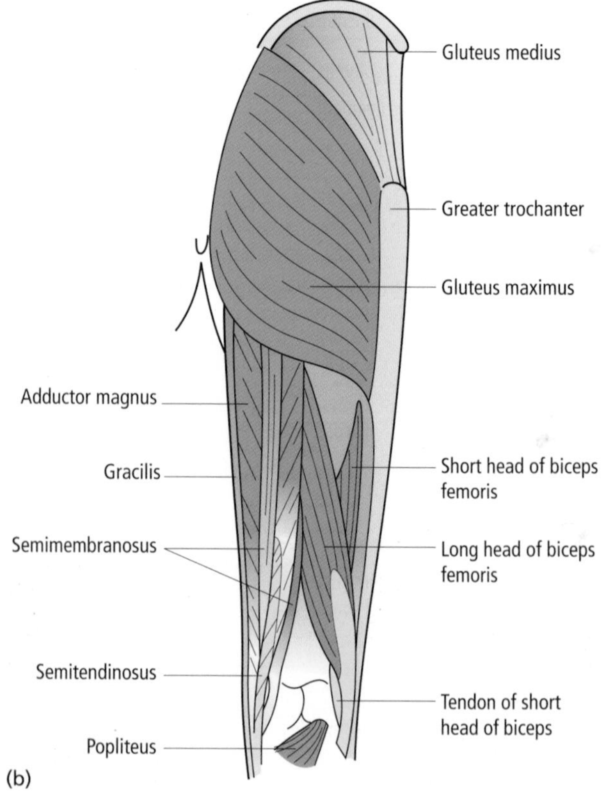

Figure 15.23 (a and b) Surface anatomy of the muscles of the right gluteal region and posterior thigh: 1, tensor fasciae latae; 2, gluteus maximus; 3, vastus lateralis; 4, long head of biceps femoris; 5, semimembranosus; 6, semitendinosus; 7, gracilis; 8, adductor magnus; 9, adductor hiatus; 10, short head of biceps femoris; 11, sciatic nerve; 12, quadratus femoris; 13, obturator internus with the gemelli above and below; 14, sacrospinous ligament; 15, piriformis; 16, sacrotuberous ligament; 17, gluteus medius

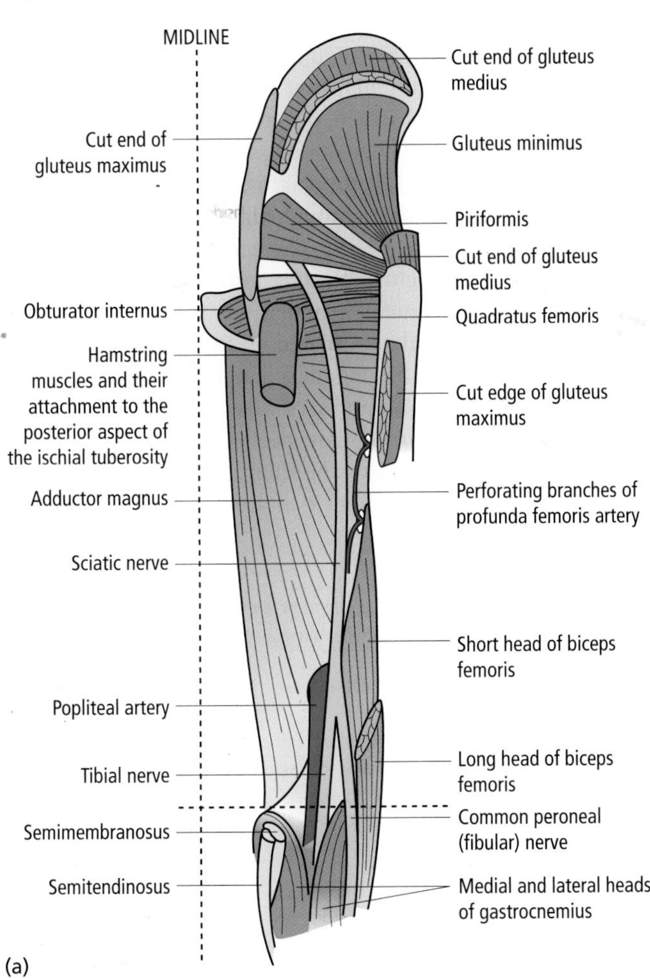

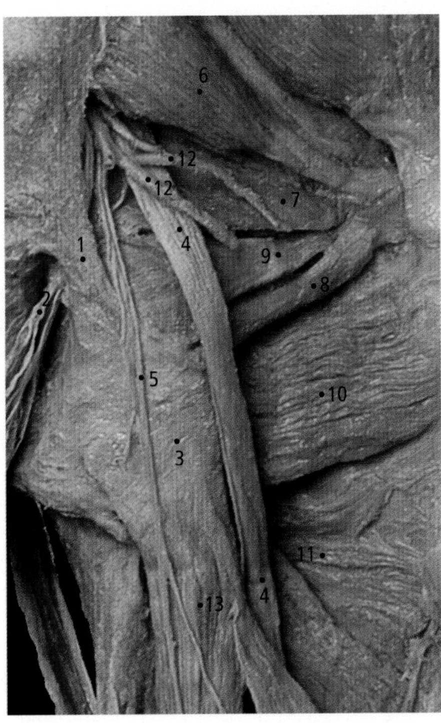

Figure 15.24 (a) Deep muscles of the posterior aspect of the right thigh (horizontal, dashed line shows level of cross section in Fig. 15.25 below). (b) Dissection of posterior thigh and gluteal region with gluteus maximus muscle removed: 1, sacrotuberous ligament; 2, pudendal nerve in ischioanal fossa; 3, ischial tuberosity; 4, sciatic nerve; 5, posterior cutaneous nerve of the thigh; 6, piriformis; 7, superior gemellus; 8, inferior gemellus, 9, obturator internus muscle and tendon; 10, quadratus femoris; 11, adductor magnus; 12, inferior gluteal artery; 13, hamstrings

THE BACK OF THE THIGH

This contains the three hamstring muscles, semimembranosus, semitendinosus and biceps femoris (Table 15.2 and Fig. 15.23), and the sciatic nerve that supplies them. There are no large vessels in the back of the thigh – its contents are supplied by a deeply placed anastomotic chain fed by the gluteal and circumflex femoral arteries above, by the perforating branches of the profunda femoris artery (p. 236), and below by the popliteal artery.

The sciatic nerve

The sciatic nerve, the largest nerve in the body, originates from the lumbosacral plexus (Fig. 15.24) on the anterior surface of piriformis. It descends through the greater sciatic foramen into the gluteal region, and thence through the posterior compartment of the thigh to end just above the popliteal fossa, by dividing into the tibial and common peroneal (fibular) nerves.

Table 15.2 Muscles of the back of the thigh

Muscle	Proximal attachment	Distal attachment	Nerve supply	Actions
Semitendinosus	Ischial tuberosity	Medial surface of upper tibia	Sciatic nerve (L5, S1)	Extends hip; strong flexor of knee. Also imparts slight medial rotation to knee
Semimembranosus	Ischial tuberosity	Posteromedial part of tibial condyle	Sciatic nerve (L5, S1)	Extends hip; strong flexor of knee. Also imparts slight medial rotation to knee
Biceps femoris	Long head: ischial tuberosity Short head: linea aspera and lateral supracondylar line of femur	The two heads join to form a tendon attached to the head of the fibula	Sciatic nerve (S1)	Extends hip; strong flexor of knee. Also imparts lateral rotation to knee

Relations

It enters the gluteal region below piriformis, lying on the ischium and obturator internus and covered by gluteus maximus. In the thigh it is covered by the hamstring muscles and descends on the posterior surface of adductor magnus.

Branches

Muscular – to the hamstrings and the ischial part of adductor magnus; *articular* – to the hip and knee joints and its terminal branches the **tibial** and **common peroneal (fibular) nerves** (Figs 15.24 and 15.25).

THE FRONT AND MEDIAL SIDE OF THE THIGH

Sartorius separates the medially placed adductor muscles (Table 15.3) from the anterior muscles, the quadriceps (Fig. 15.28). Pectineus (Fig. 15.28b) and adductor longus lie anterior to adductor brevis which, in turn, is anterior to the deeply placed adductor magnus. Gracilis lies medial to the other adductors (Fig. 15.28b). (Psoas and iliacus are described on pp. 114 and 125.) The femoral vessels pass deeply towards the femur in the adductor hiatus, leaving the anterior compartment by passing through the adductor hiatus into the popliteal fossa [Fig 15.29]. The femoral nerve has a short course in the thigh before dividing into its several branches, just inferior to the inguinal ligament.

The **femoral triangle** is situated on the front of the upper thigh bounded by the inguinal ligament superiorly, the adductor longus medially and sartorius laterally (Fig. 15.28b). It is floored by adductor longus, pectineus and iliopsoas, and its roof is the fascia lata of the thigh. The roof contains an oval **saphenous opening** about 4 cm below and 1 cm lateral to

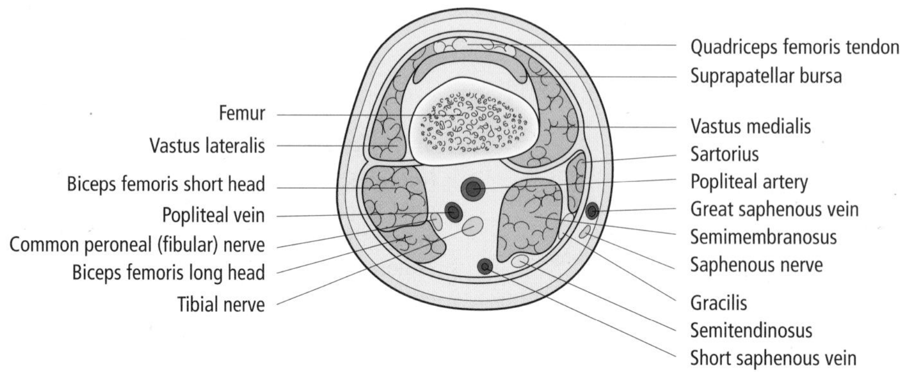

Figure 15.25 Transverse section through the right thigh at the level of the suprapatellar bursa, viewed from below (see dotted line in Fig. 15.24)

Sciatica – pain in the leg extending down from the buttock towards the heel – is caused by pressure on the sciatic nerve or its nerve roots, commonly by intervertebral disc protrusion at the L4/5 or L5/S1 level. The diagnosis is confirmed by noting that straight leg raising is diminished by the pain of the sciatica (Fig. 15.26), that the ankle reflex is absent, and that there is sensory loss over the lateral side of the leg.

'Pulled hamstrings' are very common in athletes who sprint or run explosively, e.g. footballers and squash players. The severe muscular contraction required in this sudden exertion results in tears of the attachment to the ischial tuberosity, causing intramuscular bleeding and pain.

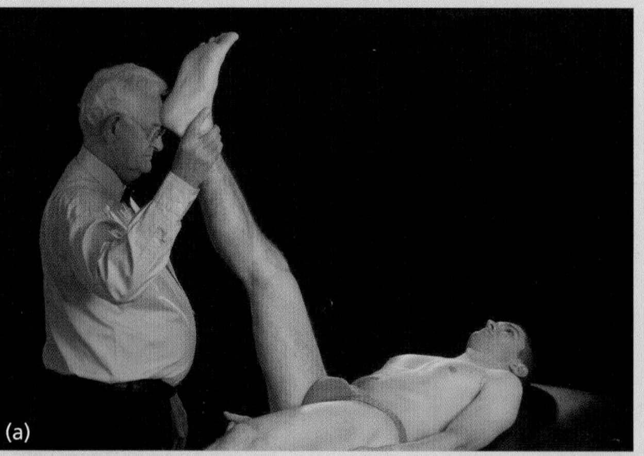

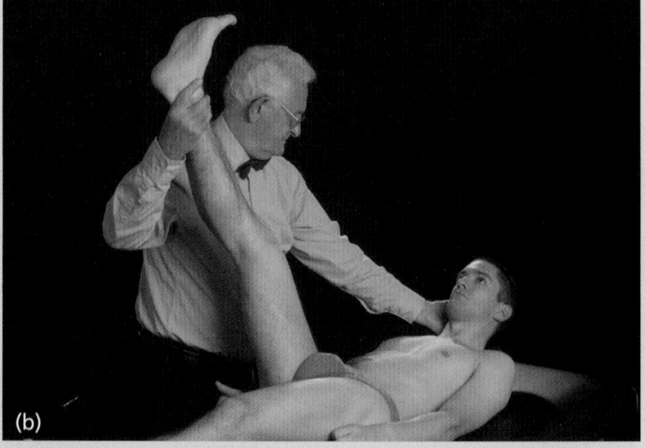

Figure 15.26 Straight leg raising: (a) The straightened leg is flexed at the hip. (b) The sciatic nerve is further stretched by extension of the ankle and neck flexion

the pubic tubercle, which conveys the great saphenous vein. In the triangle are the femoral vessels within the femoral sheath, with the femoral nerve and its branches laterally and outside the sheath. The **femoral sheath** (Fig. 15.27a) is a tube-like prolongation of transversalis fascia into the thigh, invaginated by the femoral vessels as they leave the abdomen. The sheath fuses with the vessels about 3 cm below the inguinal ligament; septa divide it into three compartments containing the femoral artery laterally and the femoral vein centrally and medially, the space known as the **femoral canal**, which contains fatty tissue and lymph nodes. The femoral canal communicates superiorly with the extraperitoneal tissue via a firm non-distensible **femoral ring**, which is bounded anteriorly by the inguinal ligament, medially by the pectineal part of the inguinal ligament, posteriorly by the thin pectineus muscle and pectineal ligament overlying the pubis, and laterally by the femoral vein.

The boundaries of the ring are of considerable clinical importance; as when herniation of abdominal contents into the femoral canal occurs the ring often provides a site of constriction for the contents of the hernial sac. Femoral herniae are rather more common in women because of their wider pelvis and larger femoral ring. They can be distinguished from inguinal herniae by their situation: they present **below** the inguinal ligament as a palpable, sometimes visible lump in the region of the saphenous opening, below and lateral to the pubic tubercle. They become subcutaneous by passing through the saphenous opening.

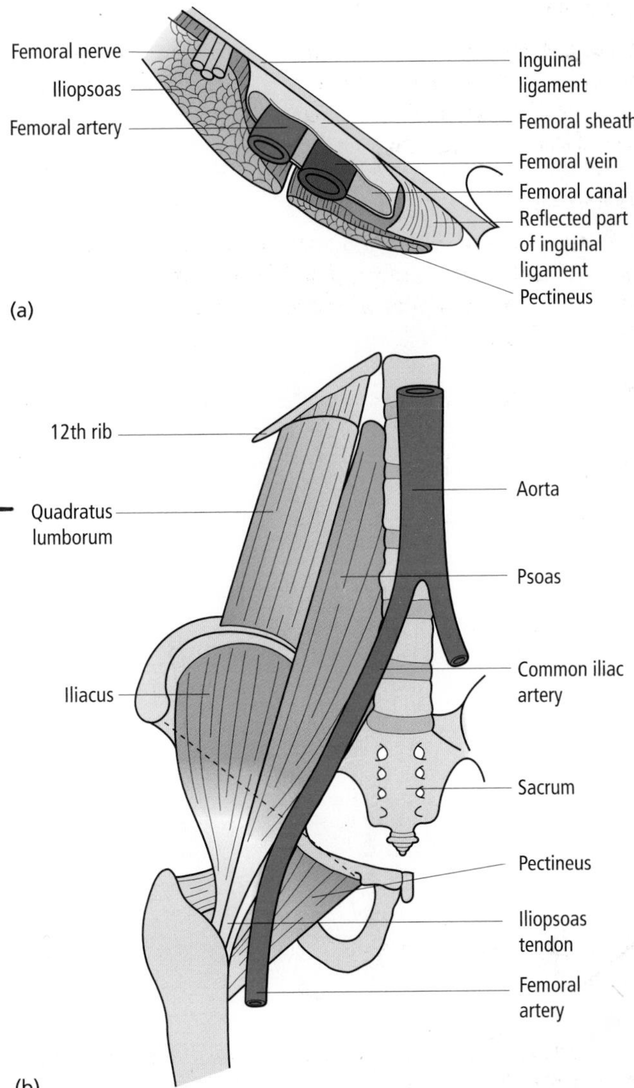

Figure 15.27 (a) Femoral sheath. (b) Deep thigh muscles showing path of femoral artery into the thigh. The dashed line marks the course of the inguinal ligament

ANTERIOR GROUP OF THIGH MUSCLES

Sartorius is a long strap-like muscle that passes obliquely and medially down the thigh. The quadriceps is a large muscle mass forming the bulk of the anterior region of the thigh. The mass is divided into four separate muscles, each of which gains attachment to the patella (Table 15.4). The four parts of quadriceps are attached to the upper border and side margins in a single musculotendinous expansion. From the

Table 15.3 The adductor muscles

Muscle	Proximal attachment	Distal attachment	Nerve supply	Actions
Pectineus	Superior aspect of pubis	Posterior femur below the lesser trochanter	Femoral nerve as well as obturator (L2, 3, 4)	A weak adductor and flexor of the hip
Adductor longus	Anterior body of pubis	Linea aspera of femur	Obturator nerve (L2, 3, 4)	Adductor of the hip, medial rotation of the femur
Adductor brevis	Body and inferior ramus of pubis	Upper half of linea aspera	Obturator nerve	Adductor of the hip, medial rotation of the femur
Adductor magnus	A wide attachment to outer surface ischiopubic ramus and ischial tuberosity	Gluteal tuberosity, whole length of linea aspera, the medial supracondylar line and, by a tendon, into the adductor tubercle of the femur	Obturator nerve	A strong adductor, medial rotation of femur; plus extension of the hip
Gracilis	Lower border of ischiopubic ramus	Upper part of medial surface of tibia	Obturator nerve	A weak adductor of the hip

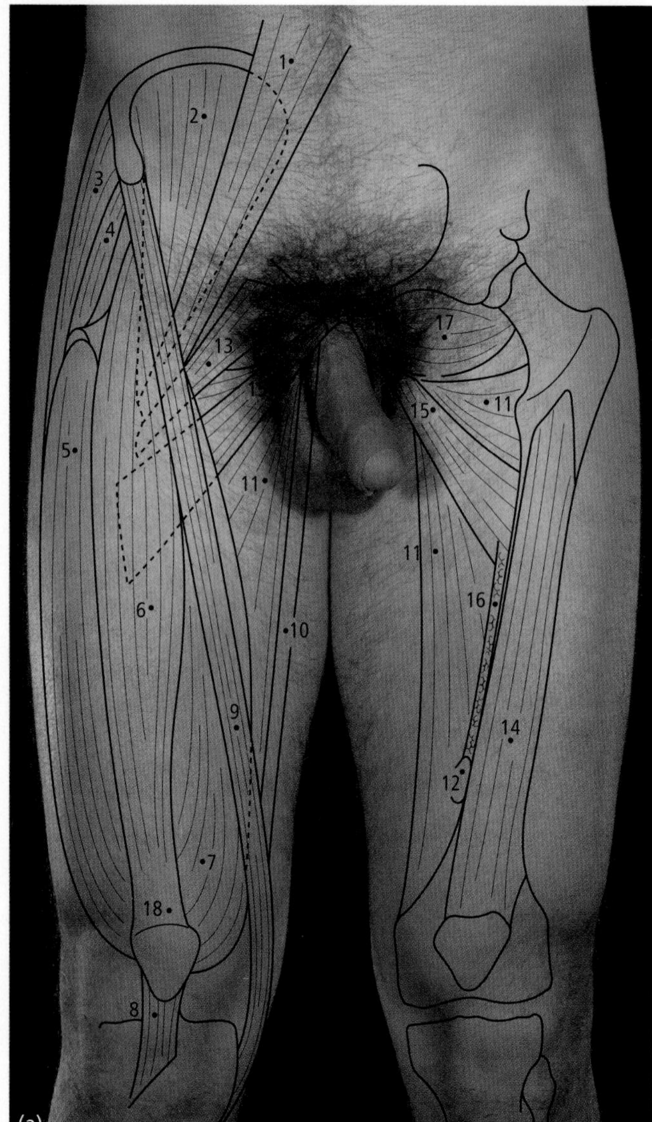

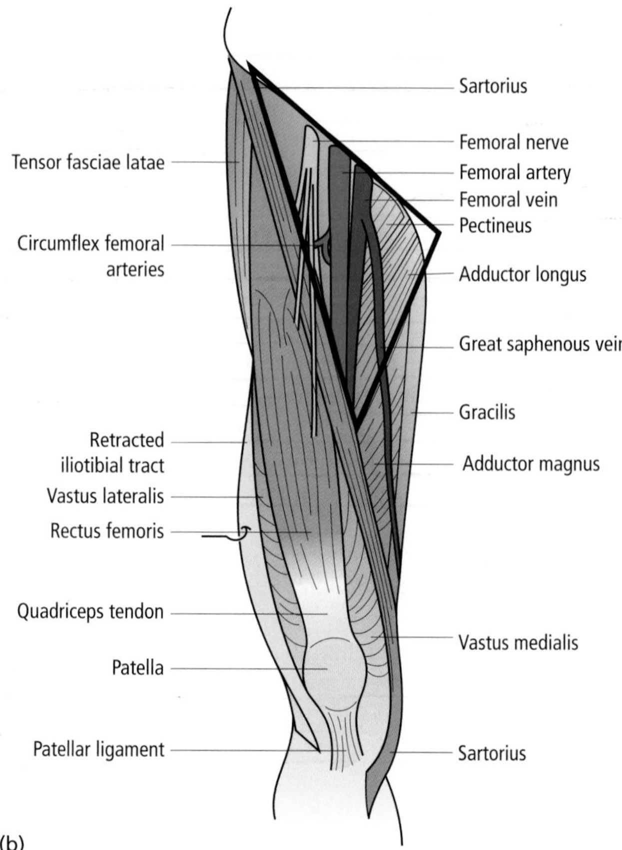

Figure 15.28 (a) Anterior aspect of thigh, showing superficial and deep muscles and femoral triangle: 1, psoas; 2, iliacus; 3, tensor fasciae latae; 4, gluteus medius; 5, vastus lateralis; 6, rectus femoris; 7, vastus medialis; 8, patellar ligament; 9, sartorius; 10, gracilis; 11, adductor magnus; 12, adductor hiatus; 13, pectineus; 14, vastus intermedialis; 15, adductor brevis; 16, adductor longus (central part of muscle excised on the left side); 17, obturator externus; 18, quadriceps tendon. (b) Anterior aspect of the thigh and femoral triangle (outlined)

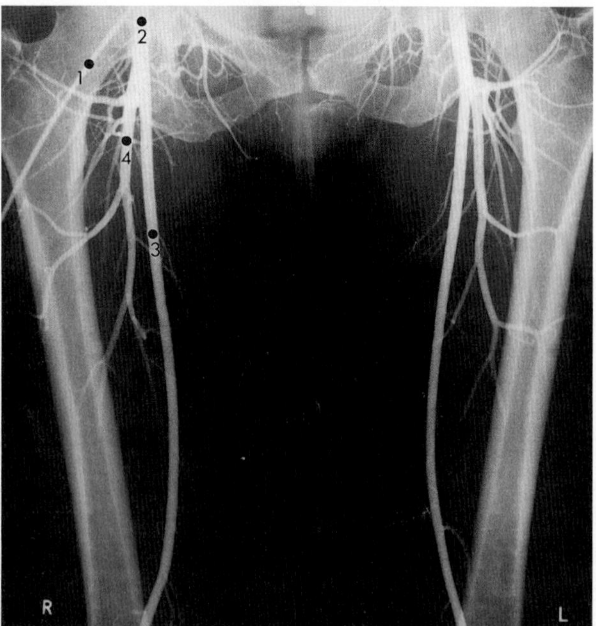

Figure 15.29 Femoral angiogram: 1, catheter; 2, femoral artery in groin; 3, femoral artery in adductor canal; 4, profunda femoris artery

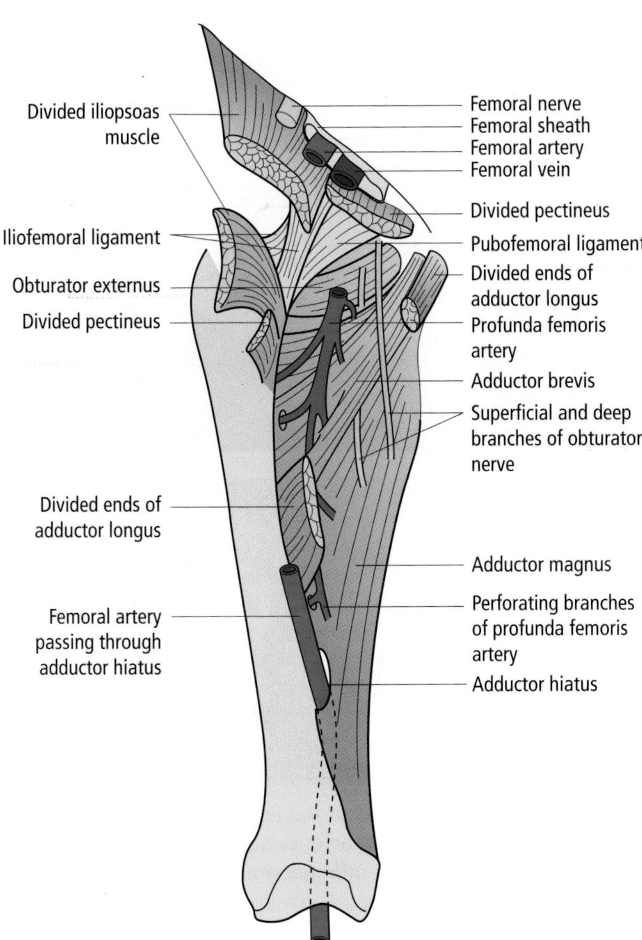

Figure 15.30 Deep aspect of medial thigh and relations of profunda femoris artery

apex of the patella the strong **patellar ligament** (ligamentum patellae) descends to become attached to the tibial tubercle. On each side of the patellar tendon the capsule of the joint is strengthened by fibrous expansions (retinacula) of the quadriceps.

BLOOD SUPPLY

The femoral artery

The femoral artery (Figs 15.27b, 15.30 and 15.31) is the continuation of the external iliac artery below the inguinal ligament. It descends vertically through the femoral triangle (Fig. 15.28b) and adductor canal to leave the latter by an opening in the adductor magnus (adductor hiatus) on the medial side of the lower femur.

Relations

At its origin it is deep to the inguinal ligament, halfway between the anterior superior iliac spine and the symphysis pubis (midinguinal point). In the femoral triangle it is palpable, being covered only by deep fascia and skin; the femoral vein lies medial to it. It leaves the triangle at its apex on adductor longus and enters the **adductor canal** with its vein and the saphenous nerve (p. 237); within the canal it is deep to sartorius. Three to four centimetres above the adductor tubercle of the femur the artery passes through the opening in the tendon of adductor magnus (adductor hiatus) to enter the popliteal fossa as the popliteal artery.

Table 15.4 Anterior thigh muscles

Muscle	Proximal attachment	Distal attachment	Nerve supply	Actions
Sartorius	Anterior superior iliac spine	Upper part of medial surface of tibia	Femoral nerve (L2, 3, 4)	Weak flexor abductor and lateral rotator of hip and knee flexor
Quadriceps				
a) Rectus femoris	By two heads:	By a single tendon into the upper border of the patella	Femoral nerve	Powerful extensor of the knee; flexor of the hip
	a) anterior inferior iliac spine			
	b) ilium, just above the acetabulum			
b) Vastus medialis	By a wide aponeurosis to lesser trochanter linea aspera and medial supracondylar line of femur	To medial side of patella; some of its lower fibres are horizontal	Femoral nerve	Powerful extensor of the knee. Prevention of lateral dislocation of the patella by its horizontal fibres
c) Vastus lateralis	The greater trochanter and the linea aspera	The lateral side of the patella	Femoral nerve	Powerful extensor of the knee
d) Vastus intermedius	The anterior and lateral surfaces of the shaft of the femur	The upper border of the patella	Femoral nerve	Powerful extensor of the knee

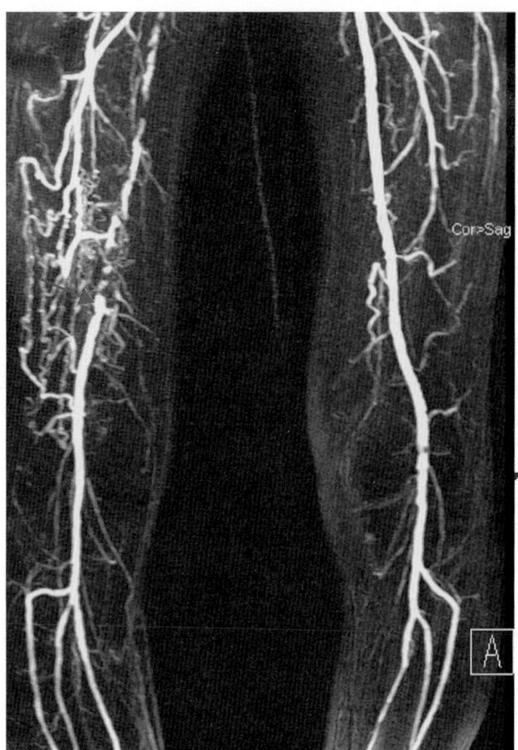

Figure 15.31 MR angiogram showing right femoral artery atherosclerosis, occlusion and narrowing, especially marked at the adductor hiatus (arrow)

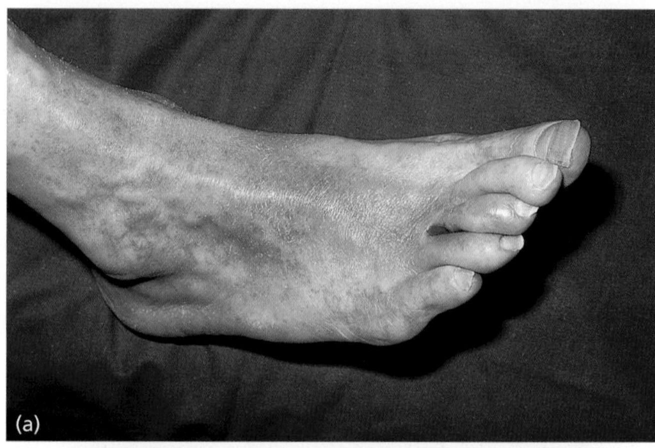

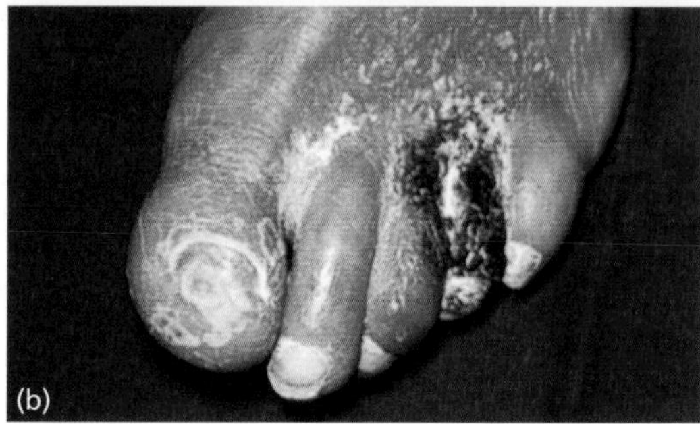

Figure 15.32 Ischaemic changes of the feet due to peripheral vascular disease blocking distal arteries: (a) ischaemic ulcer between third and fourth toes; (b) gangrenous fourth toe

Branches

Just as the artery enters the femoral triangle it gives off three small branches to the skin of the lower abdominal wall and the inguinal region. The **profunda femoris artery** (Fig. 15.30) is the largest of its branches; it arises in the femoral triangle and descends close to the femur between the adductor muscles, giving off three or four perforating branches that pierce adductor magnus and supply the posterior part of the thigh, and contribute to anastomoses with branches of the popliteal artery. The **medial** and **lateral circumflex femoral arteries** encircle the upper femur and supply muscles and the hip joint, and contribute to the anastomoses around the femur and hip joint.

The femoral artery is very accessible in the femoral triangle; its pulsation is readily found below the midinguinal point, and first-aiders are taught to use it as a pressure point for the control of haemorrhage from the leg. Radiologists frequently use it for arterial catheterization, and clinicians for sampling arterial blood.

The femoral artery is one of the commonest sites of peripheral arterial disease, the artery becoming blocked beyond the origin of profunda femoris down to the adductor hiatus (Fig. 15.31). The decrease in blood supply affects particularly the muscles of the calf, and exercise pain (intermittent claudication) may result. In more severe cases it results in ischaemic ulceration of the skin (Fig. 15.32).

The numerous branches of the femoral artery, but especially the medial circumflex femoral with contribution from the gluteal arteries, make a rich anastomosis around the hip joint, most branches of which pass to the head of femur via the retinacular fibres of the neck. A small branch of the obturator artery passes into the head of femur, and is considered more important in children.

The femoral vein

The femoral vein begins at the opening in the lower end of adductor magnus as the continuation of the popliteal vein. It ascends with the femoral artery to end under the inguinal ligament, as the external iliac vein. At first it lies behind the artery, but ends on its medial side.

The femoral vein is easily accessible on the medial side of the femoral artery. It is frequently used for venous access in shocked patients with a low blood pressure and collapsed veins.

Tributaries

The **profunda femoris vein** and the **medial** and **lateral femoral circumflex veins** have a similar course to their arteries. The **great saphenous vein,** which drains the skin and subcutaneous tissues of much of the leg and thigh (p. 220), pierces the deep fascia over the saphenous opening in the roof of the femoral triangle to enter the femoral vein.

NERVES

The **femoral nerve** (Fig. 15.28b) is a branch of the upper part (L2, 3, 4) of the lumbosacral plexus (p. 116). It descends in the pelvis between iliacus and psoas, entering the thigh under the inguinal ligament lateral to the femoral artery and outside the femoral sheath. In the femoral triangle it immediately divides into terminal branches:

- **Cutaneous nerves** – supply skin on the medial and anterior aspect of the thigh.
- **Saphenous nerve** – the longest branch of the femoral nerve (L4) accompanies the femoral artery until the adductor hiatus, at which point it emerges from the adductor canal medial to sartorius to descend on the medial side of the knee. In the leg it entwines around the great saphenous vein to pass anterior to the medial malleolus. It supplies the skin over the medial side of the leg and foot.

It is often damaged when varicose veins are stripped, causing diminished and altered sensation over the medial ankle region.

- **Muscular branches** – to pectineus, sartorius and quadriceps.

The **obturator nerve** is a branch of the lumbosacral plexus (L2, 3, 4), whose pelvic course is described on p. 116. It enters the thigh through the obturator foramen, where it divides into anterior and posterior branches to supply all the adductors and pectineus, except the lateral half of adductor magnus (sciatic nerve). Its cutaneous branches supply the skin over the medial thigh above the knee.

MCQs

1. The femoral nerve supplies: **T/F**

- **a** gluteus minimus muscle (___)
- **b** rectus femoris (___)
- **c** the skin over the lateral malleolus (___)
- **d** iliacus muscle (___)
- **e** pectineus muscle (___)

Answers

1.

a ***F*** – *Gluteus minimus is supplied by the superior gluteal nerve.*

b ***T***

c ***F*** – *The femoral nerve supplies the skin over the lower medial part of the leg and medial malleolus via its saphenous branch (L4).*

d ***T***

e ***T***

---

2. The hip joint: **T/F**

- **a** is supplied by the nerve to rectus femoris (___)
- **b** is supplied by the nerve to quadratus femoris (___)
- **c** is supplied by the obturator nerve (___)
- **d** has a posterior capsule attached to the greater trochanter (___)
- **e** is supported most strongly by the ischiofemoral ligament (___)

Answers

2.

a ***T*** – *Hilton's law states that a joint receives its nerve supply from the same nerves that innervate …*

b ***T*** – *… muscles acting across that joint. Hence the hip joint is innervated by the femoral, obturator, …*

c ***T*** – *… the sciatic, and the nerve to quadratus femoris.*

d ***F*** – *The capsule of the hip joint is attached anteriorly to the trochanters and the intertrochanteric line between but posteriorly it is attached halfway along the femoral neck.*

e ***F*** – *The ischiofemoral ligament is not as strong as the inverted Y-shaped iliofemoral ligament, which passes from the anterior inferior iliac spine to each end of the intertrochanteric line.*

---

3. In the midthigh region the: **T/F**

- **a** floor of the adductor canal is adductor magnus (___)
- **b** roof of the adductor canal laterally is the vastus medialis (___)
- **c** femoral artery lies medial to its vein (___)
- **d** iliotibial tract lies along the medial aspect (___)
- **e** gracilis muscle is often supplied by the femoral nerve (___)

Answers

3.

a ***F*** – *The adductor canal (or subsartorial canal) is found medially in the middle third of the thigh. It commences at the apex of the femoral triangle and lies on adductor longus; it finishes below at the hiatus in the adductor magnus.*

b ***T*** – *Sartorius forms the medial roof.*

c ***T*** – *The contents of this canal are the femoral artery and vein, with the terminal cutaneous branch of the femoral nerve, the saphenous nerve and, occasionally, the nerve to vastus medialis and a sensory branch of the obturator nerve. The nerves lie anterior, the artery medial and the vein laterally.*

d ***F*** – *This notable thickening of the fascia lata lies along the lateral thigh from its proximal attachment to the tensor fasciae latae muscle to its distal attachment to the lateral condyle of the tibia.*

e ***F*** – *gracilis is a member of the adductor group of muscles and innervated by the obturator nerve. It is also a weak flexor of the knee joint.*

EMQs

Each question has an anatomical theme linked to the chapter, and a list of 10 related items (A–J) placed in alphabetical order: these are followed by five statements (1–5). Match **one or more** of the items A–J to each of the five statements.

Muscles of the hip and thigh

A. Adductor longus
B. Adductor magnus
C. Biceps femoris
D. Gluteus maximus
E. Obturator externus
F. Pectineus
G. Piriformis
H. Semitendinosus
I. Tensor fascia lata
J. Vastus lateralis

Match the following statement to the muscle(s) in the above list.

1. Transmits the femoral artery
2. Forms the floor of the femoral triangle
3. Attached to the head of the fibula
4. Attached to the anteromedial upper tibia
5. Attached to the iliotibial tract

Answers

1 B; 2 AF; 3 C; 4 H; 5 DI

Nerves of the hip and thigh

A. Adductor longus
B. Adductor magnus
C. Biceps femoris
D. Gluteus maximus
E. Obturator externus
F. Pectineus
G. Piriformis
H. Semitendinosus
I. Tensor fascia lata
J. Vastus lateralis

Match the following nerves to the muscle(s) in the above list.

1. Sciatic
2. Femoral
3. Lumbar plexus
4. Obturator
5. Superior gluteal

Answers

1 CH; 2 FJ; 3 ABEFJ; 4 ABEF; 5 I

APPLIED QUESTIONS

1. A butcher's knife slips and plunges into his thigh at the apex of the femoral triangle. Why is this likely to be particularly bloody?

1. Not only are the femoral artery and vein endangered as they pass down the front of the thigh towards the subsartorial canal, but also their branches and tributaries. Midway down the thigh a knife piercing sartorius and the femoral vessels also lacerates adductor longus, a fairly thin muscle, and may damage the profunda femoris vessels on its deep surface. The injury is therefore very bloody owing to damage to two large arteries and their accompanying veins.

2. An infected cut on the heel causes tenderness in which lymph nodes?

2. Lymph from the superficial tissues of the heel runs in the lymphatics that follow one or other of the saphenous veins. Those following the great saphenous vein eventually drain to the vertically disposed groups of superficial inguinal nodes around the termination of the vein, in the groin. The lymph vessels following the small saphenous vein pierce the deep fascia in the popliteal fossa and enter the popliteal nodes. From here lymph passes to the deep inguinal nodes around the femoral vein in the femoral triangle.

16 The knee, leg and dorsum of the foot

OSTEOLOGY

The **patella** (Fig. 16.1) is a sesamoid bone, triangular in shape with its apex inferior. Its anterior surface is subcutaneous; the posterior is smooth, with a smaller medial and a larger lateral facet for articulation with the femoral condyles. The quadriceps tendon is attached to the upper border and the patellar tendon or ligament to the apex; muscle fibres from vastus medialis are attached to its medial border and tendinous expansions from the vastus medialis and lateralis (retinacula) are attached to the medial and lateral borders, and also to the neighbouring tibial condyles. In the standing position the lower border of the patella lies slightly proximal to the level of the knee joint.

The **tibia** (Fig. 16.2a–d) is a long bone possessing an upper end, a shaft and a lower end. The **upper end** is expanded by the medial and lateral condyles and flattened superiorly forming the **tibial plateau** with oval medial and lateral facets articulating with the femoral condyles. Between the articular facets is a rough intercondylar area which gives attachment to the two menisci and the anterior and posterior cruciate ligaments. The prominent anterior **tibial tuberosity** below the superior surface provides attachment for the patellar tendon; semimembranosus is attached along the side of the medial condyle. Beneath the lateral condyle is the articular facet for the head of the fibula.

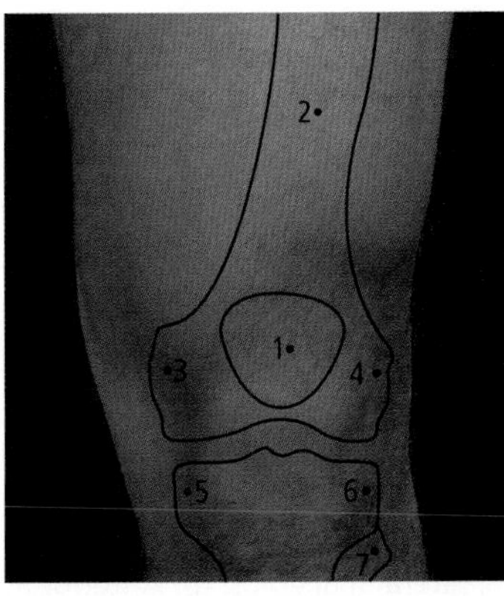

Figure 16.1 Surface anatomy of the bones of the knee: 1, patella; 2, femur; 3, medial femoral condyle; 4, lateral femoral condyle; 5, medial tibial condyle; 6, lateral tibial condyle; 7, head of fibula

The **shaft** is triangular in section with medial, lateral and posterior surfaces. The upper part of the medial surface gives attachment to the tibial collateral ligament of the knee joint and to sartorius, gracilis and semitendinosus (see Fig. 16.23b,c, p. 255); more distally the medial surface and sharp anterior border lie subcutaneously. To the lateral surface is attached tibialis anterior. The posterior surface is crossed by an oblique ridge, the **soleal line**, which gives attachment to soleus; to the surface above the line is attached popliteus, and to the area below the line tibialis posterior and flexor digitorum longus. The interosseous membrane is attached to a sharp ridge on the lateral border. The expanded lower end has a medial projection, the **medial malleolus**; its distal surface, together with the lateral surface of the malleolus, articulates with the talus. The posterior border of the lower end is grooved medially by the tendon of tibialis posterior. To the roughened lateral surface is attached the interosseous ligament of the inferior tibiofibular joint. The tibial condyles, its anterior border, the medial surface and the medial malleolus are palpable (Fig. 16.2a).

Because of the bone's subcutaneous position, tibial shaft fractures due to direct trauma are frequently associated with skin wounds (compound fractures) (Fig. 16.3a,d) and are therefore prone to infection and poor union.

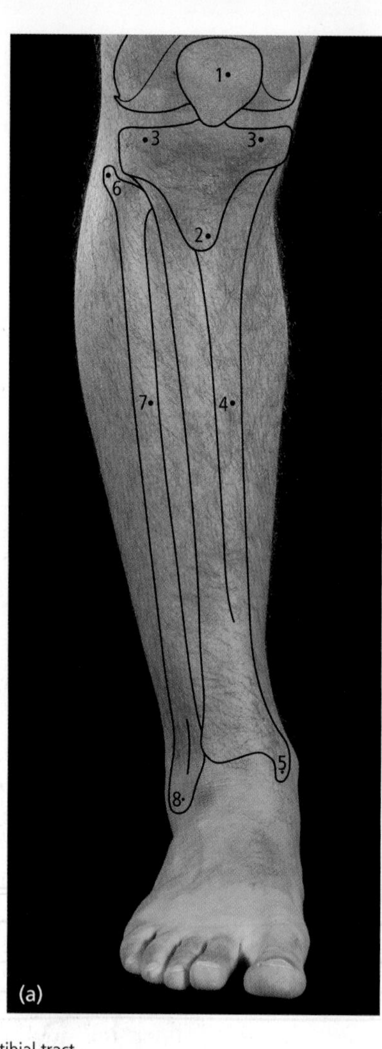

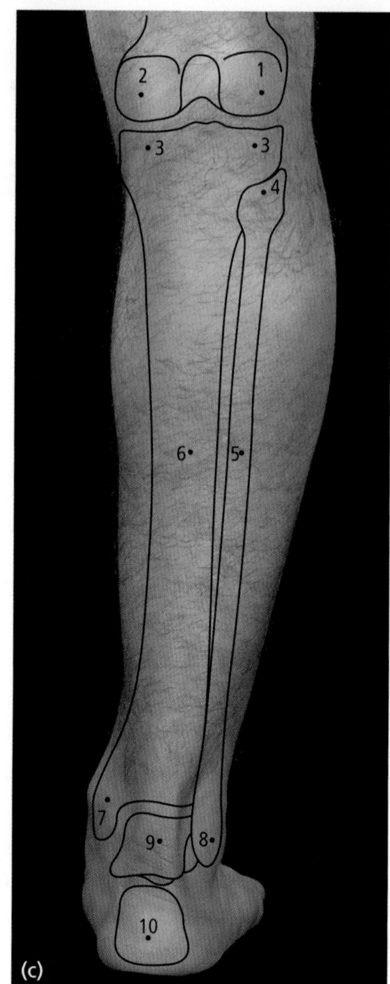

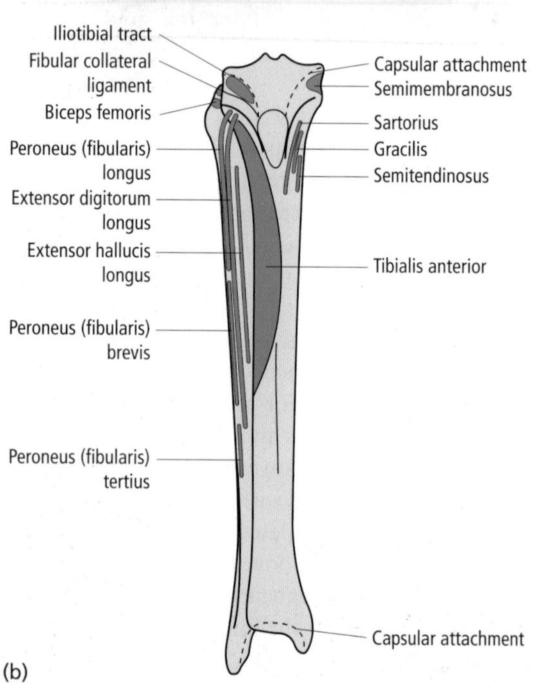

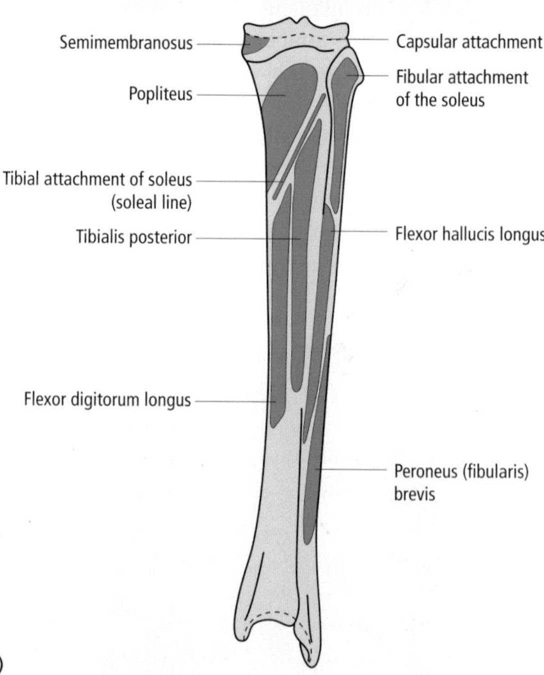

Figure 16.2 (a) Surface anatomy of bones of the leg, anterior aspect: 1, patella; 2, tibial tuberosity; 3, tibial plateau; 4, anterior subcutaneous surface of tibia; 5, medial malleolus; 6, head of fibula; 7, shaft of fibula; 8, lateral malleolus. (b) Anterior aspect of tibia and fibula: muscle and capsular attachments. (c) Surface anatomy of bones of the leg, posterior aspect: 1, lateral femoral condyle; 2, medial femoral condyle; 3, tibial plateau; 4, head of fibula; 5, shaft of fibula; 6, shaft of tibia; 7, medial malleolus; 8, lateral malleolus; 9, talus; 10, calcaneus. (d) Posterior aspect of tibia and fibula: muscle and capsular attachments

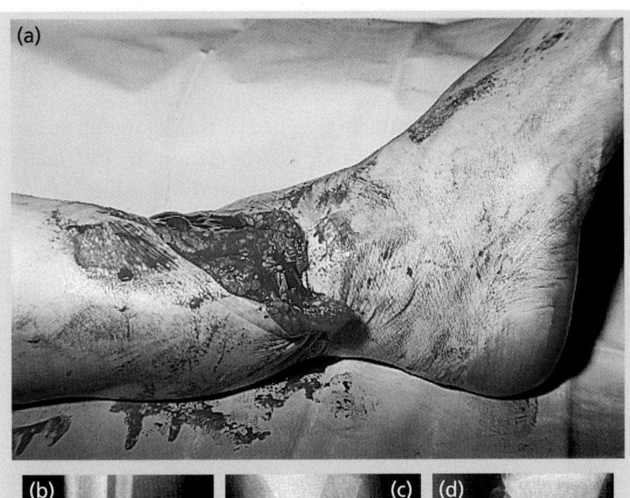

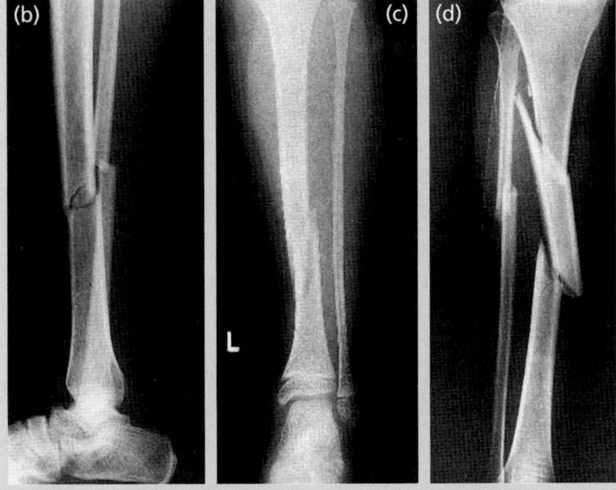

Figure 16.3 (a) Fractured shaft of tibia with compound wound. (b) Transverse fracture. (c) Spiral fracture. (d) Comminuted fracture of the tibia

The **fibula** (Fig. 16.2a,b) is a long bone with a head, a shaft and a lower end. It carries no weight but gives attachment to many muscles. The expanded **head** has an oval articular facet for the tibia; to its apex is attached the fibular collateral ligament of the knee joint and biceps tendon. The common peroneal nerve lying within peroneus longus is in close proximity to the neck of the fibula just below the head of the bone and can be palpated here. It is liable to damage by tight bandaging or a tight plaster cast. The **shaft** is long and slender; to its narrow anterior surface are attached the extensor muscles, to the posterior surface are attached the flexor muscles, and to the lateral surface the peroneal muscles. The expanded **lower end** forms the palpable **lateral malleolus** (Fig. 16.2a), which lies about 1 cm lower than the medial malleolus. Its medial side has an articular surface for the talus. Above the articular facet is the roughened area for the interosseous ligament of the inferior tibiofibular joint, and below it the bone gives attachment to the posterior talofibular ligament. The interosseous membrane is attached to its medial border. Both the head and the lateral malleolus are palpable.

A severe inversion of the ankle may result in ligamentous injury and talar pressure on the lateral malleolus severe enough to fracture the lower end of the fibula.

THE KNEE JOINT

The **knee joint** (Fig. 16.4a,b) is a synovial joint of a modified hinge variety between the lower end of the femur, the patella and the tibial plateau. The articular surface on the femur is formed of three continuous surfaces: a middle concave surface for the patella, and markedly convex medial and lateral condylar surfaces for articulation with the tibia. The posterior surface of the patella has a medial and a larger lateral facet for articulation with the femoral concavity. The upper surface of each tibial condyle is oval and slightly concave.

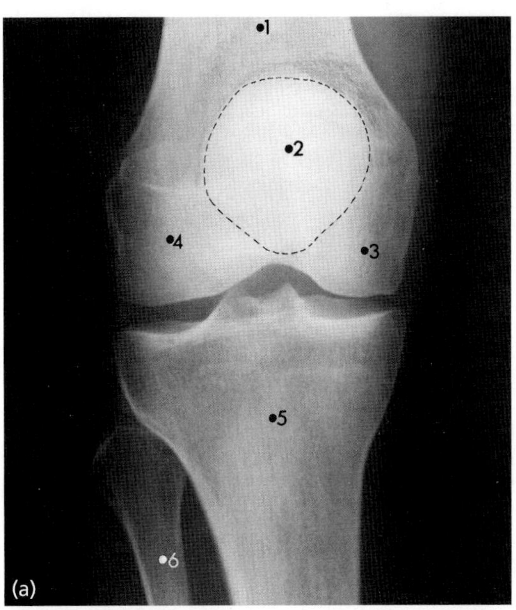

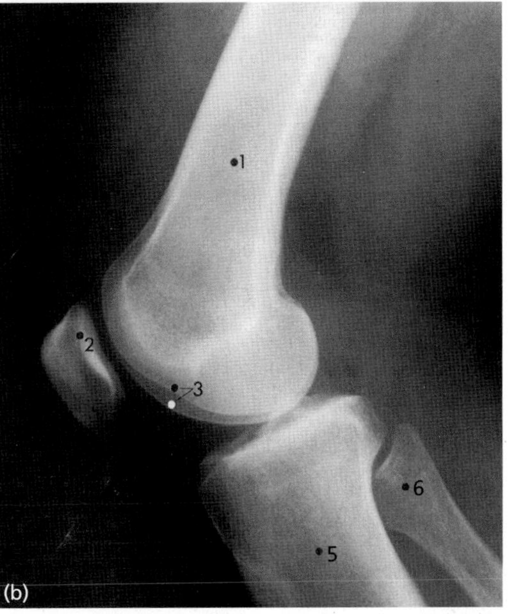

Figure 16.4 X-rays of knee. (a) Antero-posterior view. (b) Lateral view: 1, femur; 2, patella; 3, femoral condyles; 4, lateral femoral condyle; 5, tibia; 6, fibula

The lower limb

Ligaments

Capsule

This is attached on the femur close to the articular margins medially and laterally, and above the intercondylar notch (Figs 16.5a–e and 15.11b, p. 224). It is attached to the margins of the patella and to the periphery of the tibial plateau, except for anteriorly, where it descends below the tibial tuberosity, and posterolaterally where it is pierced by the tendon of popliteus.

Capsular thickenings

Coronary ligaments tether the margins of the medial and lateral menisci to the nearby margin of the tibial plateau.

Accessory ligaments

- **Patellar tendon**– from the apex of the patella to the tibial tuberosity.

The knee jerk reflex is demonstrated by hitting the mid-point of this tendon with a tendon hammer, often with the knee hanging flexed over the bed or with the knees crossed. This should elicit contraction of the quadriceps muscle, which extends the knee and tests the integrity of L3 and L4 nerve roots.

- **Patellar retinacula** – tendinous expansions of the vasti muscles passing to the patellar margins and to the tibial condyles.
- **Tibial collateral ligament** – a broad flat ligament passing from the medial epicondyle of the femur to the medial surface of the upper tibia. It is part of the capsule.
- **Fibular collateral ligament** – a round cord passing from the lateral epicondyle of the femur to the head of the fibula. It is separate from the capsule.
- **Anterior and posterior cruciate ligaments** – strong, intracapsular ligaments; the anterior passes upwards and backwards from the front of the tibial intercondylar area to the medial surface of the lateral femoral condyle (Fig. 16.5e); the posterior passes forwards and upwards from the back of the intercondylar area to the lateral surface of the medial condyle of the femur. Forward displacement of the tibia on the femur is prevented by the anterior cruciate; posterior displacement by the posterior cruciate.

Intracapsular structures

The **synovial membrane** shows signs of the knee joint's development from three separate joint cavities; the patellofemoral joint communicates with each 'tibiofemoral

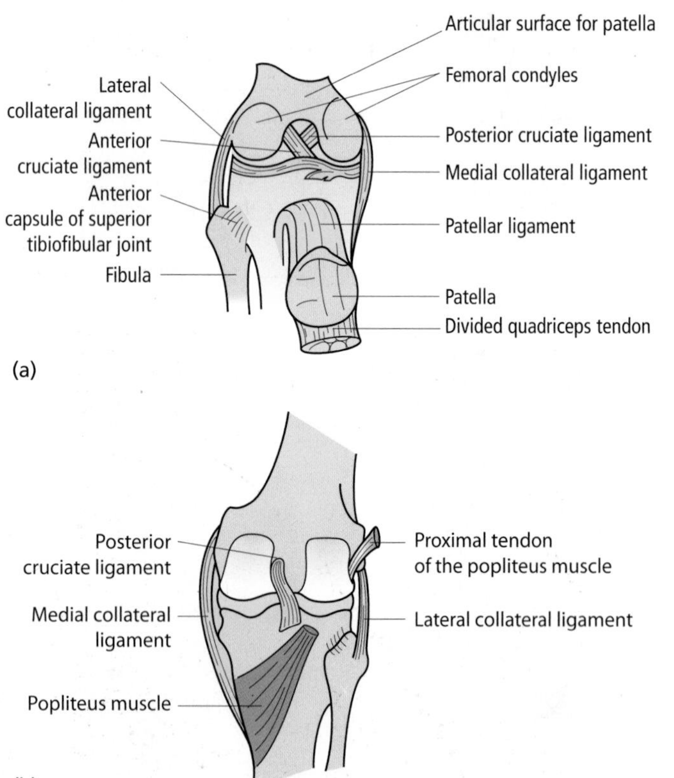

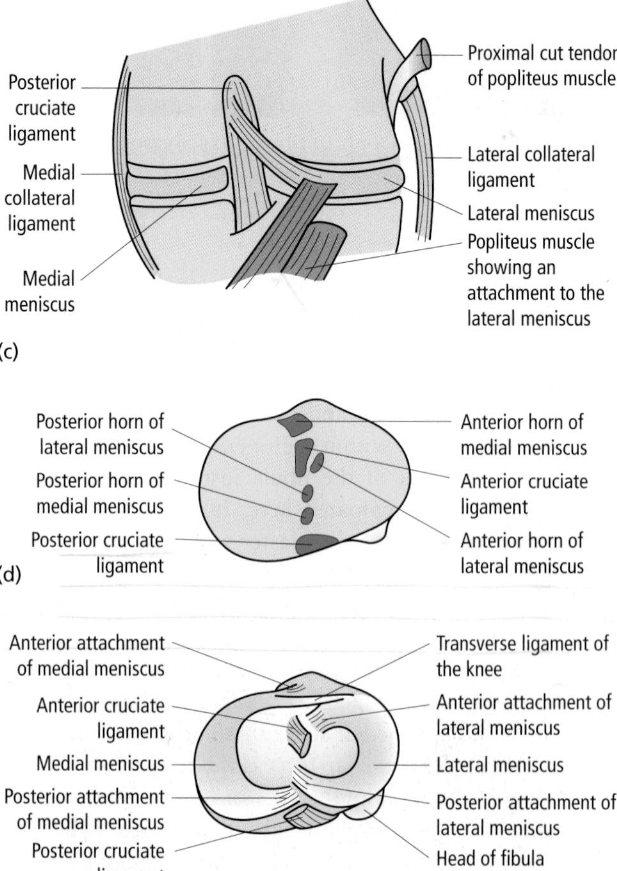

Figure 16.5 (a) Anterior aspect of knee joint with quadriceps muscle divided and patellar ligament turned inferiorly. (b) and (c) Posterior aspect of right knee joint. (d) and (e) Upper end of right tibia showing ligamentous and meniscal attachments to the intercondylar region of the tibial plateau; superior view of tibial plateau showing attachments of cruciate ligaments and menisci

joint', but there is a remnant of the patellofemoral joint's membrane persisting as the **infrapatellar fold**, connecting the lower border of the patella to the intercondylar notch. Both cruciate ligaments lie outside of the synovial cavity in the fibrous septum between the tibiofemoral joints, but a communication between the joints exists in front of the ligaments. Proximally the synovial membrane is attached to the articular margins of the femur, distally to the margins of the tibial articular facets and the front of the intercondylar area. The synovium above the patella extends between quadriceps and the femur as the suprapatellar bursa (Fig. 16.7). The joint cavity communicates with this bursa and the popliteal and gastrocnemius bursae.

Rupture of the synovia of the knee joint as a consequence of osteoarthritis, or its herniation, results in a cystic swelling in the popliteal fossa (Baker's cyst). The lump is fluctuant but not tender, but if the cyst leaks then fluid may track down the calf, which becomes swollen and tender, mimicking a calf vein thrombosis. ●

The **menisci** are two crescentic pieces of fibrocartilage with thickened outer margins. Each lies on a tibial condyle attached by its ends, the anterior and posterior horns, to the intercondylar area (Fig. 16.5e) and by its outer margin to the capsule. The medial cartilage is larger and semicircular and its central attachments embrace those of the lateral cartilage, which is smaller and forms three-fifths of a circle. The tendon of popliteus is attached to the posterior margin of the lateral meniscus.

The stability of the joint depends entirely on its ligaments and neighbouring muscles but, because it is a mobile weight-bearing joint, injuries are common and particularly so in sports involving running and physical contact such as soccer or rugby. Most injuries occur when a side force to the knee is applied whilst the leg is weight-bearing, i.e. when the foot is fixed to the ground. A blow to the lateral side may result in tearing of the medial tibial collateral ligament and, through the ligament's attachment to the medial meniscus, tearing of the medial meniscus. The knee is particularly prone to this injury when flexed for it is then that the collateral ligaments are slack and making little contribution to the stability of the knee. Rupture of the cruciate ligaments is the result of severe anterior or posterior force being applied to the knee.

Tears of the anterior cruciate ligament are seen most frequently in young sportsmen; they are usually the consequence of violent abduction and twisting of the knee, such as may occur in a sliding football tackle. The diagnosis can be supported by a positive 'drawer' sign, i.e. the demonstration of excessive anterior movement of the tibia on the femur. The drawer test indicates the integrity or otherwise of the cruciate ligaments (Fig. 16.9).

The medial meniscus is the more liable to injury because it is fixed to the tibial collateral ligament. Presenting symptoms are pain and swelling of the knee, or locking of the knee owing to the partially detached cartilage becoming wedged between the tibial and femoral condyles. Tearing of the menisci is usually caused by forceful rotation of a flexed knee. In these circumstances external rotation causes the medial meniscus to be torn by being ground between

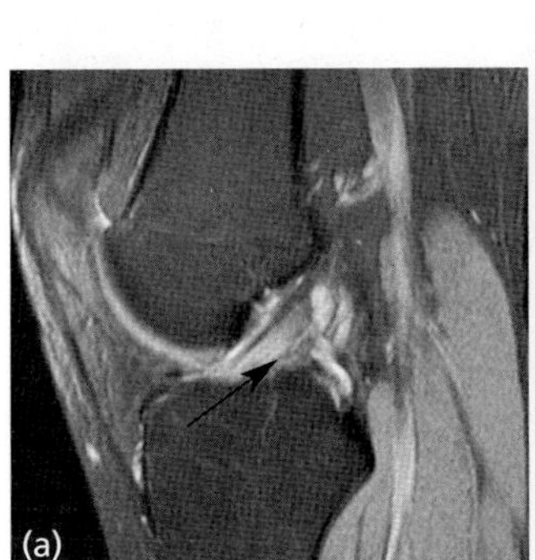

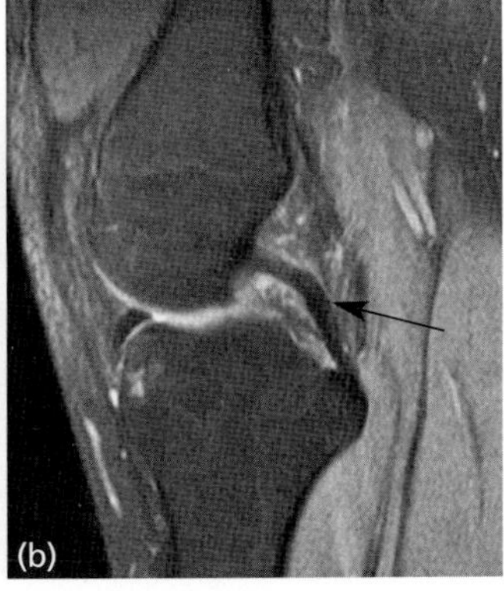

Figure 16.6 MRI of the knee, sagittal views showing: (a) anterior cruciate ligament (arrow); and (b) posterior cruciate ligament (arrow)

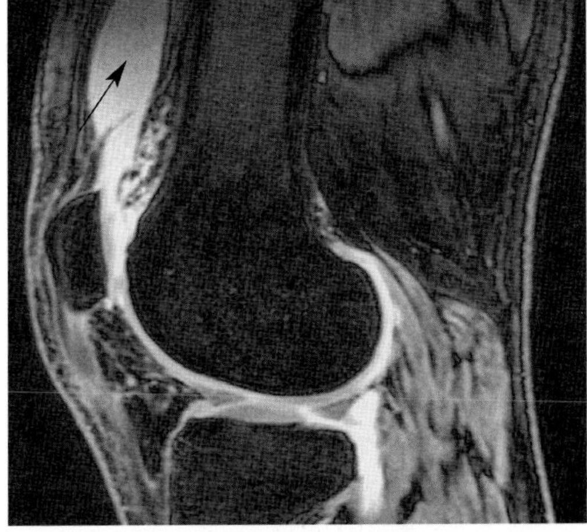

Figure 16.7 Knee MR arthrogram (the suprapatellar bursa is arrowed)

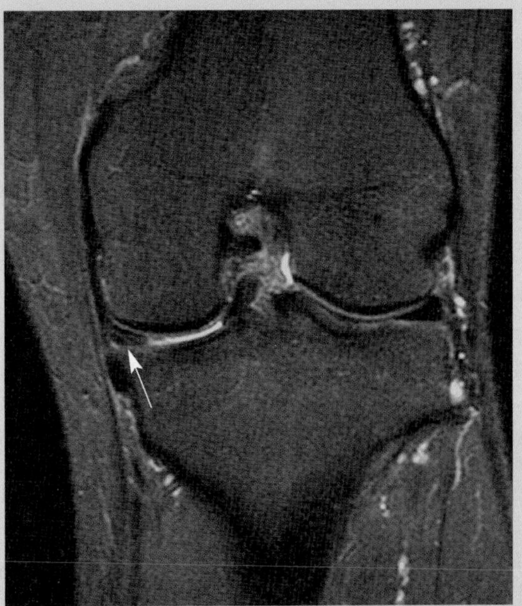

Figure 16.8 Coronal MRI of the knee showing torn medial meniscus (arrow)

the medial condyles of the femur and tibia. Internal rotation may tear the lateral meniscus. Displaced fragments of the meniscus lodged between the condyles prevent full extension of the knee.

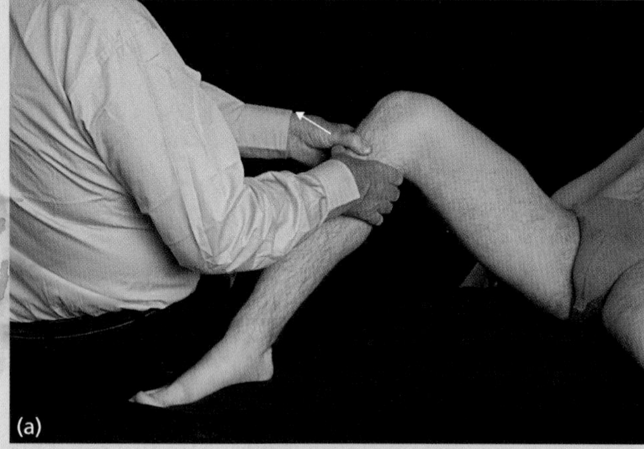

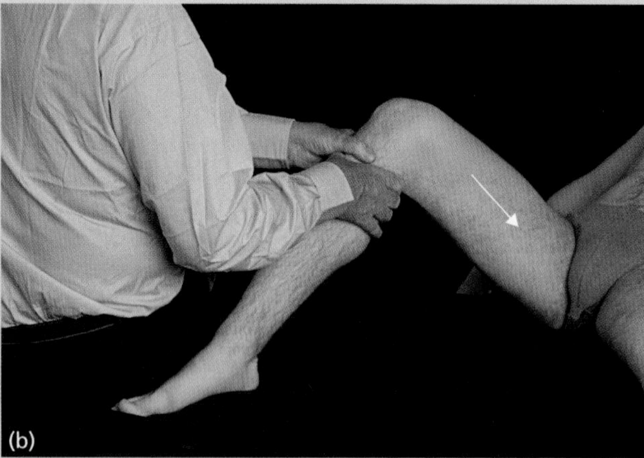

Figure 16.9 Drawer sign – testing laxity of the anterior and posterior cruciate ligaments. The lower leg is gripped around the upper tibia, with the knee flexed, and the tibia pushed backwards and pulled forwards (arrows). There should be no movement in these planes

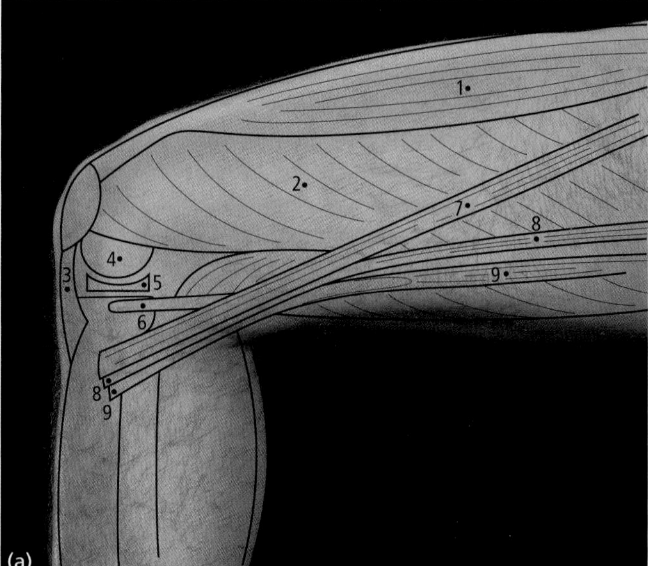

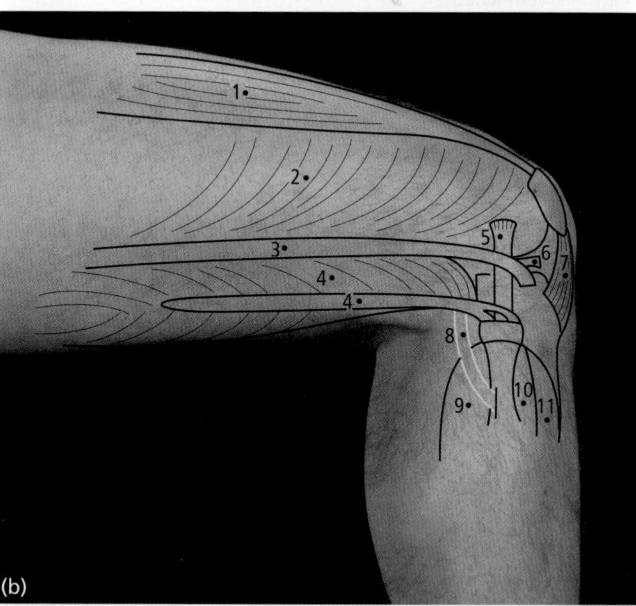

Figure 16.10 Muscles in the flexed knee. (a) Medial view: 1, rectus femoris; 2, vastus medialis; 3, patellar ligament; 4, medial condyle of femur; 5, medial meniscus; 6, tendon and muscle belly of semimembranosus; 7, sartorius; 8, gracilis muscle and tendon attachment; 9, semitendinosus muscle and tendon attachment. (b) Lateral view: 1, rectus femoris; 2, vastus lateralis; 3, iliotibial tract; 4, biceps femoris; 5, lateral collateral ligament of the knee; 6, lateral meniscus; 7, patellar ligament; 8, common peroneal (fibular) nerve; 9, peroneus (fibularis) longus; 10, extensor digitorum; 11, tibialis anterior

Functional aspects

Movements

The joint is capable of flexion, extension and a little rotation:

- **Flexion** – by hamstrings assisted by gastrocnemius.
- **Extension** – by quadriceps and the iliotibial tract (Fig. 16.10a,b). During movement the femoral condyles roll on the tibial condyles and also glide backwards. When the leg is almost straight the capsular and cruciate ligaments become taut and stop further backward gliding of the lateral femoral condyle. Further extension is only possible by backward movement of the medial condyle around the axis of the taut anterior cruciate ligament (medial rotation of the femur on the tibia). Rotation and extension are limited by the collateral ligaments of the knee. When fully extended the knee is in a 'locked' (i.e. stable) position, with almost no muscular contraction involved. At the start of flexion the femur rotates laterally on the tibia, and popliteus muscle pulls the lateral meniscus backwards, thereby preventing it being crushed between the lateral femoral and tibial condyles. This is the 'unlocking' movement of popliteus.
- **Rotation** – a small amount of rotation may be produced by the hamstrings when the knee is flexed.

Stability

The bony surfaces contribute little to the joint's stability, which is largely dependent on strong ligaments and powerful muscles. Its collateral ligaments are inextensible; the cruciate ligaments limit gliding and distraction of the bones; quadriceps anteriorly and gastrocnemius and hamstrings posteriorly stabilize the joint.

Quadriceps tends to pull the patella laterally because of the obliquity of the femur, but the displacement is limited by the projection of the lateral condyle of the femur and by the resistance provided by the horizontally attached fibres of vastus medialis into the medial border of the patella. When one stands on the extended knee the centre of gravity passes in front of the axis around which the femoral condyles roll; the posterior cruciate ligaments thus take the strain.

Blood supply

There is an extensive anastomosis around the knee, contributed to by the popliteal, femoral and anterior tibial arteries (see Fig 16.25a,b, p. 256).

Nerve supply

This is by branches of the tibial, common peroneal (fibular), obturator and femoral nerves.

Relations

The joint is mainly subcutaneous, being separated from the skin by quadriceps, the patella and patellar ligament anteriorly, the biceps tendon laterally, and semimembranosus and semitendinosus medially. To its posterior lie the popliteal vessels and, more superficially, the tibial and common peroneal (fibular) nerves in the popliteal fossa.

Usually dislocation of the patella occurs to the lateral side of the knee (Fig. 16.11a). It is often due to a flat lateral femoral condyle or weakness in the lower fibres of vastus medialis. Direct injury to the patella may cause it to fracture into several fragments, a stellate fracture (Fig. 16.11b). A transverse fracture into two fragments is more commonly the consequence of sudden acute contraction of quadriceps whilst attempting to correct a slip (Fig. 16.11c). In young adolescents the tibial tuberosity may become painful and reveal irregular ossification of the tendinous insertion at the tibial tuberosity (Osgood–Schlatter disease; Fig. 16.12).

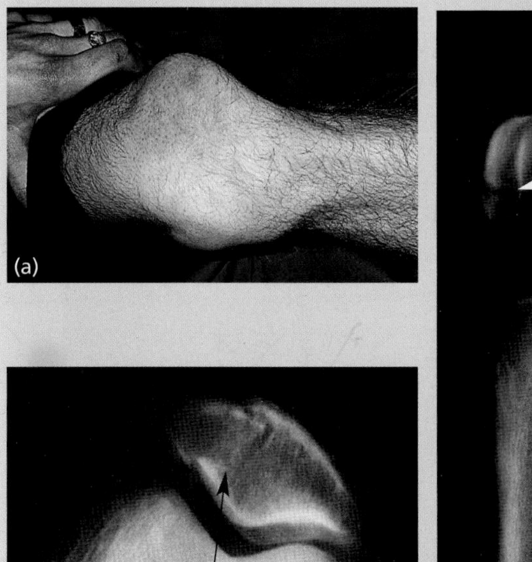

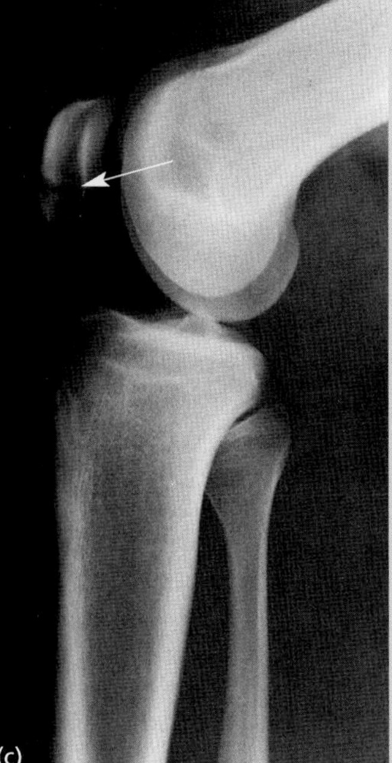

Figure 16.11 (a) Dislocated patella. (b) Stellate fracture of patella (arrow). (c) Transverse fracture of patella (arrow)

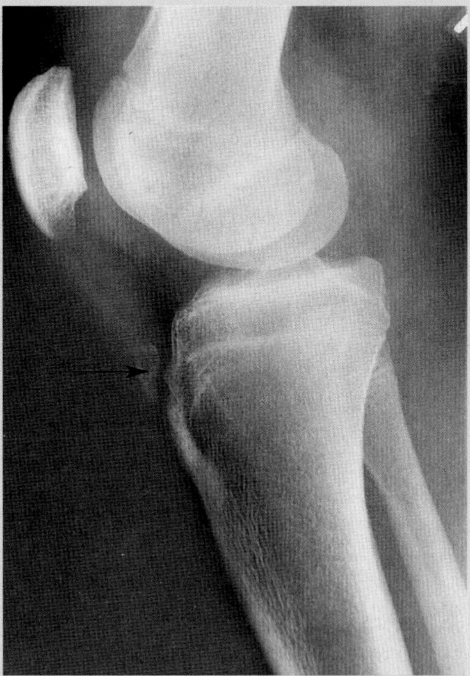

Figure 16.12 Osgood–Schlatter's disease showing irregular ossification of the bony attachment of the patellar ligament (arrow)

Bursae

These are numerous and variable. Anteriorly are the **suprapatellar**, which extends into the thigh deep to quadriceps and communicates with the knee joint, and the **prepatellar, superficial** and **deep infrapatellar**, which are related to the patellar ligament.

Posteriorly lie the **popliteal bursa**, deep to its muscle, and one associated with the **gastrocnemius** deep to its medial head. Both communicate with the knee joint and the **semimembranosus** bursa, which lies between the muscle and the medial head of gastrocnemius.

Suprapatellar 'bursitis' – Because of the communication between it and the knee joint an effusion into the knee joint also involves the suprapatellar bursa. This can be detected by the patellar tap: pushing the patella towards the femoral condyle results in a palpable contact between the two bones, which is caused by fluid separating the patella and the femoral condyles, and indicates excessive fluid in the knee joint.

Prepatellar bursitis, more commonly known as 'plumber's' or 'housemaid's knee', results from chronic irritation of these bursae caused by constant kneeling on a hard surface. A tender fluctuant swelling is found over the patella (Fig. 16.13).

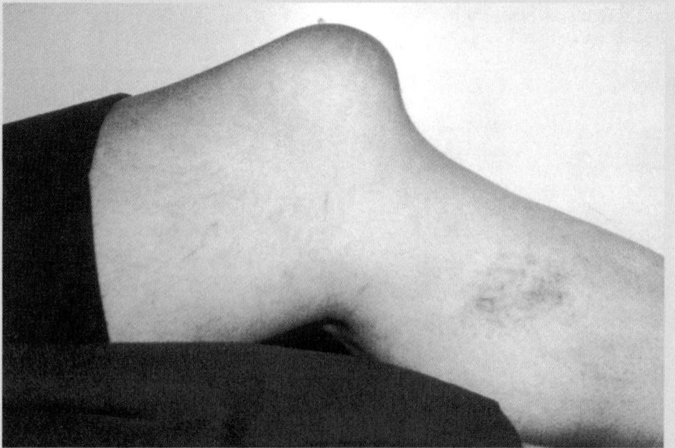

Figure 16.13 Prepatellar bursitis from constant kneeling down and scrubbing floors

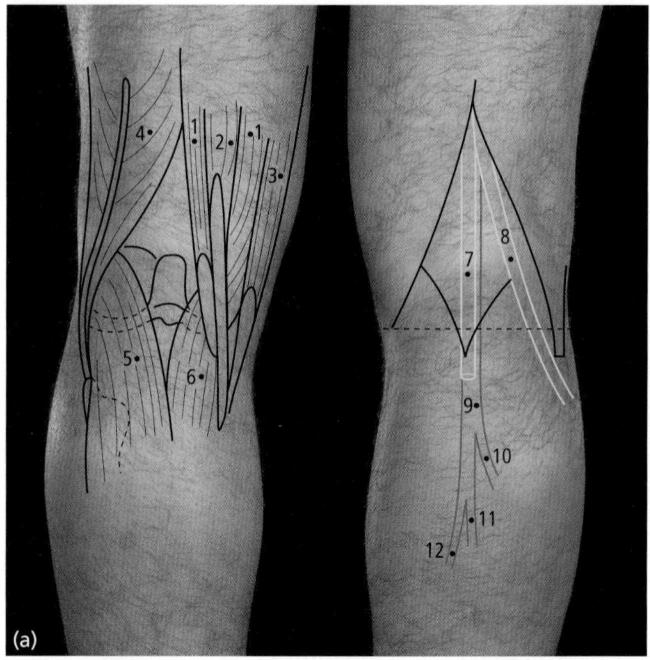

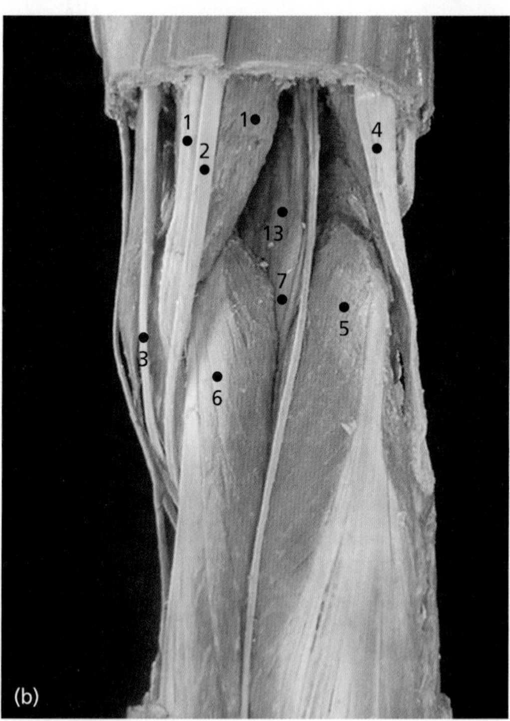

Figure 16.14 (a) Surface anatomy of the popliteal fossa: 1, semimembranosus; 2, semitendinosus; 3, gracilis; 4, biceps femoris; 5, lateral and; 6, medial head of gastrocnemius; 7, tibial nerve; 8, common peroneal (fibular) nerve; 9, popliteal artery; 10, anterior tibial artery; 11, peroneal (fibular) artery; 12, posterior tibial artery (the popliteal vein, 13, between the artery and main nerves has been omitted in the diagram) – dotted line shows level of transverse section in Fig. 16.15. (b) Dissection of the right popliteal fossa with corresponding numbers to (a)

THE TIBIOFIBULAR JOINTS

Little movement occurs between the tibia and fibula.

The **superior tibiofibular joint** is a plane synovial joint between the undersurface of the lateral tibial condyle and the articular facet of the head of the fibula. Its synovia may be continuous with that of the knee joint.

The **inferior tibiofibular joint** is a fibrous joint between the adjacent inferior surfaces of the two bones. A strong, short, interosseous tibiofibular ligament unites them.

The **interosseous membrane** unites the interosseous borders of the two bones and gives attachment to the deep flexor and the extensor muscles of the leg.

The **popliteal fossa** is a diamond-shaped fossa behind the knee joint bounded superomedially by semitendinosus and semimembranosus, superolaterally by biceps femoris, and inferiorly by the medial and lateral heads of gastrocnemius

(Figs 16.14a and 16.15). Its floor is the posterior surface of the femur, the knee joint capsule and the popliteus muscle, and it is roofed by thickened fascia lata which is here pierced by the small saphenous vein. It contains the popliteal vessels and branches, the tibial nerve, the common peroneal (fibular) nerve and branches and a few lymph nodes.

THE LEG AND DORSUM OF THE FOOT

The leg muscles are divided into anterior, lateral and posterior groups lying in fascial compartments separated by the tibia and fibula (Fig. 16.16a,b), interosseous membrane and anterior and posterior intermuscular septa, which pass inwards from

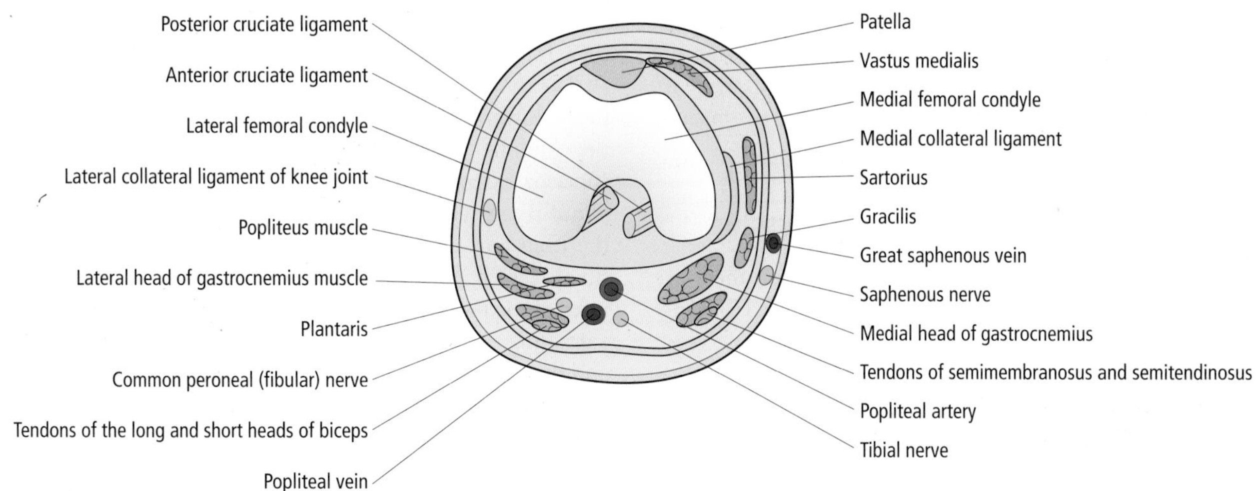

Figure 16.15 Transverse section through right knee, viewed from below (at level of dotted line in Fig. 16.14a)

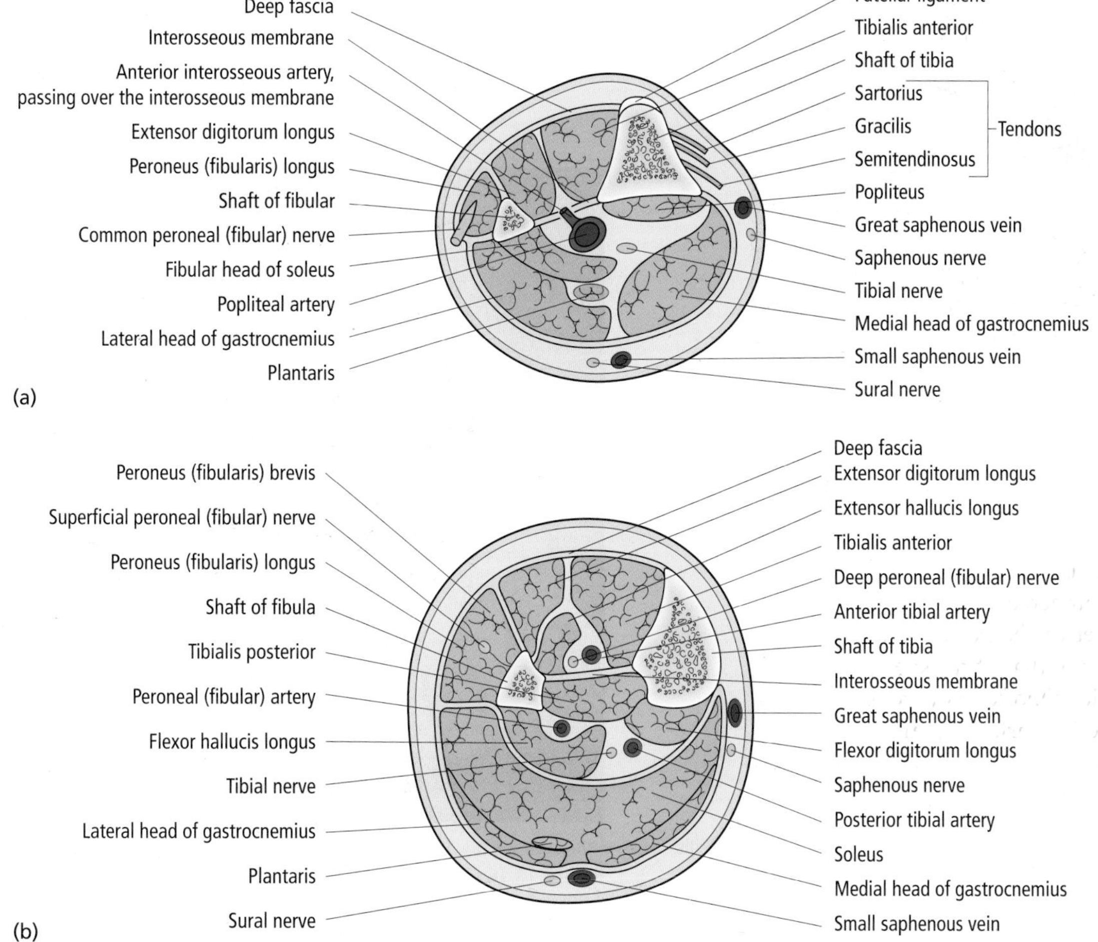

Figure 16.16 Transverse section (a) through the right leg at lower popliteal fossa, viewed from below (see dotted line A in Fig. 16.17); (b) through mid-calf, viewed from below (see dotted line B in Fig. 16.17)

the investing deep fascia of the leg. Below, the deep fascia is thickened to form the superior extensor retinaculum (see Fig. 16.19b below).

These fascial compartments are inextensible. Any swelling within the fascial compartment as a result of bleeding, infection or venous obstruction produces a rise in the intracompartmental pressure that will hinder its blood supply and produce tender, swollen muscles (**compartment syndrome**). Surgical treatment is urgently required. A fasciotomy incision the length of the compartment is necessary to reduce the pressure within the fascial compartment.

The anterior (dorsiflexor) group of muscles

Only tibialis anterior is attached to the tibia; the others are each attached to the fibula (Table 16.1 and Fig. 16.17). Only one, extensor digitorum brevis, is confined to the foot. All are supplied by branches of the common peroneal (fibular) nerve. During walking these muscles pull the leg forward over the grounded foot; when the foot is not bearing weight they dorsiflex the foot and toes (Fig. 16.18).

In the foot is the **extensor digitorum brevis,** attached proximally to the anterior part of the upper surface of the calcaneus, distally by four small tendons to the medial four toes. It extends the medial four toes.

The two **extensor retinacula** lie across the extensor tendons in the lower leg and in front of the ankle joint. They prevent the tendons 'bowstringing' (Figs 16.18b and 16.19b). The **superior extensor retinaculum** is a thickening of deep fascia, about 3 cm wide, stretching between the anterior border of the tibia and fibula over the extensor tendons, the anterior tibial vessels and the deep peroneal (fibular) nerve. The **inferior extensor retinaculum** is thicker and bifurcates, extending medially from the upper surface of the calcaneus and then splitting into two parts in front of the ankle joint; the upper part is attached to the medial malleolus and the lower blends with the plantar aponeurosis. The **synovial sheaths** of the long extensors lie deep to the inferior retinaculum; only that of tibialis anterior extends proximally to the superior retinaculum (Fig. 16.19b).

Figure 16.17 Surface anatomy of the anterior lower leg showing muscles: 1, patellar ligament; 2, sartorius; 3, gracilis; 4, semitendinosus; 5, soleus; 6, gastrocnemius; 7, tibialis anterior; 8, extensor digitorum; 9, peroneus (fibularis) longus; 10, extensor hallucis longus; 11, peroneus (fibularis) tertius; 12, subcutaneous tibial surface. Dashed lines A and B relate to transverse sections on p. 249

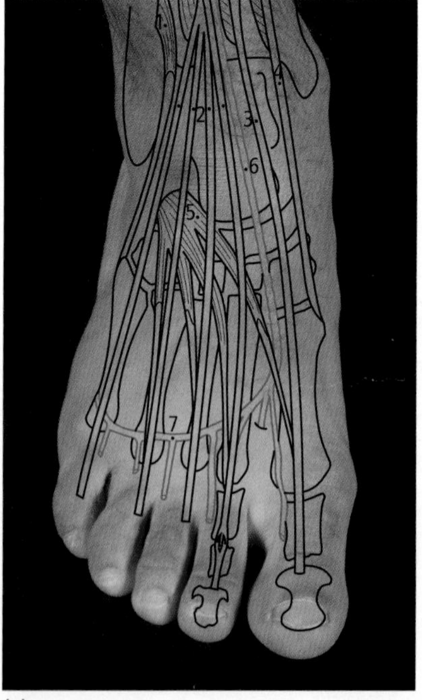

(a)

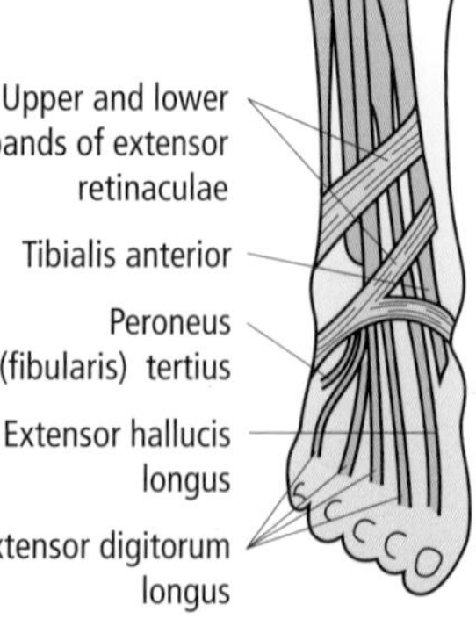

(b)

Figure 16.18 (a) Surface anatomy of the dorsum of foot showing tendon attachments: 1, peroneus (fibularis) tertius; 2, the four tendons of extensor digitorum longus; 3, extensor hallucis longus; 4, tendon of tibialis anterior; 5, extensor digitorum brevis; 6, dorsalis pedis artery; 7, arcuate artery (b) Anterior view of ankle showing extensor retinacula

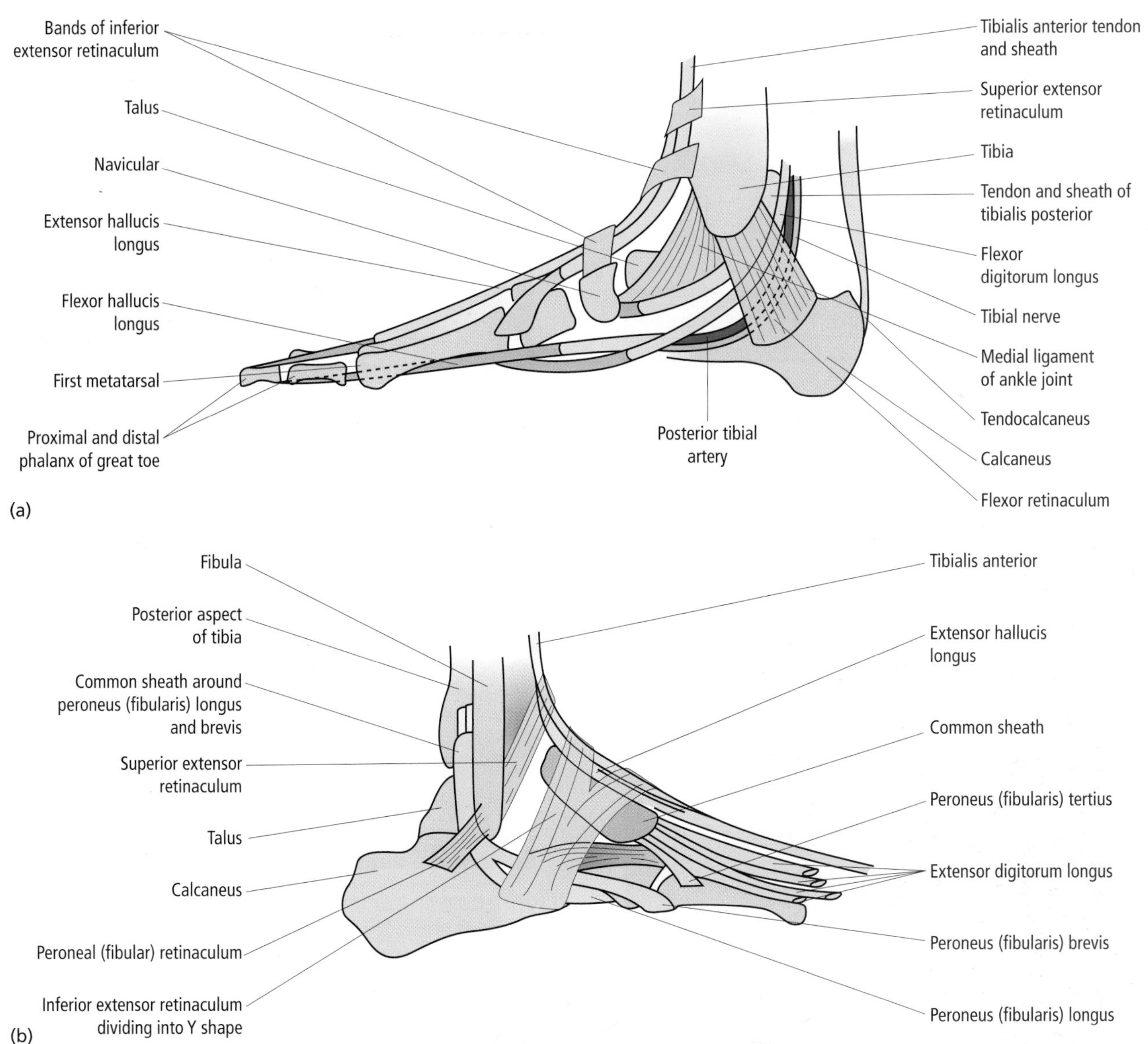

Figure 16.19 Right ankle region. (a) Medial aspect of the ankle. (b) Lateral aspect of ankle showing tendons and retinaculae

Table 16.1 Muscles of anterior (extensor) compartment of leg

Muscle	Proximal attachment	Distal attachment	Nerve supply	Functions
Tibialis anterior (Figs 16.17 and 16.18)	Lateral condyle and upper lateral surface of tibia	Medial cuneiform and base of first metacarpal	Peroneal (fibular) nerve (L4)	Dorsiflexion and inversion of foot
Extensor hallucis longus	Middle of anterior surface of the fibular and interosseous membrane	Base of distal phalanx of hallux	Peroneal (fibular) nerve (L5, S1)	Extension of hallux and dorsiflexion of ankle
Extensor digitorum longus	Lateral condyle of tibia and upper 3/4 of anterior interosseous membrane and fibula	Middle and distal phalanges of lateral four digits	Peroneal (fibular) nerve (L5, S1)	Extension of toes and dorsiflexion of ankle
Peroneus (fibularis) tertius	Lower anterior fibula and interosseous membrane	Base of 5th metacarpal	Peroneal (fibular) nerve (L5, S1)	Dorsiflexion of ankle, weak everter of foot

The lateral (evertor) group of muscles

These are important in maintaining balance during standing (Table 16.2 and Fig. 16.20a–c). Both peroneal (fibular) muscles are supplied by the superficial peroneal nerve.

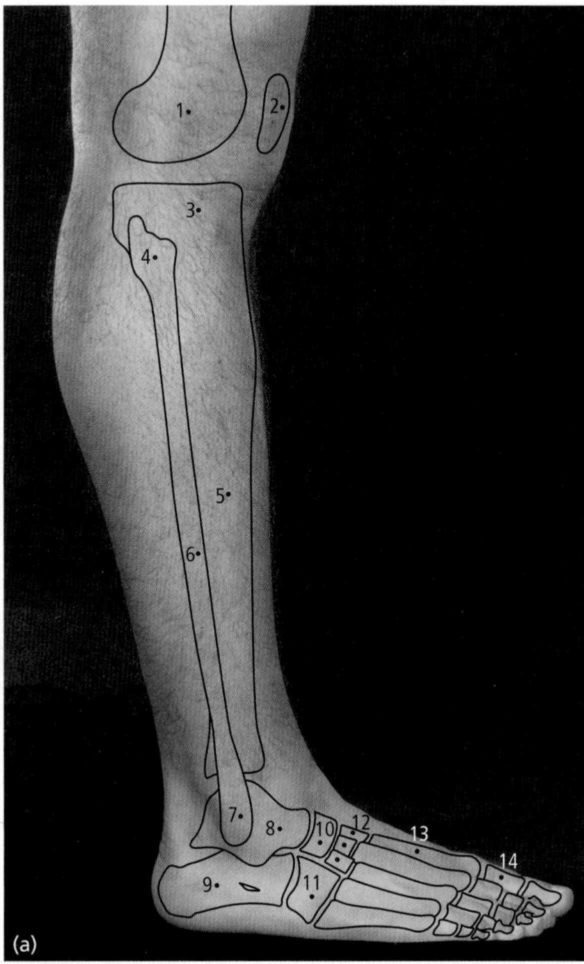

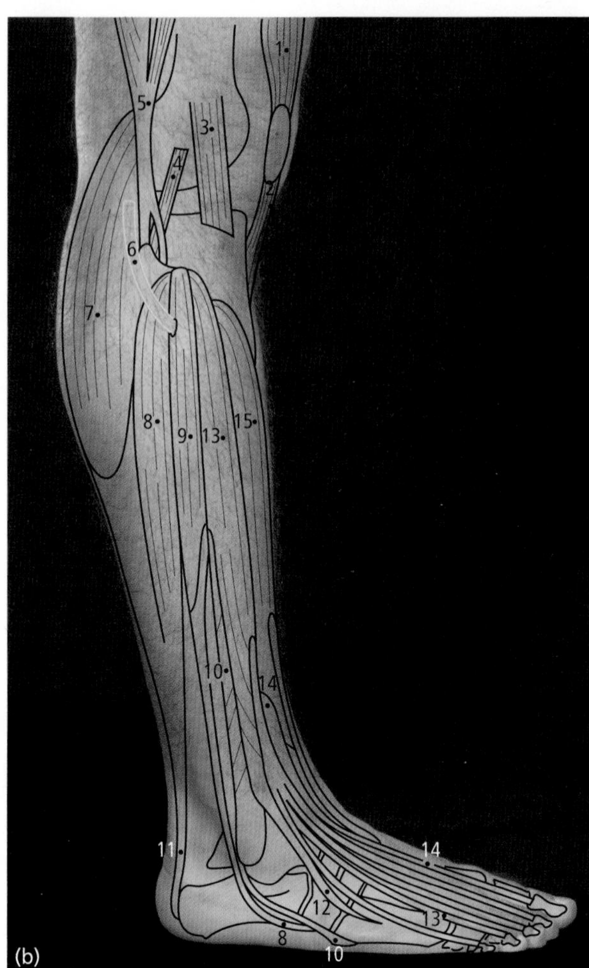

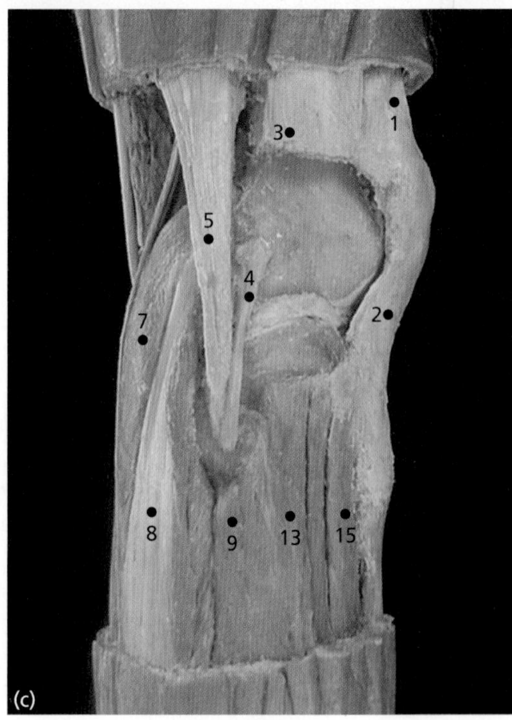

Figure 16.20 Surface anatomy and dissection of the lateral lower right leg. (a) Bones: 1, lateral condyle of femur; 2, patella; 3, tibial plateau; 4, head of fibula; 5, shaft of tibia; 6, shaft of fibula; 7, lateral malleolus; 8, talus; 9, calcaneus; 10, navicular; 11, cuboid; 12, medial, intermediate and lateral cuneiform; 13, metatarsals; 14, phalanges. (b) Muscles: 1, quadriceps; 2, patellar ligament; 3, iliotibial tract; 4, lateral collateral ligament of the knee joint; 5, biceps femoris; 6, common peroneal (fibular) nerve; 7, gastrocnemius; 8, soleus; 9, peroneus (fibularis) longus; 10, peroneus (fibularis) brevis; 11, tendocalcaneus; 12, peroneus (fibularis) tertius; 13, muscle and four tendons of the extensor digitorum longus; 14, tendon of extensor hallucis longus; 15, tibialis anterior. (c) Dissection of lateral side of upper leg region (muscles labelled as in (b))

Table 16.2 Lateral muscles of leg (peroneal (fibular) compartment)

Muscle	Proximal attachment	Distal attachment	Nerve supply	Functions
Peroneus (fibularis) longus	Head and upper 2/3 of fibula	Base of 1st metatarsal and medial cuneiform	Peroneal (fibular) nerve (L5, S1, 2)	Eversion of foot and weak plantar flexor of ankle
Peroneus (fibularis) brevis (Fig. 16.19b)	Lower 2/3 of lateral surface of fibula	Base of 5th metatarsal	Peroneal (fibular) nerve (L5, S1, 2)	Eversion of foot and weak plantar flexor of ankle

Forced inversion injuries – 'twisted ankles' – often result in avulsion of the base of the 5th metatarsal, the attachment of peroneus (fibularis) brevis (Fig. 16.21).

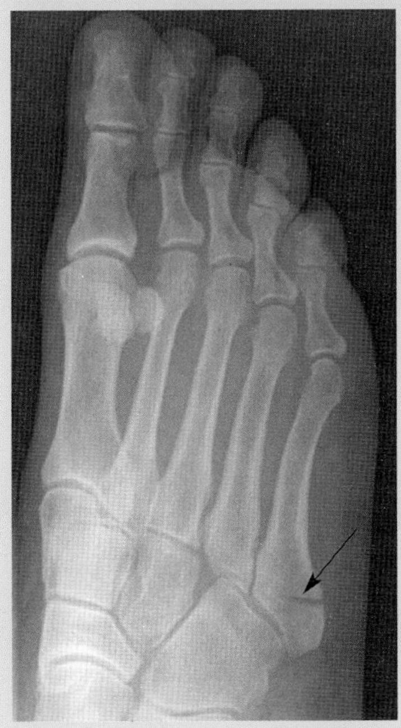

Figure 16.21 Fracture of the base of the 5th metatarsal (arrow)

The posterior (plantarflexor) group of muscles

These help in propelling the body forward during walking by plantarflexing the grounded foot (Table 16.3 and Figs 16.22a–d and 16.23a,b). Gastrocnemius is the most superficial, lying over popliteus and soleus, which in turn is superficial to flexor digitorum longus and flexor hallucis longus. Both gastrocnemius and soleus muscles are powerful plantarflexors of the foot and thus are important in posture and locomotion. Between and within the muscles are extensive deep plexuses of veins; contraction of these calf muscles pumps the blood within them towards the heart against gravity. This muscle pump is sometimes known as the 'third heart'.

Branches of the tibial nerve supply all these muscles.

Rupture of the tendocalcaneus (Achilles tendon) usually occurs as the result of acute contraction of an unexercised muscle, such as may occur during a middle-aged person's first tennis game of the season, or the father's race at a school sports day. Rupture may be partial or complete; conservative treatment is adequate for partial tears but complete tears may require surgical treatment. The ankle reflex is demonstrated by tapping the tendon with a tendon hammer, easiest shown with the patient in the kneeling position. It tests the integrity of S1 and S2 nerve roots.

Table 16.3 Posterior muscles of the leg

Muscle	Proximal attachment	Distal attachment	Nerve supply	Functions
Gastrocnemius (Fig. 16.22a)	By two heads Lateral head: lateral condyle of femur Medial head: proximal to the medial condyle of the femur	Posterior surface of calcaneus by the tendo Achilles	Tibial nerve (S1, 2)	Flexion of knee, plantar flexion of ankle
Soleus	Head of fibula (soleal), line of femur	Posterior surface of calcaneus by the tendo Achilles	Tibial nerve (S1, 2)	Plantar flexion of ankle
Plantaris	Lateral supracondylar line of femur	Posterior surface of calcaneus by the tendo Achilles	Tibial nerve (S1, 2)	Weak assist to gastrocnemius
Popliteus	Lateral condyle of femur and lateral meniscus	Upper posterior surface of tibia	Tibial nerve (L4, 5)	Weak flexion of knee and unlocking of medial meniscus
Flexor hallucis longus	Lower 2/3 of posterior surface of fibula	Distal phalanx of hallux	Tibial nerve (S2,3)	Flexion of hallux, plantar flexion of ankle, support to the medial longitudinal arch
Flexor digitorum longus	Lower posterior surface of tibia and fibula	Distal phalanges of lateral four toes	Tibial nerve (S2, 3)	Flexion lateral four toes, plantar flexion of ankle and support of longitudinal arches of foot
Tibialis posterior	Posterior tibia below soleal line, posterior surface of fibula	Tuberosity of navicular, cuneiform and cuboid; bases of 2nd, 3rd, 4th metatarsals	Tibial nerve (L4, 5)	Plantar flexion of ankle, inversion of foot

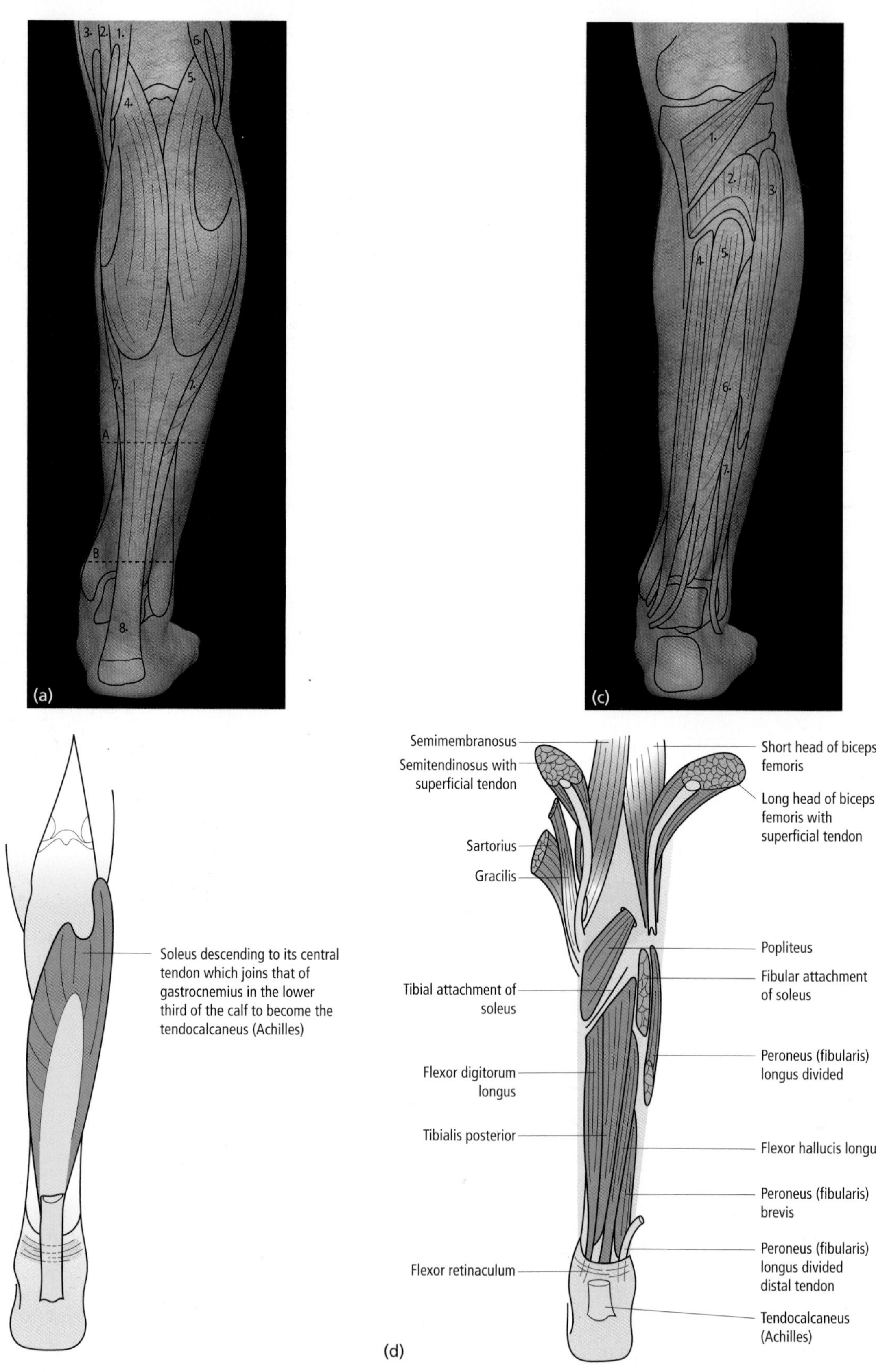

Figure 16.22 (a) Surface anatomy of the posterior aspect of right calf: 1, semitendinosus; 2, semimembranosus; 3, gracilis; 4, 5, medial and lateral heads of gastrocnemius; 6, biceps femoris; 7, soleus; 8, tendocalcaneus (the dotted lines A and B relate to the transverse sections of Fig. 16.28a,b, p. 258). (b) Posterior aspect of right calf showing soleus (gastrocnemius has been removed). (c) Surface anatomy of the posterior aspect of the calf showing: 1, popliteus; 2, soleus; 3, peroneus (fibularis) longus; 4, flexor digitorum longus; 5, tibialis posterior; 6, flexor hallucis longus; 7, peroneus (fibularis) brevis. (d) Deep aspect of posterior leg after removal of soleus and gastrocnemius

The **flexor retinaculum** (Figs 16.19a and 16.24a,b) is a thickened band of deep fascia passing from the medial malleolus to the medial side of the calcaneus, crossing from medial to lateral, the tendons of tibialis posterior and flexor digitorum longus, the posterior tibial vessels, the tibial nerve and the tendon of flexor hallucis longus. Each tendon is enclosed in a separate synovial sheath, those of flexor hallucis longus and flexor digitorum longus passing into the sole of the foot.

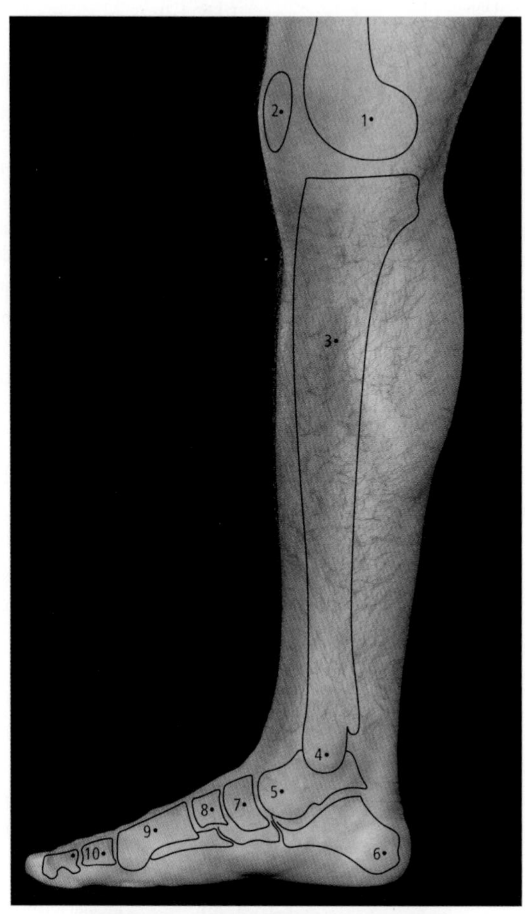

(a)

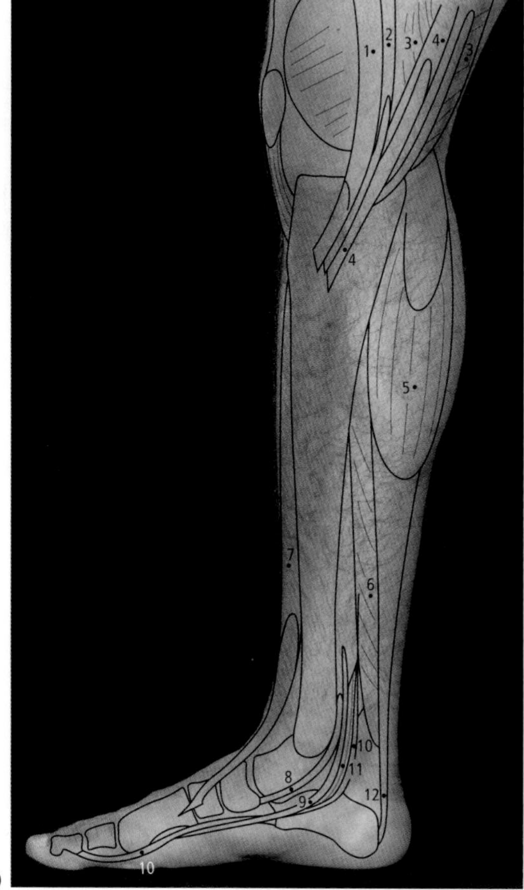

(b)

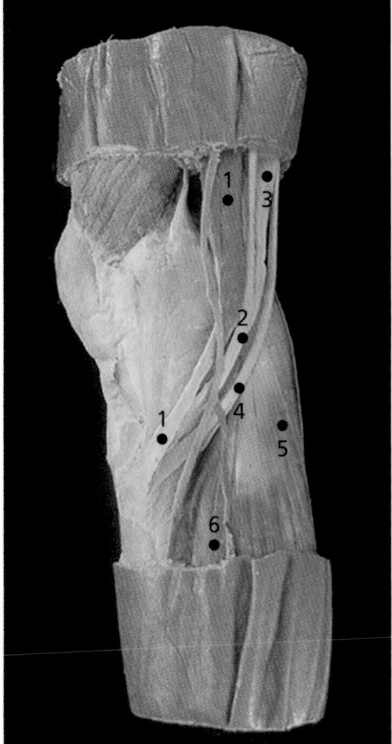

(c)

Figure 16.23 Surface anatomy and dissection of the medial aspect of right leg. (a) Bones: 1, medial femoral condyle; 2, patella; 3, shaft of tibia; 4, medial malleolus; 5, talus; 6, calcaneus; 7, navicular; 8, medial cuneiform; 9, metatarsal; 10, phalanges. (b) Muscles and tendons: 1, sartorius; 2, gracilis; 3, semimembranosus; 4, semitendinosus; 5, gastrocnemius; 6, soleus; 7, tibialis anterior; 8, tibialis posterior; 9, flexor digitorum longus; 10, flexor hallucis longus; 11, posterior tibial artery; 12, tendocalcaneus. (c) Dissection of medial aspect of upper leg (labels as in 16.23b)

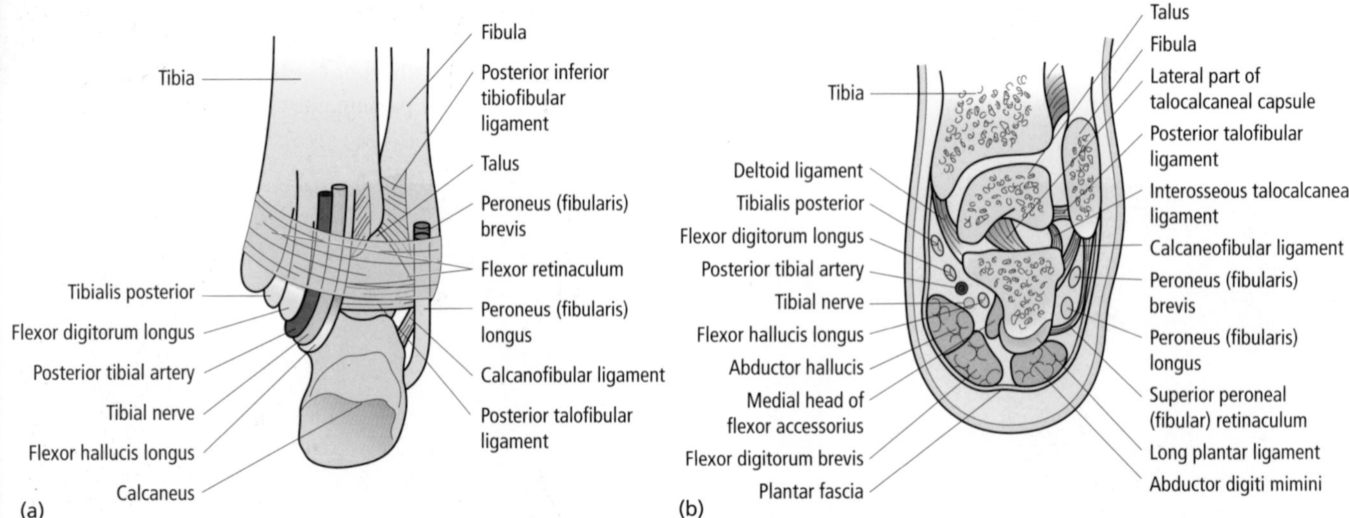

Figure 16.24 (a) Posterior aspect of ankle showing relations of structures passing behind the right ankle. (b) Oblique coronal section through the ankle and talocalcaneal joints

VESSELS AND NERVES OF THE LEG

The popliteal artery

The popliteal artery (Figs 16.25a,b and 16.26a,b) is a continuation of the femoral artery. It descends from the adductor hiatus to the lower border of popliteus, where it divides into anterior and posterior tibial arteries. Throughout its course its vein and the tibial nerve lie superficial to it.

The popliteal pulse is not easy to feel because the artery lies deep in the popliteal fossa. It is best felt in the middle of the popliteal fossa with the knee flexed.

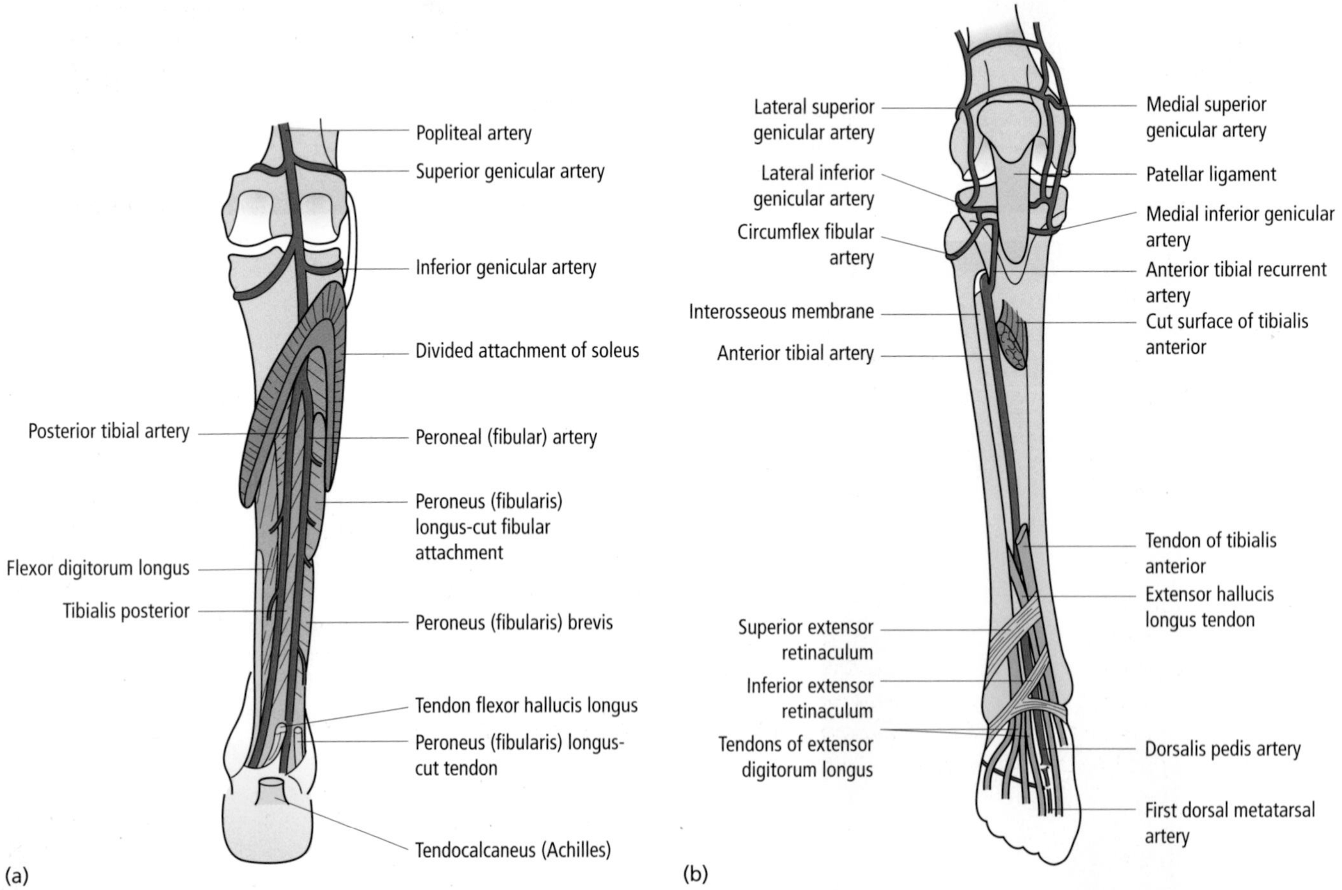

Figure 16.25 (a) Posterior aspect of knee and calf with gastrocnemius and soleus removed to show arteries. (b) Anterior dissection showing details of anastomosis around the knee joint

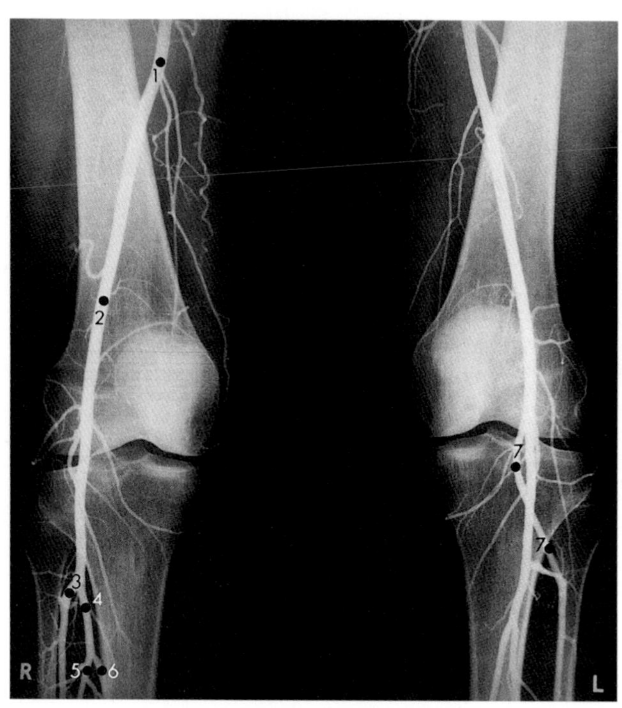

(a)

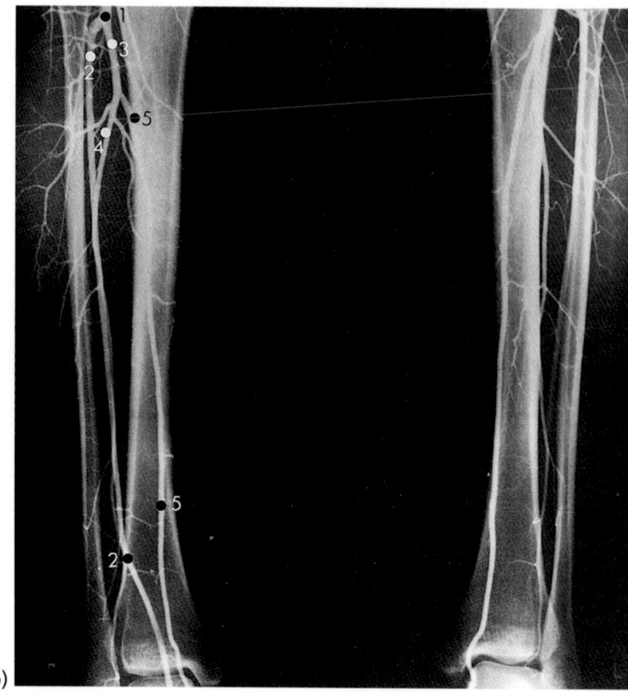

(b)

Figure 16.26 (a) Popliteal arteries filled with contrast material which has been injected into the abdominal aorta: 1, femoral artery; 2, popliteal artery; 3, anterior tibial artery; 4, tibioperoneal trunk; 5, peroneal (fibular) artery; 6, posterior tibial artery; 7, abnormally high origin of the left anterior tibial artery. (b) Arteriogram of lower leg arteries: 1, distal popliteal artery; 2, anterior tibial artery; 3, tibioperoneal trunk; 4, peroneal (fibular) artery; 5, posterior tibial artery

Branches

The **anterior tibial artery** passes forwards above the interosseous membrane and descends the extensor compartment in company with the deep peroneal (fibular) nerve. Beyond the ankle it continues as the **dorsalis pedis artery** which, in the foot, anastomoses with the lateral plantar artery. The dorsalis pedis artery can be palpated over the tarsal bones, just lateral to the extensor hallucis longus tendon. The **posterior tibial artery** descends through the flexor compartment of the leg alongside the tibial nerve. Its largest branch, the **peroneal (fibular) artery**, descends in the lateral (peroneal (fibular)) compartment. Behind the medial malleolus the posterior tibial artery divides into medial and lateral plantar arteries, which enter the sole of the foot (see Fig. 16.29). The posterior tibial artery is palpated on the medial aspect of the talus, just posterior to the medial malleolus (Fig. 16.23b).

The popliteal vein

The popliteal vein is formed by the union of the anterior and posterior tibial veins, crosses the popliteal fossa and passes through the adductor hiatus. Throughout its course it is superficial to its artery. Its tributaries correspond largely to the branches of the artery, but in addition the **small saphenous vein** (Fig. 15.3, p. 220) enters it by piercing the fascial roof of the popliteal fossa.

The tibial nerve

The tibial nerve is a terminal branch of the sciatic nerve (Fig. 16.27). Formed just above the popliteal fossa it descends through the fossa, leaving it by passing deep to soleus, where it descends through the deep flexor compartment of the leg to the back of the medial malleolus. It divides into medial and lateral plantar nerves.

Relations

In the popliteal fossa it lies superficial to the popliteal vessels. In the calf it descends deep to soleus, on tibialis posterior at first and the ankle joint later. It divides distal to the flexor retinaculum (Figs 16.24a and 16.28a).

Branches

It supplies all the muscles of the posterior compartment and sensation to the knee joint and lower leg. The **medial** and **lateral plantar nerves** are illustrated in Fig. 16.29. The **sural nerve**, a cutaneous branch, descends on gastrocnemius and unites with a branch of the common peroneal (fibular) nerve halfway down the calf to run alongside the small saphenous vein behind the lateral malleolus to the lateral side of the foot. It supplies the skin over the posterior calf, the ankle joint and the lateral surface of the foot.

The common peroneal (fibular) nerve

The common peroneal (fibular) nerve (Fig. 16.16a,b) is also a terminal branch of the sciatic nerve that originates just above the popliteal fossa. It descends along the lateral margin of the fossa and enters peroneus (fibularis) longus, where it divides into superficial and deep peroneal (fibular) nerves.

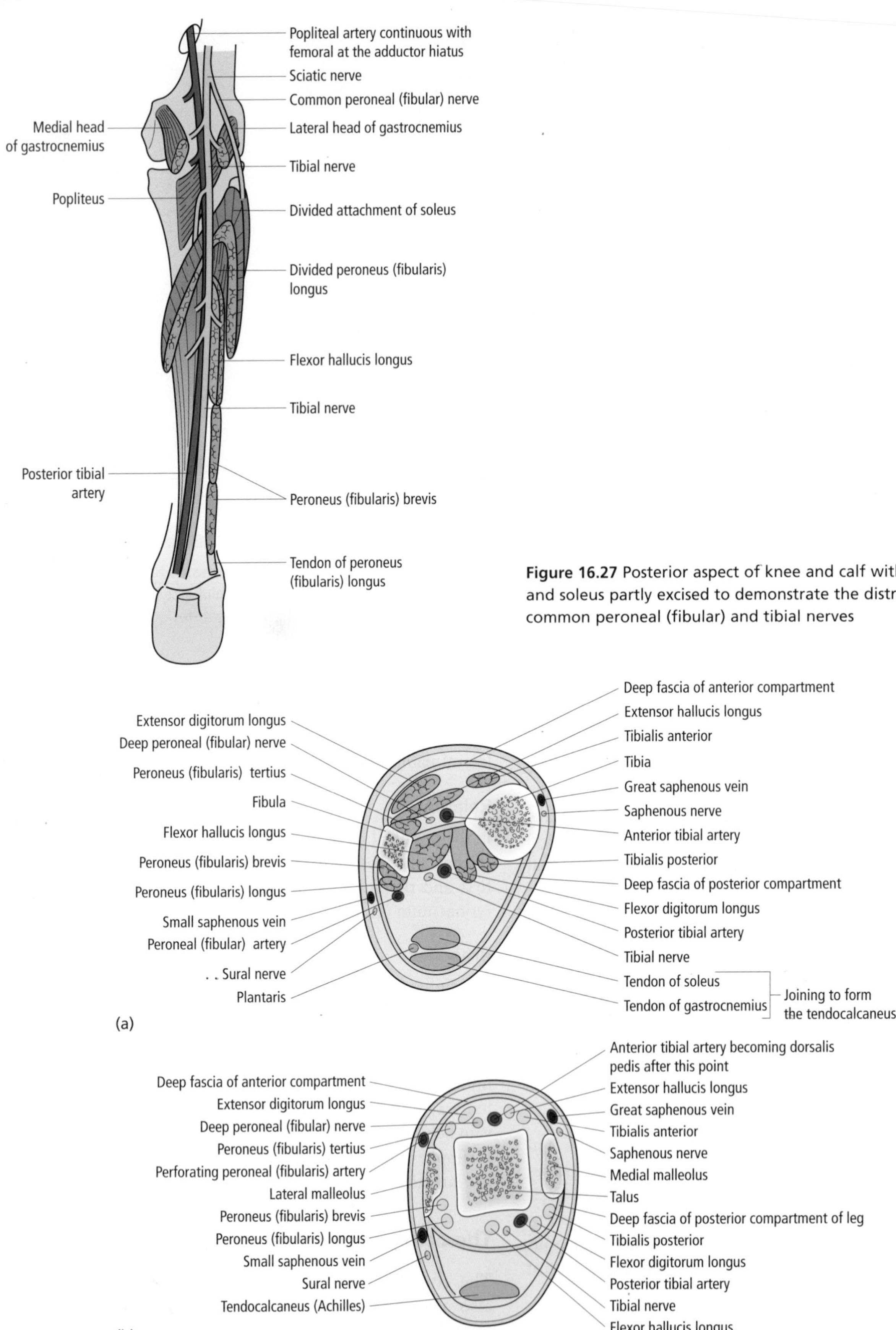

Figure 16.27 Posterior aspect of knee and calf with gastrocnemius and soleus partly excised to demonstrate the distribution of the common peroneal (fibular) and tibial nerves

Figure 16.28 (a) Transverse section of the right lower leg at junction of the middle and lower thirds, viewed from below. (b) Transverse section through the right ankle showing distribution of tendons, vessels and nerves, viewed from below. (These sections are at the levels shown by dotted lines A and B respectively in Fig. 16.22a on p. 254)

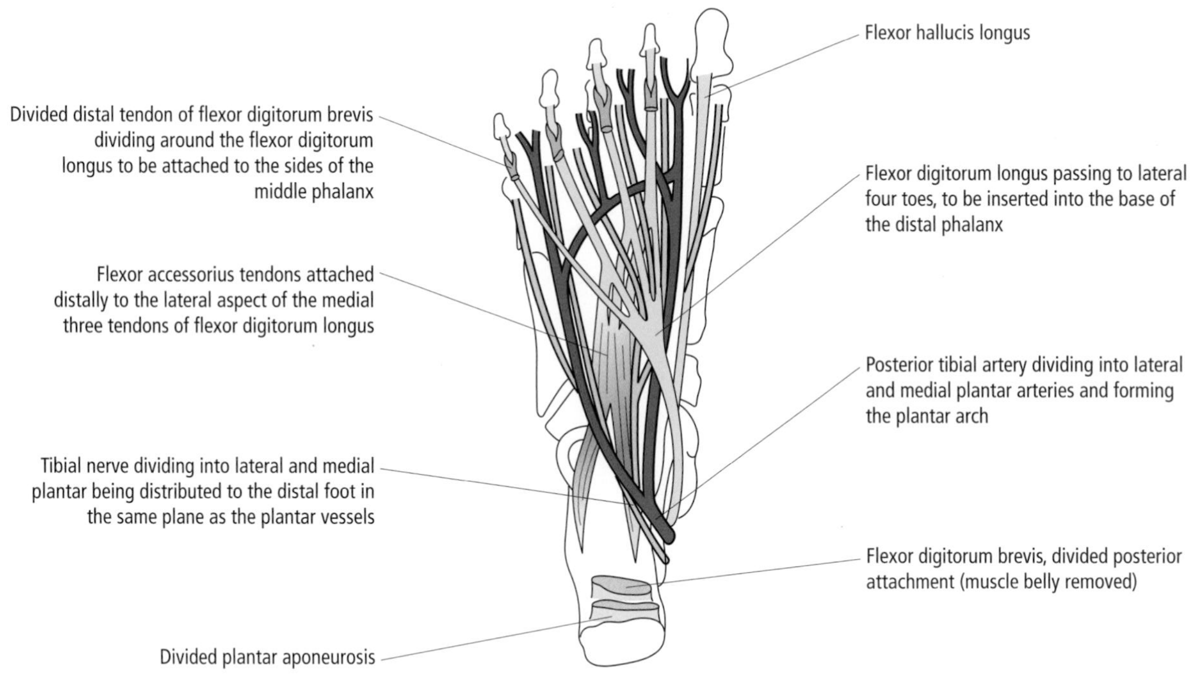

Figure 16.29 Sole of right foot; bulk of flexor digitorum brevis removed to show posterior tibial artery and tibial nerve and tendons in the sole of the foot

Relations

It is overlapped by biceps tendon in its upper course but is subcutaneous and easily palpated where it lies on the neck of the fibula (Fig. 16.20b).

Branches

- **Sural communicating branch** – pierces the roof of the popliteal fossa and joins the sural nerve halfway down the calf.
- **Lateral cutaneous nerve of leg** – supplies the lateral aspect of the leg.
- **Articular branches** – to the knee.
- **Superficial peroneal (fibular) nerve** – descends deep to peroneus (fibularis) longus and, in the lower leg, emerges through the deep fascia to divide into cutaneous branches. It supplies peroneus (fibularis) longus and brevis, cutaneous branches to the lower lateral leg and, by its dorsal cutaneous branches, which descend over the extensor retinacula, to supply the dorsum of the foot.
- **Deep peroneal (fibular) nerve** – passes around the neck of the fibula into the anterior compartment and descends in it together with the anterior tibial artery. It passes under the extensor retinacula to divide into medial and lateral terminal branches. It supplies the long dorsiflexors – extensor digitorum longus, extensor hallucis longus and tibialis anterior; its lateral terminal branch supplies extensor digitorum brevis and the ankle joint, and its medial terminal branch supplies skin in the web of the first toe on the dorsum of the foot.

Peripheral nerve injuries in the lower limb are described on p. 271.

MCQs

1. **You are invited to demonstrate the surface markings of the lower limb. Not all the landmarks you suggest are correct. Which are correct?** **T/F**
   - **a** the saphenous opening lies six finger breadths below the pubic symphysis (____)
   - **b** the tendon of adductor magnus can be palpated in the groin with the leg adducted (____)
   - **c** the site of the posterior inferior iliac spine is seen as a dimple (____)
   - **d** the common peroneal (fibular) nerve can be rolled against the head of the fibula (____)
   - **e** the lower fibres of vastus medialis lie horizontally (____)

Answers

1.

a ***F*** *– The saphenous opening lies some 3–4 finger breadths (3–4 cm) below and 1 cm lateral to the pubic tubercle.*

b ***F*** *– The tendon that is so easily felt is that of adductor longus. Adductor magnus is much more fleshy and has no obvious tendon.*

c ***F*** *– The 'dimples of Venus' seen or felt in the upper medial quadrant of the buttock are due to fascial adherence to the posterior superior iliac spines. This is also a useful landmark for the level of the 2nd sacral vertebra and the termination of the thecal sac.*

d ***F*** *– The common peroneal (fibular) nerve winds around the neck of the fibula, where it may be easily felt.*

e ***T*** *– It is these fibres that resist lateral dislocation of the patella.*

---

2. **The knee joint:** **T/F**
   - **a** can only rotate when fully extended (____)
   - **b** is reinforced by numerous ligaments, the strongest of which is the tibial collateral ligament (____)
   - **c** contains cruciate ligaments that lie within the synovial cavity (____)
   - **d** nerve supply is from the femoral and sciatic nerves only (____)
   - **e** has a meniscus to which popliteus is attached posteriorly (____)

Answers

2.

a ***F*** *– The knee joint has the ability to rotate, but only when flexed.*

b ***F***

c ***F*** *– The intracapsular cruciate ligaments, which resist anteroposterior movements of the femur on the tibia, lie extrasynovially.*

d ***F*** *– Its nerve supply follows Hilton's law and is therefore not only via the femoral and sciatic nerves but also via a branch from the obturator nerve.*

e ***T*** *– Popliteus pulls the lateral meniscus clear of the condyles at the initiation of knee flexion.*

EMQs

Each question has an anatomical theme linked to the chapter, and a list of 10 related items (A–J) placed in alphabetical order: these are followed by five statements (1–5). Match **one or more** of the items A–J to each of the five statements.

Muscles of the lower leg

A. Extensor digitorum longus
B. Extensor hallucis longus
C. Flexor digitorum longus
D. Flexor hallucis longus
E. Gastrocnemius
F. Peroneus (fibularis) brevis
G. Peroneus (fibularis) longus
H. Soleus
I. Tibialis anterior
J. Tibialis posterior

Match the following statements with the muscle(s) in the above list.

1. Attached to the femoral condyles
2. Attached to the fibula
3. Attached to the styloid process of the fifth metatarsal
4. Forms the tendocalcaneus (Achilles tendon)
5. Lies medial to the dorsalis pedis artery

Answers

1 E; 2 ABDFGHJ; 3 F; 4 EH; 5 B

Nerves of the lower leg

A. Extensor digitorum longus
B. Extensor hallucis
C. Flexor digitorum longus
D. Flexor hallucis longus
E. Gastrocnemius
F. Peroneus (fibularis) brevis
G. Peroneus (fibularis) longus
H. Soleus
I. Tibialis anterior
J. Tibialis posterior

Match the following nerves and statements with the muscle(s) in the above list.

1. Supplied by the tibial nerve
2. Supplied by the common peroneal (fibular) nerve
3. Medial to the tibial nerve at the ankle
4. Lateral to the tibial nerve at the ankle
5. Site of division of the common peroneal nerve

Answers

1 CDEHJ; 2 ABFGI; 3 CJ; 4 D; 5 G

APPLIED QUESTIONS

1. Why is a knowledge of the suprapatellar bursa clinically important?

1. The superior extension of the knee joint, known as the suprapatellar bursa, may sustain an anterior penetrating wound which, because of its connection with the knee joint, may cause a septic arthritis. Any effusion in the knee whether caused by trauma, inflammation or infection is clinically evident by detectable swelling of the suprapatellar bursa.

---

2. Why is a popliteal pulse difficult to feel even in the normal individual?

2. The popliteal pulse is difficult to palpate in most people because it is the deepest-lying structure in the popliteal fossa. Having pierced the adductor magnus at the adductor hiatus, it lies deep to its vein, which is in turn deep to the tibial nerve in the popliteal fossa. All these structures are embedded in fat, and both the artery and the vein are additionally surrounded by a tough fibrous sheath. Flexion of the knee, which allows relaxation of nerve and sheath, often facilitates palpation.

---

3. A young man is crossing the road and is knocked down by a bus. On his arrival at hospital it is noticed that he has a very swollen lateral side of the knee and lower leg, and that he cannot dorsiflex his foot. Can you explain his 'foot drop'?

3. This is a typical 'bumper-bar' injury or 'bumper fracture', which usually results in a fractured neck of the fibula and associated soft tissue damage. At this site the common peroneal (fibular) nerve winds into the lateral, and later the anterior, compartment of the lower leg, and is easily damaged. The branches of the common peroneal (fibular) nerve are the superficial and deep peroneal (fibular) nerves. The deep nerve runs with the anterior tibial artery to supply the extensor group of muscles, including tibialis anterior, whereas the superficial peroneal (fibular) nerve supplies the peroneal muscles, which are the major evertors of the foot. Damage to the deep peroneal (fibular) nerve therefore results in an inability to dorsiflex the foot, whereas an injured superficial peroneal (fibular) nerve results in an inverted foot. A combination of these is 'foot drop', i.e. an inverted plantar flexed foot which, if permanent, results in the patient catching the big toe on the swing-through and scuffing the anterolateral part of his shoes when walking.

17 The foot

The foot is an arched platform formed of separate bones bound by ligaments and muscles; it supports the body's weight, acts as a rigid lever which can propel the body forward, and yet is resilient enough to absorb the shocks resulting from impact with the ground. The foot is also important as a source of proprioceptive information essential to the maintenance of balance, during both standing and walking.

THE BONES OF THE FOOT

The skeleton of the foot comprises the tarsus, metatarsus and phalanges. The **tarsus** (Fig. 17.1a–d) comprises the talus, calcaneus, navicular, cuboid and three cuneiform bones.

The **talus** carries the whole of the body weight. It has a body, neck and head, and no muscular attachments. The **body's** upper surface is markedly convex anteroposteriorly, slightly concave from side to side, and articulates with the inferior surface of the tibia. This broad articular facet is continuous with a facet on each side of the bone for articulation with the medial and lateral malleoli; the three articular surfaces are known as the **trochlear surface** of the talus. The concave inferior surface of the body articulates with the posterior facet on the calcaneus. The posterior margin bears a posterior tubercle that gives attachment to the posterior talofibular ligament. The **neck** bears a deep groove inferiorly. The hemispherical **head** articulates with the navicular bone, the calcaneus and the plantar calcaneonavicular (spring) ligament inferomedially (see Fig. 17.7, p. 267).

The **calcaneus** (Figs 17.1 and 17.2) is an irregularly rectangular bone forming the prominence of the heel and articulating with the talus above and the cuboid anteriorly. Its upper surface has posterior, middle and anterior articular facets for the talus. The middle facet lies medially on the prominent **sustentaculum tali**, which gives attachment to the calcaneonavicular ligament (spring ligament). Behind the facet is a deep groove, the **sulcus calcanei**, which, with the sulcus tali, forms a tunnel, the **sinus tarsi**, which houses the strong talocalcaneal ligament. These articulations with the talus constitute the 'subtalar' joint that permit the movements of inversion and eversion of the ankle.

The inferior surface has an **anterior tubercle** to which is attached the short plantar ligament and, posteriorly, the **medial** and **lateral processes** on the weightbearing **tuberosity**, to which are attached the long plantar ligament, the short muscles of the sole and the plantar aponeurosis. On the lateral surface is the **peroneal (fibular) tubercle**, separating the tendons of peroneus (fibularis) longus and brevis. The posterior surface gives attachment to the tendocalcaneus and the anterior surface articulates with the cuboid bone.

The **navicular bone** lies on the medial side of the foot and articulates with the talus posteriorly and the three wedged-shaped cuneiform bones anteriorly. Its medial surface extends down to form the prominent and palpable **navicular tuberosity**, to which are attached tibialis posterior and the calcaneonavicular ligament.

The wedge-shaped **cuboid** lies laterally. It articulates with the calcaneus posteriorly, the bases of the 4th and 5th metatarsals anteriorly, and the lateral cuneiform medially. Its inferior surface gives attachment to the long plantar ligament, and it has a marked groove for the tendon of peroneus (fibularis) longus.

The three wedge-shaped **cuneiforms** articulate posteriorly with the navicular and anteriorly with the bases of the three medial metatarsals. To the medial cuneiform are attached the tendons of tibialis anterior and posterior and peroneus (fibularis) longus.

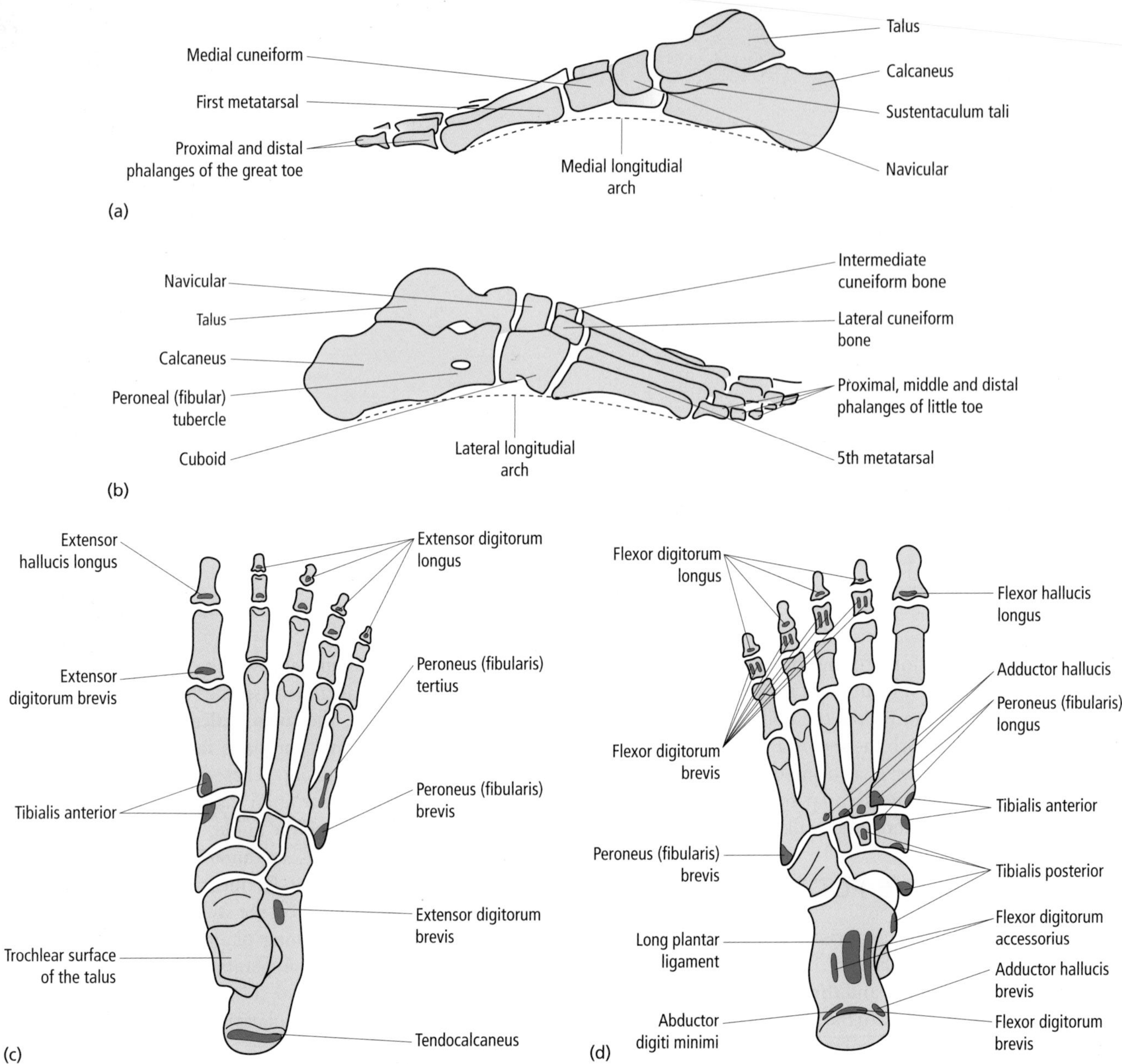

Figure 17.1 Bones of the right foot. (a) Medial aspect. (b) Lateral aspect. (c) Superior aspect and (d) plantar aspect of foot showing muscle attachments

The **metatarsals and phalanges** of the foot resemble those of the hand, but the metatarsals are longer and more slender. The first metatarsal is thick and transmits the body weight in walking. The 1st toe usually has only two phalanges.

THE ANKLE JOINT

The ankle joint is a hinged synovial joint between the mortise formed by the inferior surface of the tibia, the medial surface of the lower fibula and the trochlear surface of the talus (Fig. 17.2a,b). Its stability rests on the medial and lateral malleoli lying alongside the talus. Its capsule, attached to the articular margins, possesses capsular thickenings which contribute considerably to the strength of the joint:

- **Medial (deltoid) ligament** – this is triangular in shape, with its apex attached to the medial malleolus and its base to the navicular, the neck of the talus, the plantar calcaneonavicular ligament and the medial side of the talus (Fig. 17.3), as well as the sustentaculum tali.
- **Lateral ligament** – this has three parts: an anterior talofibular ligament from the lateral malleolus passing horizontally to the neck of the talus, the calcaneofibular ligament passing back from the malleolar tip to the lateral side of the calcaneus, and the posterior talofibular ligament passing horizontally between the malleolar fossa of the lateral malleolus and the posterior tubercle of the talus (Figs 17.4 and 17.5).

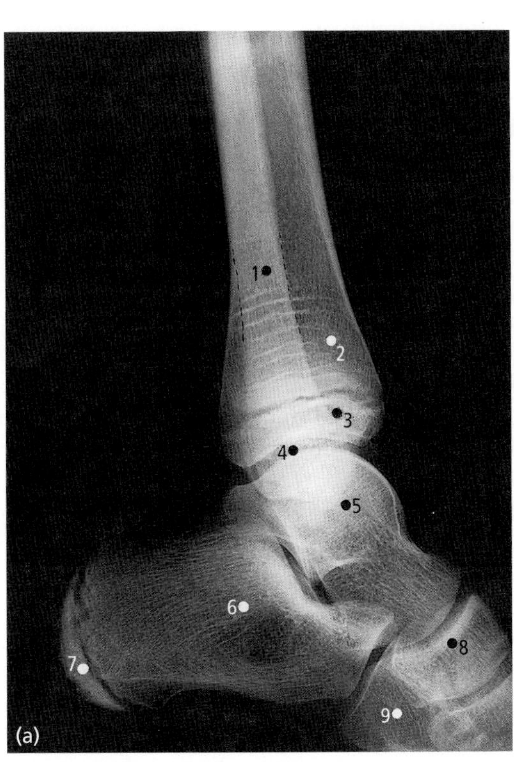

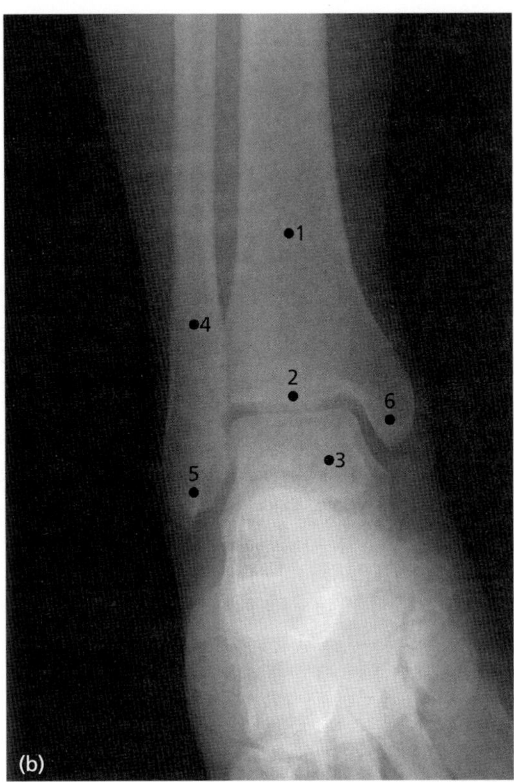

Figure 17.2 Ankle X-ray. (a) Lateral view: 1, outline of fibula overlapping tibia; 2, tibia; 3, tibial epiphysis; 4, line of the ankle joint; 5, talus; 6, calcaneus; 7, calcaneal epiphysis; 8, navicular; 9, cuboid. (b) Anteroposterior view: 1, tibia; 2, line of the ankle joint; 3, talus; 4, fibula; 5, lateral malleolus; 6, medial malleolus

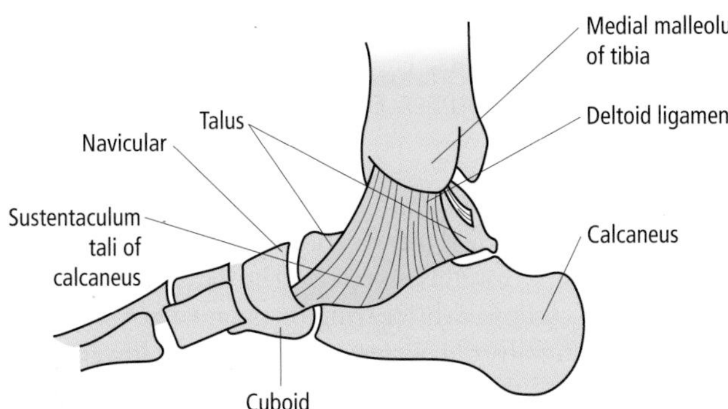

Figure 17.3 Medial aspect of the right ankle joint showing the deltoid ligament

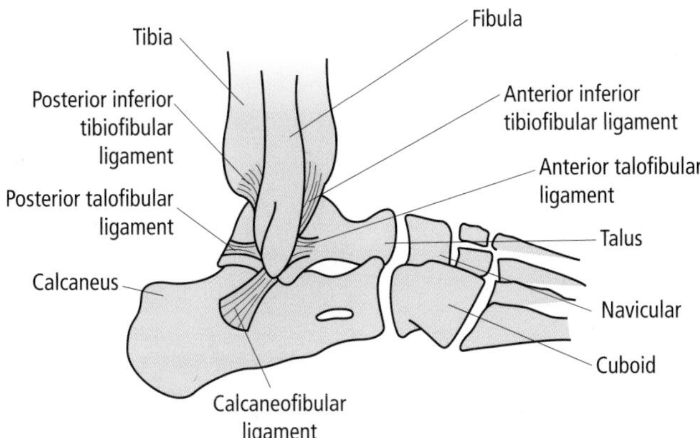

Figure 17.4 Lateral aspect of the right ankle joint showing ligaments

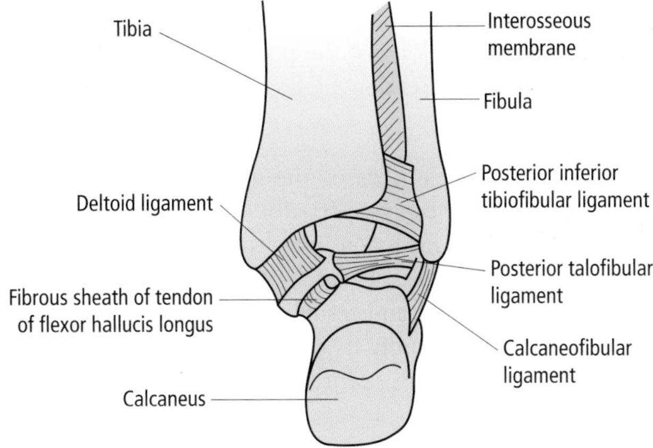

Figure 17.5 Posterior aspect of the right ankle joint showing ligaments

An accessory ligament, the **inferior transverse tibiofibular ligament**, a thick band between the two malleoli across the back of the talus, is covered with hyaline cartilage and deepens the articular surface between it and the talus.

Functional aspects

Movement

Plantar flexion (downwards movement of the foot) and dorsiflexion (upwards movement) are possible, plantar flexion by gastrocnemius and soleus, assisted by other flexor muscles and possibly the peronei. Dorsiflexion is by tibialis and other extensor muscles (plantar flexion is 'true flexion').

Stability

This is a stable joint maintained by the mortise arrangement of its bones and strong ligaments. The centre of gravity passes anterior to the joint, and as the foot is dorsiflexed on the grounded foot the tibiofibular mortise firmly grips the wider anterior talar surface, i.e. when walking up a slope. It is least stable in the plantarflexed position, for example in a ballet dancer *en pointe*.

Relations

Medially and laterally the joint is subcutaneous (Fig. 16.23a,b, p. 255). Anteriorly it is crossed, medial to lateral, by tendons of tibialis anterior and extensor hallucis longus, the anterior tibial vessels and deep peroneal (fibular) nerve, and the tendons of extensor digitorum longus. Posteromedially, from medial to lateral, it is crossed by tendons of tibialis posterior and flexor digitorum longus, the posterior tibial vessels and tibial nerve, and the tendon of flexor hallucis longus. The tendons of peroneus (fibularis) longus and brevis cross the joint posterolaterally. All the tendons are surrounded by synovial sheaths (Fig. 16.19a,b, p. 251).

The tarsal joints

The most important tarsal joints are:

- **Subtalar (talocalcaneal) joint** – a synovial joint between the inferior facet on the body of the talus and the posterior facet of the calcaneus. The capsule is partly thickened by talocalcaneal bands, but the strongest union is provided by the **interosseous talocalcaneal ligament** in the sinus tarsi which is taut in eversion.
- **Talocalcaneonavicular joint** – a synovial joint of the ball and socket variety between the hemispherical head of the talus and the concavity formed by facets on the upper calcaneus, the concavity of the navicular and the plantar calcaneonavicular ligament. The capsule is reinforced by the spring ligament, the deltoid ligament and the bifurcate ligament (see below).
- **Plantar calcaneonavicular (spring) ligament** (Fig. 17.7) – a strong thick band between the sustentaculum tali and the navicular tuberosity; it is covered by articular cartilage and contributes to the articular surface for the head of the talus. It is important in maintaining the medial longitudinal arch of the foot.
- **Calcaneocuboid joint** – a synovial joint between the reciprocal concavoconvex facets of the two bones; the capsule is reinforced by the bifurcate and the long and short plantar ligaments. The **bifurcate ligament** is attached proximally to the upper surface of the calcaneus and

The collateral ligaments of the ankle, the deltoid and the lateral ligament can be partially or completely torn by forcible eversion or inversion injuries. The severest injuries result in instability of the ankle joint. Inversion injuries are the most common and result in sprains or tears to the lateral ligament, especially its calcaneofibular and anterior talofibular components. More severe injuries result in associated bony injuries to the joint. A common fracture–dislocation of the ankle (Potts fracture) (Fig. 17.6a–d) occurs when the foot is forcibly everted. The lateral malleolus fractures first, followed by tearing of the medial collateral ligament and, finally, the posterior margin of the lower tibia shears off against the talus. The three stages are referred to as first-, second- and third-degree Potts fractures.

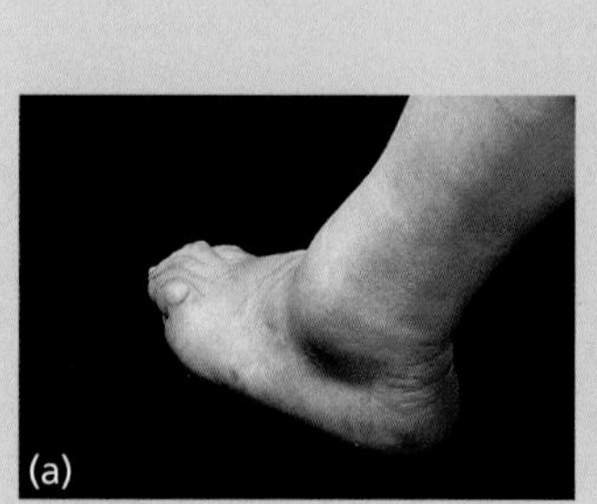

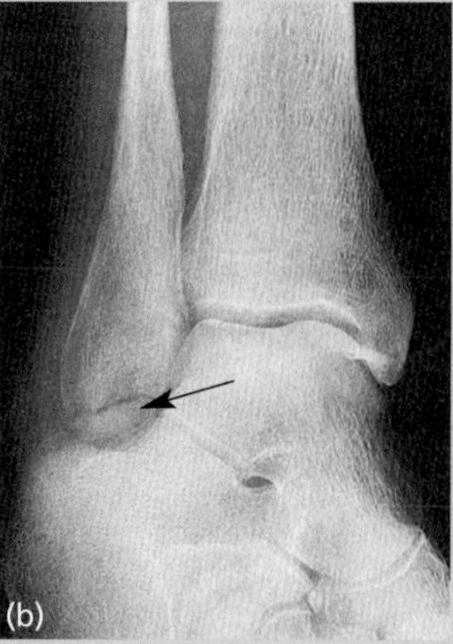

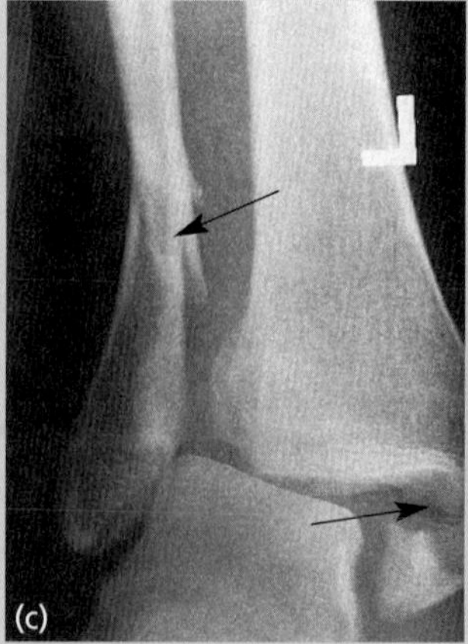

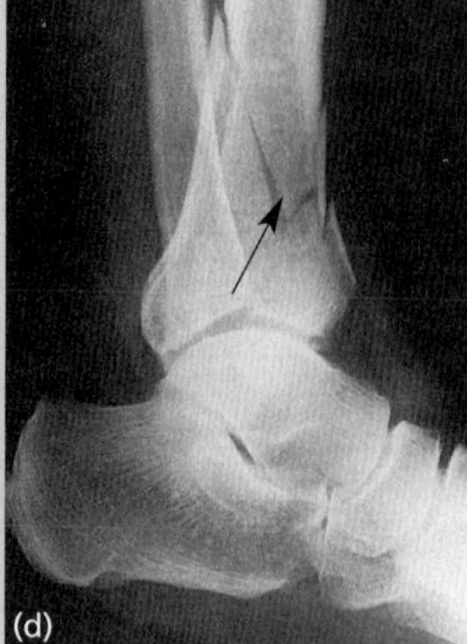

Figure 17.6 Fractures of the ankle joint (arrows): (a) shows swelling over lateral malleolus; (b) fractured lateral malleolus; (c) fractured fibula and medial malleolus; (d) fractured lower tibia

distally to the upper cuboid and navicular. The **long plantar ligament** passes between the posterior calcaneal processes to the ridges on the inferior surface of the cuboid and the bases of the lateral metatarsals. The **short plantar ligament** is more deeply placed and passes between the anterior process of the calcaneus and the adjacent cuboid (Fig. 17.7).

Functional aspects

Inversion (the sole of the foot is turned inwards and its medial border raised) and **eversion** (the sole turned outwards and its lateral border raised) are possible. Both movements occur not at the ankle joints but at the subtalar and talocalcaneonavicular joints. The calcaneus and the navicular, carrying the forefoot with them, move medially on the talus by a combination of rotary and gliding movements. The range of inversion and eversion is increased by movement at the **midtarsal (talonavicular and calcaneocuboid) joint.** Inversion is increased during plantar flexion because the narrow posterior end of the talus is not then so tightly fitted into the tibial mortise. Eversion is increased in dorsiflexion.

Inversion is produced by tibialis anterior and posterior; eversion by the peroneal (fibular) muscles. The interosseous talocalcaneal ligament limits inversion and the deltoid ligament limits eversion. These movements have been described with the foot off the ground; the same movements occurring when the foot is on the ground adjust the foot to uneven and sloping surfaces, as when walking across a steep incline or skiing down a mountain.

The **tarsometatarsal joints** and the remaining **intertarsal joints** are small plane synovial joints, capable only of slight gliding movements. They are tightly bound together by interosseous ligaments, and these are particularly strong on the **plantar aspect** of the foot.

Some children are born with the congenital deformity 'club foot' (Fig. 17.8), in which the toes most commonly point inwards and downwards (talipes equinovarus).

THE INTERPHALANGEAL JOINTS

The **metatarsophalangeal and interphalangeal joints** resemble those of the fingers but are less mobile, the metatarsal heads being bound together by deep transverse ligaments that unite all the plantar surfaces of the joint capsules. Plantar flexion and dorsiflexion occur at all these joints, as well as a very limited amount of abduction and adduction. Plantar flexion is produced by flexor hallucis longus and brevis, and flexor digitorum longus and brevis, dorsiflexion by extensor hallucis longus, and extensor digitorum longus and brevis muscles. The first metatarsophalangeal joint is much larger than the others. A sesamoid bone is often within each tendon of flexor hallucis brevis, the tendons and sesamoids being incorporated into the joint capsule. The tendon of flexor hallucis longus lies in the groove between the sesamoid bones and is thus protected from pressure.

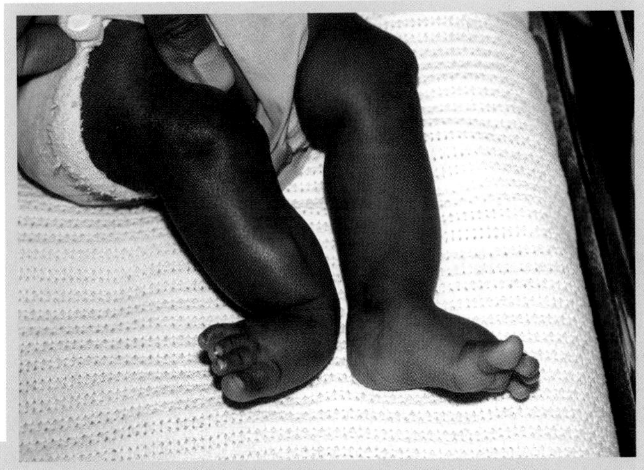

Figure 17.8 Club foot of the rare variety where the foot points outwards and upwards, known as talipes calcaneovalgus

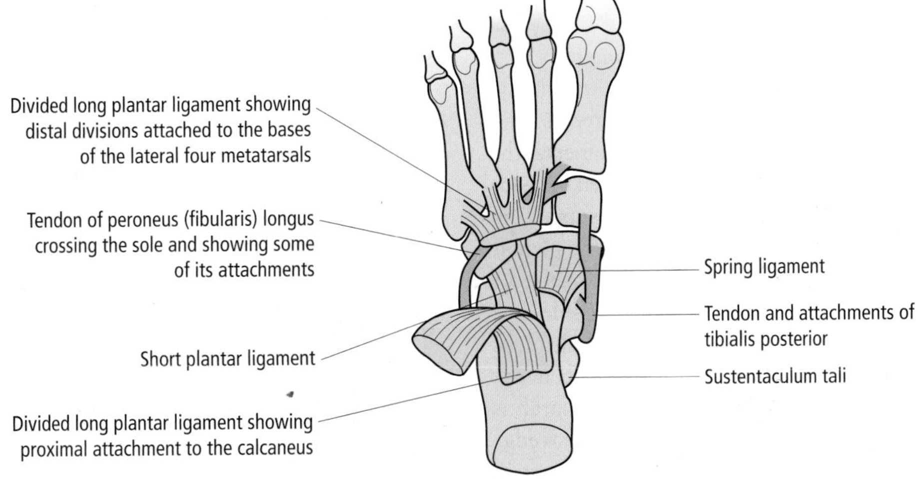

Figure 17.7 Dissection of sole of right foot showing plantar ligaments

The natural angle between the long axis of the 1st metatarsal and its proximal phalanx may be accentuated by tight shoes (**hallux valgus**) (Fig. 17.9). Hallux valgus is one of the commonest of foot deformities and is often seen in the elderly, possibly owing to loss of muscle tone. There is lateral deviation of the big toe, increased angulation of the first metatarsophalangeal joint and prominence of the metatarsal head. A protective bursa may develop on the medial side of the joint, and persistent trauma from shoes produces inflammation within it, with its attendant swelling, redness and pain (bunion). Surgical correction may be required to relieve pain or deformity.

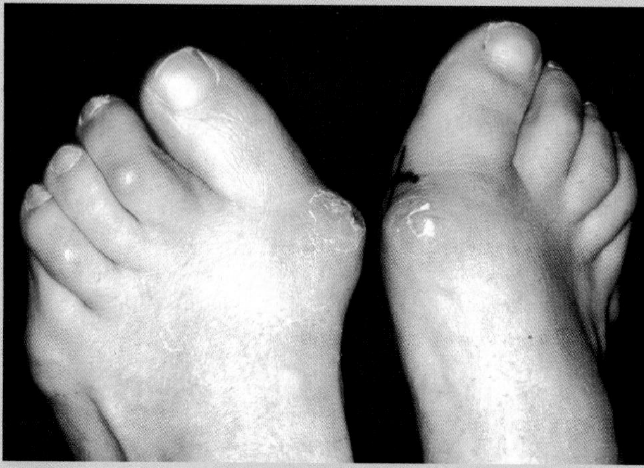

Figure 17.9 Bilateral hallux valgus

THE ARCHES OF THE FOOT

The arched foot is a human characteristic and is present from birth. Though a baby's foot appears flat because of the prominent fat pad on the sole of its foot, the skeletal basis for an arch can be seen radiologically. The arch becomes visible once the child begins to walk. The arches distribute the body weight over a larger area and prevent crushing of the vessels and nerves that cross the sole. The jointed pattern of the arch gives the foot resilience to absorb the impact of the body's weight when the foot comes into contact with the ground, yet still allows its use as a semirigid lever to propel the body forward in walking. There are medial, lateral and transverse arches, which are collectively involved in these functions.

The maintenance of each arch is dependent on bony, ligamentous and muscular factors: the short ligaments and muscles tie adjacent bones together, and the long ligaments, the plantar aponeurosis and the long muscle tendons tighten the ends of the arch together. Some long tendons act as slings, supporting the centre of the arch. The ligaments and muscles on the plantar surface are stronger and more numerous than on the dorsum.

The **medial longitudinal arch** (Fig. 17.1a) is visible and obvious; it extends from the medial process of the calcaneus via the talus, navicular and three cuneiforms to the heads of the three medial metatarsals. Some support to the arch is given by the sustentaculum tali to the talus, and by the wedge shape of some of the bones, but their contribution is not as significant as that made by the ligaments and muscles:

- The **plantar calcaneonavicular (spring) ligament** (Fig. 17.7) supports the head of the talus
- **Interosseous ligaments**
- The **plantar aponeurosis** binds the ends of the arch together
- The **short muscles** of the foot, especially abductor hallucis, flexor hallucis brevis and flexor digitorum brevis
- **Tibialis anterior** is attached to the centre of the arch
- **Flexor hallucis longus** and the medial part of **flexor digitorum longus** span across the arch
- **Tibialis posterior** ties together the posterior bones of the arch.

The **lateral longitudinal arch** (Fig. 17.1b) is lower than the medial; it extends from the lateral process of the calcaneus via the cuboid to the heads of the 4th and 5th metatarsals. Its shape is maintained largely by ligaments and to a lesser extent by muscles, namely:

- The **plantar aponeurosis**
- The **long and short plantar ligaments** unite the calcaneus, the cuboid and the bases of the 4th and 5th metatarsals
- **Interosseous ligaments**
- The **short muscles of the foot**, especially flexor digitorum brevis
- **Peroneus (fibularis) longus** passes below the centre of the arch deep to the cuboid, which it supports.

The **transverse arch** lies across the distal row of the tarsus, the cuneiform and cuboid bones, and the adjacent metatarsals. Its shape is maintained by the wedge-like shape of the cuneiform, the interosseous ligaments and the peroneus (fibularis) longus, tibialis posterior and adductor hallucis muscles.

Flat feet (pes planus) (Fig. 17.10) are caused by a flattening of the medial longitudinal arch – the result of excessive ligamentous laxity, particularly in the plantar calcaneonavicular 'spring' ligament, loss of muscle power or abnormal load distribution. Flat feet are common in older people, especially if excessive weight gain has occurred. Diagnosis is readily made by examination of wet footprints on the bathroom floor, where it is revealed that the normally raised medial arch has disappeared. The underlying cause is often inherited and the condition is usually asymptomatic, but it may cause chronic foot strain.

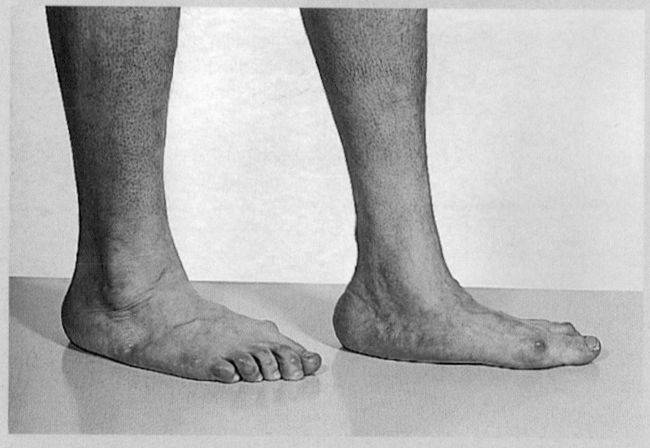

Figure 17.10 Flat feet

THE SOLE OF THE FOOT

The skin over the weightbearing areas of the heel and 'ball' of the foot is thickened in its superficial layers and firmly attached to the deep fascia. The superficial fascia is fat-filled and serves to cushion the deeper structures. The deep fascia has a thickened central portion, the **plantar aponeurosis**, and thin medial and lateral portions. The aponeurosis is attached posteriorly to the back of the undersurface of the calcaneus and divides anteriorly into five digital expansions. These are attached to the fibrous flexor sheaths and to the deep transverse ligaments between the metatarsal heads. When the toes are dorsiflexed the aponeurosis tightens and the longitudinal arch is accentuated.

Inflammation in the attachments of the plantar aponeurosis (**plantar fasciitis**) occasionally occurs and is accompanied by acute pain on pressure over the calcaneus, especially during weightbearing and standing. It is a condition often suffered by those doing a lot of walking as their job, e.g. postmen and postwomen.

Muscles of the sole

These have counterparts to those of the hand, short flexors, abductors and adductor of the great toe, lumbrical and interosseous muscles, but there is no opponens muscle (Fig. 17.11). These small muscles help to maintain the arches, and to flex and extend the toes, but have little abductor or adductor function. A sesamoid bone is present on each side of the head of the 1st metatarsal, embedded in the tendons of the short muscles passing to the phalanges of the great toe. They form a protective groove for the tendon of flexor hallucis longus.

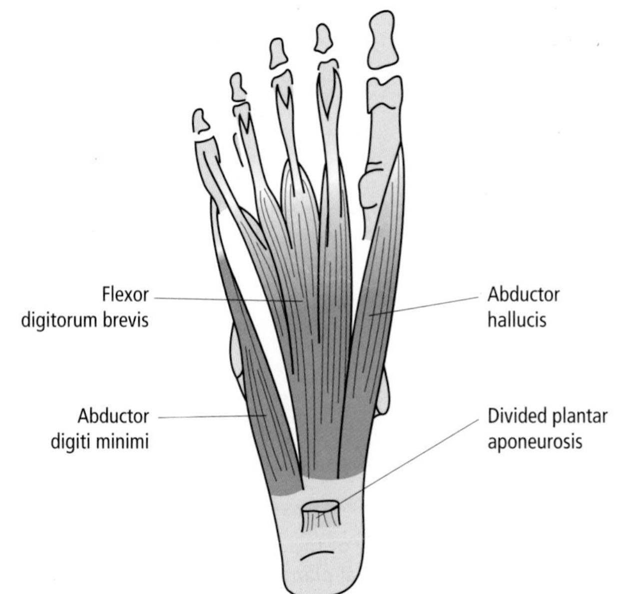

Figure 17.11 Small muscles of the right foot

Flexor accessorius has no counterpart in the hand. Attached to calcaneus posteriorly and to the tendons of flexors digitorum and hallucis longus anteriorly, it maintains tension in the long tendons and can flex the toes even when the long flexors must relax, e.g. when the leg, during the supporting phase of walking, is pulled forward over the ankle joint by tibialis anterior and the extensor muscles.

The long flexor tendons pass in the sole into the long flexor sheaths, to be attached to the terminal phalanges. Three calf muscles are inserted on the medial side of the foot: **tibialis posterior** (Fig. 17.7; see also Fig. 16.29, p. 259) to the tuberosity of the navicular, and then to most other tarsal bones and to the metatarsal bases. **Peroneus (fibularis) longus** crosses the foot inferiorly from the lateral side to attach to the medial cuneiform and the base of the 1st metatarsal, and **tibialis anterior** is attached to the same two bones. They each give much support to the arches of the foot.

The new fashion for rollerblading and inline skating often causes **tendinitis** in these long flexors as they battle to keep the feet balanced when turning corners.

Nerves of the sole

- **Medial plantar nerve** (Fig. 16.29, p. 259) – this begins under the flexor retinaculum and passes forwards, accompanied by its vessels. It supplies flexor hallucis brevis, abductor hallucis, flexor digitorum brevis and the 1st lumbrical, and supplies cutaneous branches to the medial part of the sole and the medial 3½ toes.
- **Lateral plantar nerve** – this is a terminal branch of the tibial nerve. Accompanied by its artery, it passes obliquely forwards across the sole to the base of the fifth metatarsal, to divide into deep and superficial branches which supply the remaining short muscles of the sole and cutaneous branches to the skin over the lateral side of the foot and the lateral 1½ toes.

Cutaneous nerve supply

This is outlined in Figures 17.12–17.14a,b. To summarize: we kneel on skin supplied by L3/4, and the dorsum of the foot is supplied by L5. We stand on skin supplied by S1 and sit on S3. Autonomic nerves, mainly sympathetic, are contained in the branches of the lumbosacral plexus and supply blood vessels, sweat glands and erector pili muscles.

Lower limb sensory testing (with eyes closed) of dermatomes and individual nerves:

Touch (cotton wool); Pain (sterile needle); Temperature (side of finger v cold side of tuning fork); Vibration (base of tuning fork on medial malleolus); Graphasthesia (writing numbers on shin with a blunt instrument); Position sense (recognizing direction of movement – hold sides of big toe)

Continued on p. 271

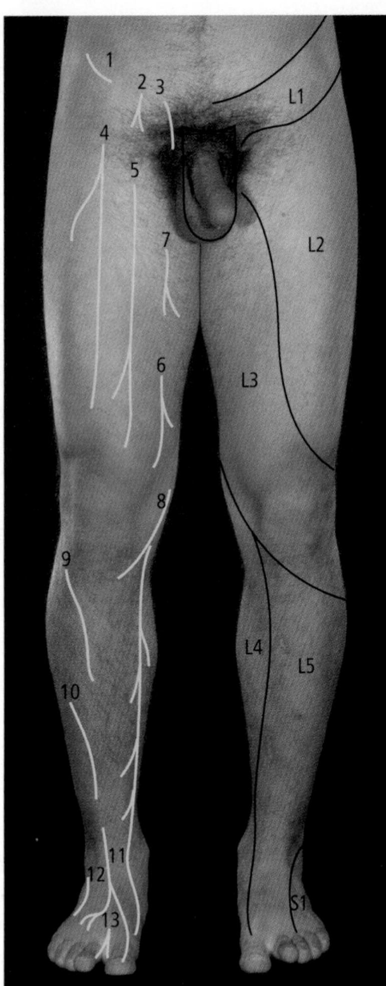

Figure 17.12 Surface anatomy showing lower leg dermatomes (left leg) and cutaneous nerves (right leg), anterior aspect: 1, subcostal; 2, femoral branch of genitofemoral; 3, ilio-inguinal; 4, lateral cutaneous of thigh; 5, intermediate cutaneous of thigh; 6, medial cutaneous of thigh; 7, obturator; 8, saphenous; 9, lateral cutaneous of calf; 10 and 11, superficial peroneal (fibular); 12, sural; 13, deep peroneal (fibular)

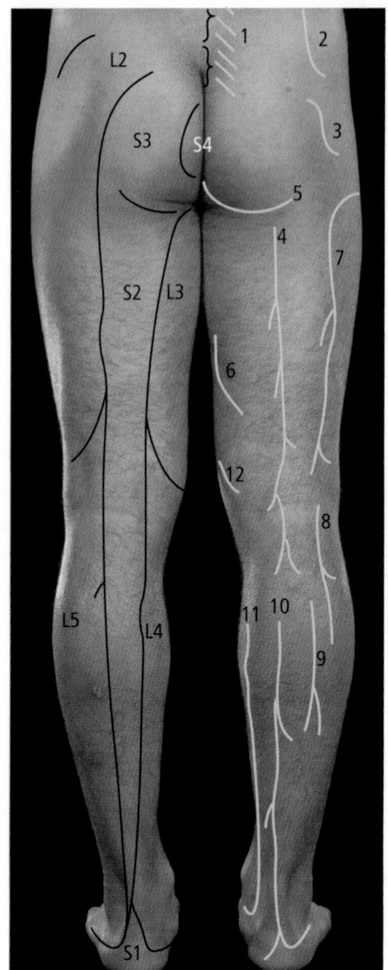

Figure 17.13 Surface anatomy of lower limb dermatomes (left leg) and cutaneous nerves (right leg), posterior aspect: 1, dorsal rami; 2, subcostal; 3, posterior lumbar rami; 4, posterior cutaneous nerve of thigh; 5, gluteal and perineal branch; 6, obturator; 7, lateral cutaneous nerve of thigh; 8, lateral cutaneous nerve of calf; 9, sural communicating; 10, sural; 11, saphenous; 12, medial cutaneous nerve of thigh

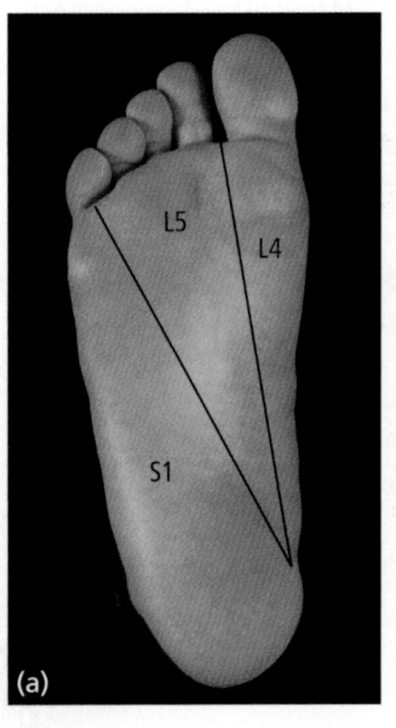

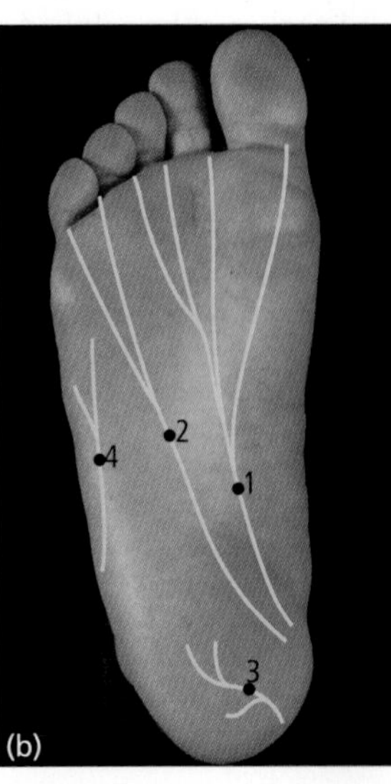

Figure 17.14 Surface anatomy of the sole. (a) Dermatomes. (b) Cutaneous nerves: 1, medial plantar; 2, lateral plantar; 3, medial calcaneal branch of the tibial nerve; 4, sural. L = lumbar, S = sacral

Motor testing

Power (dorsiflexion of foot against resistance); Tone (passive flexion and extension of relaxed knee joint); Coordination (heel up and down along opposite shin – eyes open and then closed); Reflexes (knee L3,4; ankle S1,2); note wasting and abnormal movements; individual muscles – active and passive movements, and against resistance).

PERIPHERAL NERVE INJURIES IN THE LOWER LIMB

Femoral nerve

Injuries to this nerve produce loss of knee extension (quadriceps), some loss of hip flexion (iliacus and pectineus), and loss of sensation over the front of the thigh and the medial side of the thigh, leg and foot (anterior and medial femoral cutaneous nerves and the saphenous nerves) (Fig. 17.15a–c).

Damage to the lateral femoral cutaneous nerve of the thigh, which may follow its entrapment just below the inguinal ligament close to the anterior superior iliac spine by, for example, a psoas abscess, often results in pain and sensory loss over the lateral thigh (meralgia paraesthetica).

Obturator nerve

Injury to this nerve will produce some loss in the power of adduction, but this is not complete because adductor magnus is partly supplied by the sciatic nerve. Occasionally there is an associated slight loss of sensation over the middle of the medial thigh. This is often related to lateral pelvic wall malignancy.

Sciatic nerve

A proximal injury, e.g. following a posterior dislocation of the hip, produces an almost flail limb (hip flexion is retained) but there is often no or only minimal loss of sensation (Fig. 17.16).

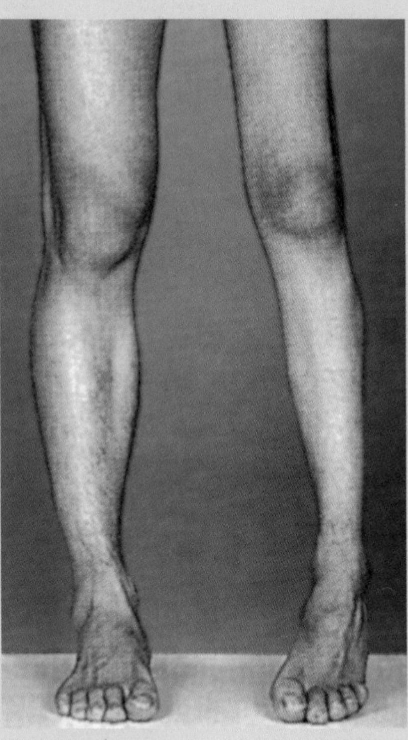

Figure 17.16 Left sciatic nerve palsy with severe muscle wasting below the knee

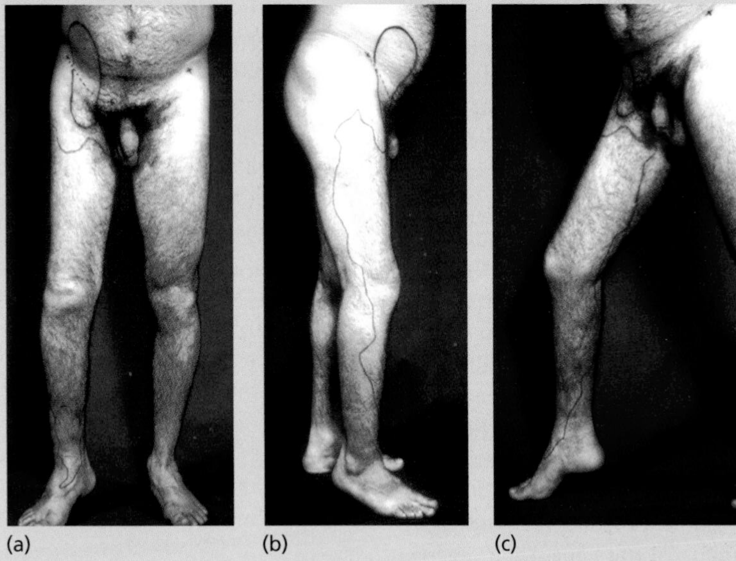

Figure 17.15 (a–c) Femoral nerve palsy caused by a haematoma within psoas muscle sheath – note the outline of the swelling marked in black across the inguinal region causing right quadriceps wasting and sensory loss over the anteromedial thigh and following the course of the saphenous nerve towards the ankle. The area of sensory loss is marked by the red line

Tibial nerve

Injury in the leg causes loss of plantar flexion and sensory loss over the sole of the foot. Injury proximal to the sural nerve produces sensory loss over the lateral side of the leg and foot similar to that produced by leprosy affecting the tibial nerve (Fig. 17.17). Injury at the ankle paralyses the small muscles of the foot, and the unopposed action of the long flexors and extensors produces a highly arched foot and claw toes.

Common peroneal (fibular) nerve

This is a relatively common injury because of its superficial and vulnerable position as it winds around the neck of the fibula. Dorsiflexion (extensor muscles) and eversion (the peronei) are lost; the foot drops and becomes inverted. There is sensory loss over the medial side of the dorsum of the foot.

Superficial peroneal (fibular) nerve

Eversion (the peronei) is lost and the foot becomes inverted. There is loss of sensation over the medial side of the dorsum of the foot.

Deep peroneal (fibular) nerve

Dorsiflexion of the foot and toes is lost and there may be sensory loss between the first and second toes.

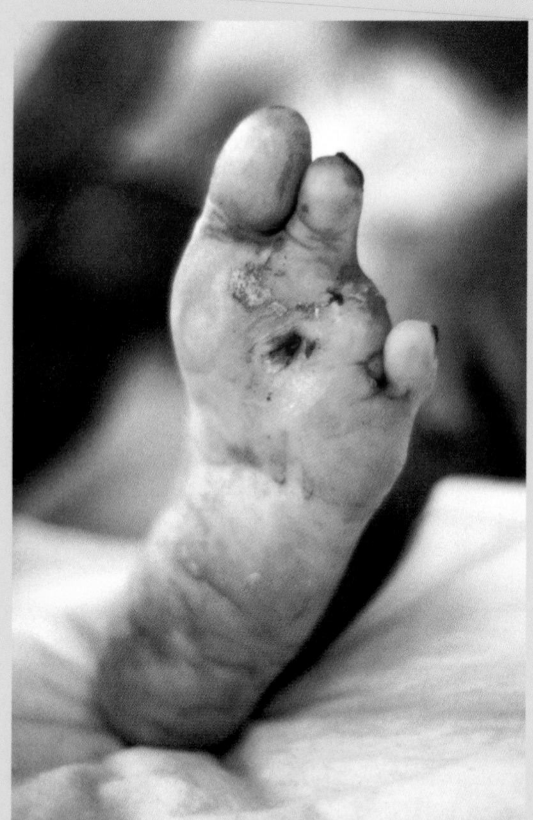

Figure 17.17 Peripheral neuropathy affecting tibial nerve causing toe loss and ulceration of sole due to loss of sensation. In the Western world this palsy is most commonly seen with diabetes mellitus

POSTURE AND WALKING

Posture

The body weight is transmitted through the pelvic girdle to both femoral heads. In each limb the weight is transmitted through bones whose internal architecture is adapted to withstand compressive stresses to the foot, whose arches distribute the weight between the calcaneal tubercles and metatarsal heads. The head of the 1st metatarsal takes more than a third of the metatarsal load.

In the normal stance the line of weight (centre of gravity) in the anatomical position lies in front of the 2nd sacral vertebra and passes slightly behind the hip joints and in front of the knee and ankle joints. The erect posture is maintained by muscles and ligaments. In the anatomical position the body's weight causes hyperextension at the hip and knee, which is resisted at the hip by the iliofemoral ligament and by contraction of iliopsoas. Hyperextension at the knee it is resisted by the collateral and cruciate ligaments and contraction of the hamstrings and gastrocnemius. The ankle joint mortise contributes more than the ligaments to the stability of the joint. Slight changes in posture may bring the line of weight behind the knee, and flexion is resisted by contraction of quadriceps. The long digital flexors help by holding the toes firmly to the ground.

Walking

In each limb the cycle of movement has a stance (supporting) phase and a swing phase. The cycle begins as the heel touches the ground and ends as the same heel touches the ground again.

In the **stance (supporting) phase** the body weight is taken on the grounded leg and muscle contraction increases the forward momentum of the body. As the heel touches the ground, extension of the hip joint gives a forward thrust and medial rotation maintains the direction of progress. Meanwhile, hip abduction by gluteus minimus, medius and tensor fasciae latae tilts the pelvis on the grounded leg, giving the swinging leg some height to move forward. The knee of the grounded leg is extended and locked, so that weight is carried by bones and ligaments, and at the end of this swing the grounded knee is unlocked by lateral rotation of the femur on the tibia. At the ankle joint plantar flexion, which is partly passive, gives way to active dorsiflexion, so that the body weight is pulled over the ankle and the foot becomes slightly everted and the body weight is transferred from the heel along the lateral border of the foot to the metatarsal heads.

The swing phase

In this, the leg swings through from a trailing to a leading position. At the hip joint, there is flexion, lateral rotation and adduction. At the knee joint, flexion occurs until the swinging foot has passed the supporting foot and then extension occurs, at the end of which some lateral rotation of the tibia may lock the knee joint in preparation for weight bearing. At the ankle joint, the foot is first dorsiflexed but becomes plantar flexed as the knee extends. The foot itself becomes inverted and the heel touches the ground (heel strike) in readiness for the next supporting phase.

Starting to **walk** involves a forward tilting of the body thus advancing the centre of gravity and the line of weight. The supporting limb is extended, the pelvis is tilted on the supporting leg, and the heel is raised by the calf muscles. The opposite limb flexes and then extends until the heel touches the ground. Thus it becomes the supporting limb after a very short swing phase. Turning to left or right involves most of the trunk muscles as well as the rotators at the hip joint. They largely determine the route followed by the swinging leg and the position of the touch-down of the swinging heel. In **running**, the centre of gravity is usually further forward due to flexion of the vertebral column, thus altering the total posture. There is considerable time between the end of the stance phase and the heel strike of the foot of the swinging leg, so that the body is clear of the ground (unsupported) for this time. In running, active plantar flexion at the ankle joint at the end of the stance phase increases the forward momentum of the body.

Although described separately, these movements merge into one another indistinguishably. Limitation of the movement at any joint results in a marked alteration in gait. The individuality of the gait depends on the length of the stride, the extent of pelvic rotation (swinging the hips) and the impetus at the end of the stance phase.

MCQs

1. In the adult foot: **T/F**

- **a** inversion is increased in plantar flexion (___)
- **b** eversion is increased in plantar flexion (___)
- **c** eversion is produced by tibialis anterior (___)
- **d** inversion is produced by the peroneal (fibular) muscles (___)
- **e** eversion is limited by tension in the deltoid ligament (___)

Answers

1.

- ***a*** ***T*** – *The movement is greatest in plantar flexion because the narrower posterior part of the talus allows more movement in the plantar flexed ankle joint.*
- ***b*** ***F*** – *The range of eversion is greatest in dorsiflexion.*
- ***c*** ***F*** – *It is produced by the peroneal (fibular) muscles.*
- ***d*** ***F*** – *It is produced by the synergistic action of tibialis anterior and posterior muscles, and limited by tension in the peroneal (fibular) muscles and the interosseous talocalcaneal ligament …*
- ***e*** ***T*** – *… and also by tension in the tibialis muscles.*

---

2. The arches of the foot: **T/F**

- **a** cause the weight of the body to be concentrated in a small area of the sole (___)
- **b** give the foot rigidity (___)
- **c** are dependent on bony factors alone (___)
- **d** are not present at birth (___)
- **e** are supported by prominent plantar capsular thickenings (___)

Answers

2.

- ***a*** ***F*** – *They allow weight to be spread over a wide area.*
- ***b*** ***F*** – *They make it resilient and well suited to absorb impacts when jumping.*
- ***c*** ***F*** – *The maintenance of the arches is dependent on muscular, ligamentous and bony factors.*
- ***d*** ***F*** – *They are present but masked by fat.*
- ***e*** ***T*** – *They are stronger and more numerous than the dorsal capsular thickenings.*

---

3. In the lower limb damage to: **T/F**

- **a** L4 results in an absent ankle jerk (___)
- **b** L2 results in weakened hip flexion (___)
- **c** the obturator nerve results in little or no sensory loss (___)
- **d** the tibial nerve results in loss of sensation on the sole of the foot (___)
- **e** S1 may result in weakness of eversion (___)

Answers

3.

- ***a*** ***F*** – *L4 is the spinal nerve involved in the knee jerk.*
- ***b*** ***T*** – *Damage to L2 affects the contraction of iliopsoas, attached to the lesser trochanter, and is a powerful flexor of the hip.*
- ***c*** ***T*** – *Remember that all cutaneous sensory supply involves much overlapping between nerves.*
- ***d*** ***T*** – *Also loss of the ankle jerk.*
- ***e*** ***T*** – *Damage to S1 also involves a loss of sensation posterior to the lateral malleolus, as well as causing problems with plantar flexion and an absent ankle jerk.*

EMQs

Each question has an anatomical theme linked to the chapter, and a list of 10 related items (A–J) placed in alphabetical order: these are followed by five statements (1–5). Match **one or more** of the items A–J to each of the five statements.

Cutaneous innervation of the lower leg

A. 1st sacral dermatome
B. 2nd lumbar dermatome
C. 3rd lumbar dermatome
D. 3rd sacral dermatome
E. 4th lumbar dermatome
F. 5th lumbar dermatome
G. Lateral cutaneous nerve of thigh
H. Obturator nerve
I. Saphenous nerve
J. Sural nerve

Match the following cutaneous innervation to the nerve(s) and dermatome(s) in the above list.

1. Front of the patella
2. Medial aspect of the ankle
3. Sole of foot
4. Buttock
5. Medial aspect of the thigh

Answers

1 C; 2 EI; 3 A; 4 D; 5 BCH

APPLIED QUESTIONS

1. Describe the anatomical basis for 'flat feet'.

1. In infants the flat appearance of feet is normal, a result of the subcutaneous fat pads in the soles. Bony arches are present at birth, but only become visible after the baby has walked for a few months. Flat feet in adolescents and adults are caused by 'fallen arches', usually the medial longitudinal. During long periods of standing, older persons, or those who rapidly gain weight, stretch the plantar ligaments and aponeurosis, which are non-elastic structures, with the loss of their important bowstringing effect in the stationary foot. The strain on the spring ligament eventually makes it unable to support the head of the talus, and as a result flattening of the medial longitudinal arch occurs, with lateral deviation of the forefoot. Fallen arches are painful owing to stretching of the plantar muscles and strained plantar ligaments. Pes planus is a true flattening from osteomuscular causes.

2. Why is it not uncommon to find that the patient with a severe sprain of the ankle has an avulsion fracture of the fifth metatarsal?

2. In severe inversion injuries tension is exerted on the laterally placed muscles and, in particular, the peronei. Peroneus (fibularis) brevis, originating from the fibula, inserts into the tuberosity of the fifth metatarsal. Tension on this insertion often results in its fracture. It is not uncommon to find, in younger patients, that the normal radiological appearances of the epiphysis in this region are wrongly thought to represent a fracture of the tuberosity.

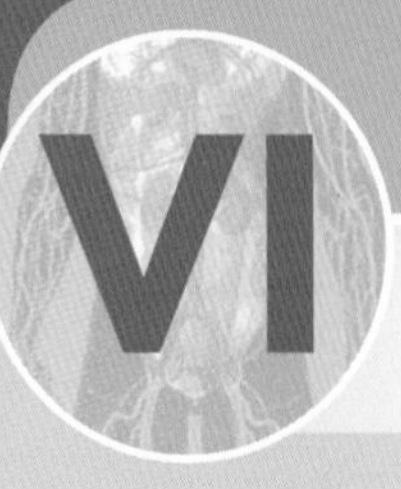

The head and neck

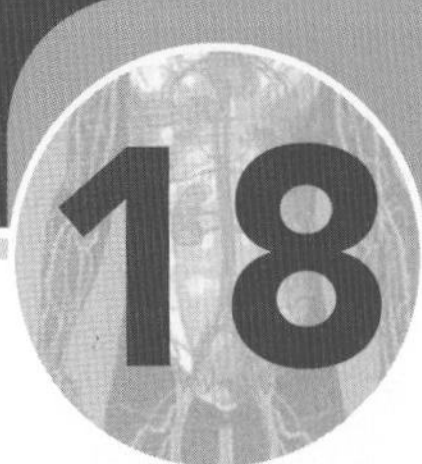

18 The skull, scalp and face

THE SKULL

The skull, a term that includes the mandible, is described viewed from above, from in front, from the side and from below.

Superior aspect

The vault (roof of the cranium) is crossed by three sutures (Fig. 18.1). The **coronal suture** separates the frontal bone from the two parietal bones posteriorly. The midline **sagittal suture** separates the two parietal bones. Its junction with the coronal suture, the **bregma**, is incompletely ossified at birth and can be felt as a diamond-shaped deficiency known as the **anterior fontanelle**. This closes at about 18 months of age. The **lambdoid suture** separates the two parietal bones and the occipital bone posteriorly, and meets the sagittal suture at the **lambda**. This, too, is not ossified at birth and presents as a small bony deficiency, the **posterior fontanelle**, which closes by the 3rd to 6th month.

Figure 18.1 Bones and sutures of vault

An early fusion of fontanelles may cause restriction to brain growth; a late closure of the fontanelles may be an indication of an increased intracranial pressure that has resulted from an accumulation of cerebrospinal fluid (CSF) (hydrocephalus) (Fig. 18.2). Hydrocephalus is the result of

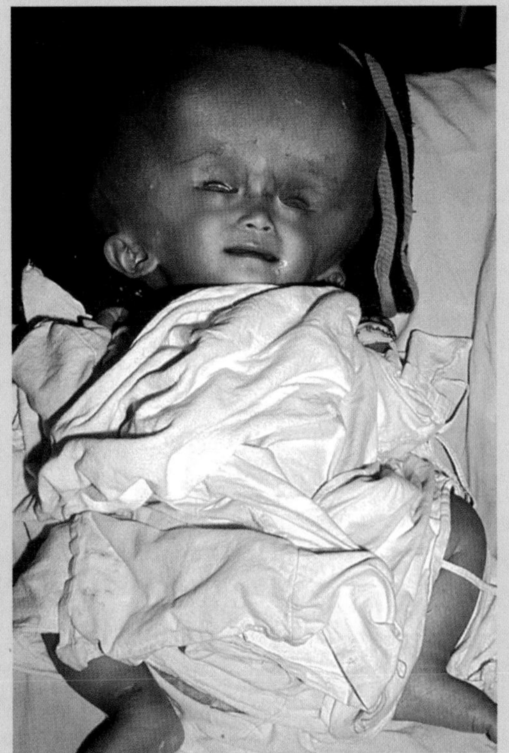

Figure 18.2 Severe untreated hydrocephalus

(a) overproduction of CSF; (b) obstruction to its flow; or (c) a decrease in its absorption. Surgical treatment usually involves draining the CSF into the venous system by means of an indwelling shunt.

Anterior aspect

The smooth convexity of the frontal bone lies superiorly; below it are the openings of the orbital, nasal and oral cavities (Fig. 18.3a–c). The **supraorbital margin** possesses a supraorbital notch or foramen in its inner third which transmits the supraorbital vessels and nerve. The lateral orbital margin is formed by the frontal and zygomatic bones (the frontozygomatic suture is subcutaneous and palpable); the medial margin by the frontal bone and the frontal process of the maxilla; the inferior margin by the maxillary bone medially; and the lateral margin by the zygomatic bone. Above the supraorbital margins are the palpable superciliary arches, between which lies the **glabella**.

The prominence of the cheek is produced by the zygomatic bone. One centimetre below the orbit on the maxilla, in line with the supraorbital notch, is the **infraorbital foramen**, from which emerge the infraorbital vessels and nerve. The **nasal aperture** is bounded above by the nasal bones, and below and laterally by the maxillae. The opening of the oral cavity is surrounded by the alveolar margins of the maxillae and mandible, which bear sockets for the teeth. The **mental foramen** on the mandible is in line with the supra- and infraorbital foramina, and from it emerge the mental vessels and nerve.

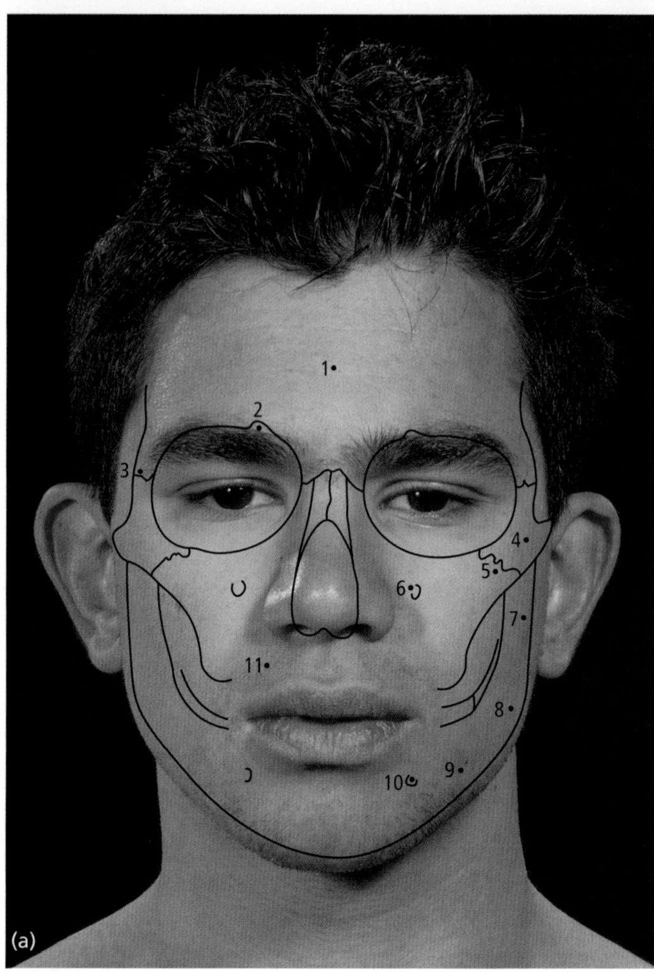

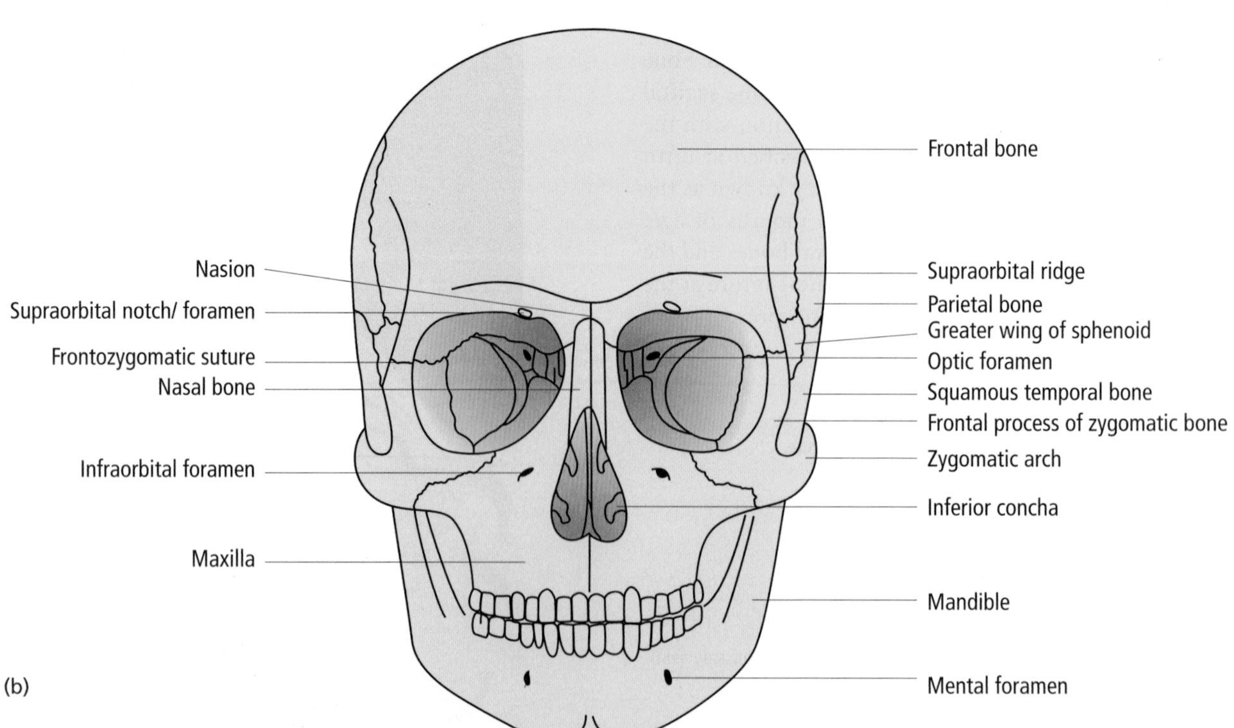

Figure 18.3 (a) Surface anatomy of the facial skeleton: 1, frontal bone; 2, supraorbital notch; 3, frontozygomatic suture; 4, zygomatic bone; 5, zygomaxillary suture; 6, infraorbital foramen; 7, ramus of mandible; 8, angle of mandible; 9, body of mandible; 10, mental foramen; 11, maxilla. (b) Skull – anterior view. (*continued*)

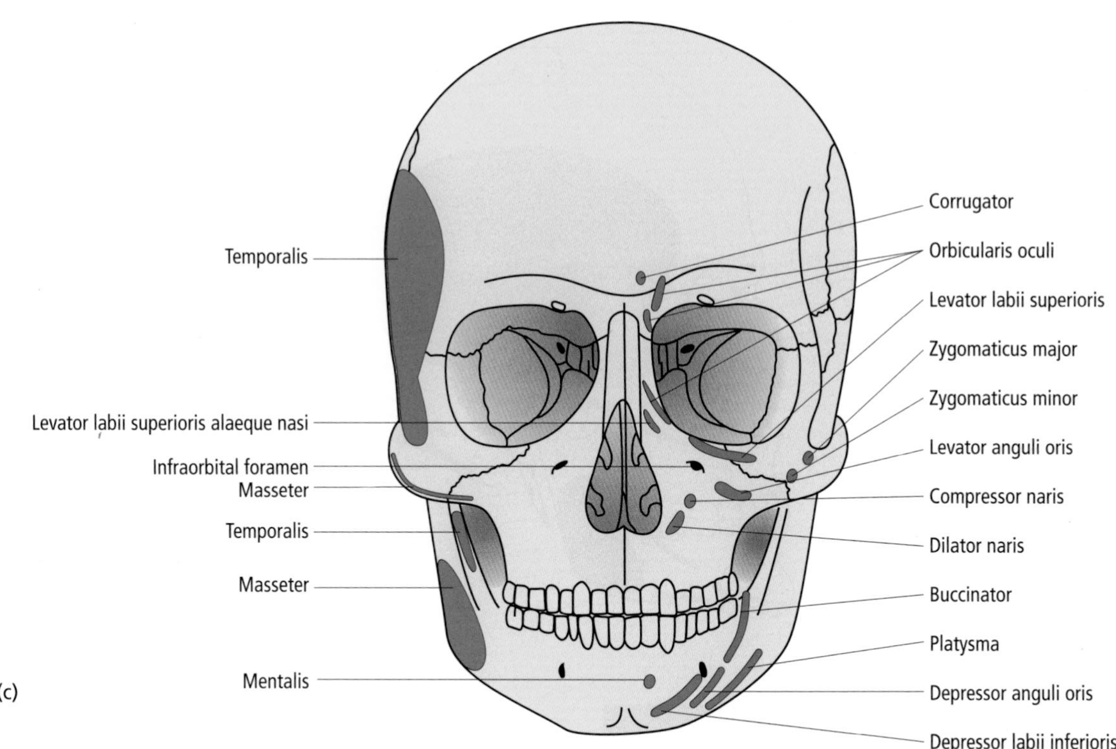

Figure 18.3 (*continued*) (c) Anterior view showing muscle attachments

Lateral aspect

The **zygomatic arch** is formed by the zygomatic process of the temporal bone and the temporal process of the zygomatic bone (Fig. 18.4a–c). The temporal superior line curves upwards and backwards from the zygomatic process of the frontal bone across the parietal bone, and then down and forwards over the squamous temporal bone to end above the external acoustic meatus. The region below the temporal line, deep to the zygomatic arch, is the **temporal fossa**, which is roofed by the temporal fascia attached to the temporal line and the upper border of the zygomatic arch. The medial wall of the fossa is formed by the frontal, parietal, temporal and greater wing of the sphenoid bones. Their H-shaped union, the **pterion,** lies about 4 cm above the midpoint of the zygomatic arch.

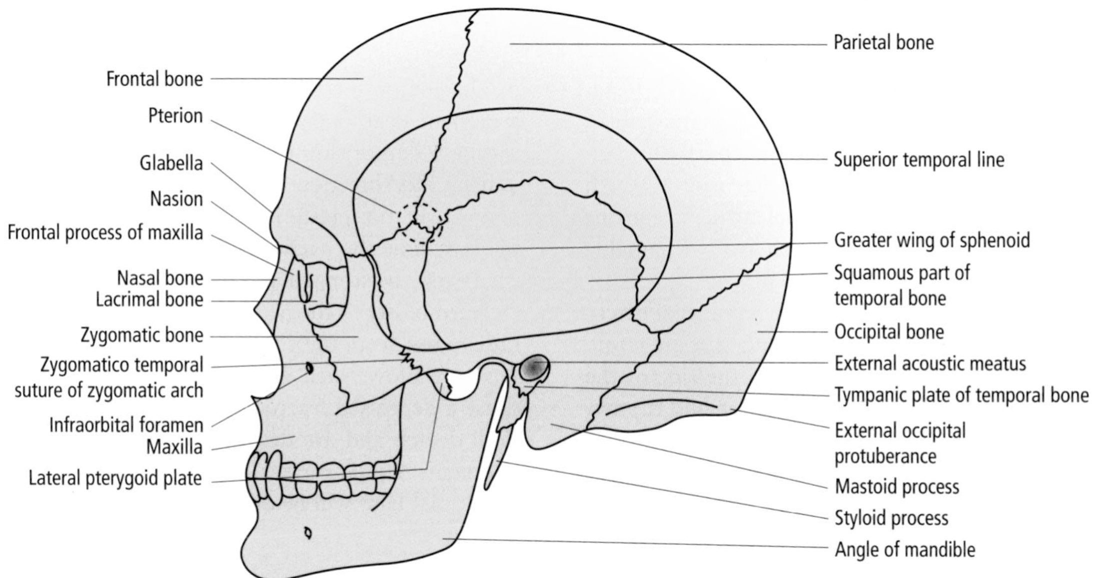

Figure 18.4 Lateral aspect of the skull: (a) Bones. (*continued*)

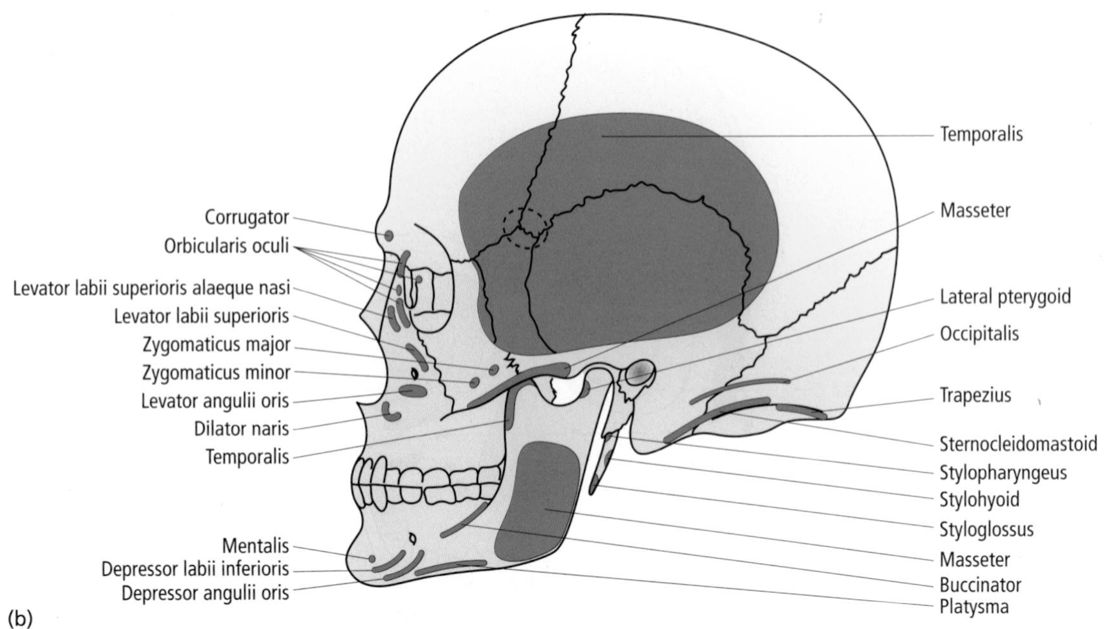

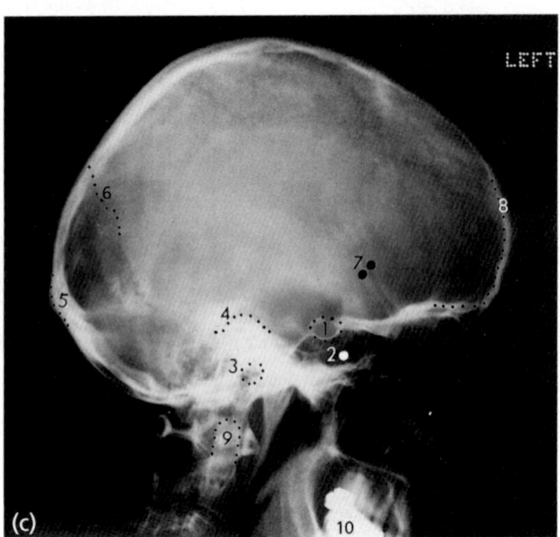

Figure 18.4 (*continued*) (b) Muscle attachments. (c) X-ray: 1, pituitary fossa; 2, sphenoidal air sinus; 3, external acoustic (auditory) meatus; 4, petrous temporal bone; 5, external occipital protuberance; 6, parieto-occipital suture; 7, meningeal vessel markings; 8, frontal bone; 9, dens of axis; 10, dental fillings

Below the temporal fossa is the **infratemporal fossa,** limited medially by the lateral pterygoid plate, which communicates with the pterygopalatine fossa through the pterygomaxillary fissure and with the orbit through the inferior orbital fissure. The **external acoustic meatus** opens below the posterior zygomatic arch and the palpable **mastoid process** is prominent behind the meatus.

The pterion overlies where the middle meningeal artery grooves the inner surface of the bone, and it is therefore an important clinical landmark. A blow to the side of the head may fracture the thin bones of the pterion and rupture the middle meningeal vessels. The resulting haematoma lies outside the dural covering of the brain but exerts pressure and compression on the underlying brain (Fig. 18.5). If the haematoma continues to grow then without surgical treatment death may follow in hours; treatment involves raising a flap of skin (whose base lies inferiorly, because it is from this direction that all vessels and nerves reach the scalp) over the pterion and drilling a burr-hole. Through the burr-hole the haemorrhage from the middle meningeal artery may be stopped and the haematoma evacuated.

Hard blows to the head result in fractures which usually radiate out from the site of impact in rather straight lines. A severe blow, such as from a hammer or a bullet, may cause a depressed fracture in which several small pieces of skull detach and are driven into the brain. The depressed fragments require surgical elevation (Fig. 18.6). Fractures of the cranial base will be discussed later (p. 287).

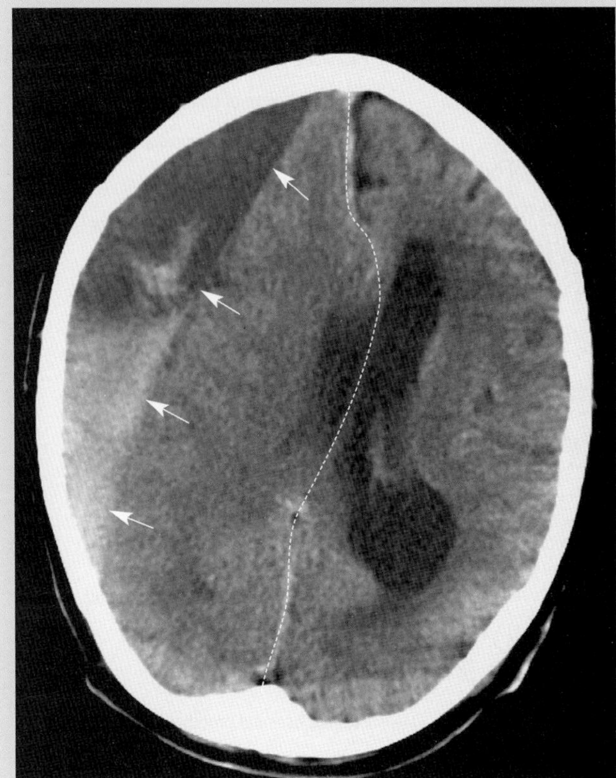

Figure 18.5 Extradural haematoma (arrowed) showing cerebral shift – the dotted line shows midline shift

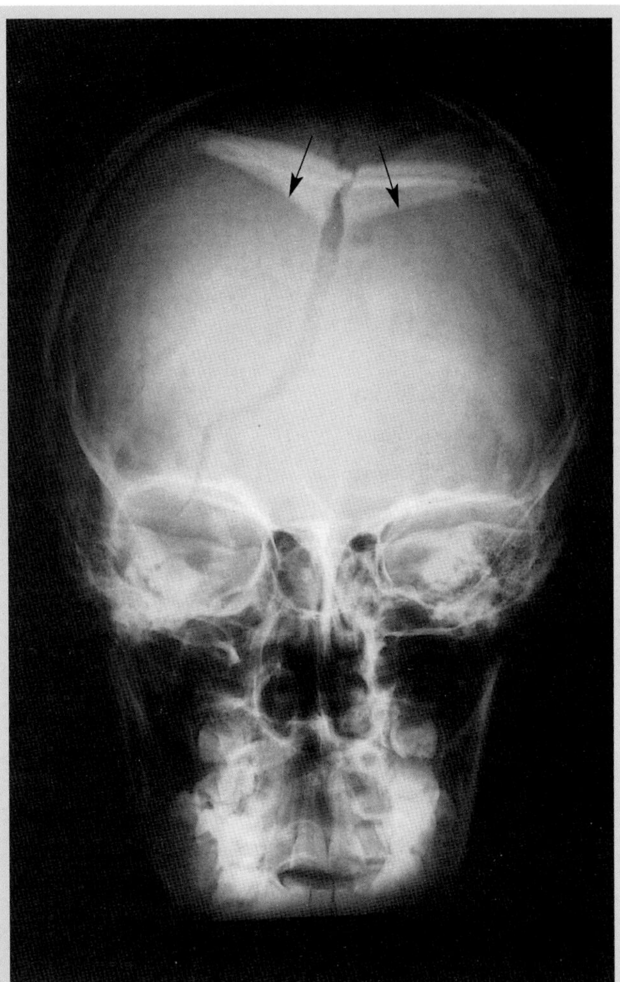

Figure 18.6 Depressed fracture of skull (arrowed)

Inferior aspect

Anteriorly is the hard palate, formed by the palatine processes of the maxillae in front of the horizontal plates of the palatine bones (Fig. 18.7a,b). It is bounded anterolaterally by the alveolar processes of the maxillae, whose rounded posterior extremity is the maxillary tuberosity. Anteriorly a midline incisive foramen communicates with the nasal cavity and transmits the greater palatine arteries and nasopalatine nerves; on the posterolateral palate are the greater and lesser palatine foramina, which convey vessels and nerves of the same name. The **posterior nasal apertures** (**choanae**) open above the palate, bounded above by the body of the sphenoid bone, below by the horizontal plates of the palatine bones, and laterally by the medial pterygoid plates. The apertures are separated by the thin, wedge-shaped midline **vomer**. From the medial pterygoid plate projects the **hamulus** (Fig. 18.8), which gives attachment to the pterygomandibular raphe. Behind the base of the lateral pterygoid process is the foramen ovale, which transmits the mandibular nerve; and posterolateral to the foramen are the spine of the sphenoid and the foramen spinosum, which transmits the middle meningeal artery. To the spine of the sphenoid is attached the sphenomandibular ligament and lateral to the spine is the **mandibular fossa**, with which the mandibular condyle articulates. The petrous temporal bone lies between the occipital and sphenoid bones and contains the carotid canal, whose inferior opening lies behind the spine of the sphenoid. Posterolateral to the carotid opening is the **jugular foramen**, which transmits the internal jugular vein and the glossopharyngeal, vagus and accessory nerves. Posterolateral to the styloid process is the stylomastoid foramen, which transmits the facial nerve. The occipital bone contains the **foramen magnum**, bounded on each side by the occipital condyles, and a foramen transmitting the hypoglossal nerve.

Posterior aspect

Behind the foramen magnum are the superior and inferior nuchal lines, between which are attached the postvertebral muscles. In the middle of the superior line is the prominent and palpable **external occipital protuberance**.

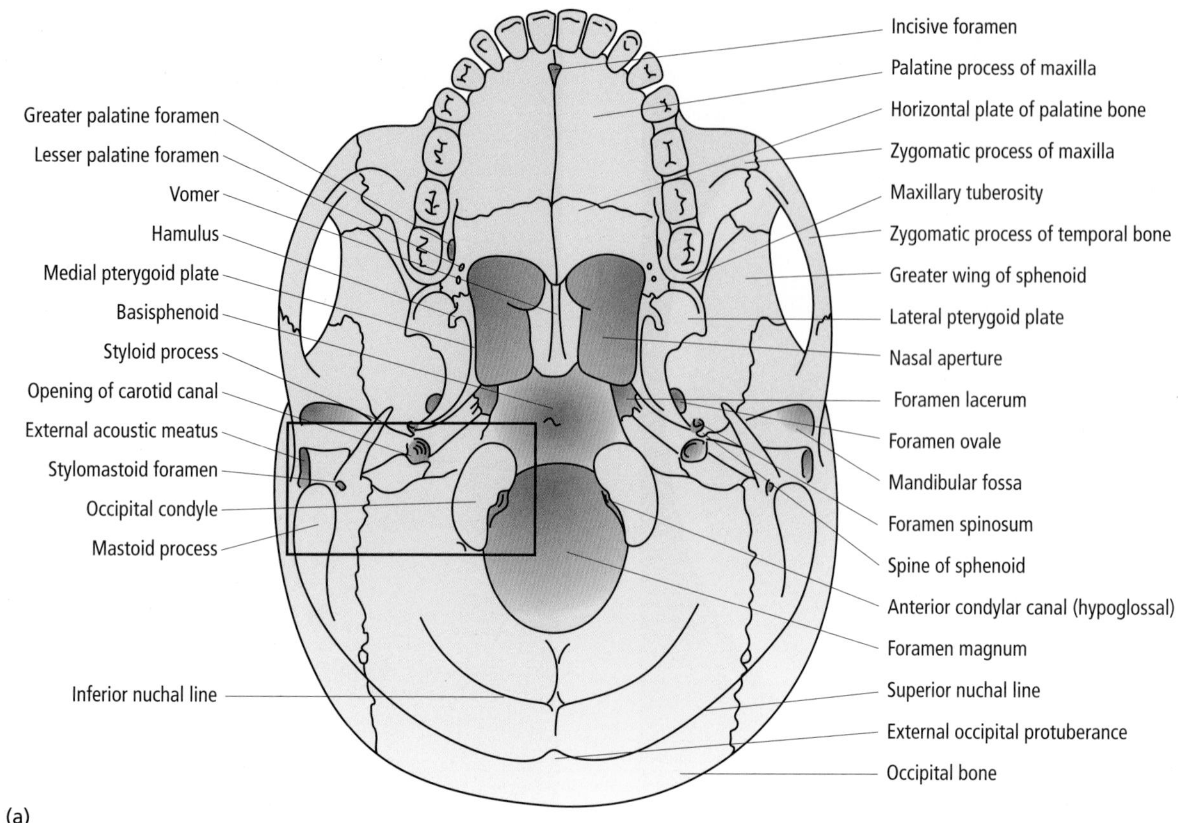
Incisive foramen
Palatine process of maxilla
Horizontal plate of palatine bone
Zygomatic process of maxilla
Maxillary tuberosity
Zygomatic process of temporal bone
Greater wing of sphenoid
Lateral pterygoid plate
Nasal aperture
Foramen lacerum
Foramen ovale
Mandibular fossa
Foramen spinosum
Spine of sphenoid
Anterior condylar canal (hypoglossal)
Foramen magnum
Superior nuchal line
External occipital protuberance
Occipital bone
Greater palatine foramen
Lesser palatine foramen
Vomer
Hamulus
Medial pterygoid plate
Basisphenoid
Styloid process
Opening of carotid canal
External acoustic meatus
Stylomastoid foramen
Occipital condyle
Mastoid process
Inferior nuchal line
(a)

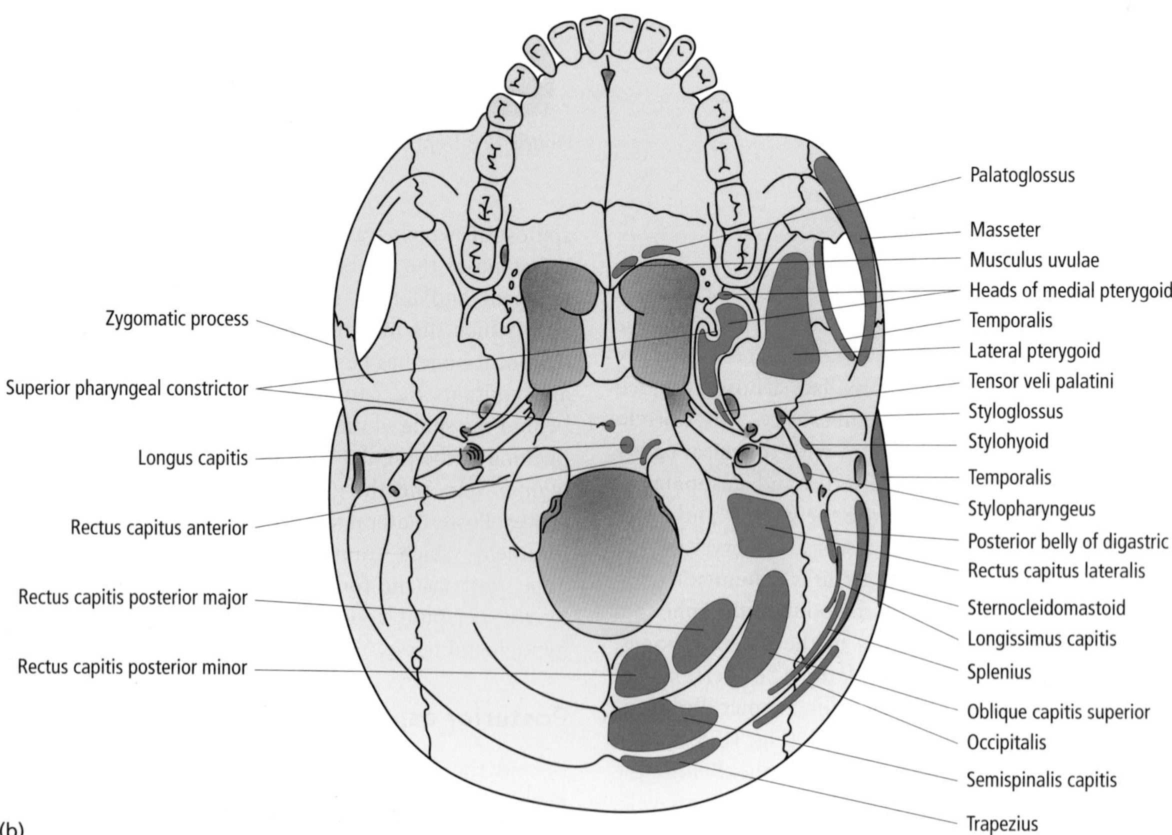
Palatoglossus
Masseter
Musculus uvulae
Heads of medial pterygoid
Temporalis
Lateral pterygoid
Tensor veli palatini
Styloglossus
Stylohyoid
Temporalis
Stylopharyngeus
Posterior belly of digastric
Rectus capitus lateralis
Sternocleidomastoid
Longissimus capitis
Splenius
Oblique capitis superior
Occipitalis
Semispinalis capitis
Trapezius
Zygomatic process
Superior pharyngeal constrictor
Longus capitis
Rectus capitus anterior
Rectus capitis posterior major
Rectus capitis posterior minor
(b)

Figure 18.7 Inferior aspect of skull: (a) bones (for boxed area see Fig. 21.17, p. 339); (b) muscle attachments

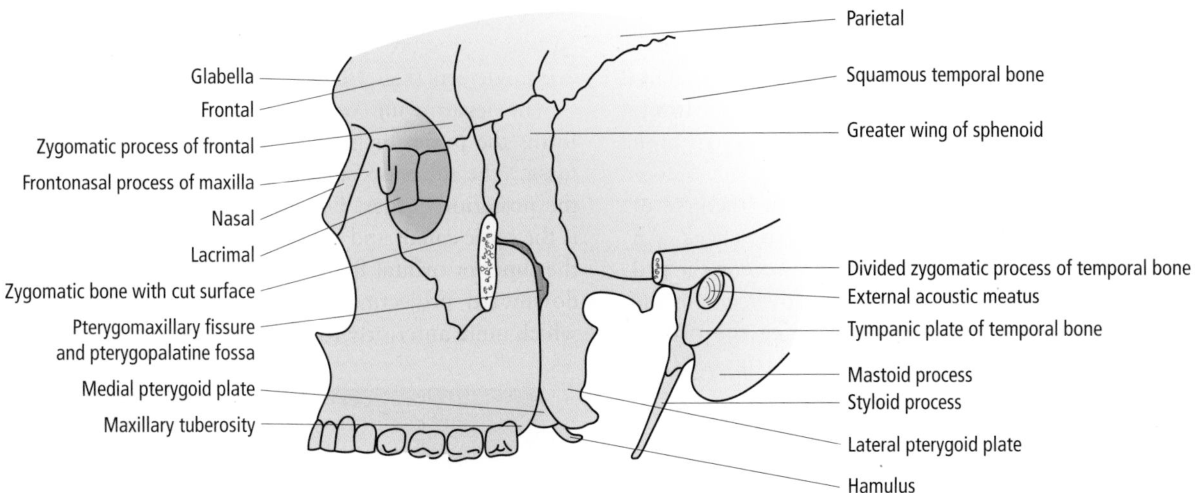

Figure 18.8 Lateral view of skull showing styloid process and pterygoid plate

THE INDIVIDUAL BONES OF THE SKULL

The mandible

The mandible (Fig. 18.9) is formed by the midline union of two halves, each with a horizontal body and a vertical ramus whose posterior junction forms the palpable **angle** of the mandible. The **ramus** is flat and rectangular. Superiorly it has two processes separated by the **mandibular notch;** the anterior **coronoid process** gives attachment to temporalis muscle, the posterior **condylar process** bears an articular head. The lateral pterygoid muscle is attached to its neck. To the lateral surface of the ramus is attached the masseter muscle. In the centre of the medial surface is the **mandibular foramen,** which transmits the inferior alveolar vessels and nerve; its lower lip, the **lingula,** gives attachment to the sphenomandibular ligament. The medial pterygoid muscle is attached below the foramen. The **body** has a smooth inferior border and an upper alveolar border containing sockets for the teeth. The **mental foramen** is on the lateral surface below the premolar teeth and it transmits the mental vessels and nerve. On the inner surface the **mylohyoid line** passes downwards and forwards to the midline and gives attachment to the mylohyoid muscle. This separates the fossa for the sublingual gland above from that for the submandibular gland below. The anterior belly of digastric muscle is attached in the midline below the mylohyoid line.

Loss of teeth in old age results in absorption of alveolar bone, so that the mental foramen, which lies midway between the upper and lower borders in adult life, is nearer to the lower border at birth and nearer to the alveolar border in old age.

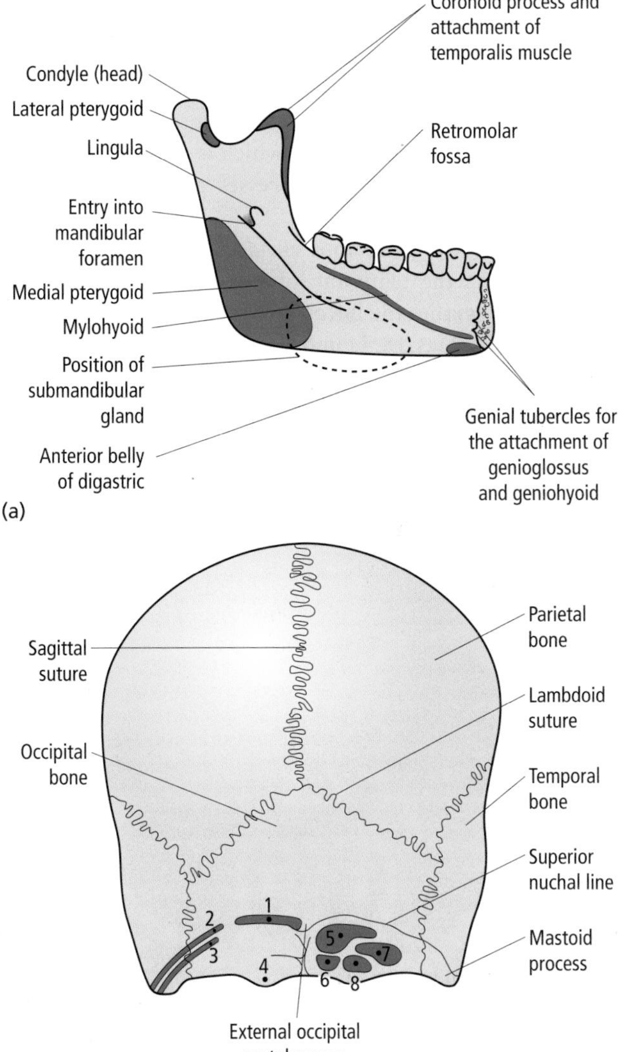

Figure 18.9 (a) Mandible – medial aspect showing muscle attachments. (b) Posterior aspect of skull, showing bones and muscle attachments: 1, trapezius; 2, sternocleidomastoid; 3, splenius capitus; 4, occipital condyle; 5, semispinalis capitis; 6, rectus capitis posterior minor; 7, superior oblique; 8, rectus capitis posterior major

Maxilla

Each maxilla (Figs 18.3, 18.4 and 18.8) consists of a body and four processes. The **body** contains the **maxillary air sinus.** Its thin superior (orbital) surface forms the larger part of the orbital floor. The **zygomatic process** (Fig. 18.7b) extends laterally to the zygomatic bone. The **alveolar process** projects downwards and bears the upper teeth, and its posterior extension forms the **maxillary tuberosity**. The horizontal **palatine process** contributes to the hard palate. The **frontal process** articulates with the frontal bone and forms part of the medial wall of the orbit.

The infraorbital nerve may be damaged in fractures of the maxilla and produce sensory loss over the cheek. An associated fracture of the zygomatic bone is common and may be marked by painful limitation of movement in the temporomandibular joint. Fractures involving the orbital floor may give rise to 'double vision' (Fig. 18.10).

The sphenoid

The sphenoid (see p. 331 and Fig. 20.10, p. 332) consists of a central body from which two pairs of processes (the greater and lesser wings) extend laterally, and two processes, the pterygoid processes, pass inferiorly. The cube-shaped **body** encloses the paired sphenoidal air sinuses. The inferior surface roofs in the nasopharynx. The superior surface is indented to form the **pituitary fossa** (sella turcica), anterior to which is the **optic groove** and posterior to which is the **dorsum sellae**, bearing the **posterior clinoid processes** projecting upwards over the fossa.

Each greater wing has four surfaces: the concave upper surface supports the temporal lobe of the brain; the lower surface which overlies the infratemporal fossa bears the **spine of the sphenoid** (Figs 18.7a and 18.8); the anterior region is the posterolateral wall of the orbit; and the lateral surface contributes to the medial wall of the temporal fossa.

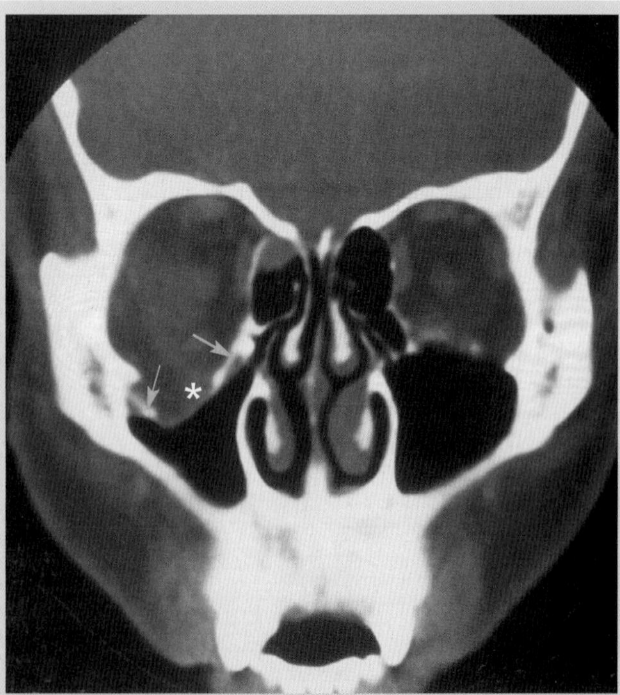

Figure 18.10 Coronal CT scan of face showing 'blow-out' orbital floor fracture (arrows) with protrusion of orbital contents into the maxillary sinus (*) – see also Fig. 19.2, p. 293

A swelling within the fossa from a pituitary tumour may produce pressure on the optic nerve or chiasma, causing visual defects (Fig. 18.11).

The lesser wing of the sphenoid extends laterally and forms the posterior limit of the floor of the anterior cranial fossa. The **anterior clinoid process** projects medially from the posterior border. Between the lesser wing and the body is the **optic canal**, and between the lesser and greater wings is the **superior orbital fissure**. From the **pterygoid process** hang downward projecting medial and lateral **pterygoid plates**, which unite anteriorly to bound the pterygoid fossa.

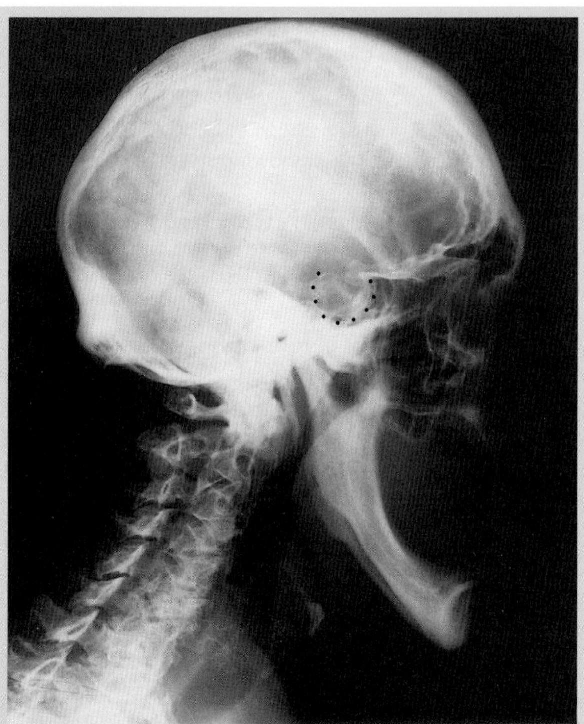

Figure 18.11 Lateral view of skull showing pituitary enlargement in a patient with acromegaly (pituitary fossa outlined with dots)

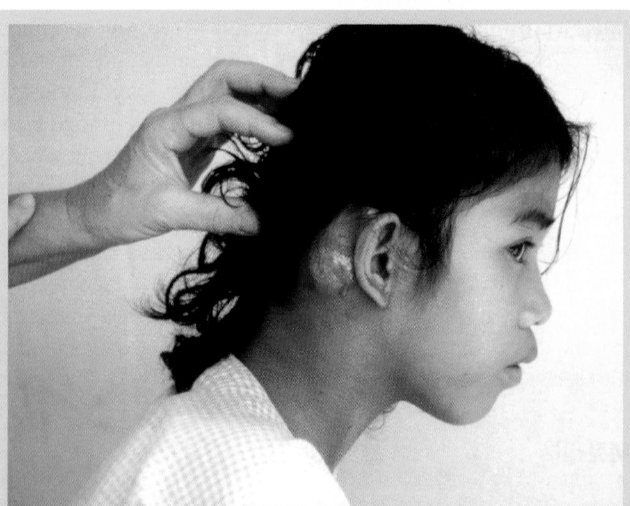

Figure 18.12 Mastoiditis in a child – note pus exuding from the swollen, inflamed mastoid process, which is pushing the pinna forwards

The temporal bones

Each **temporal bone** consists of four parts: squamous, petromastoid, tympanic and styloid. The **squamous part** (Fig. 18.4a) is a thin plate of bone on the lateral skull, articulating with the greater wing of the sphenoid, the parietal bone. Its zygomatic process extends forwards from the lateral surface and contributes to the zygomatic arch. Below the process is the **mandibular fossa** (Fig. 18.7a) for the condyle of the mandible. The thin squamous part contributes to the external acoustic meatus. The dense **petromastoid part** contains the middle and inner ears and extends medially between the sphenoid and occipital bones. Its upper surface forms part of the floor of the middle and posterior cranial fossae. The part forming the front of the posterior fossa is pierced by the **internal acoustic meatus,** which transmits the facial and vestibulocochlear nerves. The inferior surface contains the **carotid canal** for the internal carotid artery, and the **jugular fossa** lies between it and the occipital bone. The bony **auditory tube** opens anteriorly on to the inferior surface of the petrous temporal bone. The **mastoid process** (see Figs 18.4 and 18.7) is prominent posteriorly and contains the tympanic antrum and mastoid air cells.

Before the advent of antibiotics, and even nowadays in the developing world, infection in the mastoid air cells (mastoiditis) was difficult to eradicate owing to the spongy nature of this bony cavity which usually provides a barrier to easy drainage of the infection (Fig. 18.12).

Fractures of the skull base usually tear the dura and arachnoid mater and thereby cause leakage of CSF externally by the ear or nose. More rarely they may tear the internal carotid artery as it lies within the cavernous sinus to produce an acute arteriovenous fistula. This will become clinically evident as the pressure within the draining ophthalmic veins increases to produce a protruding pulsating eye. There may also be injuries to the cranial nerves lying close to the sinus, III, IV, V, and VI.

The **tympanic part** of the temporal bone is a curved plate forming the anterior wall and floor of the bony external acoustic meatus. The **styloid process** develops from the second arch cartilage (Fig. 18.8) and is a slender downward projection of the petrous part. About 2 cm long, it gives attachment to stylopharyngeus, stylohyoid, styloglossus and the stylohyoid stylomandibular ligaments. The **stylomastoid foramen** (Fig. 18.7a), between it and the mastoid process, transmits the facial nerve.

The occipital bone

The **occipital bone** (Figs 18.4, 18.7 and 18.9b) has a basilar, a squamous and two lateral portions around the **foramen magnum.** The **squamous part,** a flat plate, extends backwards and upwards to articulate with the parietal and mastoid part of the temporal bone. The outer part is marked by the **superior** and **inferior nuchal lines** and the **external occipital protuberance;** it gives attachment to the postvertebral muscles. The intracranial surface is grooved by the superior sagittal and transverse venous sinuses. The **lateral parts** bear, inferiorly, the **occipital condyles** for articulation with the atlas. Anteriorly the **hypoglossal canal** conveys the hypoglossal nerve.

The parietal bones

The **parietal bones** (Figs 18.1 and 18.4) are two convex quadrilateral plates forming the posterior skull vault. They meet at the sagittal suture and articulate anteriorly with the frontal bone at the coronal suture, and posteriorly with the occipital bone at the lambdoid suture.

The measurement across the fetal skull – the 'biparietal distance' – is used in ultrasonography to monitor intra-uterine growth.

The frontal bone

The **frontal bone** (Figs 18.1 and 18.4) has a domed superior portion forming the anterior skull vault, and its inferior horizontal **orbital plates** contribute to the roof of each orbit. It articulates superiorly with the parietal bones at the coronal suture and, inferiorly, with the sphenoid, zygomatic, nasal and ethmoid bones and the frontal process of the maxilla. The orbital plates meet the lesser wings of the sphenoid posteriorly. The paired **frontal air sinuses** are within the bone above the nose and the medial part of the orbit. In a small proportion of individuals a persistent frontal (metopic) suture remains throughout adult life and should not be mistaken for a fracture.

The zygomatic bones

The **zygomatic bones** (Figs 18.3, 18.4 and 18.7) form the prominence of each cheek. Their orbital surface contributes to the lateral wall of the orbit; the lateral surface forms the prominence of the cheek, and their temporal surface forms the anterior limit of the temporal fossa. The temporal process forms the anterior part of the zygomatic arch, the frontal process articulates with the frontal bone, and the zygoma articulates with the maxilla and with the greater wing of the sphenoid in the lateral wall of the orbit.

A fracture of this bone or the orbital plate of the maxillary bone may result in 'double vision' (diplopia) as a result of the eyeball being displaced downwards (Fig. 18.10).

The nasal bones

The **nasal bones** (Figs 18.3 and 18.4) meet anteriorly in the midline and form the skeleton of the upper part of the external nose. They articulate with the frontal bone, and with the frontal processes of the maxillae.

The **ethmoid bone** (Fig. 21.8, p. 332) consists of a midline **perpendicular plate** and a perforated horizontal **cribriform plate** uniting its two **ethmoidal labyrinths.** Between the two cribriform plates a median ridge – the crista galli – projects superiorly. The cribriform plate conveys the olfactory nerves from the forebrain to the nose.

A fracture involving the cribriform plate may result not only in loss of sense of smell (**anosmia**), but also in tearing of the dura mater that covers the nerve, resulting in a leak of cerebrospinal fluid from the nose (**CSF rhinorrhoea**).

Each ethmoidal labyrinth contains the ethmoidal air cells, which lie in the lateral wall of the nose (Figs 18.3 and 18.4) and are the immediate medial relation of the orbit.

The **lacrimal bones** (Fig. 19.1, p. 292) are small thin bones lying on the medial wall of the orbit and each, with the frontal process of the maxilla, surrounds the lacrimal sac and duct.

THE SCALP

The scalp covers the vault of the skull, extending from the supraorbital margins anteriorly to the superior nuchal line posteriorly. It consists of five layers (**SCALP**):

- Thick Skin containing many hair follicles and sweat glands.
- Fibrous Connective tissue which is adherent to the skin and to the underlying aponeurosis. It is richly supplied with vessels and nerves embedded within it.
- Musculofibrous epicranial Aponeurosis containing the **occipitalis muscle** posteriorly and the **frontalis muscle** in front. Laterally the aponeurosis is attached to the temporal fascia. Anteriorly the frontalis has no bony attachment but blends with the fibres of the orbicularis oculi muscles. Occipitalis is attached to the superior nuchal line. Occipitofrontalis draws the scalp backwards in frowning, and raises the eyebrows. It is innervated by the facial nerve.
- Loose areolar tissue allows free movement of the aponeurosis and overlying skin over the periosteum.

Scalping injuries, such as those caused by long hair catching in moving machinery, pull the outer layers of the scalp away from the skull along this layer.

- The Periosteum (pericranium) of the bones of the vault is continuous through the sutures of the vault with the endocranium.

The scalp is richly supplied by anastomosing branches of the external carotid (occipital, posterior auricular and superficial temporal arteries) and ophthalmic arteries (supraorbital and supratrochlear arteries). Veins accompany the arteries and drain to the external and internal jugular veins. They may communicate with the diploic veins of the skull via numerous emissary veins, and hence with the intracranial dural venous sinuses.

Scalp wounds bleed profusely but usually heal without hindrance or infection because of the rich blood supply. Since the vessels are supported by the surrounding connective tissue, they do not retract as readily as do other vessels. Bleeding will continue from a scalp wound until local pressure or sutures closes the vessels. Surgeons have devised numerous skin flaps based upon the vascular pedicles of the dozen or so branches that anastomose within the scalp and employ these to fashion skin flaps which, attached to an underlying segment of the cranium, allow craniotomies to be performed. Blood or pus collecting under the scalp is limited posteriorly by the attachment of occipitalis and the temporal fascia and cannot spread into the occipital or subtemporal regions. A scalp infection can spread via the diploic and emissary veins to involve the skull bones, the meninges, or even occasionally the dural venous sinuses.

The sensory innervation of the scalp is by the trigeminal, lesser and greater occipital nerves and the dorsal rami of the second and third cervical nerves (Fig. 23.9 p. 361). Lymph vessels pass to lymph nodes in the circular chain around the base of the skull; posteriorly the occipital and mastoid nodes and anteriorly to the preauricular nodes. All eventually drain to the deep cervical nodes.

THE FACE

The face contains the external openings of the mouth, nose and orbit. Facial skin is thin, sensitive and hairy. In males, facial hair is very dense over the temporal fossa, the zygomatic arch and the mandibular region. Voluntary facial muscles are attached to it. The subcutaneous tissue is very vascular and has a varying amount of fat; there is no fat in the eyelids. There is no deep fascia in most of the face, and sweat and sebaceous glands are abundant. The mucocutaneous junction around the mouth is on the facial aspect of the lips (the red margin). Mucous and small salivary glands are present on the inner aspect of the lips and cheeks.

The **facial muscles** (Figs 18.4b and 18.13) are the muscles of facial expression and are arranged as sphincters and dilators around the mouth, nose and orbit. They are all innervated by the facial nerve.

Orbicularis oris is the sphincter around the mouth and forms the greater part of the substance of the lips. Contraction produces pouting lips, as in whistling and kissing. Other muscles blend with it, such as the buccinator, and the levator and depressor muscles, which are attached to the angles of the mouth (anguli) and to the middle of the lips (labii).

Buccinator forms the greater part of the cheek. It has a continuous lateral attachment to the pterygomandibular raphé and the outer surfaces of the maxillae and mandible adjacent

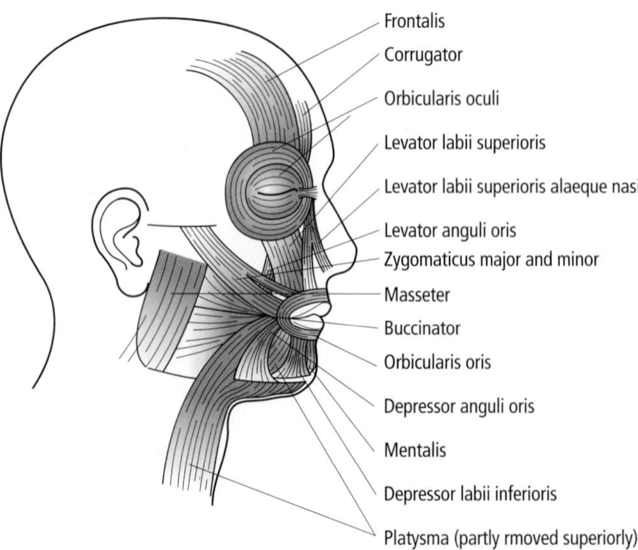

Figure 18.13 Facial muscles

to the last molar tooth. Its fibres pass forwards and medially, decussate behind the angle of the mouth and enter the lips, blending with orbicularis oris. The muscle keeps food out of the vestibule and between the teeth in chewing, and is used to increase the pressure in forced blowing (e.g. in trombone players).

Orbicularis oculi surrounds the opening of the orbit and has palpebral and orbital parts. The central palpebral fibres lie within the eyelids; the peripheral orbital fibres surround the orbital margin and are attached by the medial palpebral ligament to the frontal process of the maxilla. The fibres blend with frontalis above the orbit. The palpebral part closes the eyelid in sleep, winking and blinking; the orbital part closes the eye more forcefully and is used in frowning.

Platysma is a broad flat sheet of muscle lying in the superficial fascia on each side of the neck. Superiorly it passes over the mandible to blend with muscles around the mouth; inferiorly it blends with the superficial fascia over the upper part of the chest. It is a weak depressor of the jaw.

Vessels and nerves

The face is supplied mainly by the facial and transverse facial arteries and is drained by the facial and retromandibular veins (p. 359 and Fig. 23.6, p. 362). Lymph drainage is to the submental nodes, that of the medial part of the cheek and face to the submandibular nodes, and that of the forehead and lateral part of the cheek to the parotid nodes. Sensory nerves are conveyed by the three divisions of the trigeminal nerve and, over the jaw, by the great auricular nerve. Their distribution is illustrated in Fig. 23.9, p. 363. Motor innervation is by the facial nerve.

Table 18.1 Practical cranial nerve functions: a clinical anatomist's guide to testing

Nerve	Site of injury or disease	How to test	Abnormal signs
I. Olfactory **	Fracture across cribiform plate	Odour to each nostril	Anosmia (no sense of smell)
II. Optic ***	1 Optic foramen fracture 2 Extrasellar extension of pituitary tumour 3 Disease of optic tract and visual cortex	Shine light in affected eyes Assess visual fields Assess visual fields	Loss of direct + consensual pupil constriction Bitemporal hemianopia Homonymous hemianopia
III. Oculomotor **	Fracture across middle cranial fossae and raised intracranial pressure	Shine light in affected eye Shine light in normal eye	Direct pupil reflex absent Consensual reflex present Direct reflex present Consensual reflex absent Eye turned down and out Ptosis and dilated pupil
IV. Trochlear *	Brain stem tumour or orbital fracture	Needs specialist ocular testing	Eye fails to look down and out Patient has diplopia
V. Trigeminal **	Direct injury to the maxillary and mandibular nerves in head and neck surgery and trauma	1 Sensation to cornea 2 Sensation to cheek 3 Sensation to chin 3a Sensation to lips and cheek 4 Motor – 'Clench your teeth'	Numbness or paresthesia Masseter and temporalis fail to contract
VI. Abducens **	Fractures across both orbit and middle cranial fossae Raised intracranial pressure	Follow finger from side to side	No lateral movement Diplopia on lateral gaze
VII. Facial *****	Peripherally: 1 Malignant parotid tumours and surgery 2 Skull base fractures across the temporal bone (often bilateral) 3 Upper motor lesions	'Smile' 'Whistle' 'Wrinkle the forehead – frown'	1 Facial muscle paralysis: no forehead wrinkle 2 As 1, + loss of taste in anterior two-thirds of tongue and hearing abnormal 3 Forehead can wrinkle but otherwise facial paralysis present
VIII. Acoustic ***	Fractures of temporal bone (VII often also affected)	Clap hands near ear Tick of watch Weber test – tuning fork Rinne test – tuning fork	No hearing Sound travels to good ear only Bone/air conduction
IX. Glossopharyngeal *	Deep laceration of neck Skull base tumour Brain stem lesion	Touch anterior pillar of fauces with spatula	No gag reflex
X. Vagus **	Deep laceration of neck Skull base tumour Brain stem lesion	'Open your mouth' – look at soft palate	Uvula deviated to normal side Vocal cord paralysed – hoarse voice Cannot sing high note
XI. Spinal accessory **	Laceration or operation in posterior triangle of neck	'Shrug your shoulders' 'Push your chin against my hand' 'Take a deep breath in'	Trapezius fails to contract Sternomastoid muscle not seen nor felt to contract
XII. Hypoglossal *	Laceration, surgery and tumours in region of carotid bifurcation	'Stick your tongue out'	Tongue protrudes to side of lesion Difficulty in speaking (dysarthria)

Range: * = very rare; ***** = very common

MCQs

1. In the skull: T/F

- **a** the sutures are all fibrous joints (____)
- **b** the sagittal suture separates the frontal from the parietal bones (____)
- **c** the lambda (posterior fontanelle) lies between the sagittal and lambdoid sutures (____)
- **d** the anterior fontanelle is usually closed at birth (____)
- **e** the posterior fontanelle usually closes 18 months after birth (____)

Answers

1.

- **a** *T – And after middle age they begin to ossify from the cranial surface.*
- **b** *F – At birth the frontal bone is separated from the parietal by the coronal suture.*
- **c** *T – The lambda (posterior fontanelle) is in this position. The bregma (anterior fontanelle) is between the sagittal, coronal and frontal sutures.*
- **d** *F – The diamond-shaped anterior fontanelle is usually open until 18 months after birth.*
- **e** *F – The posterior fontanelle usually closes between the third and sixth months.*

---

2. The scalp: T/F

- **a** is attached by the occipitalis muscle to the skull (____)
- **b** is attached by the frontalis muscle to the skull (____)
- **c** receives sensory innervation from the dorsal rami of the second and third cervical nerves (____)
- **d** is supplied, in part, by the ophthalmic artery (____)
- **e** drains directly to the subcutaneous lymph nodes at the base of the skull (____)

Answers

2.

- **a** *T – Occipitalis is attached to the superior nuchal line.*
- **b** *F – Frontalis is attached to orbicularis oculi and not to bone.*
- **c** *T – These nerve fibres, conveyed in the greater and lesser occipital nerves, supply the posterior scalp.*
- **d** *T – Through its supraorbital and supratrochlear branches.*
- **e** *T – A superficial circle of lymph nodes around the base of the skull receives all lymph from the scalp.*

EMQs

Each question has an anatomical theme linked to the chapter, and a list of 10 related items (A–J) placed in alphabetical order: these are followed by five statements (1–5). Match **one or more** of the items A–J to each of the five statements.

Bones of the skull

A. Frontal
B. Mandible
C. Maxilla
D. Nasal
E. Occipital
F. Palatine
G. Parietal
H. Sphenoid
I. Temporal
J. Zygomatic

Match the following statements with the bone(s) in the above list.

1. Gives passage to the mandibular branch of the trigeminal nerve
2. Surrounds the foramen magnum
3. Gives passage to the middle meningeal artery
4. Crossed by the superficial temporal artery
5. Contains the middle ear

Answers

1 H; 2 E; 3 H; 4 I; 5 I

APPLIED QUESTIONS

1. A fracture in the region of the pterion may have serious consequences. What structure is at greatest risk in this injury?

1. The pterion is the meeting point of temporal, parietal and frontal bones with the greater wing of the sphenoid bone. In the fetal skull it is occasionally seen as a fontanelle. In the adult it lies some 4 cm above the midpoint of the zygomatic arch. The bone is relatively thin in this area, and it overlies the anterior division of the middle meningeal artery, which may be lacerated in a fracture at this site. Thus an extradural haematoma and cerebral compression may follow a direct hit.

---

2. A full sailor's beard overlies which bones?

2. The normal beard overlies the zygomatic portion of the temporal bone, zygomatic bone, the ramus, angle and body of the mandible and the maxilla. A very long beard may overlie the manubrium and body of the sternum.

19 The orbit, nose and mouth

THE ORBITAL CAVITY AND EYEBALL

The two pyramid-shaped **orbital cavities** (Fig. 19.1) lie within the facial skeleton. Each has a roof, a floor and medial and lateral walls, and contains the eyeball, extraocular muscles, vessels, nerves, lacrimal gland and fat. The periosteum of the orbit is continuous at the back of the orbit with the dura mater and sheath of the optic nerve.

The relations of the orbit are important for the clinician. The **roof**, formed by the orbital plate of the frontal bone and, posteriorly, the lesser wing of the sphenoid, separates the orbit from the anterior cranial fossa. The **floor**, formed largely by the maxilla and zygoma, separates the orbit from the maxillary air sinus and has an inferior orbital fissure posteriorly. The **lateral wall**, formed by the zygomatic bone and the greater wing of the sphenoid, separates the orbit from the temporal fossa. The **medial wall** consists of, from anterior to posterior, the maxilla, the lacrimal bone, the orbital plate of the ethmoid and the body of the sphenoid. It separates the orbit from the ethmoidal air sinuses and the nasal cavity.

Figure 19.1 Bones of the orbital cavity

The **orbital cavity** has three posterior openings, the superior and inferior orbital fissures laterally and the optic canal medially.

The **superior orbital fissure** (Figs 19.8 and 19.9), between the greater and lesser wings of the sphenoid, opens into the middle cranial fossa and is divided by the tendinous attachment of the extraocular muscles into a narrow lateral and a wider medial part. The lateral part transmits the lacrimal, trochlear and frontal nerves, the medial, the superior and inferior divisions of the oculomotor, the nasociliary, and the abducent nerves. Ophthalmic veins pass posteriorly to enter the cavernous sinus.

The **inferior orbital fissure**, between the floor and lateral wall, opens into the pterygopalatine fossa medially and the infratemporal fossa laterally. It transmits the maxillary nerve, which in the canal becomes the infraorbital nerve, and its zygomatic branch, together with communicating veins.

The **optic canal** opens into the apex of the cavity and conveys the optic nerve and ophthalmic artery from the middle cranial fossa. Anteriorly a wide canal passes downward from the cavity's inferomedial angle to the nose; it contains the nasolacrimal duct. Superolaterally is the fossa for the lacrimal gland.

A blow to the eye may, because of the thinness of the medial and inferior orbital walls, fracture the orbit. A fracture of the medial wall may involve the ethmoidal and sphenoidal sinuses; a fracture of the lower margin may involve the maxillary sinus and infraorbital nerve, resulting in loss of sensation over the cheek (Fig. 19.2). Diplopia may also occur.

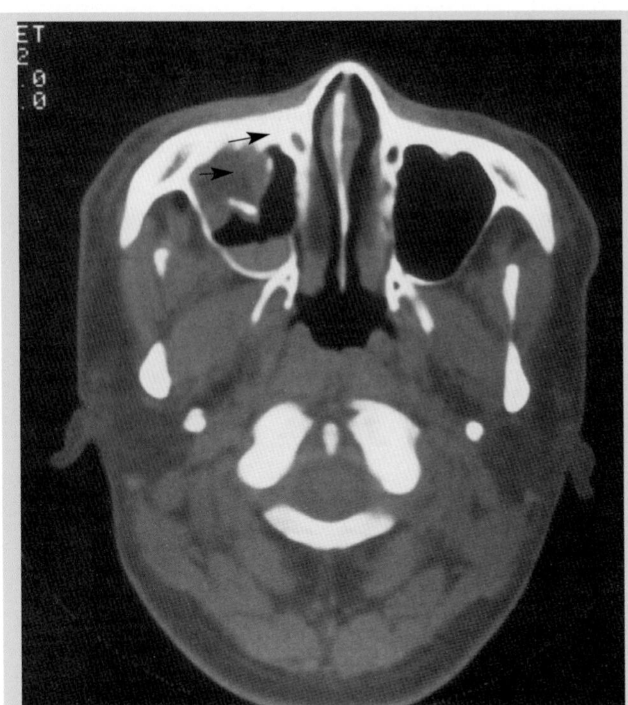

Figure 19.2 Axial CT scan of 'blow-out' orbital fracture – arrows show bony fragments pushed by orbital contents that have sunk into the maxillary air sinus below – see also Fig. 18.10, p. 284

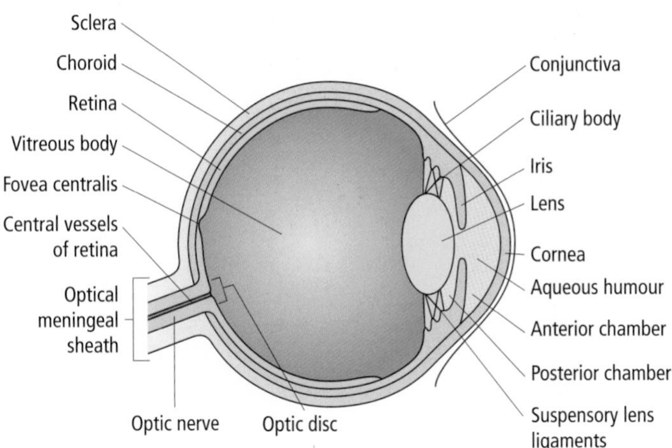

Figure 19.3 Cross-section through the eyeball

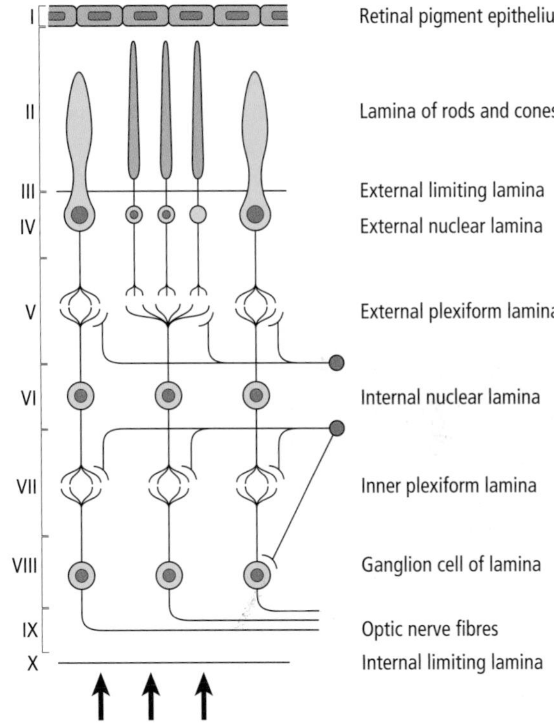

Figure 19.4 Diagram of retina – light (arrows), passes through numerous layers as shown before impinging on the photoreceptors (rods and cones)

THE EYEBALL

The eyeball is situated in the anterior orbital cavity and is almost spherical, but is distorted anteriorly by the projecting cornea (Fig. 19.3). The optic nerve leaves it posteromedially. The wall of the eyeball has three coats. From without inwards these are:

- An outer fibrous coat forming the dense white **sclera,** which covers the posterior five-sixths of the eyeball and the transparent **cornea** anteriorly.
- The pigmented **choroid** which, anteriorly, has a circular thickening, the **ciliary body,** containing the ciliary muscle. In front of the ciliary body the choroid thins to form the **iris,** with its central aperture, the **pupil.** The iris contains the circular sphincter pupillae and the radial dilator pupillae muscles.
- The **retina** contains the light receptors, which relay impulses along the optic nerve. There are several layers of nervous elements (Fig. 19.4). Medially on the posterior wall is a pale area, the **optic disc,** where the optic nerve leaves the eyeball. About 3 mm lateral to the disc, at the visual axis, is a small depression, the **fovea centralis.** The area around it, the **macula,** is used mainly for daylight vision (Fig. 19.5).

Detachment of the retina – trauma to the eye may cause fluid to track between the deeper pigmented layer and the overlying neural layer of the retina resulting in detachment of the inner layer. The patient complains of 'star burst' flashes of light and urgent laser treatment is required to prevent permanent loss of vision.

The biconvex **lens** divides the eyeball cavity into a posterior part filled with the jelly-like **vitreous body** and an anterior part filled with the more fluid **aqueous humour.** The iris further divides the anterior part into an anterior chamber between the iris and cornea and a posterior chamber between the iris and lens. These two chambers are in continuity through the pupil. The lens is held in position by its suspensory ligament passing from its periphery to the ciliary body. Accommodation, the process by which near objects are focused on the retina, is achieved by contraction of the ciliary muscle drawing forward the ciliary body and relaxing the suspensory ligament. The lens, because of its inherent elasticity, then becomes more convex.

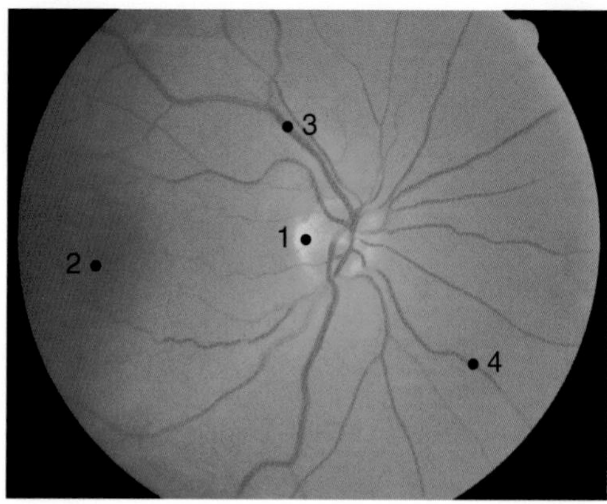

Figure 19.5 Ophthalmoscopy of normal retina: 1, optic disc; 2, macula; 3, superior temporal branches of central vein and artery; 4, inferior nasal vessels

The lens becomes harder and less elastic with age and there is a gradual loss of focusing power in the elderly (**presbyopia**). Loss of transparency of the lens occurs in some people (**cataract**) (Fig. 19.6), a condition that can be cured by lens extraction or a lens implant. In a proportion of elderly people the reabsorption of aqueous humour diminishes and the accumulation of the contents of the eye increases intraocular pressure and with it some compression of the retina with the effect that there is then a slow but progressive loss of visual acuity (**glaucoma**).

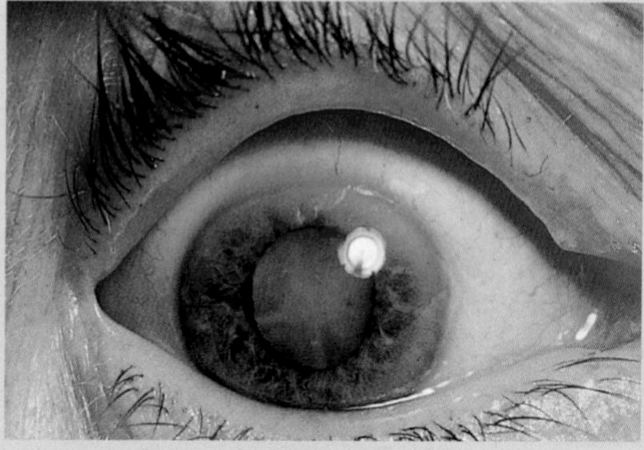

Figure 19.6 Cataract – note milky opacity of the lens behind the pupil

Blood supply

This is by the central artery of the retina and ciliary branches, both branches of the ophthalmic artery. Veins pass to the ophthalmic veins.

Occlusion of the central artery of the retina may occur as the result of arterial disease or because of embolism (the trapping of free-floating clots) in the artery. It produces permanent blindness.

Ophthalmoscopy allows examination of the retina (Fig. 19.5) and its structures: the optic disc, the macula, radiating retinal vessels and the fovea centralis. Abnormalities such as **papilloedema** (swelling of the optic disc; Fig. 19.7), which results from an increase in intracranial pressure, aneurysms, and exudates along the path of the arterial branches and 'nipping' of the veins by the arteries in patients with hypertension, can be identified ophthalmoscopically. In diabetes mellitus after some years it is not uncommon to find deterioration of eyesight that may be due to the accumulation of protein exudates covering the macula region as seen in Fig. 19.7a.

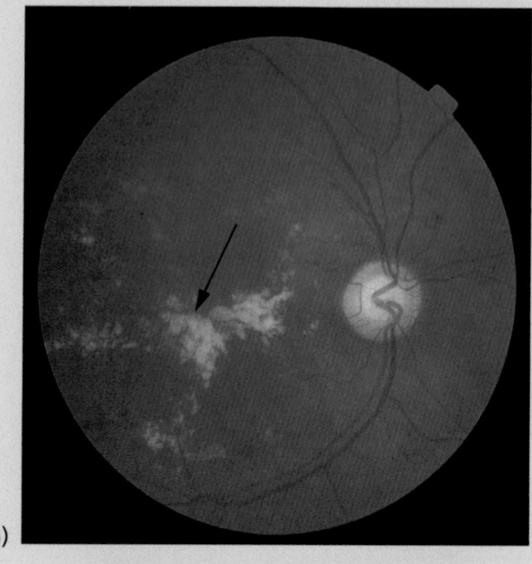

(a)

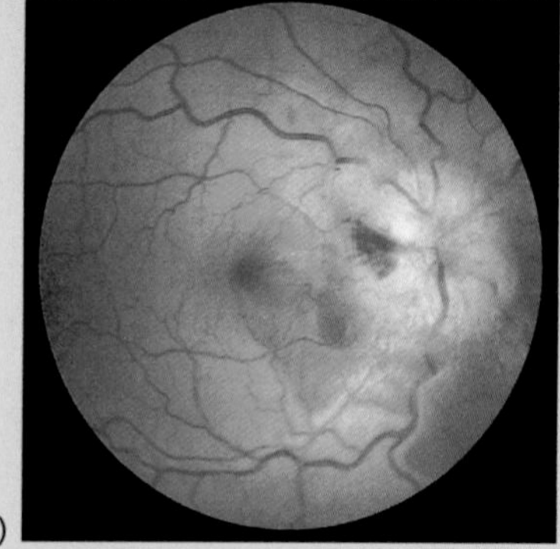

(b)

Figure 19.7 (a) Retinoscopy of diabetes mellitus with the macula destroyed by exudates (arrow). (b) Papilloedema – note and compare with Fig. 19.5. In this case, the patient has no clear optic disc due to vascular congestion and swelling

Nerve supply

The optic nerve carries sensory fibres from the retina. Ciliary nerves carry autonomic fibres to the muscles of the iris and the ciliary muscles, and sensory fibres from the conjunctiva; the long ciliary nerves carry sympathetic fibres and arise from the nasociliary nerve. The short ciliary nerves arise from the ciliary ganglion, carrying postganglionic parasympathetic fibres.

The **corneal reflex**, the 'blink reflex' when a speck of dirt touches the cornea, is mediated by trigeminal sensory fibres causing facial nerve activity to close the eyes. The **pupillary reflex** is a constriction of the pupil on exposure to bright light. The sensory component is the optic nerve and the motor component are parasympathetic fibres carried within the oculomotor nerve. The sympathetic fibres cause pupillary dilatation related to fear and excitement.

THE ORBIT

Orbital (bulbar) fascia

The eyeball behind the cornea is closely surrounded by the orbital fascia, which separates it from the orbital fat. Thickenings of the fascia attached to the lacrimal and zygomatic bones form the medial and lateral **check ligaments** of the eye, and a thickening below the eyeball forms the **suspensory ligament** that provides a hammock-like support for the eye.

Extraocular muscles

The four **rectus muscles** (Fig. 19.8) – superior, inferior, medial and lateral – are attached posteriorly to the common tendinous ring surrounding the optic canal and the medial end of the superior orbital fissure. Anteriorly the muscles pass forwards, in positions implied by their names, to be attached to the sclera just in front of the equator of the eyeball.

The **superior oblique** is attached posteriorly above the common tendinous ring (Fig. 19.9), and passes forwards for its tendon to hook around a fibrocartilaginous pulley, the **trochlea**, on the superomedial border of the front of the orbit. It then passes backward and laterally to gain attachment to the posterolateral surface of the eyeball, behind the equator.

The **inferior oblique** is attached anteriorly to the anteromedial floor of the orbit and passes backward to be attached to the posterolateral surface of the eyeball behind the equator.

Nerve supply

Lateral rectus is served by the abducent nerve, superior oblique by the trochlear nerve, and all the remaining muscles by the oculomotor nerve.

Functions

The muscles of each eye work together in a coordinated manner so as to fix both eyes on to an object. There is an angle between the visual or optic axis and the orbital axis, and all movements other than horizontal involve some rotation as well as angular deviation of the eyeball. Looking left involves contraction of the left lateral rectus and right medial rectus; looking down and to the right involves the left superior oblique and the right inferior rectus; looking up and to the left

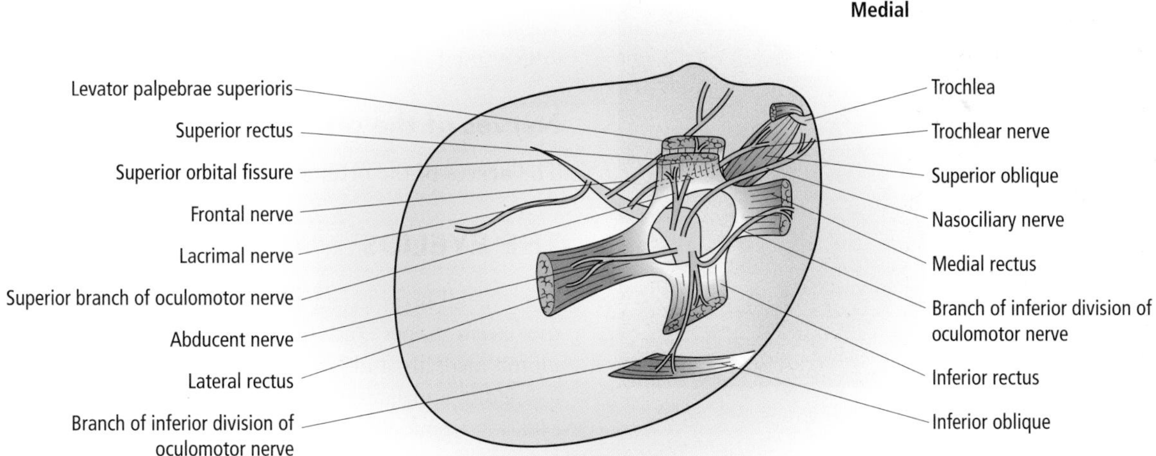

Figure 19.8 Extraocular muscles

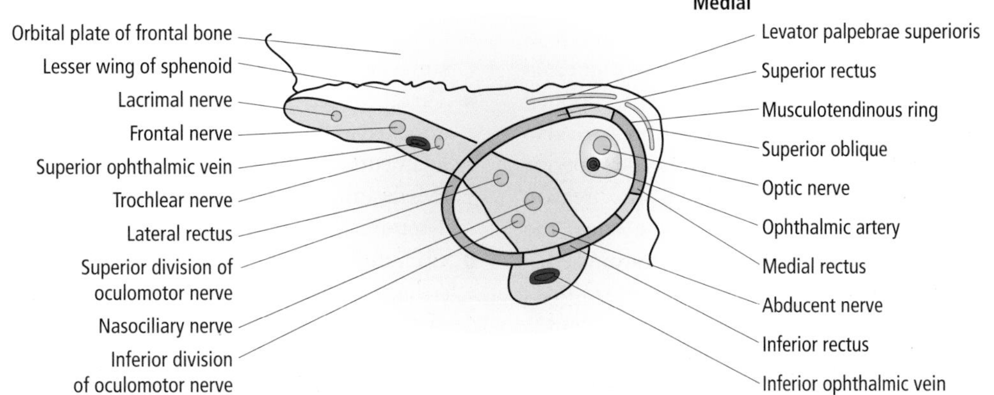

Figure 19.9 Extraocular tendinous ring and relations in the right eye

involves the left inferior oblique and the right superior rectus. An easy way to remember these complex vectors is that the CN IV (trochlear nerve formally known as the pathetic nerve) makes you look 'down and out'.

Incoordination of the muscles of the two eyes results in a squint and 'double vision' (diplopia). **Oculomotor palsy,** when complete, results in paralysis of most of the eye muscles, together with levator palpebrae superioris and the sphincter pupillae. Consequently the upper lid droops (ptosis), there is a fully dilated pupil, and the eyeball tends to look downwards and outwards owing to the unopposed action of lateral rectus and superior oblique muscles, which are not paralysed (Fig. 21.13a, p. 335). **Abducent nerve palsy** (Fig. 19.10) results in paralysis of the lateral rectus muscle and the eye cannot be moved laterally in the horizontal plane. The palsy may result from viral infection, but occasionally it may be a non-localizing sign of increased intracranial pressure, (because the long intracranial course of the nerve renders it particularly susceptible to stretching by the raised pressure). **Trochlear nerve palsy** is rare; patients attempt to minimize the diplopia it causes by tilting the head.

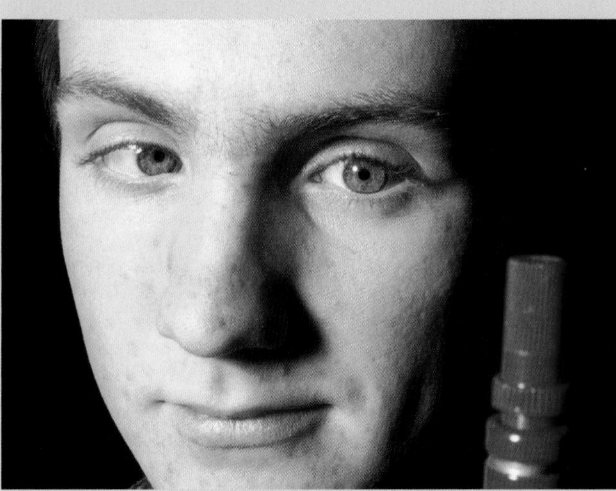

Figure 19.10 Left sixth nerve palsy – the patient is looking at the red marker: the left eye cannot abduct but the right eye movement is normal

Levator palpebrae superioris

Levator palpebrae superioris raises the upper eyelid. It is attached posteriorly above the common tendinous origin and anteriorly to the conjunctiva and tarsal plate. It is supplied by the oculomotor nerve. Some smooth muscle fibres are also present, and are innervated by sympathetics from the superior cervical ganglion (Muller's muscle). This is the reason why there is a mild ptosis in Horner's syndrome when the sympathetic fibres to the Muller's muscle are compromised.

Sympathetic denervation, which usually follows trauma or neoplastic infiltration of the cervical sympathetic trunk, causes a partially drooped eyelid (ptosis), a small pupil due to paralysis of dilator pupillae, and a hot, flushed and dry face on that side (Horner's syndrome) (Fig. 19.11).

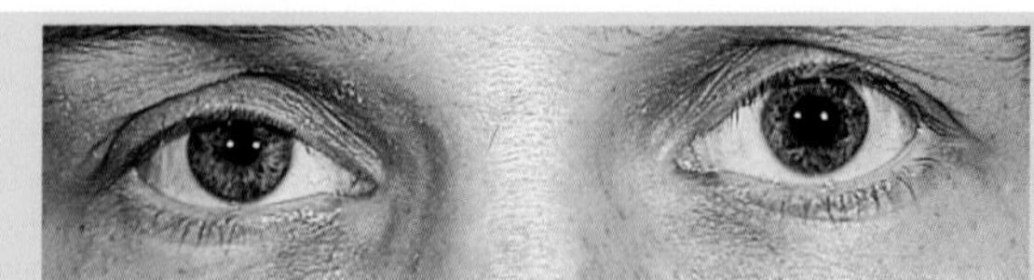

Figure 19.11 Right Horner's syndrome

Blood supply of the orbit

The **ophthalmic artery** arises as the first branch of the internal carotid artery in the middle cranial fossa above the cavernous sinus. It enters the orbit through the optic canal, and gives ciliary branches, the central artery of the retina and muscular branches before ending behind the medial side of the upper eyelid by dividing into supratrochlear, supraorbital and dorsal nasal branches.

Superior and inferior **ophthalmic veins** drain the orbit and pass through the superior orbital fissure to the cavernous sinus. They communicate through the inferior orbital fissure with the pterygoid venous plexus posteriorly, and with the facial vein anteriorly near the medial angle of the eye.

Thus infection may pass from the central part of the facial skin to involve the cavernous sinus, for example the spread of an infection from a squeezed pimple on the face may lead to a thrombosis in the cavernous sinus, with a resultant oedema of the conjunctiva and possible damage to the cranial nerves traversing the sinus (Fig. 24.8c, p. 374).

Nerves of the orbit

The **nerves of the orbit** are described more fully on p. 333.

THE EYELIDS

The eyeball is protected anteriorly by two movable skin folds, the larger upper and the smaller lower eyelids, which are united medially and laterally and limit the **palpebral fissure** at its medial and lateral angles. Within the medial angle of each eyelid is a pink elevation, the **lacrimal caruncle**. On the medial margin of each lid is a small elevation, the **lacrimal papilla,** on the apex of which is the **lacrimal punctum**, the opening of the lacrimal canaliculus (Fig. 19.12a,b). Each eyelid has five layers:

- Skin
- Superficial fascia, devoid of fat
- Palpebral fibres of orbicularis oculi and levator palpebrae superioris (Fig. 18.13, p. 287)
- Tarsal plate, an elliptical plate of dense fibrous tissue attached to the orbital margin by medial and lateral palpebral ligaments (Fig. 19.12b). On the plate's deep surface lie tarsal (Meibomian) glands, which are modified sebaceous glands. Their ducts open on to the lid margin (Fig. 19.13)
- Conjunctiva, a thin layer of epithelium lining the inner surface of both lids and which is reflected over the front of the eyeball. When the lids are closed the conjunctiva encloses a narrow sac containing a small amount of lacrimal fluid. The upper and lower pouches between the lids and the eyeball are known as the conjunctival fornices.

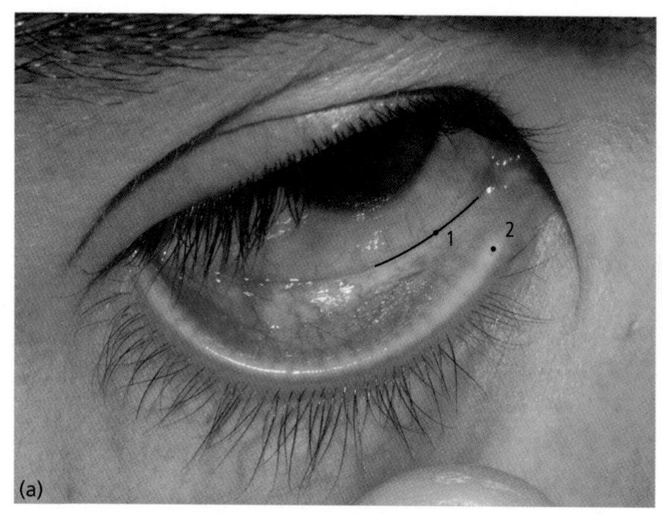

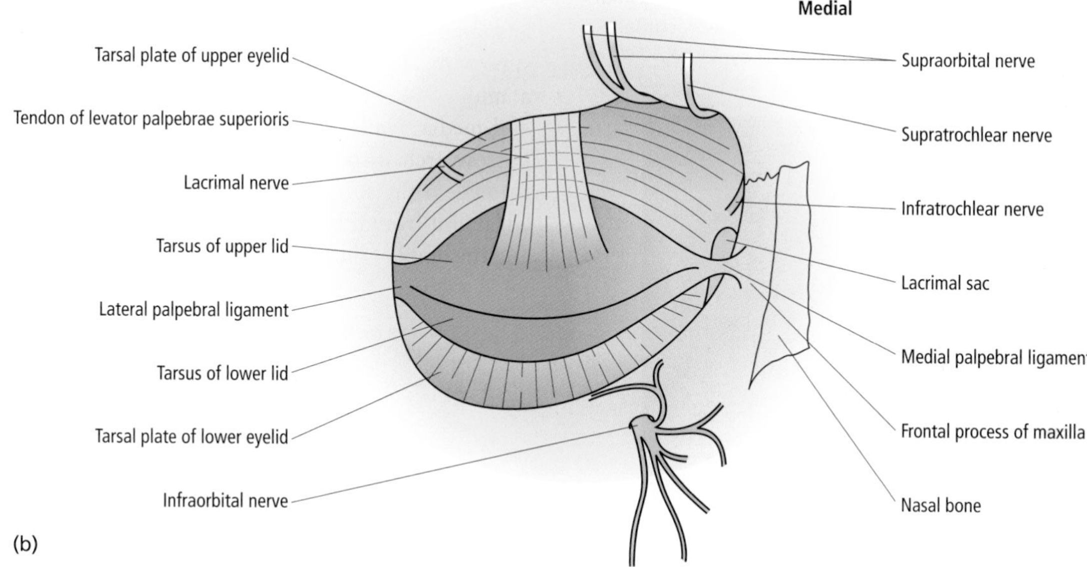

Figure 19.12 (a) Right lower eyelid everted to show lacrimal punctum: 1, conjunctival fornix; 2, lacrimal punctum. (b) Diagram of tarsal plates in closed right eye – skin, superficial fascia and palpebral muscles removed

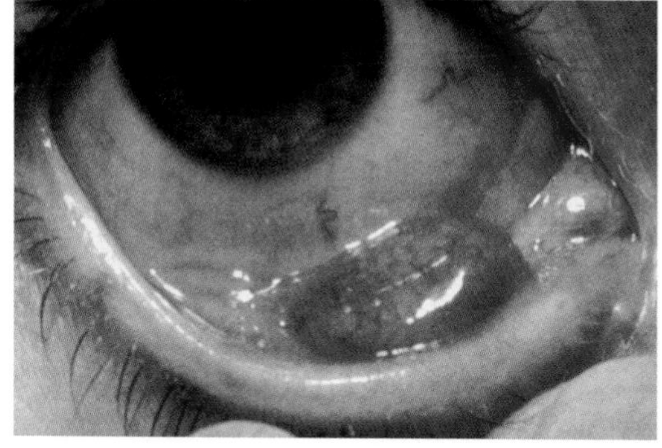

Figure 19.13 Chalazion (blocked meibomian cyst), known also as greater tarsal glands – these open on the inside of the lid and are easily misdiagnosed as a stye

The eyelashes emerge through the skin of the lid margin and small sebaceous glands are associated with them.

Eye closing is effected by orbicularis oculi and the upper lid is raised by levator palpebrae superioris.

When the sensory innervation of the cornea, the trigeminal nerve, is damaged and the cornea thus anaesthetic, it is prone to injury by particles that may cause corneal ulcers. The rash of herpes zoster (shingles) infection of the fifth cranial nerve will produce corneal ulcers.

THE LACRIMAL APPARATUS

The structures producing and removing tears are collectively termed the lacrimal apparatus (Fig. 19.14). They comprise the lacrimal gland and its ducts, the conjunctival sac, the lacrimal sac and the nasolacrimal duct. The front of the eyeball and its conjunctival covering is constantly washed by tears that are essential to ensure that the conjunctiva remains moist and viable. These are drained by blinking, when the increased intraconjunctival pressure produced by the closed lids forces the fluid into the lacrimal puncta and thence into the lacrimal sacs (Figs 19.12a and 19.15).

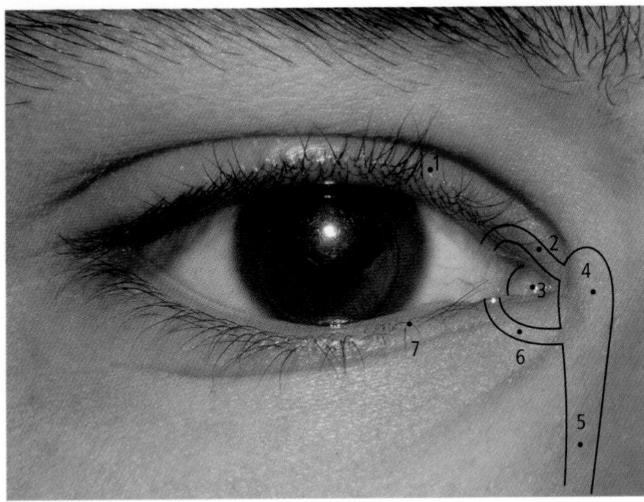

Figure 19.14 Lacrimal apparatus: 1, upper lid; 2, superior lacrimal canaliculus; 3, lacrimal caruncle; 4, lacrimal sac; 5, nasolacrimal duct; 6, inferior lacrimal canaliculus; 7, lower lid eyelashes

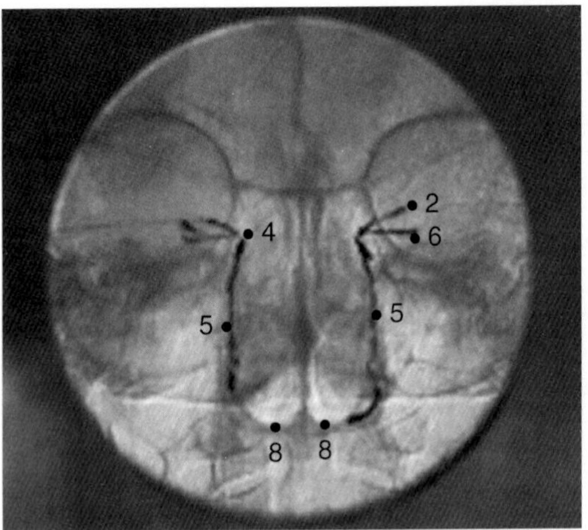

Figure 19.15 Macrodacryocystogram – this contrast medium study outlines both lacrimal apparatus (labels correspond to those in Fig. 19.14 above, with 8, hard palate)

The **lacrimal gland** is a serous gland in the superolateral angle of the orbit behind the upper lid. It is almond shaped, with a palpebral process between the conjunctiva and the tarsal plate, and it has 6–12 ducts opening into the superior conjunctival fornix. It is supplied by a branch of the ophthalmic artery and innervated by the facial nerve through the pterygopalatine ganglion; postganglionic parasympathetic secretomotor fibres pass in the lacrimal and zygomatic nerves. Its lymph drains to the parotid nodes. Each **lacrimal canaliculus** is about 10 mm long and passes from the lacrimal punctum in each eyelid to the **lacrimal sac**. This is a thin fibrous sac on the medial side of the orbit in the lacrimal fossa; it receives both lacrimal canaliculi and drains to the **nasolacrimal duct**. The duct descends in the medial wall of the orbit and opens into the inferior meatus of the nasal cavity. Its opening is guarded by a flap of mucous membrane preventing air passing up the duct when the nose is blown.

The first action one takes when crying is to blow the nose as a response to increased secretions pouring into the inferior meatus.

THE NOSE

The nose warms and moistens inspired air and has olfactory receptors. It comprises the external nose and the two nasal cavities. The **external nose** bears the anterior nostrils (nares). Its skeleton is formed superiorly by nasal bones, which articulate with the frontal bone, the frontal process of the maxillae, and inferiorly by several cartilages that surround the anterior nares. The skin covering the external nose is firmly attached over these cartilages. Just within the external nose is the **vestibule**, from which project coarse hairs (vibrissae) whose function is to keep dirt particles from entering the upper airways (Fig. 19.16).

The **nasal cavities**, between the anterior nares and the nasopharynx, are lined by ciliated columnar epithelium and, superiorly, by olfactory epithelium. They are separated by a midline septum and each possesses a roof, floor, lateral and medial walls, and anterior and posterior apertures. The narrow arched **roof** lies below the anterior cranial fossa. It is formed, from anterior to posterior, by the nasal cartilages, nasal and frontal bones, the cribriform plate of the ethmoid, and the body of the sphenoid (Fig. 19.17). The horizontal **floor**

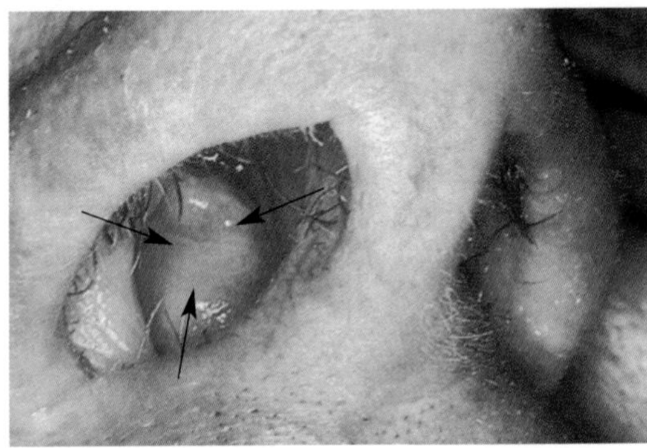

Figure 19.16 View through anterior nostrils showing polyp (arrowed)

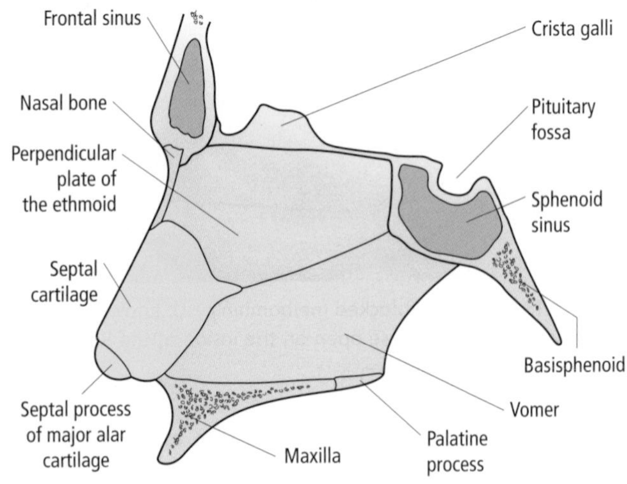

Figure 19.17 Bones of the nasal septum

The head and neck

forms part of the roof of the oral cavity and is formed by the palatine process of the maxilla and the horizontal plate of the palatine bone. Anteriorly the midline incisive canal transmits the greater palatine artery and the nasopalatine nerve. The **medial wall** of the cavity is the nasal septum. It is largely formed, from anterior to posterior, by the septal cartilage, the perpendicular plate of the ethmoid and the vomer. The **lateral wall** (Fig. 19.18) lies medial to the orbit, the ethmoid and maxillary air sinuses and the pterygopalatine fossa. Its surface area is greatly increased by three horizontal bony projections, the superior, middle and inferior **nasal conchae** (turbinates), and by diverticula, the **paranasal air sinuses**. The inferior concha is the largest and lies about 1 cm above the floor of the nose. Beneath each concha is a **meatus**, and above the superior concha the **sphenoethmoidal recess**. The sphenoid air sinus opens into the recess, the posterior ethmoidal air cells into the superior meatus, and the nasolacrimal duct opens into the inferior meatus. The middle meatus possesses the **bulla ethmoidalis**, which contains the middle ethmoidal air cells. A semicircular groove below the bulla, the **hiatus semilunaris**, has openings for the frontal, anterior ethmoidal and maxillary air sinuses (Fig. 19.19).

Nerve supply

Branches of the maxillary nerve and the anterior ethmoidal branch of the ophthalmic nerve supply the nose. The olfactory mucosa – the sensory organ of smell – is in the upper cavity, supplied by the olfactory nerves (Fig. 19.20a,b).

Blood supply

The ophthalmic, palatine and maxillary arteries are the main supply, but the anterior inferior part of the cavity receives additional branches from the facial artery. The veins drain to the pterygoid venous plexus and the facial vein.

Lymphatic drainage

The anterior cavity drains to the submandibular nodes, the posterior part to the retropharyngeal nodes.

THE PARANASAL AIR SINUSES

Paired frontal and maxillary sinuses, numerous ethmoidal and sphenoidal air sinuses lie within the corresponding bones.

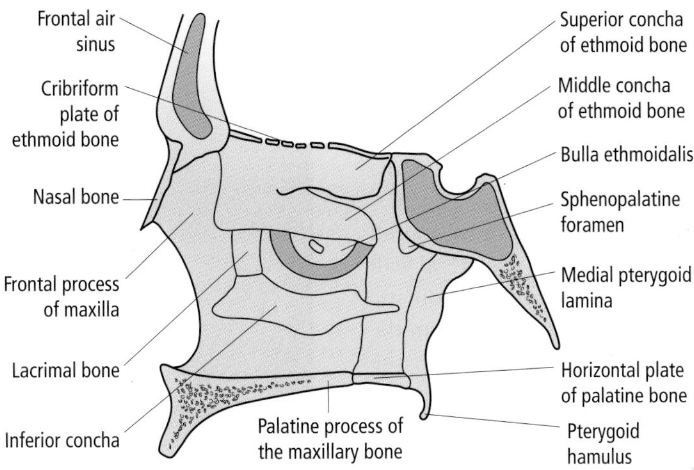

Figure 19.18 Bones of the lateral wall of nasal cavity

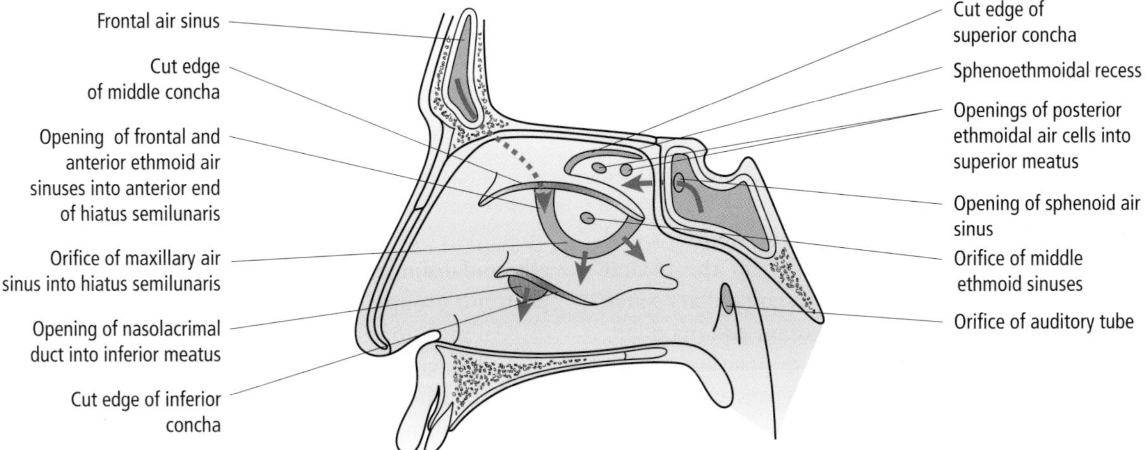

Figure 19.19 Lateral wall of nasal cavity showing openings of the paranasal air sinuses (arrows indicate directions of mucus drainage)

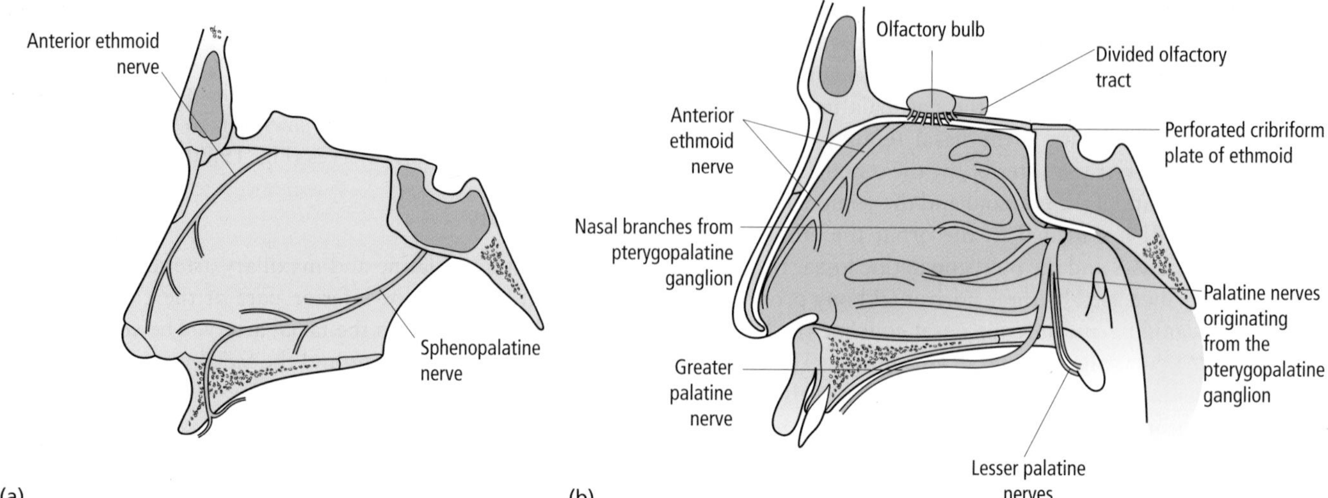

Figure 19.20 Nerve supply of: (a) septum; (b) lateral wall of nose

They develop as diverticula from each nasal cavity and are lined by its mucoperiosteum. They are small at birth and enlarge during the eruption of the second dentition, to reach adult size after puberty. They lighten the front of the skull and may increase the resonance of the voice. Their lymphatics drain mainly to the deeply placed retropharyngeal nodes.

The **frontal sinus**, situated above the medial end of the superciliary arch, is separated by a bony septum from its fellow. It lies anterior to the anterior cranial fossa and above the orbit. Each sinus opens into the middle meatus of the nasal cavity through the long frontonasal duct (Fig. 19.19).

The **maxillary sinus** (Fig. 19.21) – the largest of the paired air sinuses – is pyramidal. Its base forms part of the lateral wall of the nose, and its apex projects laterally into the zygomatic process of the maxilla. The roof separates the sinus from the orbit and conveys the infraorbital vessels and nerve in the infraorbital canal. The floor is the alveolar margin, containing molar teeth, the roots of which project into the cavity. The posterior wall contains the posterior superior alveolar nerve and lies in front of the infratemporal and pterygopalatine fossae. The anterior wall forms the facial surface of the maxilla and is covered in part by mucous membrane of the vestibule of the mouth.

The sinus opens into the hiatus semilunaris from high on its medial wall. Its lymph drains to the submandibular and retropharyngeal nodes.

The maxillary sinuses are the most commonly infected because their openings, well above the floor of the sinus, are not well positioned for natural drainage.

Because of the close relationship between frontal and maxillary sinus openings an infection in the frontal sinus will often drain by gravity into the maxillary sinus (sinusitis). The most effective way to drain the maxillary sinus is to kneel in the Muslim praying position, which brings the opening of the sinus into a dependent position for drainage. Infection of a carcinoma of the maxillary sinus may, because of the close relation of the sinus floor to the upper teeth, produce pain referred to those teeth.

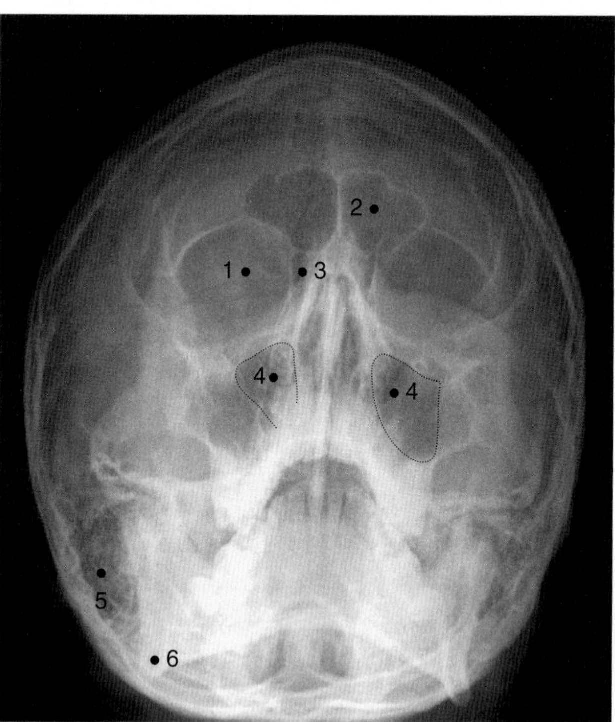

Figure 19.21 X-ray (an upwardly oblique view) showing paranasal air sinuses: 1, orbital cavity; 2, frontal sinus; 3, ethmoidal sinus; 4, maxillary sinus; 5, mastoid air cells; 6, angle of mandible

Each ethmoidal labyrinth, lying between the orbit and the upper part of the nasal cavity, contains numerous air cells, the **ethmoidal sinuses**; these are divided into anterior, middle and posterior groups.

An infection or abscess in these cells may readily invade the thin medial wall of the orbit and optic canal, causing optic neuritis and the risk of blindness.

The **sphenoidal sinuses** are contained within the body of the sphenoid and usually communicate with each other through an incomplete bony septum. They lie below the sella